New Insights into Alzheimer's Disease

New Insights into Alzheimer's Disease

Edited by Trevor Cornfield

AMERICAN
MEDICAL PUBLISHERS
www.americanmedicalpublishers.com

American Medical Publishers,
41 Flatbush Avenue,
1st Floor, New York,
NY 11217, USA

Visit us on the World Wide Web at:
www.americanmedicalpublishers.com

ISBN: 978-1-63927-441-3

Cataloging-in-Publication Data

New insights into alzheimer's disease / edited by Trevor Cornfield.
p. cm.
Includes bibliographical references and index.
ISBN 978-1-63927-441-3
1. Alzheimer's disease. 2. Alzheimer's disease--Diagnosis. 3. Alzheimer's disease--Treatment.
4. Dementia. 5. Brain--Diseases. I. Cornfield, Trevor.
RC523 .A49 2022
616.831--dc23

Table of Contents

Preface VII

Chapter 1 **Microglia limit the expansion of β-amyloid plaques in a mouse model of Alzheimer's disease** 1
Ruohe Zhao, Wanling Hu, Julia Tsai, Wei Li and Wen-Biao Gan

Chapter 2 **Tetraspanin 6: a pivotal protein of the multiple vesicular body determining exosome release and lysosomal degradation of amyloid precursor protein fragments** 12
Francesc X. Guix, Ragna Sannerud, Fedor Berditchevski, Amaia M. Arranz, Katrien Horré, An Snellinx, Amantha Thathiah, Takaomi Saido, Takashi Saito, Sundaresan Rajesh, Michael Overduin, Samir Kumar-Singh, Enrico Radaelli, Nikky Corthout, Julien Colombelli, Sébastien Tosi, Sebastian Munck, Isabel H. Salas, Wim Annaert and Bart De Strooper

Chapter 3 **Increased acetylation of Peroxiredoxin1 by HDAC6 inhibition leads to recovery of Aβ-induced impaired axonal transport** 33
Heesun Choi, Haeng Jun Kim, Jisoo Kim, Soohyun Kim, Jinhee Yang, Wonik Lee, Yeonju Park, Seung Jae Hyeon, Dong-Sup Lee, Hoon Ryu, Junho Chung and Inhee Mook-Jung

Chapter 4 **Diurnal oscillation of CSF Aβ and other AD biomarkers** 47
Brendan P. Lucey, Anne M. Fagan, David M. Holtzman, John C. Morris and Randall J. Bateman

Chapter 5 **The novel RAGE interactor PRAK is associated with autophagy signaling in Alzheimer's disease pathogenesis** 50
Yoonhee Kim, Chaeyoung Kim, Sung Min Son, Hyundong Song, Hyun Seok Hong, Sun-ho Han and Inhee Mook-Jung

Chapter 6 **3D culture models of Alzheimer's disease: a road map to a "cure-in-a-dish."** 61
Se Hoon Choi, Young Hye Kim, Luisa Quinti, Rudolph E. Tanzi and Doo Yeon Kim

Chapter 7 **Vitamin D interacts with Esr1 and Igf1 to regulate molecular pathways relevant to Alzheimer's disease** 72
Véréna Landel, Pascal Millet, Kévin Baranger, Béatrice Loriod and François Féron

Chapter 8 **Neurotrophic factor small-molecule mimetics mediated neuroregeneration and synaptic repair: emerging therapeutic modality for Alzheimer's disease** 94
Syed Faraz Kazim and Khalid Iqbal

Chapter 9 **Pim1 inhibition as a novel therapeutic strategy for Alzheimer's disease** 110
Ramon Velazquez, Darren M. Shaw, Antonella Caccamo and Salvatore Oddo

Chapter 10 **Functional alterations of myeloid cells during the course of Alzheimer's disease** 124
Aaron D. Thome, Alireza Faridar, David R. Beers, Jason R. Thonhoff, Weihua Zhao, Shixiang Wen, Belen Pascual, Joseph C. Masdeu and Stanley H. Appel

Chapter 11 **Modifying Rap1-signalling by targeting Pde6δ is neuroprotective in models of Alzheimer's disease** 135
Michael Dumbacher, Tom Van Dooren, Katrien Princen, Koen De Witte, Mélissa Farinelli, Sam Lievens, Jan Tavernier, Wim Dehaen, Stefaan Wera, Joris Winderickx, Sara Allasia, Amuri Kilonda, Stéphane Spieser, Arnaud Marchand, Patrick Chaltin, Casper C. Hoogenraad and Gerard Griffioen

Chapter 12 **Molecular and functional signatures in a novel Alzheimer's disease mouse model assessed by quantitative proteomics** 156
Dong Kyu Kim, Joonho Park, Dohyun Han, Jinhee Yang, Ahbin Kim, Jongmin Woo, Youngsoo Kim and Inhee Mook-Jung

Chapter 13 **Abnormal dendritic calcium activity and synaptic depotentiation occur early in a mouse model of Alzheimer's disease** 175
Yang Bai, Miao Li, Yanmei Zhou, Lei Ma, Qian Qiao, Wanling Hu, Wei Li, Zachary Patrick Wills and Wen-Biao Gan

Chapter 14 **Prevention of C5aR1 signaling delays microglial inflammatory polarization, favors clearance pathways and suppresses cognitive loss** 190
Michael X. Hernandez, Shan Jiang, Tracy A. Cole, Shu-Hui Chu, Maria I. Fonseca, Melody J. Fang, Lindsay A. Hohsfield, Maria D. Torres, Kim N. Green, Rick A. Wetsel, Ali Mortazavi and Andrea J. Tenner

Chapter 15 **Depletion of adult neurogenesis exacerbates cognitive deficits in Alzheimer's disease by compromising hippocampal inhibition** 208
Carolyn Hollands, Matthew Kyle Tobin, Michael Hsu, Kianna Musaraca, Tzong-Shiue Yu, Rachana Mishra, Steven G. Kernie and Orly Lazarov

Permissions

List of Contributors

Index

Preface

Alzheimer's disease (AD) is a chronic neurodegenerative condition. It is the leading cause of dementia. The major symptom of AD is the difficulty in remembering recent events. The course of the disease can be divided into four stages that are characterized by a progressive decline of cognitive and functional abilities- pre-dementia, early, moderate and advanced. A diagnosis of the condition is based on the history of the illness, examination of brain tissue, blood tests and cognitive testing with medical imaging. There exists no cure for AD and therapies are mostly palliative. Exercise, art, music and pet therapies, and other recreational activities offer some support in improving mood and behavior. Caregiving is essentially the treatment for people with Alzheimer's disease. The objective of this book is to give a general view of the different aspects of this condition. It includes some of the vital pieces of work being conducted across the world, on various topics related to Alzheimer's disease. This book is a vital tool for all studying and researching this disease.

This book is the end result of constructive efforts and intensive research done by experts in this field. The aim of this book is to enlighten the readers with recent information in this area of research. The information provided in this profound book would serve as a valuable reference to students and researchers in this field.

At the end, I would like to thank all the authors for devoting their precious time and providing their valuable contribution to this book. I would also like to express my gratitude to my fellow colleagues who encouraged me throughout the process.

Editor

1

Microglia limit the expansion of β-amyloid plaques in a mouse model of Alzheimer's disease

Ruohe Zhao[1,2], Wanling Hu[1], Julia Tsai[2], Wei Li[1,2*] and Wen-Biao Gan[1,2*]

Abstract

Background: Microglia are known as resident immune cells in the brain. β-amyloid (Aβ) plaques in the brain of Alzheimer's disease (AD) are surrounded by microglia, but whether and how microglia affect the formation and maintenance of plaques remains controversial.

Methods: We depleted microglia by injecting diphtheria toxin (DT) in $CX_3CR1^{CreER/+}$:$R26^{DTR/+}$ (*CX₃CR1-iDTR*) mice crossed with *APPswe/PSEN1dE9* (*APP/PS1*) mice. Intravital time-lapse imaging was performed to examine changes in the number and size of Congo Red-labeled amyloid plaques over 1–2 weeks. We also examined spine density and shaft diameter of dendrites passing through plaques in a *PSAPP* mouse model of AD ($PS1_{M146L}$ line 6.2 × Tg2576) crossed with *Thy1* YFP H-line mice.

Results: We found that DT administration to *CX_3CR1-iDTR* mice efficiently ablated microglia within one week and that microglia repopulated in the second week after DT administration. Microglia depletion didn't affect the number of amyloid plaques, but led to ~13% increase in the size of Aβ plaques within one week. Moreover, microglia repopulation was associated with the stabilization of plaque size during the second week. In addition, we found dendritic spine loss and shaft atrophy in the distal parts of dendrites passing through plaques.

Conclusion: Our results demonstrate the important role of microglia in limiting the growth of Aβ plaques and plaque-associated disruption of neuronal connection.

Keywords: Alzheimer's disease, Aβ plaque, Microglia depletion, Two-photon imaging, APP/PS1, $CX_3CR1^{CreER/+}$:$R26^{DTR/+}$

Background

Accumulation of β-amyloid (Aβ) in the brain is a hallmark of Alzheimer's disease (AD) [1, 2]. Studies of postmortem AD brains have revealed dystrophic neurites inside and surrounding Aβ plaques [3–6]. Studies in AD mouse models have also shown that Aβ deposition is associated with various neuronal abnormalities, including the formation of dystrophic neurites [5, 7, 8], dendritic spine loss [5, 7, 9, 10], synaptic dysfunction [11, 12] and abnormal neuronal firing [13, 14]. The variety of neuronal deficits associated with Aβ deposition likely contribute to memory loss and cognitive decline in AD patients [15–19].

Microglia are the resident immune cells in the central nervous system [20, 21]. They are clustered around amyloid plaques in both human AD brains [22, 23] and the brains of AD mouse models [24, 25]. Mutations in genes such as *CD33* and *TREM2* have been linked to microglia dysfunction and increased risks for AD [26–28]. Knockout of *CX_3CR1* [29, 30], *CD33* [27], or *TREM2* [31, 32] leads to altered plaque load, suggesting that microglia are involved in Aβ deposition. Activated microglia have been shown to phagocytose Aβ through scavenger receptor-mediated mechanisms [33–35]. Furthermore, in vivo imaging studies have shown that microglia volume surrounding plaques correlated with the decrease of plaque size [25]. Microglia processes enveloping plaque surface are suggested to constitute a barrier to prevent plaque expansion [36, 37], and the disruption of this barrier in *TREM2* deficiency mice is associated with the increase of

* Correspondence: liwei@pkusz.edu.cn; gan@saturn.med.nyu.edu
[1]Drug Discovery Center, Peking University Shenzhen Graduate School, Shenzhen 518055, China
Full list of author information is available at the end of the article

dystrophic neurites [32, 37]. Together, these studies lead to a view that microglia are involved in the clearance of Aβ and limiting the expansion of plaques.

Although many lines of evidence suggest a role of microglia in restricting the growth of amyloid plaques, several studies have shown that microglia depletion does not affect the number and size of plaques in mouse models of AD. It has been reported that chronic microglia depletion for one month by activating suicide gene *HSVTK* under *CD11b* promoter has no effects on the formation or maintenance of plaques [38]. In another study, microglia are depleted by inhibiting colony-stimulating factor 1 receptor (CSF1R) with PLX3397 from Plexxikon. PLX3397 treatment for 4 weeks results in nearly complete depletion of microglia, but has no effects on plaque load in a mouse model of AD [39]. Thus, in contrast to the view that microglia are beneficial to limiting amyloid deposits, these depletion studies suggest that microglia have no significant effect on the formation and growth of amyloid plaques.

To better understand the role of microglia in Aβ deposition, we examined the number and size of plaques after depleting microglia by administration of diphtheria toxin (DT) to $CX_3CR1^{CreER/+}$:$R26^{DTR/+}$ (*CX$_3$CR1-iDTR*) mice crossed with *APPswe/PSEN1dE9* (*APP/PS1*) mice. Using two-photon time-lapse imaging of Aβ plaques in mice more than 12 months old, we found that Aβ plaque size, but not plaque number, showed a significant increase over 7 days after microglia depletion. In addition, we found a significant reduction in dendritic spine density and dendritic diameter in the distal segments of dendrites passing through plaques. Taken together, our results suggest that microglia play an important role in limiting the growth of Aβ plaques and reducing neuronal damage associated with Aβ deposition.

Methods

Transgenic mice

APPswe/PSEN1dE9 (*APP/PS1*) were purchased from Guangdong Medical Laboratory Animal Center, China. C57BL/6 mice expressing YFP in layer-V pyramidal neurons (*Thy1* H-line) and *Rosa26-stop-iDTR* (*DTR*) mice were purchased from the Jackson Laboratories, US. CX_3CR1^{CreER} mice were generated in New York University School of Medicine [40]. These mice were crossbred and litters were genotyped by PCR using the following primers: for *APP/PS1* mice, 5′- TCATGACTATCCT CCTGGTGG-3′ and 5′- CGTTATAGGTTTTAA ACACTTCCCC-3′; for CX_3CR1^{CreER} mice, 5′- AAGAC TCACGTGGACCTGCT-3′, 5′- CGGTTATTCAACTT GCACCA-3′ and 5′- AGGATGTTG ACTTCCG AGTTG-3′; for *DTR* mice, 5′- CTGGCTTCTGAG-GACCG-3′ and 5′-CGAAGAGTTTGTCCTCAACCG-3′. 12–24 months old quadruple transgenic mice were used for microglia depletion experiment and in vivo imaging. Age-matched animals with *APP/PS1* mutation but no *CreER* or *DTR* gene were used as controls.

For studies of dendritic abnormalities near plaques, mutant human amyloid precursor protein (FAD $APP_{670/671}$ line Tg2576) and mutant human Presenilin 1 ($PS1_{M146L}$ line 6.2) mice were obtained from Taconic and the University of South Florida, respectively. All experiments were done in accordance with the institutional guidelines.

Labeling amyloid plaques in vivo

Mice were anesthetized with pentobarbital sodium (100 mg/kg) 24–48 h before imaging. Congo Red was injected into the subarachnoid space using a fine glass electrode guided by a micromanipulator. The electrode was backfilled with Congo Red (3 μl, 0.5% in artificial cerebral spinal fluid (ACSF), filtered through a 0.20 μm syringe filter before use, Sigma) and inserted through the thinned skull. After subarachnoid space was reached (as evidenced by free dye diffusion), Congo Red was then pressure injected with a picospritzer (20 p.s.i., 20 ms, 0.8 Hz) over 20–30 min. Dye labeling of amyloid plaques was typically observed within 30 min of injection.

In vivo two-photon imaging of Aβ plaques

The procedure of transcranial two-photon imaging was described previously [7, 41]. Briefly, after exposing the skull surface and gluing the skull to a custom-made steel plate, a small region ~1 mm in diameter was thinned with a highspeed drill, and a microsurgical blade was then used to continue thinning until the skull area ~500 μm in diameter was ~20 μm in thickness. A picture of the brain vasculature in the thinned region was taken with a CCD camera and used as a landmark for future relocation. Animals were placed under a two-photon microscope, and image stacks of plaques within a depth of 300 μm from the pial surface were obtained in the step size of 1 μm with a 1.05 N.A. 25× water-immersion objective and with two-photon laser tuned to 880 nm. For each frame, a 512 × 512 pixel, zoom 1× image was taken from a 508 × 508 μm ROI. Image stacks from motor, somatosensory and visual cortices yielded a full three-dimensional data set of Aβ plaques labeled with Congo Red in these cortical regions. After imaging, the plate was gently detached from the skull and the scalp was sutured, and the animals were returned to their home cages until the next viewing.

Microglia depletion

Depletion of microglia was performed according to previously published studies [40]. Animals received two doses of 10 mg of tamoxifen (20 mg/ml, dissolved in corn oil, Sigma) to induce Cre-mediated recombination and DTR expression, with a separation of 48 h between doses. Diphtheria toxin (Sigma) was diluted in PBS (50 μg/ml) and 1 μg of toxin was given i.p. for three consecutive days for depletion of microglia.

Immunohistochemistry

Mice were anesthetized and perfused with 0.9% PBS. CNS tissue was removed and fixed in 4% PFA, rinsed with PBS and sectioned at 150 μm with a vibratome. Sections were permeabilized in 1% Titron X-100 in PBS for 3 h and blocked with 5% normal goat serum for 1 h. Sections were incubated overnight with primary antibodies against Iba1 (Wako, 1:500). Sections were then washed with PBS/ 0.05% Tween-20, and then incubated with Alexafluor-conjugated goat anti-rabbit IgG secondary antibodies (Life Technologies, 1:500) for 2 h. Sections were washed as before and mounted for imaging. Confocal images were obtained on a Biorad Radiance 2000 confocal microscope.

Labeling and imaging fixed brain slice

Transversal slices (150–200 μm thick) of fixed brains were cut on a vibratome. Congo Red was used to visualized fibrillary amyloid in triple *YFP/APP/PS1* transgenic mice. Fixed brain slices were incubated in 0.5% Congo Red for 30 min and then rinsed with 0.1 M PBS. Slices were then mounted between two glass cover-slips in Vectashield (Vector Laboratories) and sealed with dental wax.

Labeled brain slices were imaged by laser scanning confocal microscopy using either a N.A. 1.25 40× or a N.A. 1.3 60× oil-immersion objective. Neuronal structures labeled with YFP and fibrillar amyloid deposits with Congo Red were scanned sequentially using 488 nm and 568 nm laser excitation, respectively. Image stacks at 0.3–1.0 μm steps were acquired to generate three-dimensional data sets of neuronal structures and amyloid plaques.

Image analysis

To analyze the in vivo images of Aβ plaques, all images were processed using a custom-written Matlab algorithm. For each plaque, the frame with highest mean fluorescence intensity out of the entire image stack was identified as the center frame of this plaque. 2 additional frames above and below the center (5 frames combined) were used to analyze plaque size. In each image frame, plaque border was determined by setting a threshold of 3 times of standard deviation of the background fluorescence (mean value of the lowest 10% fluorescence intensity of the entire image) of the current frame. The averaged plaque area with the border was used as the plaque size.

To quantify fluorescence surrounding a plaque, fluorescence intensity across a radial line from the center point towards the outer area of a plaque was extracted. This radial line was drawn in a randomized direction and was kept in the same direction in analyzing the same plaque between different imaging sessions. This radial line was separated into the "inside" part and the "outside" part by the border of plaque. Fluorescence intensity across the line was normalized to a 0–100% scale with the highest value across the line as 100%. Normalized fluorescence intensity within 5 μm surrounding plaque border in the "outside" part was used as the measurement of fluorescence intensity surrounding the plaque.

To quantify changes of dendritic structures near Aβ deposits in fixed brain slices, dendritic spine densities and shaft diameters were measured with Metamorph software. Spine density and shaft diameter were measured for the proximal or distal dendritic segment (proximal or distal dendritic segments had comparable length, ranging from 20 to 80 μm), depending on the region in which the segment was located. Segments close to the soma and before the plaques were defined as proximal segments. Segments far away from the soma and after plaques were defined as distal segments. The border of Aβ deposits was determined as the position in which a sharp increase in fluorescence intensity was observed.

Statistics

All data were presented as mean ± S.E.M. Kolmogorov-Smirnov test was used to test normality of sample's distribution. Student's t-test (two-tailed) was used to test for differences between groups whose distributions passed Kolmogorov-Smirnov test. Independent-samples Mann-Whitney test and related-samples Wilcoxon Signed rank test was used to compare differences between groups whose distributions did not pass Kolmogorov-Smirnov test. Significant levels were set at $P \leq 0.05$. All statistical analyses were performed using the IBM SPSS Statistics 23.

Result

Cre-dependent microglia depletion in the brain

Previous studies have reported that microglia depletion by activating suicide gene *HSVTK* or by inhibiting CSFR1 had no significant effect on the number and size of amyloid plaques in mouse models of AD [38, 39]. To better understand the role of microglia in amyloid deposition, we took advantage of a recently-developed method to deplete microglia by administrating diphtheria toxin (DT) into *CX$_3$CR1-iDTR* mice [40]. Two-month-old *CX$_3$CR1-iDTR* mice first received 10 mg of tamoxifen by gavage both on Day 1 and Day 3 to induce Cre-mediated recombination and DTR expression under *CX$_3$CR1* promoter. 1 μg DT was then administrated by intraperitoneal injections for three consecutive days on Day 10–12. The effect of DT administration on microglia depletion was examined 1 to 14 days after DT administration (Fig. 1a). We found that *CX$_3$CR1-iDTR* mice had a marked reduction of microglia 1 day after DT

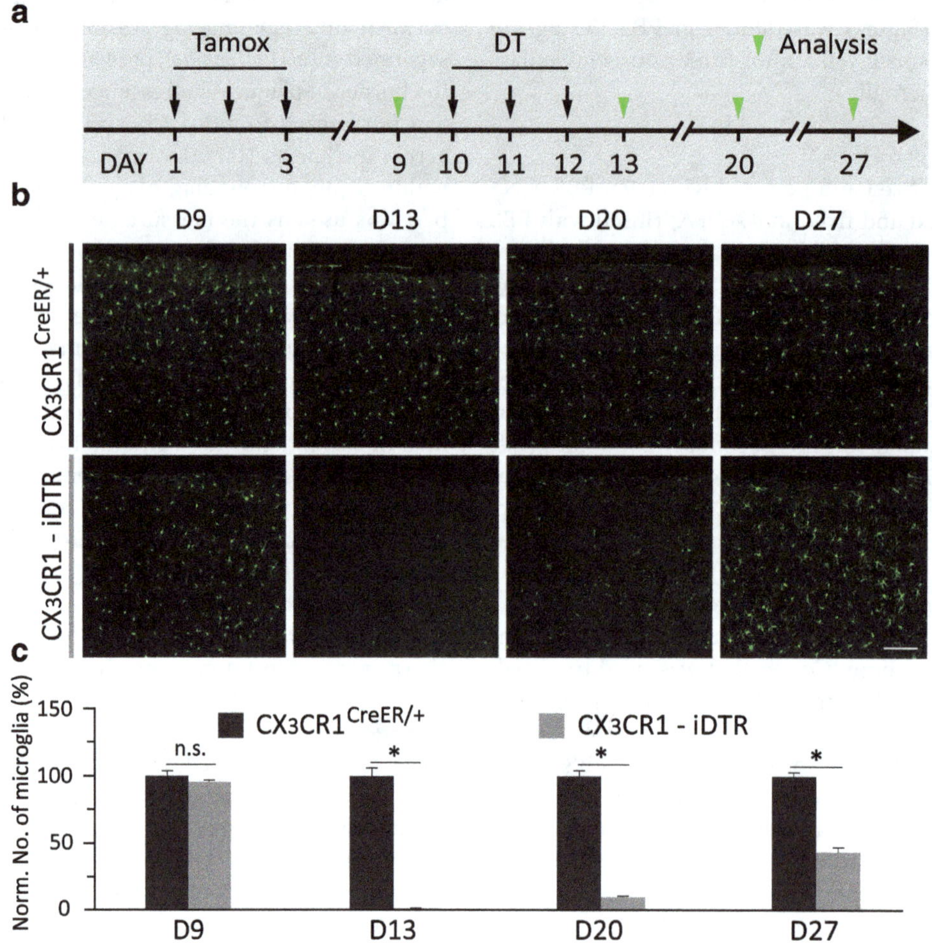

Fig. 1 Microglia are depleted in *CX_3CR1-iDTR* mice over 1–7 days after DT administration and repopulate within 2 weeks after DT administration. **a**. Timeline of tamoxifen administration, DT administration and analysis of microglia number. Microglia were examined by Iba1 staining before (D9), 1 day after (D13), 1 week after (D20) and 2 weeks after DT administration (D27). **b**. Coronal sections of the cortex stained for Iba1 from $CX_3CR1^{CreER/+}$ and *CX_3CR1-iDTR* mice on D9, D13, D20 and D27, respectively. Scale bar, 100 μm. **c**. Quantification of Iba1 positive cells showing that the majority of microglia were depleted in the first week after DT administration and ~50% of microglia were repopulated during the second week in *CX_3CR1-iDTR* mice ($n = 4$, * $P < 0.05$, Mann-Whitney test)

administration (Day 13) and the surviving microglia number was 0.8 ± 0.8% compared with control mice without DTR expression. Microglia remained largely absent in the cortex 7 days after DT administration (Day 20, 13.1 ± 1.3%). 2 weeks after DT administration, 57.4 ± 4.6% of microglia were found in the cortex of *CX_3CR1-iDTR* mice, indicating microglia repopulation occurred at this stage (Fig. 1b, c). Similar dynamics of microglia depletion and repopulation following DT administration were observed in the cortex of *APP/PS1/CX_3CR1-iDTR* mice at 15 month of age (Additional file 1: Figure S1). Thus, consistent with previous findings [40], these results show that after DT administration, microglia are efficiently depleted from the cortex of *CX_3CR1-iDTR* mice or *APP/PS1/CX_3CR1-iDTR* mice within one week, but start to repopulate during the second week.

Microglia depletion over 2 weeks has no effect on the number of plaques

To investigate whether microglia depletion affects Aβ deposition, we crossed *APP/PS1* mice with *CX_3CR1-iDTR* mice and depleted microglia in mice more than 12 months old (17 ± 2 months old). We first examined the effect of microglia depletion on the number of amyloid plaques over 1–2 weeks after DT administration (Fig. 2a). To label Aβ plaques, Congo Red was injected into the subarachnoid space 24–48 h before each imaging session (see Methods). Congo Red-labeled Aβ plaques were imaged through thinned-skull window using two-photon microscopy. Time-lapse imaging of the same cortical regions was performed 1 day (Day 13), 1 week (Day 20) and 2 weeks (Day 27) after DT administration (Fig. 2b, d). We found that the average plaque density in *APP/PS1/CX_3CR1-iDTR* mice before DT administration was 515 ± 63 mm^{-3},

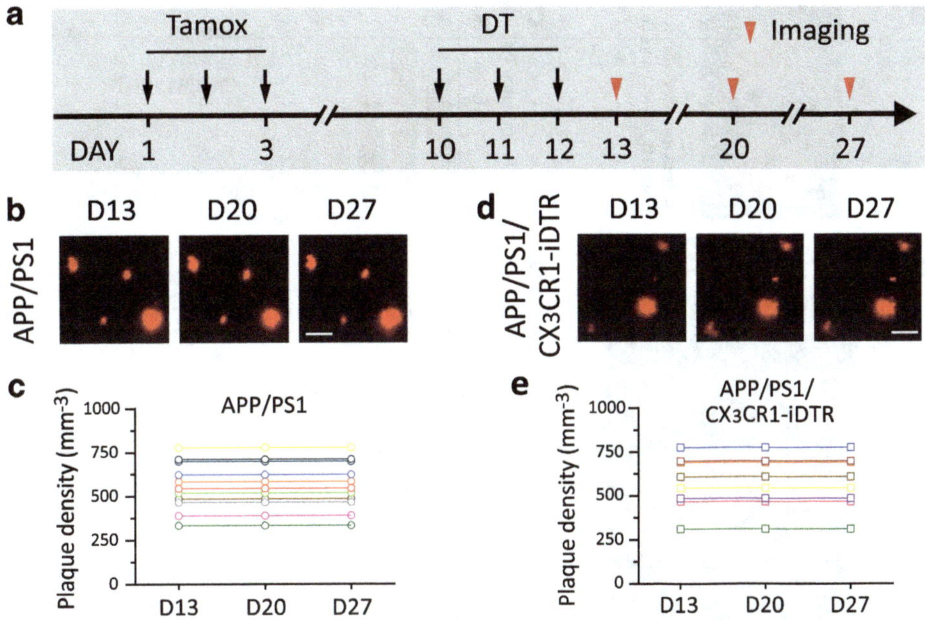

Fig. 2 Ablation of microglia by DT administration has no effect on the number of amyloid plaques. **a**. Timeline of tamoxifen administration, DT administration and in vivo imaging of Congo Red-labeled plaques. Time-lapse imaging was performed 1 day after (D13), 1 week after (D20) and 2 weeks after DT administration (D27). **b**. Images of the same ROIs in *APP/PS1* mice over 1–2 weeks. **c**. Quantification of plaque density in *APP/PS1* mice in each ROI. **d**. Images of the same ROIs in *APP/PS1/CX$_3$CR1-iDTR* mice over 1–2 weeks. Neither elimination of existing Aβ plaques nor formation of new plaques occurred in *APP/PS1* or *APP/PS1/CX$_3$CR1-iDTR* mice. **e**. Quantification of plaque density in *APP/PS1/CX$_3$CR1-iDTR* mice in each ROI

comparable to that in *APP/PS1* mice (574 ± 42 mm^{-3}, $P > 0.05$). Consistent with the previous study showing no formation of new plaques over weeks in *APP/PS1* mice older than 9 months [42], we found that in >12 month-old *APP/PS1* mice, no disappearance of existing plaques or appearance of new plaques was detected over 1–2 weeks (Fig. 2b, c). Notably, the number of Aβ plaques also remained the same over 1–2 weeks in mice when microglia were depleted by DT administration (Fig. 2d, e). No new plaques or disappearance of existing plaques was observed during this period. Thus, consistent with the previous study reporting microglia depletion has no significant effect on the number of plaques [38, 39], our findings suggest that ablation of microglia by DT administration does not affect the number of Aβ plaques over 1–2 weeks.

Microglia depletion leads to enlargement of Aβ plaques

In addition to examining the effect of microglia depletion on plaque number, we also compared the size of plaques over time in mice with or without microglia by two-photon time-lapse imaging. The Congo Red-labeled area of plaque was used as the measurements of plaque size. The border of amyloid plaques was determined such that the fluorescence intensity of amyloid plaques was above 3 times of standard deviation of the background fluorescence (Fig. 3a, see Methods). The size of Aβ plaques identified in *APP/PS1* (308.9 ± 27.6 μm^2) and *APP/PS1/CX$_3$CR1-iDTR* mice (343.3 ± 35.5 μm^2) were comparable before DT administration (P = 0.23, Fig. 3b). Consistent with previous studies [42–44], we found that the size of plaques showed no significant change over 1–2 weeks in *APP/PS1* mice older than 12 months (Fig. 3c–f). In contrast to the stable size of amyloid plaques in *APP/PS1* mice, we found that after DT administration plaques showed a significant increase (12.8 ± 3.2%, $P < 0.001$) in size from Day 13 to Day 20 in *APP/PS1/CX$_3$CR1-iDTR* mice (Fig. 3d, e). Furthermore, during the second week after DT administration when microglia repopulated (Fig. 1b, c), we found that *APP/PS1/CX$_3$CR1-iDTR* mice showed no additional increase of plaque size from Day 20 to Day 27 (P = 0.32, Fig. 3d, f). Taken together, these results strongly suggest that microglia have an important role in limiting the growth of amyloid plaques.

To further understand how the absence of microglia affects amyloid deposition, we examined Congo Red fluorescence intensity surrounding plaques. Fluorescence intensity across a radial line from plaque center towards outer area was measured (Fig. 4a) and separated into the "inside" part and the "outside" part by the border of plaque (Fig. 4b, see Methods). By examining fluorescence intensity within 5 μm surrounding plaque border in the "outside" part, we found a significant increase of Congo Red fluorescence intensity from Day 13 to Day 20 (43.7%, $P < 0.001$, Fig. 4c). In the following second week when microglia repopulated (Day 20 to Day 27),

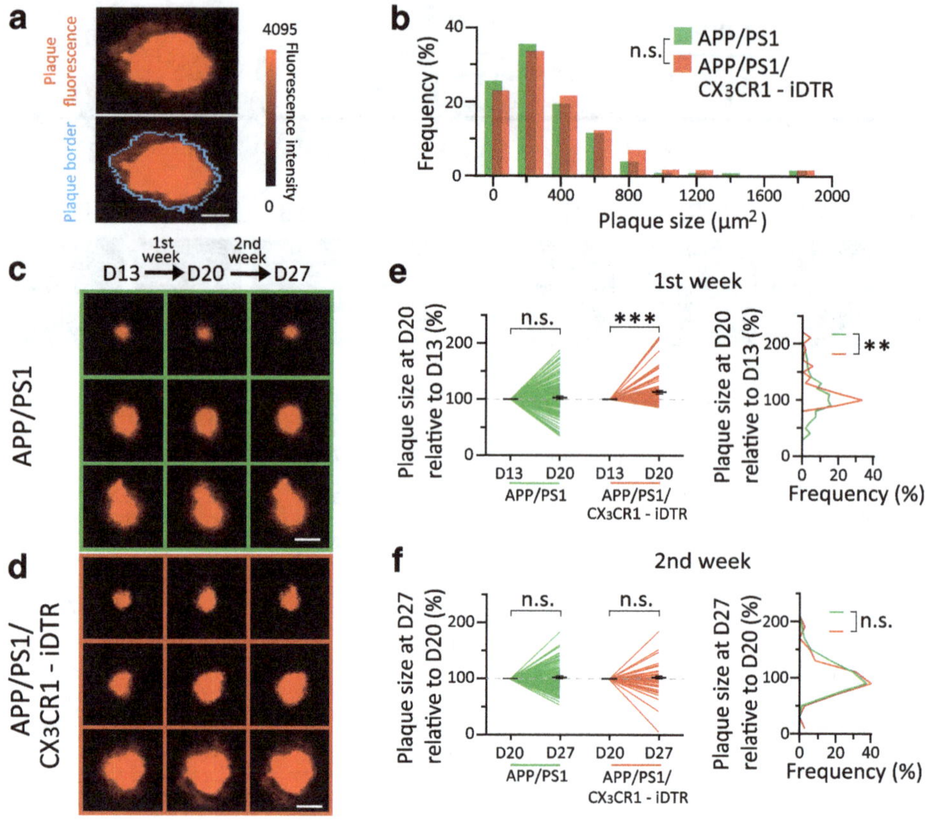

Fig. 3 Microglia depletion induces increase in plaque size. **a**. *Blue curve* in the bottom panel indicates the identified plaque border for the example in the upper panel. The border of amyloid plaque was determined such that the fluorescence intensity of amyloid plaques was above 3 times of s.d. **b**. Distribution of plaque size on Day 13 in the cortex of *APP/PS1* mice (*green bars*, n = 129 plaques from 5 mice) and *APP/PS1/CX₃CR1-iDTR* mice (*red bars*, n = 75 plaques from 4 mice) (P = 0.23, Mann-Whitney test). **c**. Three examples of plaques imaged over 1–2 weeks in *APP/PS1* mice. **d**. Three examples of plaques imaged over 1–2 week in *APP/PS1/CX₃CR1-iDTR* mice. **e**. Change of plaque size in the first week after DT administration. No significant change in plaque size was detected within one week in *APP/PS1* mice (n = 129 plaques from 5 mice, P = 0.16, Wilcoxon matched-pairs signed rank test). Microglia depletion induced a significant increase in plaque size in *APP/PS1/CX₃CR1-iDTR* mice (n = 75 plaques from 4 mice, ***P < 0.001, Wilcoxon matched-pairs signed rank test). The distribution of plaque size at D20 relative to D13 is significantly different between these two groups (right panel, ** P < 0.01, Mann-Whitney test). **f**. Change of plaque size in the second week after DT administration. No significant change in plaque size was detected in *APP/PS1* mice (n = 92 plaques from 5 mice, P = 0.52, Wilcoxon matched-pairs signed rank test). Aβ plaques in *APP/PS1/CX₃CR1-iDTR* mouse cortex didn't continue to grow from D20 to D27 (n = 40 plaques from 4 mice, P = 0.32, Wilcoxon matched-pairs signed rank test). The distribution of plaque size at D27 relative to D20 is not significantly different between these two groups (right panel, P = 0.52, Mann-Whitney test). Scale bar in a, c and d, 20 μm

fluorescence intensity in the surrounding area didn't continue to increase (P = 0.84, Fig. 4d). The change and stabilization of Congo Red fluorescence surrounding plaques after microglia depletion and repopulation provide further evidence that microglia are involved in limiting plaque growth.

Aβ deposits cause abnormalities in dendrites passing through plaques

Our findings in *APP/PS1/CX₃CR1-iDTR* mice showed that microglia depletion resulted in ~13% increase in plaque size within one week. Based on the averaged plaque size in *APP/PS1* mice (308.9 ± 27.6 μm^2, Fig. 3b), we estimated that for each plaque the cortex area covered by Aβ accumulation increase by ~40 μm^2 over one week in the absence of microglia. Previous studies have shown various abnormalities of axons and dendrites inside or near plaques [5, 7–10]. It is possible that ~13% expansion of plaques after microglia depletion may lead to more extensive damage in neuronal circuits. To better understand neuronal damage associated with plaques, we examined spine density and shaft diameter of dendrites passing through and outside plaques in fixed brain slices. In this experiment, *PS1* mutant mice (*PS1*$_{M146L}$ line 6.2) were first crossed with *APP* mutant mice (FAD *APP*$_{670/671}$ line Tg2576). This mouse model of AD (*PSAPP* mice) was further crossed with *Thy1* YFP H-line mice to visualize dendrites and dendritic spines of pyramidal neurons in fixed brain slices from 6 to 10-month-old mice. Amyloid plaques were labeled with Congo Red (Fig. 5a). When dendritic segments passing through plaques were divided into "proximal" segments

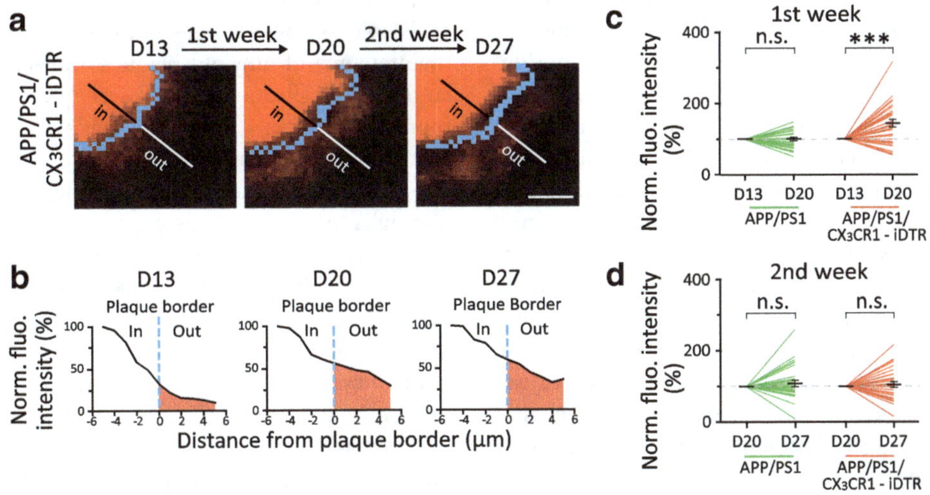

Fig. 4 Absence of microglia induces increase of Congo Red-labeled Aβ fluorescence surrounding plaques. **a**. An example of an Aβ plaque in *APP/PS1/CX₃CR1-iDTR* mice at D13, D20 and D27, with blue curves indicating plaque border. A radial line from the center point towards the outer area of a plaque is separated by the plaque border, with the inside part representing area in the plaque ("in", black) and the outside part representing the area surrounding the plaque ("out", white). Scale bar, 5 μm. **b**. Fluorescence intensity across the line in a, with 5 μm inside the plaque and 5 μm outside the plaque. Shadow area represents fluorescence intensity surrounding plaques. **c**. Normalized fluorescence intensity surrounding plaques from D13 to D20. Microglia depletion in *APP/PS1/CX₃CR1-iDTR* mice induced a significant increase of fluorescence in the area surrounding plaque ($n = 30$ plaques, $^{***}P < 0.001$, Wilcoxon matched-pairs signed rank test). **d**. In the second week after DT administration (from D20 to D27), fluorescence surrounding plaques showed no additional increase in *APP/PS1/CX₃CR1-iDTR* mice ($n = 30$ plaques, $P = 0.84$, Wilcoxon matched-pairs signed rank test)

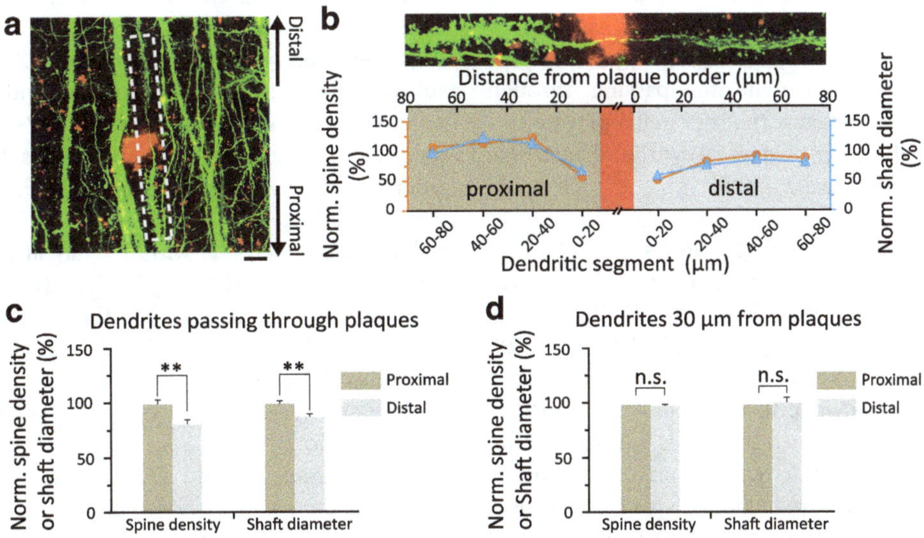

Fig. 5 Aβ plaques cause spine loss and shaft atrophy in the distal segments of dendrites passing through plaques **a**. Confocal image of YFP labeled dendrites passing through and near Aβ plaques in the fixed brain slice of *PSAPP* mice crossed with *Thy1* YFP H-line mice. Aβ plaques were labeled with Congo red (*red*). A yellow fluorescent protein-labeled dendrite (*green*) showed a significant reduction in spine density and dendritic diameter after entering the plaque. Scale bar, 20 μm. **b**. Upper panel shows the dendritic branch passing through the plaque in dashed area in a. Bottom panel shows the quantification of spine density (*orange curve*) and shaft diameter (*blue curve*) in every 20 μm long of dendritic segments, ranging from 0 to 80 μm from plaque border. **c**. Distal segments of dendrites passing through Aβ plaques showed reduced spine density and shaft diameter compared to proximal segments. ($n = 22$ dendrites from 4 mice, $^{**}P < 0.01$, student t-test). **d**. Spine density and shaft diameter of dendrites located greater than 30 μm away from plaque deposits showed no difference in the proximal and distal segments ($n = 22$ dendrites from 4 mice, $P > 0.05$, student t-test)

(segments between the cell body and the plaque) and "distal" segments (remaining segments after exiting the plaque, Fig. 5a, b), we found that distal segments of dendrites passing through plaques showed 19.4 ± 2.8% reduction in spine density and 11.1 ± 1.3% reduction in shaft diameter ($P < 0.01$) as compared to proximal segments (Fig. 5c). In contrast, dendrites that did not pass through plaques and were located > 30 μm away from plaque border showed no significant difference in spine density and shaft diameter between the corresponding distal and proximal segments (Fig. 5d). These findings show that amyloid plaque formation not only leads to dendritic abnormalities inside plaques, but also causes more global changes in distal segments of dendrites passing through plaques. The alterations of distal parts of dendrites passing through plaques suggest that ~13% expansion of amyloid plaques after microglia depletion could cause sizable damage in neuronal connectivity.

Discussion

It is generally believed that microglia are involved in regulating Aβ deposition, a key hallmark of Alzheimer's disease. However, the precise role of microglia in plaque formation and maintenance remains unclear. There are conflicting views on whether microglia are critical for limiting Aβ plaques, or microglia have no effect on plaque deposition. In this work, we examined the function of microglia in Aβ deposition by depleting microglia and imaging Aβ plaques in the living cortex of an *APP/PS1* mouse model. Our findings indicate the size of amyloid plaques increases in the absence of microglia. We further show that Aβ plaques are associated with dendritic spine loss and shaft atrophy in dendrites passing through plaques. These findings suggest that microglia play an important role in limiting Aβ plaques growth and neuronal damage in Alzheimer's disease.

Microglia limit the expansion of Aβ plaques

Mutations of *CD33* and *TREM2* genes expressed in microglia have been linked to increased risks of AD [26, 27, 37]. Altered Aβ load has been observed in $CX_3CR1^{-/-}$ [29, 30], $TREM2^{-/-}$ and $CD33^{-/-}$ mice [27]. In vitro studies have shown that microglia phagocytose Aβ [33–35]. Furthermore, in vivo studies have shown that Aβ is localized within microglial lysosomes and microglia volume surrounding plaques correlates with the reduction of plaque size over one month [25]. Together, these studies strongly suggest a role of microglia in Aβ clearance and/or regulating d Aβ deposition. However, previous studies of depleting microglia by introducing suicide gene *HSVTK* or inhibiting CSFR1 have shown that microglia depletion has no effect on both formation and maintenance of plaques [38, 39]. In the present study, using Cre-dependent microglia depletion and time-lapse imaging, we have now provided direct evidence that in the AD mouse model older than 12 months, microglia depletion over 1 week does not affect the formation or maintenance of amyloid plaques, but leads to a ~13% enlargement of plaque size in the cortex (Fig. 3d, e). Furthermore, 2 weeks after DT administration, microglia repopulation was associated with the stabilization of plaque size (Fig. 3d, f). Our findings strongly suggest the role of microglia in restricting the expansion of plaques.

It is important to point out several differences between previous studies and our work on the effect of microglia depletion. One difference is that previous studies examined the number and size of amyloid plaques using fixed brain tissues from different animals with or without microglia depletion [38, 39]. The variability in plaque number and size between different animals may make it difficult to detect relatively small changes in plaque size after microglia depletion. Taking advantage of time-lapse imaging, we have been able to track the same plaques over time and reveal the relative small changes (~13% over one week) of plaque size in response to microglia depletion. It is also important to note that microglia depletion in previous studies may take longer to occur than in our studies. The prolonged process of microglia depletion might cause compensatory responses such as astrocyte activation, which could lead to degradation of Aβ [45, 46]. Further studies are needed to address these possibilities in order to better understand the role of microglia in amyloid plaque deposition.

In addition to microglia in the brain, peripheral myeloid cells also express CX_3CR1 and therefore could be depleted by DT administration in *APP/PS1/CX₃CR1-iDTR* mice. However, microglia and peripheral CX_3CR1^+ cells have substantially different turnover rates and are derived from different precursor populations [40, 47–50]. Microglia are long-lived population [47] and it has been shown that when tamoxifen is administrated ~30 days prior to the administration of DT, *CX₃CR1-iDTR* mice have a dramatic reduction of microglia within 1 day after DT administration [40]. On the other hand, CX_3CR1^+ cells in the spleen or blood are not affected as these peripheral CX_3CR1^+ myeloid cells in *CX₃CR1-iDTR* mice are replenished through a CX_3CR1^- bone marrow precursor [47–50] and no longer express DT receptors 30 days after tamoxifen administration [40]. In our experiment, the time period between tamoxifen and DT administration was 7 days. Based on the rapid turnover of peripheral CX_3CR1^+ cells (Fig. 2 in ref. [40]), we expect that over this 7 day period the majority of peripheral CX_3CR1^+ cells would be replenished through a CX_3CR1^- bone marrow precursor and do not express DT receptors. A small fraction of peripheral myeloid cells would still express DT receptors and would be depleted following DT administration. Therefore, we could not completely rule out the possibility that in addition to microglia depletion, the depletion of some peripheral CX_3CR1^+ myeloid cells may also affect the growth of amyloid plaques. Future studies to specifically deplete peripheral CX_3CR1^+ myeloid cells using bone marrow transplantation are needed to determine the potential contribution of peripheral CX_3CR1^+ cell population in amyloid plaque formation.

Plaque growth may cause extensive neurite damage

A variety of studies have shown that abnormal spine density, spine turnover and diameter of dendritic shaft are associated with Aβ plaques [5, 7–9, 51]. In the current study, we found dendritic spine loss and shaft atrophy in the distal segments of dendrites passing through plaques when compared with proximal segments in the *PSAPP* mouse model of AD (Fig. 5a–c). This distal effect was not found in the dendrites which did not pass through plaques and were 30 μm away from Aβ plaques (Fig 5d). These results suggest that the expansion of Aβ plaques could cause damage not only in the local position but also to the entire distal segments of dendrites passing through. In this way, amyloid deposits might disrupt the signal propagation and protein transportation generated from soma and further lead to the degeneration of distal segments. The distal effect in dendrites passing through plaques also implies that extensive damage of neurites could be caused by enlargement of Aβ plaques when microglia are absent or microglia function is altered. These findings underscore the role of microglia in restricting the enlargement of plaques and limiting the neuronal damage in Alzheimer's disease. The expansion of amyloid plaques after microglia depletion and plaque-associated dendritic abnormalities likely contribute to memory loss and cognitive decline in AD [15–19]. However, it is worth mentioning that microglia in AD mice also likely have impacts on the function of neuronal circuits and animal's behaviors beyond their role in amyloid deposition and associated dystrophic neuritis [40, 52]. Thus, the depletion of microglia and resulting plaque expansion may or may not indicate disease worsening in AD mice. Future studies are needed to examine the impact of microglia depletion on neuronal network activity and plaque-associated synaptic abnormalities in the living mouse cortex in order to better understand microglia functions in AD. Furthermore, while plaque-associated dystrophic neurites have been shown in several AD mouse models and AD patients [4, 5, 7, 9, 51, 53], whether similar effects of amyloid plaques on distal dendrites observed in *PSAPP* mice also occur in other mouse models of AD remains to be investigated.

Conclusion

Our data highlight that microglia play an important role in limiting the growth of Aβ plaques. Microglia depletion does not affect plaque numbers, but causes a significant increase of plaque size over one week. Furthermore, microglia repopulation is associated with the stabilization of plaque size. Restricting the growth of plaques by microglia could have a significant impact on reducing abnormalities in dendrites passing through amyloid plaques. Taken together, our studies reveal an important role of microglia in limiting the growth of Aβ deposition and neuronal damage in the pathogenesis of AD.

Additional file

Additional file 1: Microglia are depleted in *APP/PS1/CX₃CR1-iDTR* mice over 1–7 days after DT administration and repopulate within 2 weeks after DT administration. **a**. Timeline of tamoxifen administration, DT administration and two-photon (2P) imaging. Microglia were examined before (D9), 1 day after (D13), 1 week after (D20) and 2 weeks after DT administration (D27). **b**. Time-lapse imaging in the same region in *APP/PS1/CX₃CR1-iDTR* mice and microglia morphology is revealed by CreER-IRES-EYFP under *CX₃CR1* promoter. The effects of DT administration over 1–2 weeks are similar to the effects on *CX₃CR1-iDTR* mice (Fig. 1b).

Abbreviations

ACSF: artificial cerebral spinal fluid; AD: Alzheimer's disease; APP/PS1: APPswe/PSEN1dE9; Aβ: β-amyloid; CX_3CR1-iDTR: $CX_3CR1^{CreER/+}$:$R26^{DTR/+}$; DT: diphtheria toxin; DTR: diphtheria toxin receptor; PSAPP: $PS1_{M146L}$ line 6.2 × Tg2576; ROI: region of interest

Acknowledgement

We thank members of Gan lab for critical comments and helpful discussions on this manuscript.

Funding

This work was supported by NIH 5R01 NS087198 and the Investigator Initiated Research Grant from Alzheimer's Association (IIRG-08-92101) to W.-B. G., Shenzhen Science and Technology Innovation Funds KQTD2015032709315529, JSGG20140703163838793, JSYJ20160428154351820 and ZDSYS201504301539161 to W. L.

Authors' contributions

RZ, WL and WG designed the experiments and wrote the manuscript; RZ and WL performed in vivo imaging; JT performed confocal imaging; WH bred quadruple transgenic mice and performed genotyping; RZ and JT analyzed the data; All authors read and approved the final manuscript.

Authors' information

Information for all the co-authors is listed in the title page.

Competing interests

The authors declare that they have no competing interests.

Author details

[1]Drug Discovery Center, Peking University Shenzhen Graduate School, Shenzhen 518055, China. [2]Skirball Institute, New York University School of Medicine, New York, NY 10016, USA.

References

1. Querfurth HW, LaFerla FM. Alzheimer's disease. N Engl J Med. 2010;362:329–44.
2. Scheltens P, Blennow K, Breteler MM, de Strooper B, Frisoni GB, Salloway S, et al. Alzheimer's disease. Lancet. 2016;388:505–17.
3. Cummings BJ, Su JH, Geddes JW, Van Nostrand WE, Wagner SL, Cunningham DD, et al. Aggregation of the amyloid precursor protein within degenerating neurons and dystrophic neurites in Alzheimer's disease. Neuroscience. 1992;48:763–77.
4. Knowles RB, Wyart C, Buldyrev SV, Cruz L, Urbanc B, Hasselmo ME, et al. Plaque-induced neurite abnormalities: implications for disruption of neural networks in Alzheimer's disease. Proc Natl Acad Sci U S A. 1999;96:5274–9.
5. Grutzendler J, Helmin K, Tsai J, Gan WB. Various dendritic abnormalities are associated with fibrillar amyloid deposits in Alzheimer's disease. Ann N Y Acad Sci. 2007;1097:30–9.
6. Serrano-Pozo A, Betensky RA, Frosch MP, Hyman BT. Plaque-associated local toxicity increases over the clinical course of Alzheimer disease. Am J Pathol. 2016;186:375–84.
7. Tsai J, Grutzendler J, Duff K, Gan WB. Fibrillar amyloid deposition leads to local synaptic abnormalities and breakage of neuronal branches. Nat Neurosci. 2004;7:1181–3.
8. Adalbert R, Nogradi A, Babetto E, Janeckova L, Walker SA, Kerschensteiner M, et al. Severely dystrophic axons at amyloid plaques remain continuous and connected to viable cell bodies. Brain. 2009;132:402–16.
9. Spires TL, Meyer-Luehmann M, Stern EA, McLean PJ, Skoch J, Nguyen PT, et al. Dendritic spine abnormalities in amyloid precursor protein transgenic mice demonstrated by gene transfer and intravital multiphoton microscopy. J Neurosci. 2005;25:7278–87.
10. Bittner T, Burgold S, Dorostkar MM, Fuhrmann M, Wegenast-Braun BM, Schmidt B, et al. Amyloid plaque formation precedes dendritic spine loss. Acta Neuropathol. 2012;124:797–807.
11. Walsh DM, Klyubin I, Fadeeva JV, Cullen WK, Anwyl R, Wolfe MS, et al. Naturally secreted oligomers of amyloid beta protein potently inhibit hippocampal long-term potentiation in vivo. Nature. 2002;416:535–9.
12. Akhtar MW, Sanz-Blasco S, Dolatabadi N, Parker J, Chon K, Lee MS, et al. Elevated glucose and oligomeric beta-amyloid disrupt synapses via a common pathway of aberrant protein S-nitrosylation. Nat Commun. 2016;7:10242.
13. Busche MA, Eichhoff G, Adelsberger H, Abramowski D, Wiederhold KH, Haass C, et al. Clusters of hyperactive neurons near amyloid plaques in a mouse model of Alzheimer's disease. Science. 2008;321:1686–9.
14. Busche MA, Kekus M, Adelsberger H, Noda T, Forstl H, Nelken I, Konnerth A. Rescue of long-range circuit dysfunction in Alzheimer's disease models. Nat Neurosci. 2015;18:1623-1630.
15. Terry RD, Masliah E, Salmon DP, Butters N, DeTeresa R, Hill R, et al. Physical basis of cognitive alterations in Alzheimer's disease: synapse loss is the major correlate of cognitive impairment. Ann Neurol. 1991;30:572–80.
16. Masliah E, Ellisman M, Carragher B, Mallory M, Young S, Hansen L, et al. Three-dimensional analysis of the relationship between synaptic pathology and neuropil threads in Alzheimer disease. J Neuropathol Exp Neurol. 1992;51:404–14.
17. Spires-Jones TL, Hyman BT. The intersection of amyloid beta and tau at synapses in Alzheimer's disease. Neuron. 2014;82:756–71.
18. Hardy JA, Higgins GA. Alzheimer's disease: the amyloid cascade hypothesis. Science. 1992;256:184–5.
19. Jack CR Jr, Lowe VJ, Weigand SD, Wiste HJ, Senjem ML, Knopman DS, et al. Serial PIB and MRI in normal, mild cognitive impairment and Alzheimer's disease: implications for sequence of pathological events in Alzheimer's disease. Brain. 2009;132:1355–65.
20. Prinz M, Priller J, Sisodia SS, Ransohoff RM. Heterogeneity of CNS myeloid cells and their roles in neurodegeneration. Nat Neurosci. 2011;14:1227–35.
21. Gomez Perdiguero E, Schulz C, Geissmann F. Development and homeostasis of "resident" myeloid cells: the case of the microglia. Glia. 2013;61:112–20.
22. Rozemuller JM, Eikelenboom P, Stam FC. Role of microglia in plaque formation in senile dementia of the Alzheimer type. An immunohistochemical study. Virchows Arch B Cell Pathol Incl Mol Pathol. 1986;51:247–54.
23. Mattiace LA, Davies P, Yen SH, Dickson DW. Microglia in cerebellar plaques in Alzheimer's disease. Acta Neuropathol. 1990;80:493–8.
24. Meyer-Luehmann M, Spires-Jones TL, Prada C, Garcia-Alloza M, de Calignon A, Rozkalne A, et al. Rapid appearance and local toxicity of amyloid-beta plaques in a mouse model of Alzheimer's disease. Nature. 2008;451:720–4.
25. Bolmont T, Haiss F, Eicke D, Radde R, Mathis CA, Klunk WE, et al. Dynamics of the microglial/amyloid interaction indicate a role in plaque maintenance. J Neurosci. 2008;28:4283–92.
26. Hollingworth P, Harold D, Sims R, Gerrish A, Lambert JC, Carrasquillo MM, et al. Common variants at ABCA7, MS4A6A/MS4A4E, EPHA1, CD33 and CD2AP are associated with Alzheimer's disease. Nat Genet. 2011;43:429–35.
27. Griciuc A, Serrano-Pozo A, Parrado AR, Lesinski AN, Asselin CN, Mullin K, et al. Alzheimer's disease risk gene CD33 inhibits microglial uptake of amyloid beta. Neuron. 2013;78:631–43.
28. Jonsson T, Stefansson H, Steinberg S, Jonsdottir I, Jonsson PV, Snaedal J, et al. Variant of TREM2 associated with the risk of Alzheimer's disease. N Engl J Med. 2013;368:107–16.
29. Lee S, Varvel NH, Konerth ME, Xu G, Cardona AE, Ransohoff RM, et al. CX3CR1 deficiency alters microglial activation and reduces beta-amyloid deposition in two Alzheimer's disease mouse models. Am J Pathol. 2010;177:2549–62.
30. Liu Z, Condello C, Schain A, Harb R, Grutzendler J. CX3CR1 in microglia regulates brain amyloid deposition through selective protofibrillar amyloid-beta phagocytosis. J Neurosci. 2010;30:17091–101.
31. Wang Y, Cella M, Mallinson K, Ulrich JD, Young KL, Robinette ML, et al. TREM2 lipid sensing sustains the microglial response in an Alzheimer's disease model. Cell. 2015;160:1061–71.
32. Wang Y, Ulland TK, Ulrich JD, Song W, Tzaferis JA, Hole JT, et al. TREM2-mediated early microglial response limits diffusion and toxicity of amyloid plaques. J Exp Med. 2016;213:667–75.
33. Paresce DM, Ghosh RN, Maxfield FR. Microglial cells internalize aggregates of the Alzheimer's disease amyloid beta-protein via a scavenger receptor. Neuron. 1996;17:553–65.
34. Koenigsknecht J, Landreth G. Microglial phagocytosis of fibrillar beta-amyloid through a beta1 integrin-dependent mechanism. J Neurosci. 2004;24:9838–46.
35. Herber DL, Mercer M, Roth LM, Symmonds K, Maloney J, Wilson N, et al. Microglial activation is required for Abeta clearance after intracranial injection of lipopolysaccharide in APP transgenic mice. J Neuroimmune Pharmacol. 2007;2:222–31.
36. Condello C, Yuan P, Schain A, Grutzendler J. Microglia constitute a barrier that prevents neurotoxic protofibrillar Abeta42 hotspots around plaques. Nat Commun. 2015;6:6176.
37. Yuan P, Condello C, Keene CD, Wang Y, Bird TD, Paul SM, et al. TREM2 Haplodeficiency in mice and humans impairs the microglia barrier function leading to decreased Amyloid compaction and severe axonal dystrophy. Neuron. 2016;90:724–39.
38. Grathwohl SA, Kalin RE, Bolmont T, Prokop S, Winkelmann G, Kaeser SA, et al. Formation and maintenance of Alzheimer's disease beta-amyloid plaques in the absence of microglia. Nat Neurosci. 2009;12:1361–3.
39. Spangenberg EE, Lee RJ, Najafi AR, Rice RA, Elmore MR, Blurton-Jones M, et al. Eliminating microglia in Alzheimer's mice prevents neuronal loss without modulating amyloid-beta pathology. Brain. 2016;139:1265–81.
40. Parkhurst CN, Yang G, Ninan I, Savas JN, Yates JR 3rd, Lafaille JJ, et al. Microglia promote learning-dependent synapse formation through brain-derived neurotrophic factor. Cell. 2013;155:1596–609.
41. Yang G, Pan F, Parkhurst CN, Grutzendler J, Gan WB. Thinned-skull cranial window technique for long-term imaging of the cortex in live mice. Nat Protoc. 2010;5:201–8.
42. Hefendehl JK, Wegenast-Braun BM, Liebig C, Eicke D, Milford D, Calhoun ME, et al. Long-term in vivo imaging of beta-amyloid plaque appearance and growth in a mouse model of cerebral beta-amyloidosis. J Neurosci. 2011;31:624–9.
43. Yan P, Bero AW, Cirrito JR, Xiao Q, Hu X, Wang Y, et al. Characterizing the appearance and growth of amyloid plaques in APP/PS1 mice. J Neurosci. 2009;29:10706–14.
44. Burgold S, Bittner T, Dorostkar MM, Kieser D, Fuhrmann M, Mitteregger G, et al. In vivo multiphoton imaging reveals gradual growth of newborn amyloid plaques over weeks. Acta Neuropathol. 2011;121:327–35.
45. Wyss-Coray T, Loike JD, Brionne TC, Lu E, Anankov R, Yan F, et al. Adult mouse astrocytes degrade amyloid-beta in vitro and in situ. Nat Med. 2003;9:453–7.
46. Koistinaho M, Lin S, Wu X, Esterman M, Koger D, Hanson J, et al. Apolipoprotein E promotes astrocyte colocalization and degradation of deposited amyloid-beta peptides. Nat Med. 2004;10:719–26.
47. Ajami B, Bennett JL, Krieger C, Tetzlaff W, Rossi FM. Local self-renewal can sustain CNS microglia maintenance and function throughout adult life. Nat Neurosci. 2007;10:1538–43.
48. Lawson LJ, Perry VH, Gordon S. Turnover of resident microglia in the normal adult mouse brain. Neuroscience. 1992;48:405–15.
49. van Furth R, Cohn ZA. The origin and kinetics of mononuclear phagocytes. J Exp Med. 1968;128:415–35.

50. Fogg DK, Sibon C, Miled C, Jung S, Aucouturier P, Littman DR, et al. A clonogenic bone marrow progenitor specific for macrophages and dendritic cells. Science. 2006;311:83–7.
51. Kirkwood CM, Ciuchta J, Ikonomovic MD, Fish KN, Abrahamson EE, Murray PS, et al. Dendritic spine density, morphology, and fibrillar actin content surrounding amyloid-beta plaques in a mouse model of amyloid-beta deposition. J Neuropathol Exp Neurol. 2013;72:791–800.
52. Miyamoto A, Wake H, Ishikawa AW, Eto K, Shibata K, Murakoshi H, et al. Microglia contact induces synapse formation in developing somatosensory cortex. Nat Commun. 2016;7:12540.
53. Bittner T, Fuhrmann M, Burgold S, Ochs SM, Hoffmann N, Mitteregger G, et al. Multiple events lead to dendritic spine loss in triple transgenic Alzheimer's disease mice. PLoS One. 2010;5:e15477.

2

Tetraspanin 6: a pivotal protein of the multiple vesicular body determining exosome release and lysosomal degradation of amyloid precursor protein fragments

Francesc X. Guix[1,2*], Ragna Sannerud[1,2†], Fedor Berditchevski[3†], Amaia M. Arranz[1,2], Katrien Horré[1,2], An Snellinx[1,2], Amantha Thathiah[4], Takaomi Saido[5], Takashi Saito[5], Sundaresan Rajesh[3], Michael Overduin[6], Samir Kumar-Singh[7], Enrico Radaelli[1,2], Nikky Corthout[1,2], Julien Colombelli[8], Sébastien Tosi[8], Sebastian Munck[1,2], Isabel H. Salas[1,2], Wim Annaert[1,2] and Bart De Strooper[1,2,9*]

Abstract

Background: The mechanisms behind Aβ-peptide accumulation in non-familial Alzheimer's disease (AD) remain elusive. Proteins of the tetraspanin family modulate Aβ production by interacting to γ-secretase.

Methods: We searched for tetraspanins with altered expression in AD brains. The function of the selected tetraspanin was studied in vitro and the physiological relevance of our findings was confirmed in vivo.

Results: Tetraspanin-6 (TSPAN6) is increased in AD brains and overexpression in cells exerts paradoxical effects on Amyloid Precursor Protein (APP) metabolism, increasing APP-C-terminal fragments (APP-CTF) and Aβ levels at the same time. TSPAN6 affects autophagosome-lysosomal fusion slowing down the degradation of APP-CTF. TSPAN6 recruits also the cytosolic, exosome-forming adaptor syntenin which increases secretion of exosomes that contain APP-CTF.

Conclusions: TSPAN6 is a key player in the bifurcation between lysosomal-dependent degradation and exosome mediated secretion of APP-CTF. This corroborates the central role of the autophagosomal/lysosomal pathway in APP metabolism and shows that TSPAN6 is a crucial player in APP-CTF turnover.

Keywords: Alzheimer's disease, Amyloid precursor protein, Intraluminal vesicles, Multivesicular bodies, Tetraspanin-6

Background

Alzheimer's disease (AD) is a devastating neurodegenerative disease and the first cause of human dementia [1]. Quantitative and qualitative alterations of the amyloid Aβ peptides together with tau-pathology, initiate a long cycle of cellular action and reaction eventually leading to severe neuronal loss [2]. Aβ peptides are generated from the transmembrane protein Amyloid Precursor Protein (APP) by proteolytic activities exerted by the β-secretase BACE1 and members of the γ-secretase family [3]. While mutations in APP and presenilins (the catalytic components of the γ-secretases complexes) alter Aβ production in familial AD cases [4], the mechanisms by which Aβ-peptide production, clearance and aggregation are altered in non-familial cases is of varied etiology [5–11].

Detergent resistant membrane (DRM) and tetraspanin-enriched microdomains (TEMs) play important roles in the regulation of the proteases that generate Aβ [12–17]. TEMs represent molecular assemblies of proteins and lipids based on multiple interactions involving four-transmembrane-domain proteins of the tetraspanin superfamily [18, 19]. In an unbiased proteomic analysis, our laboratory found that tetraspanins CD9 and CD81 (also known as TSPAN28 and TSPAN29) interact with components of the γ-secretase complex and modulate its activity towards APP [20]. Two other tetraspanins

* Correspondence: fguixrafols@gmail.com; Bart.destrooper@cme.vib-kuleuven.be
†Equal contributors
[1]VIB Center for Brain and Disease research – VIB, Leuven, Belgium
Full list of author information is available at the end of the article

(TSPAN33 and TSPAN5) promote Notch activity [21]. Tetraspanins also play a role in the maturation and trafficking of ADAM10, one of the enzymes involved in the non-amyloidogenic cleavage of APP [22–24] and finally, interact with the γ-secretase complexes and ADAM10 or BACE1 to form supramolecular complexes in the membrane [17]. Beyond their involvement in the regulation of these proteolytic enzymes, tetraspanins play a crucial role in many other cellular processes, from the control of the endocytic trafficking to autophagic-induced cell death [18, 25–28]. Specifically, our interest in the role of tetraspanin-6 (TSPAN6) in sporadic AD was supported by observations from several independent groups which indicate that the mRNA levels of TSPAN6 are increased in the prefrontal cortex of AD patients and correlate with Braak stage progression [29–31]. Therefore, we decided to focus our studies on the role that TSPAN6 plays in the molecular pathogenesis of sporadic AD.

We demonstrate here that overexpression of TSPAN6 affects APP metabolism, but unexpectedly, this effect does not involve the γ-secretases. In contrast, we determined that TSPAN6 is enriched in multivesicular bodies (MVBs) and intraluminal vesicles (ILVs). Increasing TSPAN6 levels enhances endosomal size and leads to an increased number of intraluminal vesicles (ILVs) and increased secretion of exosomes containing the APP-CTF. TSPAN6 recruits the cytosolic adaptor syntenin through its PDZ1 domain which explains the increased exosome release, while the impaired degradation of proteins is due in part to the decreased fusion between autophagosomes and lysosomes caused by TSPAN6 expression. Thus the accumulation of APP-CTF is caused by a dual mechanism putting TSPAN6 in a pivotal point in the pathway of ILV towards exosomes or lysosomal degradation. The cellular pathology resembles the wide spread endolysosomal disturbances observed in neurons from patients suffering from sporadic AD.

Methods

Western blots

Total cell lysates were prepared in lysis buffer containing 50 mM HEPES pH 7.4, 150 mM NaCl, 1% TritonX100 (unless otherwise indicated) and complete protease inhibitors (Roche Applied Science). Post-nuclear fractions were taken, and protein concentrations were determined using standard BCA assay (Pierce Biotechnology). Proteins were separated on NuPAGE 4–12% Bis–Tris gels (Invitrogen) and transferred to nitrocellulose membranes for Western blot analysis. After blocking the membrane with 1% non-fat milk in T-TBS 1× (0.05 M Tris, pH 7.5; 0.15 M NaCl; 0.1% Tween20), the proteins were detected with the commercial antibodies: polyclonal anti-TSPAN6 antibody (1/500; Abgent), monoclonal MAB5232 anti-CTF-PS1 and monoclonal MAB1563 anti-NTF-PS1 (1/5000; Chemicon/Millipore), monoclonal 9C3 anti-Nct (1/5000), monoclonal 6E10 anti-Aβ (SIGNET), monoclonal anti-LC3β (D11) XP (1/1000; Cell Signalling), polyclonal anti-sAPPβ (1/1000; Covance), monoclonal anti-BACE1 D10E5 (1/1000; Cell Signalling), polyclonal anti-p62 (1/1000), monoclonal anti-FlagM2 antibody (1/4000; Sigma-Aldrich), monoclonal anti-βactin (1/5000; Sigma), polyclonal anti-APLP2 (1/1000; W2CT donated by Dominic Walsh), monoclonal anti-LRP1 EPR3724 (1/15000; Epitomics), monoclonal anti-Tsg101 (1/1000; Santa Cruz). The following in-house made antibodies: B63 for APP (1/10,000), B80 for Aph1a (1/1000) and B126 for Pen2 (1/2000).

Signals were detected using the chemiluminescence detection with Renaissance (PerkinElmer Life Sciences). Quantifications were performed by densitometry with the software AIDA

Generation of the Tspan6 knockout mice and genotyping

For this KO line, ES cells derived from the 129/OlaHsd mouse substrain were used to generate chimeric mice. F1 mice were generated by breeding with C57BL/6 females. F2 homozygous mutant mice were produced by intercrossing F1 heterozygous males and females. The KO line has subsequently been backcrossed several times to C57BL/6.

In order to genotype the *Tspan6 KO* mice, tails were lyzed with KAPA Genotyping Kit (KAPA Biosystems) following the instructions of the company. For the PCR, 3 different primers were used: 5'- TGTGATCAAGG ACTCAAGCTTGTAC-3', 5'-CTTACTCACCAGTTTCA GCATCCAG-3' and 5'-GGGTGGGATTAGATAAATG CCTGCTCT -3'.

Immunohistochemistry on brain sections

Immunohistochemistry was performed as described in [32]. Briefly, antigen retrieval was performed in citrate buffer (0.018 M citric acid.H_2O, 0.082 M sodium citrate, pH = 6) using microwave heating. Endogenous peroxidases and non-specific antigens were blocked by incubating sections in 0.3% H_2O_2 for 20 min followed by a 1:5 diluted normal horse serum block for 30 min. Sections were incubated overnight at 4 °C with primary antibodies: polyclonal anti-Tspan6 C-terminus (Abgent, 1:50 dilution), mouse monoclonal (mAb) anti-vGlut2 (Abcam, 1:2000 dilution) and mAb anti-GAD67 (Millipore, 1:500 dilution). Sections were further incubated with biotin conjugated secondary antibodies and extravidin conjugated HRP, each for 30 min at room temperature, and detected with 5, 5' diaminobenzidine (Dako, Heverlee, Belgium). Images were captured using 40x objective and Olympus UC30 colour camera (Olympus, Antwerp, Belgium).

For double immunohistochemistry staining, combinations of anti-Tspan6 C-terminus antibody (Abgent, 1:50 dilution) with either anti-vGlut2 mouse monoclonal (Abcam, 1:2000 dilution) or anti-GAD67 mouse monoclonal (Millipore, 1:500 dilution) were incubated overnight and detected with DAG-Cy3 and DAM-Cy5 (Jackson Immunoresearch). Sections were counterstained with 5 μg/mL DAPI (Sigma-Aldrich, Diegem, Belgium) for 5 min and visualized with a dual spinning disk confocal microscope (Ultra*View* VoX, PerkinElmer, Seer green, UK) and images analysed using Volocity (PerkinElmer) essentially as described earlier [32].

Mouse brain homogenates for western blot

Pieces of cerebral cortices of 1 year old *Tspan6*$^{+/Y}$ ($n = 7$) and *Tspan6*$^{-/Y}$ ($n = 7$) mice or 1 year old App$^{NL/F}$ x *Tspan6 wt* ($n = 5$) and App$^{NL/F}$ x *Tspan6 KO* mice ($n = 6$) were homogenized on ice in 0.5 M sucrose PKM buffer (100 mM Potassium phosphate; 5 mM $MgCl_2$; 3 mM KCl; pH 6.5) containing 1% TritonX100 and 0.1% SDS. After removal of the debris by 30 minuts centrifugation at 14.000 rpm and 4 °C, 40 μg of total protein per sample was loaded on NuPAGE 4-12% Bis-Tris gels (Invitrogen).

Mouse brain homogenates for ELISA

Pieces of mice cerebral cortices coming from 1 year old *Tspan6*$^{+/Y}$ ($n = 7$) and *Tspan6*$^{-/Y}$ ($n = 7$) mice were weighted and homogenized in 5 volumes of pre-filtered extraction buffer (0.4% diethanolamine, 50 mM NaCl, 1x Protease inhibitors (Roche)) with Fastprep (45 s at 6 m/s). The homogenates were centrifuged at 14.000 rpm for 5 min at 4 °C and the supernatants were ultracentrifuged at 90.000 rpm for 30 min at 4 °C. A 10% volume of neutralization buffer (0.5 M Tris-HCl, pH = 6.8) was added to the new supernatants before determination of the $A\beta_{40}$ and $A\beta_{42}$ content by ELISA. For normalization purposes, protein concentration was measured by standard BCA assay (Pierce Biotechnology).

Primary neurons

Primary cultures of mouse cortical neurons were obtained from *Tspan6 KO* mice at E14.5. The procedure was carried out in accordance with the Ethic Committee of K. Leuven University (Ethische Commissie Dierproeven, KULeuven). Briefly, the cortical region of the brain was aseptically dissected and trypsinized for 15 min. Cells were seeded in phenol-red MEM with L-glutamine (Invitrogen) plus 10% horse serum and 0.6% glucose into 0.1 mg/ml poly-l-lysine coated plates. After 120 min, medium was removed and neurobasal medium containing B27 supplement (NB-B27) was added.

ELISA

For detection of human and mouse Aβ, an in-house ELISA sandwich was carried out. Briefly, 96-wells Nunc-Immuno plates (Nunc, Denmark) were coated overnight at 4 °C with JRF AB038 antibody for Aβ1-38, JRF cAb040/28 antibody for Aβ40 or JRF Ab042/26 antibody for Aß42 (Janssen Pharmaceutica), all used at 1.5 mg/ml in PBS containing 0.1% casein (Casein Buffer). Plates were washed 5 times with Washing Buffer (PBS-0.05% Tween 20) before the addition of the samples or the standard curve made with consecutive dilutions (from 100 to 0.0003 ng/ml) of human or mouse Aβ40 and Aβ42 (rPeptide). Detection antibody was obtained from Janssen; huAB25-HRPO. After overnight incubation at 4 °C and 5 time washes with the Washing Buffer, the samples were developed with a 0.02% TMB (tetramethylbenzidine) solution in Sodium Acetate (100 mM pH 4.9) containing 0.03% H_2O_2. The reaction was stopped with 0.2 N H_2SO_4 and read at 450 nm on a Perkin Elmer Envision 2103 multilabel reader.

Immunoisolation of late compartments

Late compartments were isolated from HEK293 cells co-expressing an empty vector or myc-TSPAN6 together with LAMP1 fused to mRFP and to a double Flag-tag (LAMP1-mRFP-Flag) as previously described in Zoncu et al. [33] with small variations. Briefly, cells were harvested from 2 x T175 flasks per condition through scraping in cold PBS, spun down and resuspended in 1 ml of fractionation buffer: 50 mM KCl, 90 mM K-Gluconate, 1 mM EGTA, 5 mM $MgCl_2$, 50 mM Sucrose, 20 mM HEPES, pH 7.4, supplemented with 2.5 mM ATP, 5 mM Glucose and protease inhibitors. Cells were mechanically broken by passing them through a 23G needle attached to a 1 ml syringe, then spun down at 2000 g for 10 min, yielding a post nuclear supernatant (PNS). The PNS was brought to 2 ml with fractionation buffer and subjected to immunoprecipitation with 50 μl of anti-FlagM2 affinity beads for 3 h at 4 °C. Late-compartments were in this way captured by the beads while the rest of organelles were washed out by 3 consecutive washes with fractionation buffer. Late-compartments bound to the beads were re-suspended in loading buffer and proteins were separated on a 4-12% SDS-PAGE gel. After transferring proteins onto a nitrocellulose membrane by western blot, the enrichment of late compartments were analyzed with an anti-LAMP1 antibody, the content of APP and APP-CTF was evaluated with a polyclonal anti-APP antibody (B63) and the overexpression of TSPAN6 was determined by a polyclonal TSPAN6 antibody.

Pulse-chase

HEK293 cells were seeded on 6-well plates and co-transfected with FlagAPP-C99 and an empty vector or

TSPAN6. After 24 h cells were starved for 45 min and labeled with radioactive methionine/cysteine [35S] for 15 min. Cells were chased for indicated time points and lyzed in lysis buffer (1% TritonX100 in 100 mM NaCl, 50 mM HEPES pH 7.2 and protease inhibitors). FlagAPP-C99 was immunoprecipitated from the cell lysates using FlagM2-Sepharose beads (Sigma-Aldrich) and submitted to SDS-PAGE/western blot. Radiolabeled proteins were visualized with phosphoimaging.

Proximity ligation assay (PLA)

PLA was carried out with the DuoLink In Situ Kit according to the manufacturer guidelines (Olink Bioscience). Briefly, HEK293 cells transfected with myc-TSPAN6 or left untransfected (technical control) were fixed in 4% paraformaldehyde on coverslips and blocked with blocking solution (0.3% TritonX100 and 5% goat serum in PBS) for 15 min at RT. A mouse monoclonal anti-myc antibody (9E10) and a rabbit monoclonal anti-APP antibody (Y188) were diluted 1/200 in PBS and applied to the samples for 2 h at RT in a humidity chamber. After removing the primary antibodies by 3 consecutive washes with PBS (5 min each), the samples were incubated for 1 h at 37 °C with the PLA Probes diluted 1/5 in PBS. After the incubation time, the unbound PLA probes were removed by consecutive washes with Buffer A (provided by the manufacturer), followed by the incubation of the samples for 30 min at 37 °C with the ligase. Buffer A was used to wash the samples before the addition of the polymerase-amplification solution. After 100 min incubation at 37 °C in a humidity chamber, the samples were washed with buffer B (provided by the manufacturer) and mounted for analysis by confocal microscopy.

γ-Secretase assay with endogenous substrate

HEK293-APPwt cells were transfected with myc-TSPAN6, and 24 h post-transfection cell membranes were prepared. Cells were harvested and resuspended in hypotonic buffer (10 mM Tris, pH 7.3, 10 mM MgCl2, 1 mM EDTA and 1 mM EGTA) for 10 min on ice. Cells were then homogenized by passing 15 times through a 21G needle and centrifuged for 10 min at 100 g to pellet nuclei. The resulting supernatant was centrifuged 30 min at 16 000 g. Pelleted membranes were resuspended in citrate buffer (150 mM sodium citrate, adjust pH 6.4 with citric acid, complete protease inhibitors) and incubated at 4 °C (as negative control) or at 37 °C for 2 h. Analysis of γ-secretase products was performed with standard SDS-PAGE/western blot.

γ-Secretase assay with exogenous substrate

HEK293 cells were transfected with myc-TSPAN6 for 24 h or treated with *siRNA-TSPAN6* for 48 h. Cell were homogenized in Buffer A (20 mM pipes pH7, 140 mM KCl, 0.25 M sucrose, 5 mM EGTA) with complete protease inhibitors (Roche Applied Science) and the microsomal membrane fraction was obtained by ultracentrifugation at 55.000 rpm at 4 °C. Cell-free assays were performed as described by Kakuda and colleagues [34] with some minor modifications. Briefly, microsomal membrane fractions solubilized in Buffer B (50 mM pipes, pH7, 0.25 M sucrose, 1 mM EGTA) containing 1% CHAPSO were mixed with recombinant APP-C99-3 × FLAG substrate (0.5 μM final concentration), 0.0125% phosphatidylethanolamine, 0.1% phosphatidylcholine, and 2.5% DMSO. Reactions were incubated at 37 °C for 4 h. Aβ species produced during the reaction were measured by ELISA and the levels of AICD produced were determined by SDS-PAGE electrophoresis and western blot with a mouse anti-FlagM2 and goat anti-mouse IR800 antibody. Infrared signals were detected using the Odyssey Infrared Imaging System.

Exosomes isolation and quantification

HEK293 cells non-overexpressing (control) or overexpressing TSPAN6 were incubated for 2 days under growing conditions (at 37 °C and 5% CO_2) with Exosomes-depleted medium obtained by overnight ultracentrifugation of 20% FBS-supplemented DMEM/F12 at 100.000 g and 4 °C and diluted 1:2 in FBS-free DMEM/F12. After 2 days the medium was collected and the death cells and other debris were removed by consecutive centrifugations at 4 °C at 200 g for 10 min, 2000 g for 10 min and 12000 g for 45 min. Finally the exosomes were obtained by ultracentrifugation of the supernatant at 110.000 g for 1 h at 4 °C. The pellet containing the exosomal fraction was washed once with pre-filtered PBS and posterior ultracentrifugation at 110.000 g for 1 h at 4 °C. The quality of the exosomal fraction obtained by this method was determined by comparing the protein expression of exosomal markers and non-exosomal proteins between total lysate and the exosomal fraction after electrophoretic separation of the samples on 4-12% SDS-PAGE and posterior western blot analysis with specific antibodies against the ER marker calnexin, Tsg101, TSPAN6 and actin. Determination of the number of exosomes present in the exosomal fraction was carried out by Nanosight.

Electron microscopy

HEK cells and primary neurons grown on aclar coverslips were rinsed briefly and fixed in 1.3% glutaraldehyde in 66 mM cacodylate buffer for 2 h at RT before processing for electron microscopy. Then the cells were washed for 30 min in 0.1 M cacodylate buffer and post-fixed for 2 h at RT in 1% OsO_4, 1.5% $K_4Fe(CN)_6$ in 0.1 M cacodylate buffer. Cells were rinsed again in 0.1 M cacodylate buffer and stained with 3% uranyl acetate for 1 h. Dehydration was performed at RT by transferring the cells to 35%, 50%, 70%, 90% and two steps of 100% ethanol for 10 min each. The cells were then embedded in EMbed812 and resin blocks were sectioned on an ultramicrotome (Leica Ultracut UCT, Leica Mycrosystems). Ultrathin sections (70 nm) were mounted on copper grids and imaged using a JEM-1400 transmission electron microscope (JEOL), equipped with an 11Mpixel Olympus SIS Quemesa camera. Quantifications of the area and number of subcellular compartments were performed with the image processing software ImageJ (Fiji distribution).

Lentiviral vectors production and transduction of neurons in culture

The vectors psPAX2 and pMD2.G were constructed and provided by D. Trono (Geneva, Switzerland); the vector pLVx-puro was used to subclone *Tspan6*.

Lentiviral particles were produced by using TransIT-LT1 transfection protocol on 60% confluent HEK293. Cells were transfected with a plasmid mix containing the vector pLVx encoding Tspan6 (LV-Tspan6) or empty pLVx (LV-cnt), the packaging construct psPAX2 and the envelope plasmid pMD2G-VSVG (at the following ratio 1.5:2:1). After 4 h post-transfection, the medium was replaced by fresh growth medium and cells were left for 24 h to produce viral particles. The 24 h-medium was harvested and fresh growth medium was added to the cells for additional viral production. After another 24 h the medium was harvested and mixed with the first 24 h medium. The medium was ultracentrifugated at 50.000 g for 2 h at 16 °C to pellet down the viral particles. Finally, the lentiviral vesicles were resuspended in sterile 100 μL PBS.

Primary cortical neurons derived from $Tspan6^{+/Y}$ and $Tspan6^{-/Y}$ E14.5 embryos were plated in 12-wells plates and transduced at DIV 6 by replacing the growth medium (NB-B27) by fresh neurobasal medium without B27 (NB) containing 3 μL of LV-TSPAN6 or LV-cnt. After 4 h the medium was replaced by the original NB-B27 and the neurons were left for 2 days to express the gene of interest. At DIV 9 the medium was replaced by experimental medium (NB containing only glutamate) and 24 h later it was collected for Aβ determination and neurons were lyzed in lysis buffer for western blot analysis or fixed in 1.3% glutaraldehyde in 66 mM cacodylate buffer for EM analysis.

Confocal laser scanning microscopy and quantification

Cells were plated on glass coverslips, transfected 24 h and processed for indirect immunolabeling the next day as in [35]. Images were captured on a confocal microscope (Leica TCS SP5 II, Leica Microsystems) connected to an upright microscope, using an oil-immersion plan Apo 60x A/1.40 NA objective lens. Image acquisition was performed with LAS (Leica Microsystems Gmbh, Wetzlar, Gemany) and further processed with ImageJ (Rasband, W.S., ImageJ, U. S. National Institutes of Health, Bethesda, Maryland, USA, http://imagej.nih.gov/ij/, 1997–2016). The ImageJ plugin JACoP (Fabrice P. Cordelieres, Institut Curie, Orsay, France. Susanne Bolte, IFR 83, Paris, France) was used for signal colocalization by overlap quantification (Manders coefficients). Images were acquired with identical settings and regions of interest covering whole cells were used for quantification [36]. Data are expressed as mean ± s.e.m. from n cells

Study of autophagic flux

HEK293 cells were seeded on 12-well plates and transfected with an empty vector or TSPAN6. After 24 h the cells were washed once with *Earle's Balanced Salt Solution* (EBSS) medium and incubated with EBSS medium for the time indicated with or without 10 μM Bafilomycine A1. After the incubation time, the cells were lyzed in lysis buffer at 4 °C and proteins were analyzed by SDS-PAGE electrophoresis and western blot. The activation of autophagy was analyzed with a polyclonal antibody anti-LC3β (Cell Signalling) and a polyclonal antibody against p62. The effect of the activation of autophagy on the degradation of APP-CTF or PS1-CTF (negative control) was evaluated with a polyclonal antibody against APP (B63) and a monoclonal antibody against PS1-CTF (Millipore). The overexpression of TSPAN6 was evaluated with a polyclonal antibody against TSPAN6 (Abgent).

Cell-based assay for Notch

HEK293 cells were seeded on 6-wells plates (800.000 cells/well). For the evaluation of the effect of TSPAN6 overexpression on the γ-secretase-mediated cleavage of Notch, cells were co-transfected with NotchΔE and an empty vector or TSPAN6. For the study of the effect of TSPAN6 downregulation on Notch processing, cells were co-transfected with siRNA against TSPAN6 (*siRNA-TSPAN6*) or a scrambled siRNA (siRNA-cnt) and NotchΔE. The cells were treated with 10 μM lactacystine overnight to allow the accumulation of the NICD product before lyzing the cells in lysis buffer for 20 min. After lysis, the samples were spun down for 14.000 rpm for 15 min at 4 °C and 30 μg of total protein of the supernatant was run on a 12% MES gel and transferred to a nitrocellulose membrane by western blot. Analysis of NotchΔE cleavage was evaluated with a monoclonal antibody against cleaved Notch1 (Val1744; 1/1000) and a monoclonal antibody against myc (9E10; 1/15000). Goat anti-mouse IR700 antibody and goat anti-rabbit IR800 antibody were used to analyze the infrared signals of the bands with the Odyssey Infrared Imaging System.

Real-time PCR

Total RNA was extracted from HEK293 cells expressing an empty vector or TSPAN6 with the miRVana kit (Thermo Fisher Scientific). Briefly, cells were collected in 1 ml ice-cold Trizol after a brief wash in ice-cold PBS and homogenized with a 23G syringe needle on ice. After the addition of 200 µL chloroform the homogenate was centrifuged at 12,000 g for 1 min at RT and the aqueous phase (~400 µL) was transferred to a new tube and mixed with 1.25 volumes of ethanol 100% at RT. The mixture was loaded onto a column and spun at 12,000xg for 40 s at RT. After several washes of the column with washing solutions, total RNA was eluted with RNA-free water (50 ng/µL). To obtain the cDNA, the reverse transcription mix contained 4 µl of total RNA (200 ng), 4 µl of 5× reaction buffer, 2 µl of enzyme mix and 10 µl of water. The reactions were incubated at 42 °C for 1 h followed by inactivation at 95 °C for 5 min.

For real-time PCR determination of the APP and BACE1 mRNA levels, samples were diluted 40x and 5 µl product was assessed in a PCR reaction mix containing 10 µl of SYBR Green master mix. Real-time PCR was performed on 96-wells plates using the LightCycler 480 Real-Time PCR system (Roche, Indianapolis, IN, USA). The PCR conditions were 95 °C, 10 min followed by 45 cycles at 95 °C, 10 s and 55 °C, 20 s. The crossing point (Cp) was determined by using the second derivative method and data were normalized with actin. Fold changes and statistical significance were calculated using one-way ANOVA.

NMR spectroscopy and C-terminal peptide ligand titration

For the heteronuclear magnetic resonance spectroscopy (NMR) analysis of syntenin-1 and TSPAN6 interaction, uniformly 15 N-labeled syntenin-1 PDZ tandem domain (113 to 273), referred to as "syntenin-1 PDZ12," was expressed as a GST fusion in Escherichia coli BL21 (DE3) at 25 °C in M9 minimal medium using 15NH4Cl as the sole nitrogen source. The purification of GST-fused protein was performed as reported previously [37]. The NMR samples contained 200 µM protein, 150 mM NaCl, 500 µM TCEP [Tris(2-carboxyethyl)phosphine], and 50 µM AEBSF in 50 mM Tris buffer (pH 7.5). All NMR spectra were recorded at 30 °C on a Varian Inova 800-MHz spectrometer equipped with a room temperature 5-mm 1H/13C/15 N z-axis pulse field gradient probe, with data processed using the Azara package and analyzed using Ansig [38]. Synthesized C-terminal TSPAN6 peptide was purchased from Sigma-Genosys and contained an extra Arg residue at the N terminus, to improve peptide solubility. Titrations of syntenin-1 PDZ12 proteins with C-terminal TSPAN6 peptide were conducted by recording a series of 1H,15N HSQC spectra of 15 N-labeled protein (200 µM), with increasing molar concentrations of the peptide ligand, up to a protein-to-peptide ratio of 1:8. The combined backbone 1H and 15 N chemical shift changes, $\Delta\delta$, were calculated as reported earlier [39].

Syntenin contructs

Constructs expressing syntenin wt and mutants were obtained as described previously [40].

Brain clearing and 3D Lightsheet imaging

The App$^{NL\text{-}F/NL\text{-}F}$ mice were generated before [41]. Fixed brains from 1 year old App$^{NL/F}$ x *Tspan6 KO* and App$^{NL/F}$ x *Tspan6 Wt* mice were permeabilized with 1% Triton X-100 at room temperature for 24 h. Amyloid plaques were stained in 0.1% Thioflavin-S solution for 24 h. Then we rinsed them 2 times in PBS and dehydrated the tissue in an ethanol series (30%, 50%, 70%, 80%, 96% and 2 times in 100%, 1 day incubation time each) at room temperature. We rinsed the brains in 100% hexane for 1 h and then transferred them into a clearing solution of 1 part Benzyl Alcohol (Sigma) in 2 parts Benzyl Benzoate (Sigma), aka BABB. We stored whole brains in the clearing solution for at least 2 days at room temperature before imaging.

After clearing of intact mouse brains, imaging was achieved using a custom made Lightsheet microscope. The detection unit is equipped with a Nikon Macroscope AZ100M (Nikon Europe, The Netherlands), an ORCA R2 camera (Hamamatsu, Japan) and single bandpass and longpass filters (SemRock, Rochester, NY). The magnification used to resolve amyloid plaques was in a range of 9x-12x and cortical volumes of about Illumination was achieved with a 50 mm focal length cylindrical lens providing a lightsheet thickness in the order of 5–10 microns, with a slitted and collimated beam of 488 nm and 561 nm solid state lasers.

Image analysis of 3D volume

A custom ImageJ macro was used to extract, count and measure the individual volumes of the amyloid plaques in the acquired image Z-stacks. The macro performs the detection of candidate plaques (hits) by extracting 3D objects around significant intensity maxima. It then displays local volumes (boxes) cropped around hit locations, both in Thiaflovin and control (autofluorescence) channels, into an image montage. The user can navigate to hit locations within the full volume by interacting with the montage and discards invalid hits based on visual inspection. Intensity Z-projections of the cropped volumes is also displayed to quickly guide the user to suspicious hits. Validated amyloid plaques are finally automatically counted and their individual volumes exported to coma separated text files for further statistical analysis.

Results

TSPAN6 alters cellular proteostasis

Given that several studies [29–31] show that *TSPAN6* transcripts increase in late Braak stages of the Alzheimer's disease brain, we first overexpressed a myc-tagged form of TSPAN6 (myc-TSPAN6) in human embryonic kidney (HEK293) cells. As we anticipated that tetraspanins affect γ-secretase activities, we selected APP and two other known substrates of γ-secretases, i.e. APLP2 and LRP1 for further analysis. Levels of APP, APLP2 and LRP1 full length proteins were not affected upon TSPAN6 overexpression in HEK cells stably expressing APP (HEK-APPwt) (Fig. 1a). However a strong accumulation of their respective CTFs (APP-CTF, APLP2-CTF and LRP1-CTF; Fig. 1a,b) was seen. $A\beta_{40}$ but not $A\beta_{42}$ was increased in the conditioned medium of TSPAN6 transfected cells (Fig. 1c), suggesting a preserved γ-secretase activity. The increased levels of substrate (APP-CTF) might explain the increased $A\beta_{40}$ but some effects on the processivity of the enzyme cannot be excluded given the selective effect on $A\beta_{40}$. γ-Secretase expression was not affected by TSPAN6 overexpression Additional file 1: Figure S1a) and no effects were seen in vitro in γ-secretase activity assays using microsomal fractions of control, TSPAN6-overexpressing or TSPAN6-downregulated HEK-APPwt cells (Additional file 2: Figure S2a,b). Interestingly, the expression levels of BACE1 and the consequent generation of sAPPβ in early endosomes (EE) [35] were elevated by TSPAN6 while no changes in the levels of ADAM10 and sAPPα were found (Additional file 1: Figure S1a-c). In contrast, downregulation of endogenous TSPAN6 in HEK-APPwt cells using siRNA gave the opposite results: reduced CTF levels of APP, APLP2, LRP1 (Fig. 1d,e) and reduced BACE1- and sAPPβ-levels (Additional file 1: Figure S1d-f), with no change in the levels of the γ-secretase components.

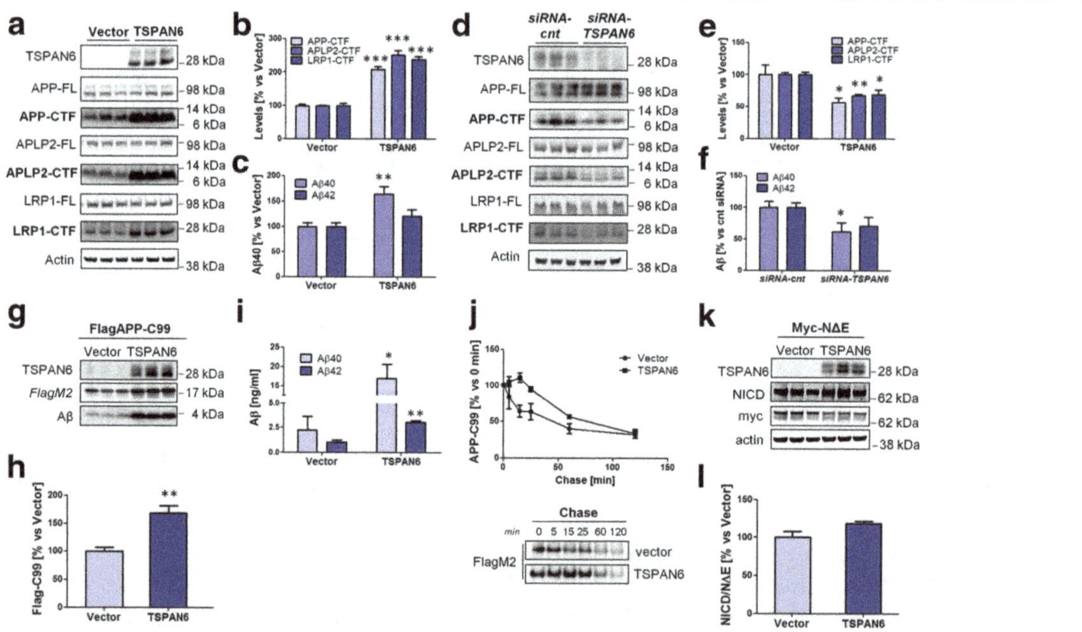

Fig. 1 TSPAN6 affects the normal proteostasis of the cell. **a** TSPAN6 was transfected in HEK-APPwt ($n = 3$ technical repeats) and analyzed by western blot using antibodies against APP, APLP2 and LRP1. The CTF levels of APP (APP-CTF), APLP2 (APLP2-CTF) and LRP1 (LRP1-CTF) were elevated by overexpressing TSPAN6. No changes in the levels of full-length proteins for APP (APP-FL), APLP2 (APLP2-FL) and LRP1 (LRP1-FL) were observed. **b** Quantification of bands in panel **a** confirmed the increase in CTF levels of APP, APLP2 and LRP1. **c** Aβ determination by ELISA in the 24 h conditioned medium of HEK-APPwt cells like those in panel **a** shows increased $A\beta_{40}$ levels ($n = 3$ experiments). **d** Cell lysates of HEK-APPwt cells treated 48 h with a scrambled siRNA (siRNA-cnt) or a siRNA against *TSPAN6* (*siRNA-TSPAN6*) were analyzed by western blot as in panel **a** ($n = 3$ experiments). In contrast to panel **a**, the levels of APP-CTF, APLP2-CTF and LRP1-CTF were strongly reduced in siRNA-*TSPAN6*-treated cells. **e** Quantification of bands in panel **d.** **f** Aβ levels determined by ELISA in the 24 h-conditioned medium of the cells in panel **d** show a significant decrease in $A\beta_{40}$ levels. **g** HEK293 cells were co-transfected with FlagAPP-C99 and TSPAN6 or an empty vector and lysates analyzed by western blot with antibodies against FlagM2 and 6E10 ($n = 3$ experiments). **h** Quantification of FlagAPP-C99 from panel **g.** **i** Aβ in the 24 h conditioned medium of the cells from panel **g** measured by ELISA. TSPAN6 overexpression increases $A\beta_{40}$ and $A\beta_{42}$ levels. **j** Transfected HEK293 analyzed by pulse-chase labeling. Cells were incubated for two hours with ^{35}S-Met/Cys and FlagAPP-C99 was immunoprecipitated at specific time-points with FlagM2-affinity gel. The density of the bands in the autoradiography was quantified and plotted ($n = 3$ experiments). This shows a slower disappearance of FlagAPP-C99 during the first 30 min in cells overexpressing TSPAN6. **k** HEK293 cells co-transfected with myc-tagged NotchΔE and TSPAN6 or an empty vector ($n = 3$ experiments). TSPAN6 overexpression do not change myc-NΔE levels. **l** Quantification of panel **k** shows no differences in terms of NICD production in TSPAN6. Statistical significance was determined by *t*-test (*$p < 0.05$, **$p < 0.01$, ***$p < 0.001$)

To gain insight into the cellular mechanism of the altered proteolysis we focused on the accumulation of the APP-CTFs which are generated by α- or β-secretases (APP-C83 and APP-C99, respectively). We co-transfected HEK293 cells with similar amounts of Flag-tagged APP-C99 (FlagAPP-C99) and an empty vector (negative control) or TSPAN6 (Fig. 1 g). Both FlagAPP-C99 and secreted Aβ levels were enhanced by TSPAN6 (Fig. 1 g-i), consistent with the altered proteolysis of the APP-CTF fragments. We also tested the effect of TSPAN6 on myc-tagged Notch-ΔE, a synthetic fragment from Notch that is used as a direct substrate for γ-secretase, and which can be compared to APP-CTF. The Notch-CTF did not change and generation of the Notch intracellular domain (NICD) by γ-secretase was not affected following overexpression or down regulation of TSPAN6 (Fig. 1 k,l; Additional file 2: Figure S2c,d), indicating specificity of the TSPAN6-mediated effect on APP-CTF, APLP1-CTF and LRP1-CTF relative to the Notch-CTF.

The turn-over of FlagAPP-C99 was further investigated with pulse-chase experiments. Cells were radiolabeled with ^{35}S-Met/Cys. At the time points indicated, FlagAPP-C99 was immunoprecipitated and analyzed by SDS-PAGE and autoradiography. TSPAN6-overexpression resulted in a delay in the degradation of FlagAPP-C99 which was overcome after 30 min (Fig. 1j). The endogenous protein can accumulate in presence of high TSPAN6 levels assuming that APP-C99 is continuously being produced and considering the delayed start of its degradation. Altogether these data strongly suggest that TSPAN6 affects specifically the degradation of some proteins, including APP-CTF, APLP2-CTF and LRP-CTF.

APP-CTFs accumulate in endosomal compartments in TSPAN6-overexpressing cells

We next investigated the subcellular compartmentalization and accumulation of APP-CTF upon TSPAN6 overexpression. As shown in Fig. 2, TSPAN6 is mainly present in LAMP1 positive organelles and to a lesser extent in EEA1 positive organelles. By contrast, we found no-colocalization with the Golgi marker GM130. APP-CTFs show strong co-localization with TSPAN6 in LAMP1 cellular compartments (Fig. 3a,b). This co-localization was specific for the CTFs of APP since N-terminal epitopes of APP show only a weak co-localization with myc-TSPAN6 (Additional file 3: Figure S3). Remarkably, overexpression of myc-TSPAN6 increases the co-localization of endogenously expressed APP-CTF with LAMP1 by threefold and with EEA1 by twofold (Fig. 3a,b). We confirmed the enrichment of APP-CTFs in LAMP1 positive organelles by immunoisolation of these compartments after expression of Flag-tagged LAMP1 (Flag-LAMP1) and using Flag-tag antibody coupled to beads [33]. APP-CTF was found to enrich in the immunoprecipitated LAMP1 positive organelles when cells overexpressed TSPAN6 (Fig. 3c), confirming that TSPAN6 increases the levels of APP-CTFs in these compartments.

TSPAN6 favors the generation of exosomes

These studies indicate that TSPAN6 impairs degradation of the APP-CTF that accumulates in endosomal compartments. Thus we decided to study these organelles at the ultrastructural level on HEK293 cells overexpressing TSPAN6 by Transmission electron microscopy (EM). EM analysis revealed that expression of TSPAN6 led to a duplication of the number of endosomal structures. These were moreover 40% larger than those observed in control cells (Fig. 4a-c). Furthermore, in TSPAN6-expressing cells intraluminal vesicles (ILVs) of multivesicular bodies (MVBs) were somewhat larger when compared to control cells (Fig. 4 ac-af). These data were further confirmed by stereological analysis that demonstrated that the ILVs present in cells overexpressing TSPAN6 have a larger surface compared to the largest ILVs found in control cells and also appear to display more empty space in EM (Fig. 4d).

APP-CTF degradation can occur via sorting into ILVs from the rim of the MVB followed by fusion to lysosomal or autolysosomal compartments. Given the altered ILVs morphology found by EM analysis, we explored a possible defect in this pathway as a TSPAN6-induced mechanism leading to APP-CTF accumulation. We expressed the constitutively active GTP-locked mutant form of the early endosomal marker Rab5 (Rab5^{Q79L}). Rab5^{Q79L} blocks recycling from EEs resulting in enlarged EEs through fusion events without affecting the formation of ILVs [42]. As shown in Fig. 5, TSPAN6 co-localizes with Rab5^{Q79L} at the rim of such enlarged endosomes but is also found in the lumen (Fig. 5a). Interestingly APP-CTF distribution between the rim and the lumen of MVBs was not different between TSPAN6-overexpressing and control cells (Fig. 5a,b), indicating that TSPAN6 does not interfere with the sorting of APP-CTF into ILVs (Fig. 5b). The enlarging effect of Rab5^{Q79L} on endosomes is however significantly enhanced in the presence of TSPAN6 (Fig. 5c).

Ubiquitinated proteins are recognized by ESCRT-proteins and sorted to ILVs in MVB. Further degradation occurs when the latter fuse to autophagosomes and lysosomes. Alternatively cargo sorted to tetraspanin-enriched microdomains in the limiting membrane of the endosome may go to ILVs destined for exosome release in an ESCRT-independent manner [43]. APP-CTF accumulates in TSPAN6-enriched microdomains, as demonstrated by sucrose gradient fractionation of CHAPSO-solubilized lysates from TSPAN6-overexpressing cells (Additional file 4: Figure S4a) and a proximity ligation assay of APP-CTF and myc-TSPAN6 (Additional file 4:

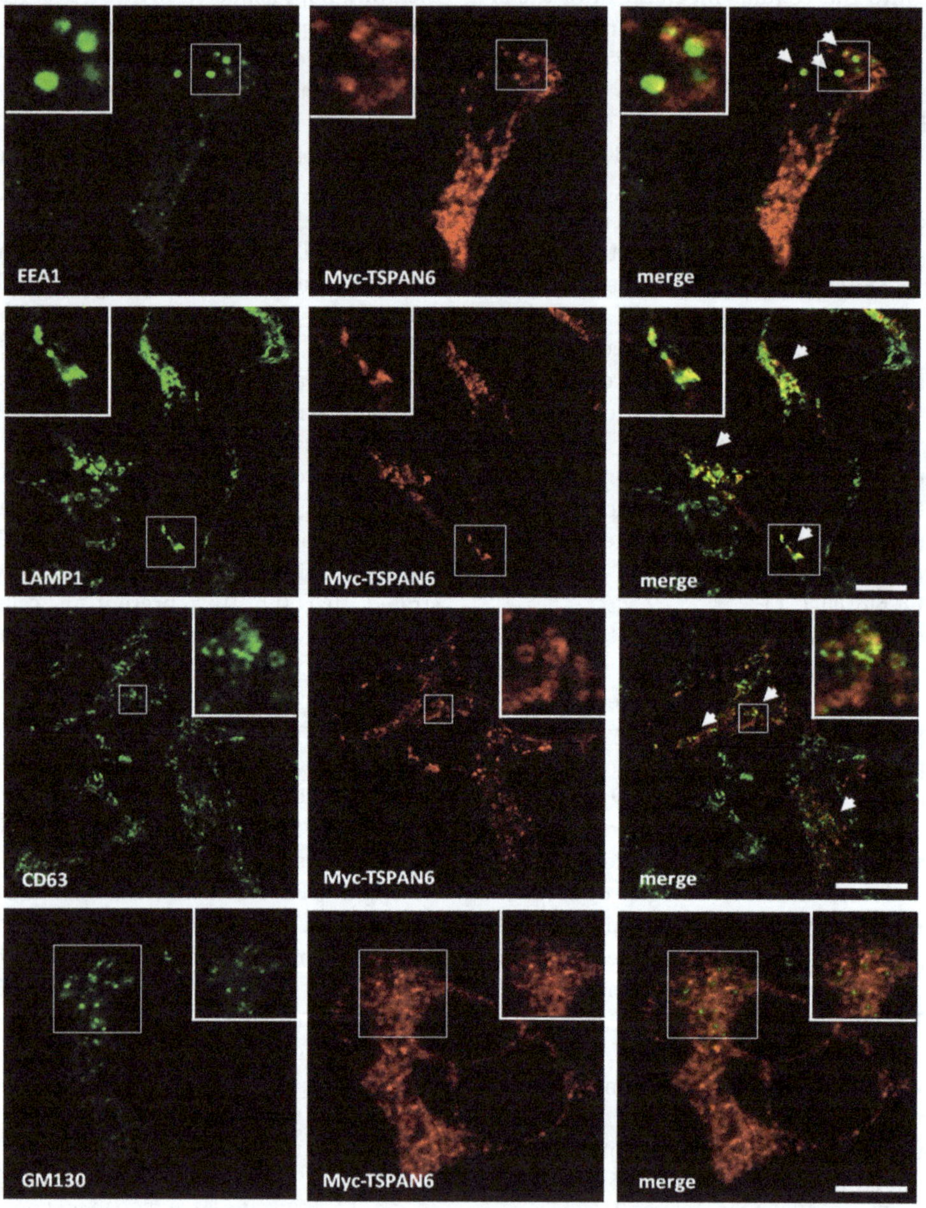

Fig. 2 Subcellular localization of TSPAN6 in HEK293 cells. HEK293 cells were transfected with myc-tagged TSPAN6 (myc-TSPAN6), fixed and immunostained for EEA1 as an early-endosomes marker (upper panels), LAMP1 and CD63 as markers for late-compartments (middle panels), and GM130 to visualize the Golgi organelle (lower panels). Myc-TSPAN6 (detected with a rat monoclonal anti-myc antibody) shows a high degree of co-localization (arrows) with late-compartments (detected with a mouse monoclonal antibody against LAMP1 and a rabbit polyclonal antibody against CD63), and a lower co-localization with early endosomes (detected with a mouse monoclonal antibody against EEA1). Low co-localization was observed with the Golgi organelle (detected with a monoclonal antibody against GM130). Scale bars = 10 μm

Figure S4b). Interestingly, cells overexpressing TSPAN6 show larger ILVs (Fig. 4a-d), resembling those generated by the ESCRT-independent pathway [44]. We therefore compared the number of exosomes secreted from TSPAN6-overexpressing HEK293 cells and from control cells (Fig. 5d-g). We used the particle tracking system Nanosight to count and to determine the size of the vesicles present in the conditioned medium. TSPAN6 overexpression increased the average (μ) number of exosomes ($\mu_{vector} = 1280 \times 10^6$; $\mu_{Tspan6} = 2139 \times 10^6$; Fig. 5, f,g), which shows an average size of about 120 nm (Fig. 5 g). Both TSPAN6 and APP-CTF were present in exosomes isolated from HEK293 cells (Fig. 5e). Thus, TSPAN6 significantly affects the generation of exosomes, and although the amount of APP-CTF per exosome remains equal (Fig. 5e), the total pool of APP-CTF in exosomes is thus increased by 60%, partially explaining the APP-CTF accumulation in TSPAN6 overexpressing cells.

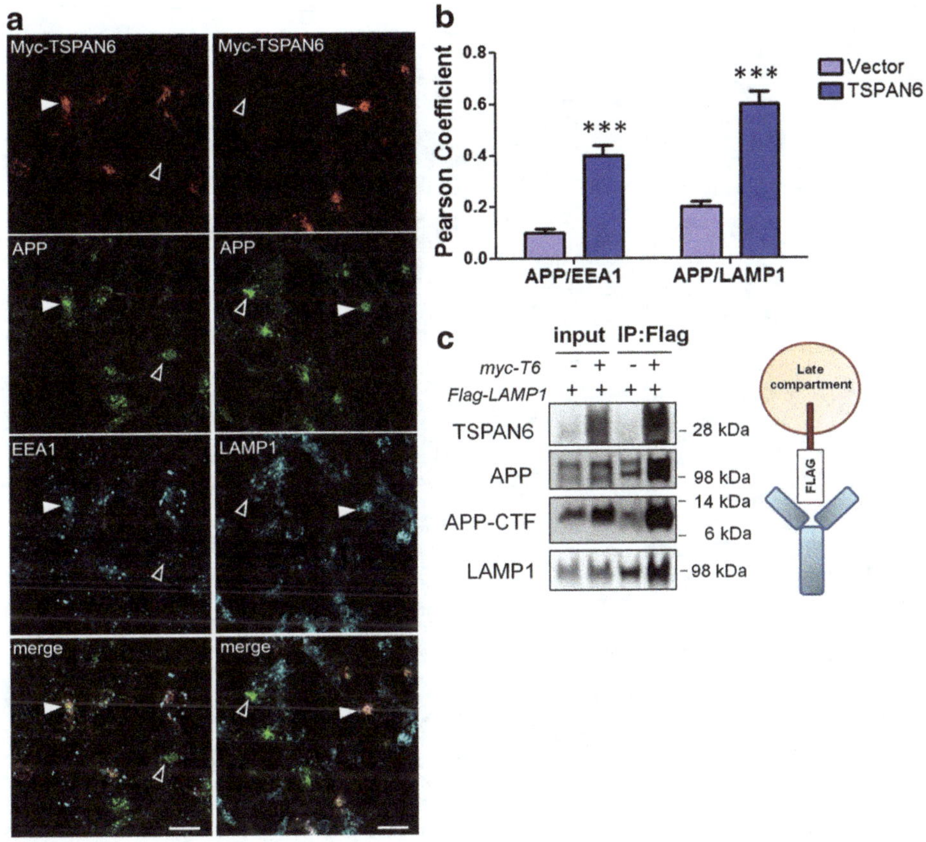

Fig. 3 APP-CTF accumulates in endosomal compartments in TSPAN6-overexpressing cells. **a** Immunofluorescence microscopy of HEK293 cells overexpressing myc-tagged TSPAN6, fixed and probed with a rat monoclonal antibody against myc, a rabbit monoclonal antibody against APP-CTF (Y188), and mouse monoclonal antibodies against EEA1 and LAMP1 to visualize early and late endosomal compartments, respectively. Cells overexpressing myc-TSPAN6 show more APP co-localizing with EEA1 and LAMP1 (filled arrowheads) compared to non-overexpressing cells (empty arrowheads). **b** Quantification of the number of cells non-overexpressing or overexpressing TSPAN6 showing co-localization of APP-CTF with early (EEA1) or late endosomal (LAMP1) compartments. **c** Immunoisolation of LAMP1-containing compartments as described [33], after overexpressing Flag-tagged LAMP1 in non-overexpressing or overexpressing myc-tagged TSPAN6. The total inputs and the immunoisolated compartments were analyzed by western blot with specific antibodies against APP, APP-CTF, TSPAN6 and LAMP1. Statistical significance was determined by *t*-test (****p* <0.001)

The cytosolic adapter syntenin interacts with TSPAN6 and mediates the increased formation of ILVs fated for exosome secretion

The syndecan-syntenin-alix pathway triggers the biogenesis of ILVs destined to be secreted as exosomes, bypassing the degradative pathway [45]. These effects resemble those observed here in TSPAN6-overexpressing cells. In addition, syntenin interacts with the carboxy-terminal end of tetraspanin CD63 [39]. Thus we investigated if syntenin mediates the TSPAN6-induced generation of ILVs destined to exosomes and whether it might be involved in the decreased APP-CTF degradation.

Syntenin is an adapter protein that consists of an N-terminal domain, followed by a tandem PDZ module and a C-terminal domain. The PDZ module recognizes short sequences at the C-terminus of transmembrane proteins [46]. We investigated if the C-terminus of TSPAN6 contains a canonical PDZ-binding motif that can interact to syntenin. We therefore generated a series of mutants at the C-terminus of myc-tagged TSPAN6 (Fig. 6a) substituting each time a single amino acid residue for glycine. While Flag-tagged syntenin co-immunoprecipitates myc-TSPAN6, the substitution of one of the last two C-terminal amino acids by glycine disrupted this interaction (Fig. 6a,b). In addition we found that the immobilized C-terminal peptide of TSPAN6 and CD63 (positive control) but not the corresponding regions of some other tetraspanins (i.e., CD81, Net-5, Net-2 and CD231) can retain syntenin from cell lysates (Fig. 6c), confirming the specificity of this interaction.

To further demonstrate the interaction between TSPAN6 and syntenin in vitro, we co-transfected HEK293 cells with Flag-TSPAN6 and HA-tagged wt syntenin (SYNwt-HA) or HA-tagged syntenin lacking the first 101 N-terminal (SYNΔN-HA) or the last 17

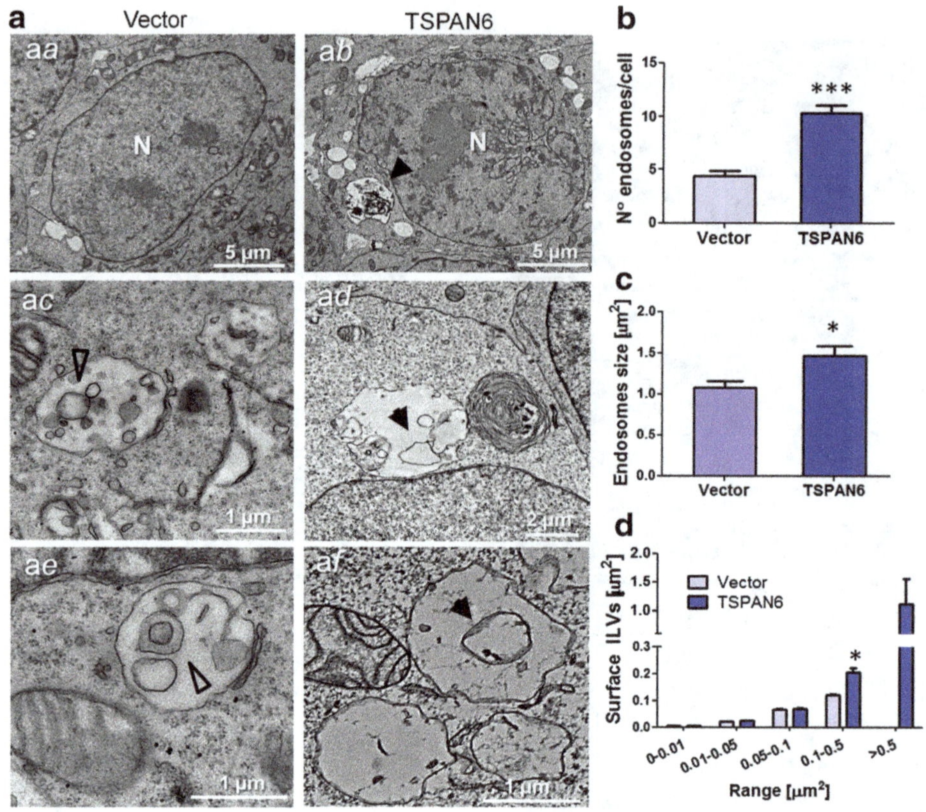

Fig. 4 Endosomal alterations in TSPAN6-overexpressing cells. **a** EM images showing enlarged compartments in HEK293 cells overexpressing TSPAN6. HEK293 cells expressing an empty vector (control) present endosomes (**a***a*) showing a normal aspect and multivesicular bodies (MVBs; **a***c* and **a***e*) containing normal-sized intraluminal vesicles (ILVs, empty arrowheads). In comparison, HEK293 cells overexpressing TSPAN6 show a higher number of endosomal compartments (**a***b*), some of them with non-degraded material in the lumen (**a***b*, arrowheads) and MVBs with enlarged ILVs (**a**d and **a***f*; arrowheads). The nucleus is indicated with an N. **b** Quantification of the number of endosomes from TEM images of HEK293 cells like those shown in panel **a**. Overexpression of TSPAN6 increases the number of endosomal compartments per cell ($n = 72$ control cells; $n = 59$ TSPAN6-transfected cells; 2 independent experiments). **c** Analysis of the size of endosomal compartments from TEM images. Larger endosomal compartments are found in HEK293 cells overexpressing TSPAN6 in comparison to controls cells expressing an empty vector ($n = 167$ endosomes for control cells; $n = 267$ for TSPAN6-transfected cells; 2 independent experiments). **d** Determination of the surface of ILVs from TEM images like those shown in panel **a**. All the ILVs from the control or the TSPAN6-overexpressing cells were grouped according to their size in μm^2 ($n = 202$ ILVs from control cells; $n = 204$ ILVs from TSPAN6-overexpressing cells; 2 independent experiments). This demonstrates enrichment for larger structures in the TSPAN6 overexpressing cells. The mean of the surface plotted for each range shows larger ILVs in cells overexpressing TSPAN6 when comparing ILVs larger than 0.1 μm^2. Statistical significance was determined by t- test (*$p < 0.05$, ***$p < 0.001$)

C-terminal amino acids (SYNΔC-HA). Flag-TSPAN6 immunoprecipitated SYNwt-HA and SYNΔN-HA but not SYNΔC-HA, suggesting that, like CD63, the C-terminus of syntenin is necessary for the stabilization of the interaction with TSPAN6 (Fig. 7a). In order to investigate the role played by the PDZ1 and PDZ2 domains of syntenin in the interaction, we performed NMR titration analysis of ^{15}N-labeled syntenin PDZ1&2 with unlabeled C-terminal peptide of TSPAN6 consisting of the last 10 amino acids of the human protein (TSPAN6-C). The chemical shift perturbations were used to map the binding sites, revealing a contact surface for TSPAN6-C predominantly in the PDZ1 domain binding pocket (Fig. 7b).

In order to evaluate the relevance of the TSPAN6-syntenin interaction for exosome production, we compared the number of these vesicles secreted by HEK293 cells after stable knock down of syntenin (HEK-Syn KD) and transfected with an empty vector or with a vector expressing TSPAN6 (Fig. 7c). The total number of exosomes generated by HEK-Syn KD is dramatically lower compared to the wild type HEK293 cells, in agreement with the role that syntenin, together with syndecan and alix, plays in the biogenesis of exosomes [45]. Interestingly, in HEK-Syn KD cells, and as opposed to HEK293 wt cells (Fig. 5f,g), overexpression of TSPAN6 did not increase the total number of exosomes (compare Fig. 5f,g with Fig. 7c), nor the size distribution (Fig. 7d). This

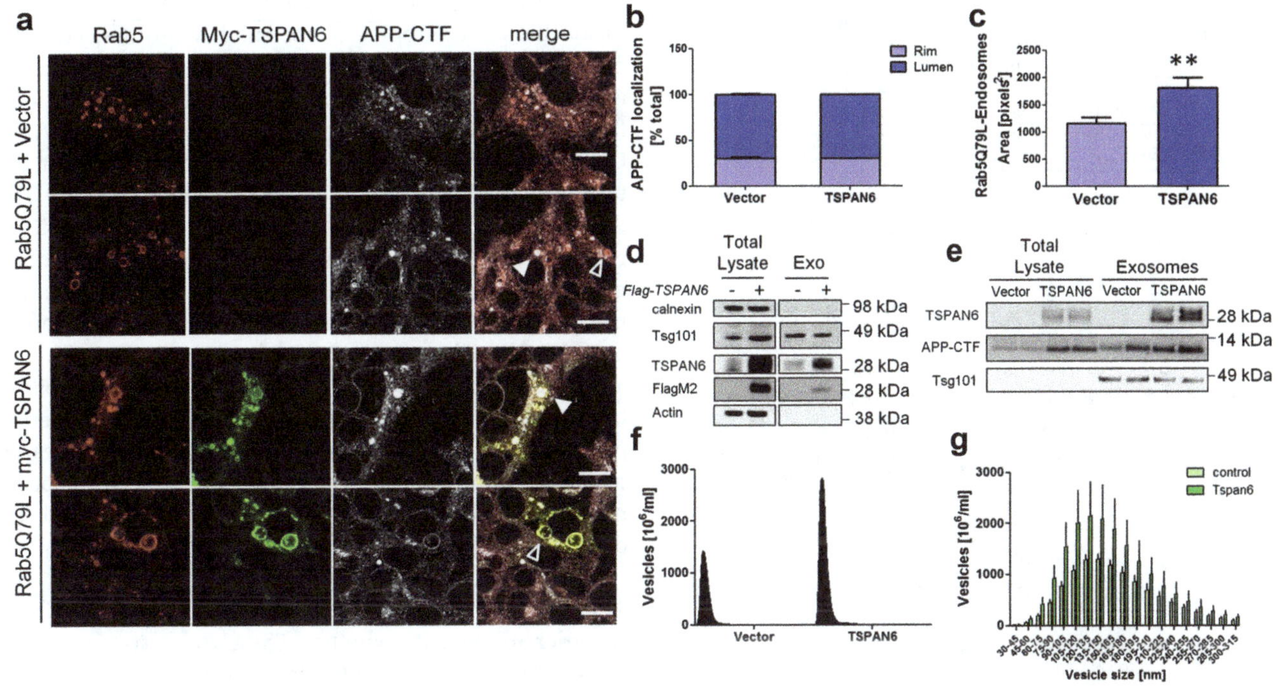

Fig. 5 TSPAN6 is found in ILVs and enhances the formation of exosomes. **a** Representative staining of 2 independent experiments showing HEK293 cells overexpressing the Rab5^{Q79L} mutant together with an empty vector (upper panels) or myc-TSPAN6 (lower panels). Immunofluorescence studies were carried out with monoclonal antibodies against myc (to detect TSPAN6), APP-CTF and Rab5. APP-CTF is observed in the lumen (filled arrowheads) and the limiting membrane (empty arrowheads) of endosomes in both conditions; however, cells overexpressing myc-TSPAN6 show enlarged endosomes. Scale bar = 10 μm. **b** Percentage of APP-CTF in the lumen or the rim of endosomes in cells overexpressing an empty vector ($n = 109$ endosomes; 2 independent experiments) or myc-TSPAN6 ($n = 106$ endosomes; 2 independent experiments). **c** The average area (pixels^2) of Rab5^{Q79L} endosomes in cells overexpressing myc-TSPAN6 ($n = 75$ endosomes; 2 independent experiments) was increased in comparison to control cells expressing an empty vector ($n = 65$ endosomes; 2 independent experiments). **d** Western blot analysis of total HEK293 lysates (transfected with Flag-TSPAN6 or left untransfected) or the exosomal fraction (Exo) isolated from their conditioned medium. The blot was probed with a monoclonal antibody against FlagM2 and a polyclonal antibody against TSPAN6 to assess the overexpression of protein, a monoclonal antibody against calnexin (non-exosomal protein), a polyclonal antibody against Tsg101 (exosomal protein) and a monoclonal antibody against actin. **e** The western blot of total HEK293 lysates and their exosomal fractions shows no differences in the APP-CTF levels for the same amount (2.5 μg) of exosome lysates when TSPAN6 is overexpressed. **f** Quantification of the concentration of secreted exosomes (vesicles/ml) by the nanovesicles tracking system Nanosight from control HEK293 cells or overexpressing TSPAN6 (3 independent experiments per condition), shows that TSPAN6 increases the secretion of exosomes. **g** Graph showing the distribution of the concentrations of the vesicles grouped by size (nm) and found in the exosomal fractions of TSPAN6-overexpressing HEK293 cells and control cells (data from panel **f**). TSPAN6-overexpressing cells show a higher concentration for all the vesicle sizes. Statistical significance was determined by *t*-test (**p <0.01)

clearly suggests that the TSPAN6-syntenin interaction is necessary in the formation of ILVs destined to exosomes. We next investigated whether TSPAN6-triggered accumulation of APP-CTF occurs in HEK-Syn KD cells. The western blot analysis shows that TSPAN6 can induce the same APP-CTF accumulation in both wt and KD cells (Fig. 7e,f), suggesting that syntenin is largely dispensable for the effect. This conclusion was supported by the observation that the same amount of APP-CTF accumulated in HEK293 after co-expressing TSPAN6 together with syntenin wt (Syn-wt) or a syntenin mutant which is unable to interact with TSPAN6 (Syn-PDZ1*) (Fig. 7 g,h). The results thus suggest that TSPAN6 stabilizes APP-CTF by an additional mechanism upstream of syntenin-induced exosome formation.

TSPAN6 overexpression impairs the fusion of autophagosomes to lysosomes

TSPAN6 induces the accumulation of enlarged endosomal compartments (Fig. 4a-c) suggesting an impairment of the downstream degradative pathways. In addition we found that autophagosomal and multilamellar compartments, (Fig. 8aa-ad) together with enlarged endosomes filled with heterogeneous material (Fig. 8ab-ac) are more commonly found in HEK293 cells overexpressing TSPAN6.

Hence we investigated whether TSPAN6 overexpression affects the degradation of APP-CTF by impairing the autolysosomal pathway. Firstly, we determined how the autophagic flux affects APP-CTF degradation in non-transfected (control) or TSPAN6-transfected HEK293 cells (Fig. 8b-d). Autophagy was induced by starvation of

a

Mutant name	C-terminal mutation
TSPAN6-Wt	NH_2-...yclsraitnnqyeiv-COOH
TSPAN6(-1)	NH_2-...yclsraitnnqyeiG-COOH
TSPAN6(-2)	NH_2-...yclsraitnnqyeGv-COOH
TSPAN6(-4)	NH_2-...yclsraitnnqGeiv-COOH
TSPAN6(-5)	NH_2-...yclsraitnnGyeiv-COOH
TSPAN6(-7)	NH_2-...yclsraitGnqyeiv-COOH

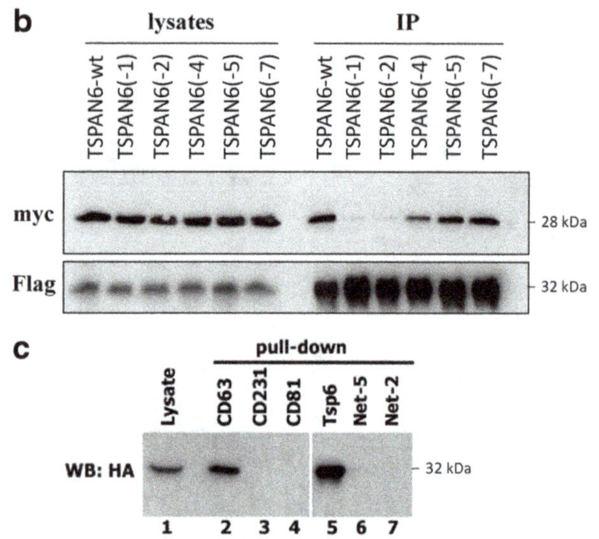

Fig. 6 The C-terminal cytoplasmic region mediates the interaction of TSPAN6 with syntenin-1. **a** Table illustrating the location of the point mutations on the myc-tagged TSPAN6 mutants used in the co-immunoprecipitation experiment shown in **b. b** Co-expression of Flag-tagged syntenin in HEK293 cells together with myc-tagged TSPAN6-wt or lacking one of the last c-terminal amino acids (TSPAN6(-1) to TSPAN6(-7)). After immunoprecipitation of Flag-tagged syntenin, the interaction with the different TSPAN6 mutants was evaluated by western blot with an anti-myc antibody. The last 2 amino acids of TSPAN6 are essential for the interaction with syntenin. **c** N-terminally biotinylated peptides corresponding to the indicated C-termini of tetraspanins were synthesized and conjugated to avidin-agarose beads. HEK293 cells ectopically expressing HA-tagged syntenin were lysed in immunoprecipitation buffer (0.5% Brij 98-0.5% Triton X-100-PBS), incubated with the avidin-immobilized peptides and the interaction to syntenin was analyzed by western blot. TSPAN6 (Tsp6) and CD63 (positive control) C-terminal peptides also interacted with syntenin. Net-5, Net 2 (negative controls reported not to interact to syntenin), CD231 or CD81 did not interact to syntenin

cells cultured in serum free Earle's Balanced Salt Solution (EBSS) medium for 2 h and 4 h, as previously reported [47–49]. The lysosome inhibitor bafilomycin A1 was added to the medium of 4 h starved cells as a positive control to estimate maximal APP-CTF accumulation. In control cells, APP-CTF levels decreased by about 40% after 4 h of starvation while the levels remained unchanged in TSPAN6-overexpressing cells (Fig. 8b,c). The levels of p62, a protein involved in the recognition of ubiquitinated proteins by the autophagosome, were also less decreased during autophagy induction in TSPAN6-overexpressing cells (Fig. 8b-d), though the impairment on p62 degradation was not so pronounced as for APP-CTF.

In order to test the hypothesis that TSPAN6 impairs the fusion between autophagosomes and lysosomes, HEK293 cells were co-transfected with the autophagosome-associated protein LC3 double-tagged with GFP and RFP (LC3-GFP-RFP) and an empty vector or myc-TSPAN6. Cells were put into starvation with EBBS medium for 3 h to induce the formation of autophagosomes (Fig. 8e). The fusion of newly formed autophagosomes with lysosomes is reflected in loss of green fluorescence of the GFP protein due to the low pH of lysosomes. Cells overexpressing myc-TSPAN6 (blue) showed a decreased ratio of the number of red vesicles versus the total number of vesicles (red and green) per cell (Fig. 8f). This, together with the parallel increased number of autophagosomes in cells overexpressing myc-TSPAN6 (Fig. 8 g), suggests a decreased fusion of autophagosomes to lysosomes. Cells kept in normal growth medium in similar circumstances did not display autophagosomes (Additional file 5: Figure S5).

APP processing is altered in neurons of *Tspan6* KO mice

In order to evaluate whether TSPAN6 exerts similar effects on the amyloidogenic pathway in a physiologically relevant context we investigated the effect of a loss of function mutation on APP processing in the cerebral cortex of adult *Tspan6 wt* or *Tspan6 KO* mice. As shown in Fig. 9a, Tspan6 is expressed in neuronal bodies of the cerebral cortex of *Tspan6 wt* mice but not in *Tspan6 KO* mice. We observed a moderate to intense Tspan6 reactivity in brain regions with neurons expressing glutamate decarboxylase (GAD)-67, an enzyme involved in GABA synthesis, and in neurons expressing the vesicular glutamate transporter 1 (vGLUT1), a glutamate transporter that transports cytoplasmic glutamate into vesicles (Additional file 6: Figure S6). We then compared the expression levels of App and Bace1 in the cerebral cortex of 1 year old *Tspan6 wt* and *Tspan6 KO* mice by western blot (Fig. 9b). App expression levels were significantly decreased in *Tspan6 KO* mice, while App-CTF and Bace1 showed minimal effects (Fig. 9b,c). *Tspan6 KO* mice show also lower levels of $A\beta_{40}$ and $A\beta_{42}$ peptides in the cerebral cortex (Fig. 9d). We also cultured primary cortical neurons from *Tspan6 wt, het,* or *KO* E14.5 embryos. The expression levels of App-CTFs were decreased in *Tspan6 het* and *Tspan6 KO neurons* compared to *Tspan6 wt* neurons (Fig. 9e,f). The protein levels of App, App-CTFs, Bace1, and the secretion of sAppβ were decreased in *Tspan6 KO* neurons (Fig. 9e, f). *Tspan6 KO* neurons produced less $A\beta_{40}$ compared to *Tspan6 wt* neurons (Fig. 9 g), while $A\beta_{42}$ was only minimally affected. Finally overexpression of Tspan6 in *Tspan6 wt* and *KO neurons* increased the protein levels of App and p62, indicating a deficit in autophagy, and the secretion of $A\beta_{40}$ and $A\beta_{42}$ to the media (Additional file 7: Figure S7a,b). However no effects on App-CTF

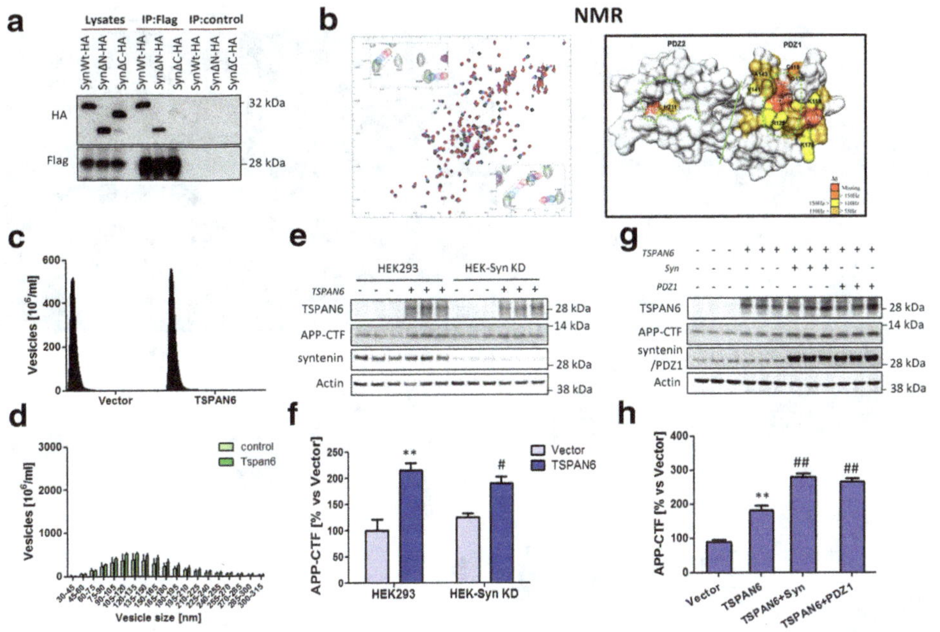

Fig. 7 The interaction of syntenin with TSPAN6 mediates the enhanced formation of exosomes. **a** Flag-tagged TSPAN6 (Flag-TSPAN6) and HA-tagged syntenin (SynWt-HA) or syntenin lacking either the N-terminal fragment (Syn**Δ**N-HA) or the C-terminal fragment (Syn**Δ**C-HA) were co-transfected in HEK293 cells. Flag-TSPAN6 was immunoprecipitated with an anti-Flag antibody from cell lysates and the interaction was evaluated by western blot using an anti-HA antibody. Total lysates (first 3 lanes) show that the 3 syntenin constructs were expressed. However only SynWt-HA and Syn**Δ**N-HA but not Syn**Δ**C-HA were immunoprecipitated with Flag-TSPAN6. The absence of anti-Flag antibody gives no bands (negative control, last 3 lanes). **b** Nuclear magnetic resonance spectroscopy (NMR) analysis of syntenin-1 and TSPAN6 interaction. The left panel shows the superposition of six two-dimensional 1H-15 N-HSQC spectra of uniformly 15 N-labeled syntenin-1 PDZ domain (200 μM) titrated with increasing concentrations of C-terminal peptide of TSPAN6. The right panel shows the locations of syntenin PDZ residues involved in binding. **c** Exosomes isolated from the conditioned medium of HEK293 cells stably knocked down for syntenin (HEK-Syn KD) and overexpressing an empty vector (control) or TSPAN6 were analyzed by Nanosight. Overall, the number of exosomes is lower in HEK-Syn KD cells compared to HEK293 wt cells (Fig. 5**f**). Overexpression of TSPAN6 in HEK-Syn KD did not alter the number of exosomes secreted. **d** Same plot as in Fig. 5 **g** but for HEK293 cells stably knocked down for syntenin (HEK293-KD Syntenin). Neither number of exosomes nor size distribution change between TSPAN6-overexpressing and control cells (data from panel **c**). **e** HEK293 or HEK-Syn KD were co-transfected with an empty vector (control) or with TSPAN6 ($n = 3$ technical replicates). TSPAN6 overexpression increases the APP-CTF levels in both HEK293 and HEK-Syn KD cells. **f** Quantification of the western blots of panel **e. g** HEK293 cells were transfected with an empty vector (control), TSPAN6 alone or with either syntenin (Syn) or syntenin with a point mutation in PDZ1 domain (PDZ1) that prevents the interaction to TSPAN6. Lysates were analyzed by western blot ($n = 3$ technical replicates). Overexpression of TSPAN6 increases the APP-CTF levels. This effect is potentiated by co-expression of Syn or PDZ1 mutant. **h** Quantification of APP-CTF levels from the western blot shown in panel **g**. Statistical analysis was carried out with *t*-test (** $p < 0.01$ vs vector; ## p0.01;vs TSPAN6 alone)

and Bace1 levels were observed. The impairment of autophagy was confirmed by EM analysis of *Tspan6 wt* neurons overexpressing Tspan6, which show enlarged vesicles with undegraded material in the lumen (Fig. 10), resembling those found in TSPAN6-overexpressing HEK cells. These data demonstrate that Tspan6 is physiologically involved in neural APP metabolism.

Finally, we investigated the consequences of Tspan6 loss in an AD mouse model by crossing *Tspan6 KO* mice with mice expressing endogenous levels of the human APP gene with the Swedish and Iberian mutations ($App^{NL/F}$) that trigger the formation of amyloid plaques [41]. When we examined by western blot total lysates of the cerebral cortex of 1 year old $App^{NL/F}$ x *Tspan6 KO*, we observe a decrease in the levels of App-CTF, Bace1, Aβ and p62 in comparison to $App^{NL/F}$ x *Tspan6 wt* mice. However we did not find differences in terms of amyloid plaque content by using a combination of a brain clearing methodology with Thioflavin-S staining (Additional file 8: Figure S8c).

Discussion

We demonstrate here that TSPAN6 is localized in endosomal and lysosomal structures and plays a critical role in the complex housekeeping of MVBs in the cell. Overexpression of TSPAN6 dramatically altered the morphology of these structures, causing alterations in the turnover of several proteins including APP-CTF, BACE1 and Aβ involved in AD. The increased secretion of Aβ peptide seems to be a direct consequence of the increment in the levels of APP-CTF due to TSPAN6 overexpression, as supported by the parallel increase in the levels of secreted Aβ and transfected FlagAPP-C99 in cells overexpressing TSPAN6. This was corroborated

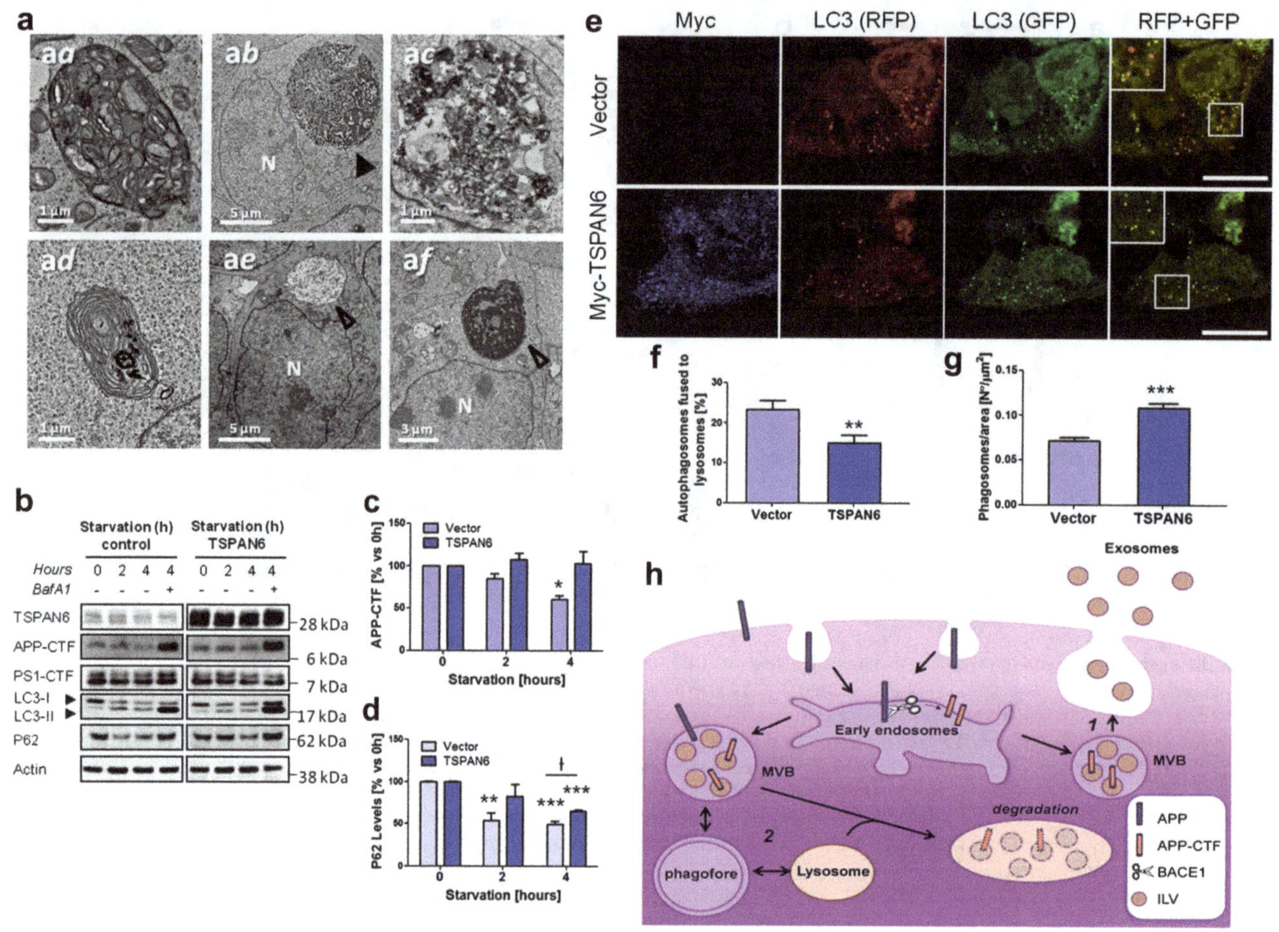

Fig. 8 Overexpression of TSPAN6 compromises autophagy. **a** HEK293 cells overexpressing TSPAN6 analyzed by TEM show phagosomes (*aa*) multilamellar bodies (*ad*) and large vacuoles containing undegraded heterogeneous material in the lumen (*ab-ac*, arrowheads). In comparison, HEK293 cells expressing an empty vector present a reduced number of enlarged vesicles with homogeneous luminal material (*ae-af*, empty arrowheads). Nucleus is indicated with an N. **b** Representative experiment showing autophagy induction in control (empty vector) or TSPAN6-overexpressing HEK293 cells by 2 h and 4 h starvation. Lysates were analyzed by western blot with antibodies against TSPAN6, APP, P62, LC3β, PS1-CTF and actin. TSPAN6-overexpressing cells show no degradation of APP-CTF after 4 h starvation compared to control cells. Activation of autophagy was assessed by conversion of LC3-I into LC3-II and the degradation of P62. The levels of PS1-CTF and actin were used as negative controls. **c** Quantification of APP-CTF levels from western blots like in panel **b** ($n = 3$ experiments). **d** Quantification of P62 levels from western blots like in panel **b** ($n = 3$ experiments). **e** HEK293 cells co-transfected with LC3-GFP-RFP and an empty vector or myc-TSPAN6 were starved for 3 h to induce autophagy. The fusion of autophagosomes (red and green) with lysosomes (red) is reflected in the loss of the fluorescence of GFP protein due to the low pH found in lysosomes. TSPAN6 overexpression is detected with an anti-myc antibody (blue) (scale bar = 10 μm). **f** Ratio between the number of autophagosomes fused to lysosomes versus the total number of autophagosomes (2 independent experiment; $n = 43$ autophagosomes for control; $n = 43$ autophagosomes for TSPAN6). **g** The number of phagosomes not fused to lysosomes (red and green) per cell is increased in cells overexpressing TSPAN6 (2 independent experiments, $n = 59$ cells for control; $n = 80$ cells for TSPAN6). **h** Scheme showing the cellular pathways affected by TSPAN6. 1-Increased levels of TSPAN6 increment the secretion of exosomes by a syntenin-dependent mechanism. 2-TSPAN6 impairs the fusion between autophagosomes and lysosomes affecting the cellular proteostasis. Statistical significance was determined by t- test (*$p < 0.05$, **$p < 0.01$, ***$p < 0.001$), ƚ $p < 0.05$)

in TSPAN6-overexpressing primary neurons, were an accumulation of transduced FlagAPP-C99 is observed (Additional file 9: Figure S9). On the other hand we could not demonstrate APP-CTF accumulation at endogeneous levels of APP expression in neurons, in contrast to HEK cells. Apparently, as we see still increased Aβ secretion in TSPAN6 overexpressing neurons, the neurons have additional capacity to turn-over APP-CTF. (Additional file 7: Figure S7b).

It is clear that the effects of TSPAN6 on APP-CTF and Aβ generation are complex. Apart from a decreased turn-over (which makes more APP-CTF available for γ-secretase cleavage), and an increased secretion of APP-CTF containing exosomes, there is also an increase of BACE1 levels by TSPAN6 in HEK 293 cells. While this also might contribute to the increased generation of secreted Aβ, the fact that APP-CTFs are stabilized when overexpressed, indicates a BACE-1 independent mechanism.

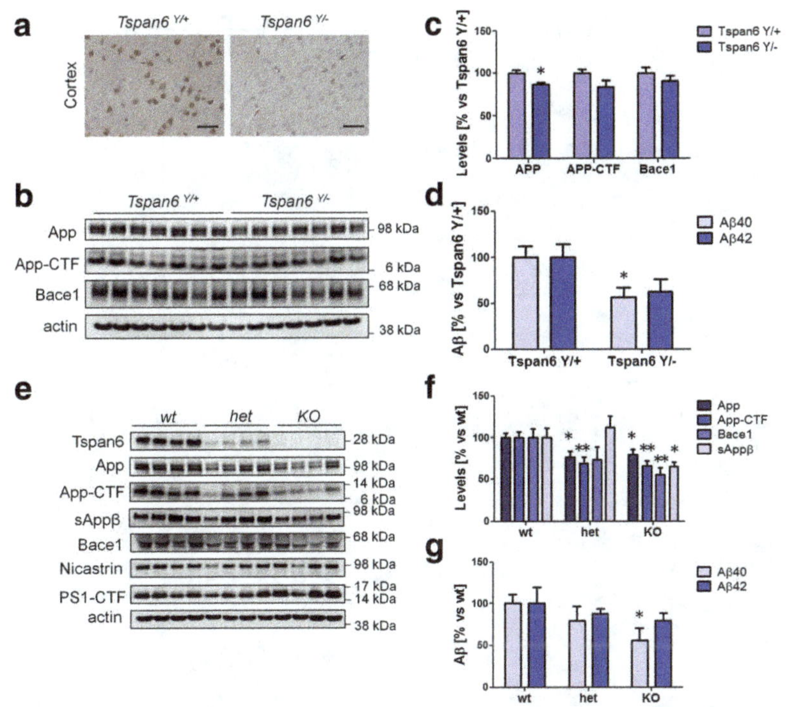

Fig. 9 TSPAN6 controls neural protein homeostasis in vivo. **a** Immunohistochemistry on cerebral sections of the cortex (layer 4) of *Tspan6* $^{Y/+}$ and *Tspan6* $^{Y/-}$ adult mice (1 year old, scale bar = 40 μm). Sections were probed with a polyclonal anti-Tspan6 antibody. Only neuronal bodies of Tspan6 $^{Y/+}$ were positive. **b** Western blot analysis of the cerebral cortex of *Tspan6* $^{Y/+}$ and *Tspan6* $^{Y/-}$ adult mice (7 x *Tspan6* $^{Y/+}$ and 7 x *Tspan6* $^{Y/-}$ 1 year old mice). **c** Quantification of bands shown in panel **b** shows a statistically significant decrease of the App levels in *Tspan6* $^{Y/-}$ mice and slightly decreased levels of App-CTF and Bace1 that do not reach statistical significance. **d** ELISA determinations of the Aβ content in the cerebral cortex of the mice in panel **b**. $A\beta_{40}$ levels were significantly decreased in *Tspan6* $^{Y/-}$ mice. **e** Western blot analysis of lysates of *Tspan6 wt (Tspan6* $^{+/+}$ *or Tspan6* $^{Y/+}$*)*, *Tspan6 het* (*Tspan6* $^{+/-}$) and *Tspan6 KO* (*Tspan6* $^{-/-}$ or *Tspan6* $^{Y/-}$) E15 primary neuronal cultures showing a reduction in the protein levels of App, App-CTF, sAppβ and Bace1 in *Tspan6 het* and *KO* cultures. **f** Quantification of the intensity of the bands of western blot experiments as in panel **e** show a statistically significant reduction in the protein levels of App, App-CTF, sAppβ and Bace1 in *Tspan6 KO* primary neuronal cultures ($n = 8$ for *wt*, $n = 8$ for *het*, $n = 8$ for *KO*). **g** Aβ levels measured by ELISA in 24 h conditioned medium show a statistical significant reduction of $A\beta_{40}$ levels in *Tspan 6 KO* neurons ($n = 8$ for *wt*, n = 3 for *het*, and $n = 4$ for *KO*). Statistical significance was determined by *t*-test (*$p < 0.05$, **$p < 0.01$)

The effect of TSPAN6 on APP-CTF, decreasing its degradation and increasing exosome release, suggests that TSPAN6 affects the lysosomal-MVB-exosome system at the level of ILVs destined either for degradation or biogenesis of exosomes. The sorting of proteins to ILVs is a crucial step in the proper degradation of proteins (including APP) as MVBs fuse to lysosomes but also determines the secretion of proteins via exosomes. At least two molecular signals have been involved in determining the type of ILVs generated: the ESCRT-dependent pathway drives the degradation of the cargo via lysosomes/autophagosomes while ESCRT-independent pathways, such as ceramide-rich membrane microdomains or tetraspanins, are thought to generate ILVs destined to exosomes. Our results show that overexpression of TSPAN6 in HEK293 cells induces enlarged endosomes with ILVs morphologically resembling those of ESCRT-depleted cells. In addition this is accompanied by an increased secretion of exosomes which depends on the specific interaction of TSPAN6 with syntenin. Syntenin allows syndecans and associated molecules to escape degradation by facilitating their translocation to the exosomal route [45]. Thus, our data suggest that TSPAN6 induces an ESCRT-independent formation of ILVs destined for the biogenesis of exosomes in disfavor of an ESCRT-dependent pathway destined to degradation, which explains the stabilization of APP-CTF. Although TSPAN6 interaction with syntenin is required for the increased formation of exosomes, we found that TSPAN6 overexpression increased APP-CTF levels even in the absence of syntenin. These results suggest that TSPAN6 exerts an additional proteostatic effect on APP-CTF. However, it is interesting to notice that in low syntenin conditions, TSPAN6-triggered APP-CTF accumulation is less pronounced, suggesting that syntenin is responsible for at least part of the effect observed. In turn, the PDZ mutant of syntenin can per se induce the

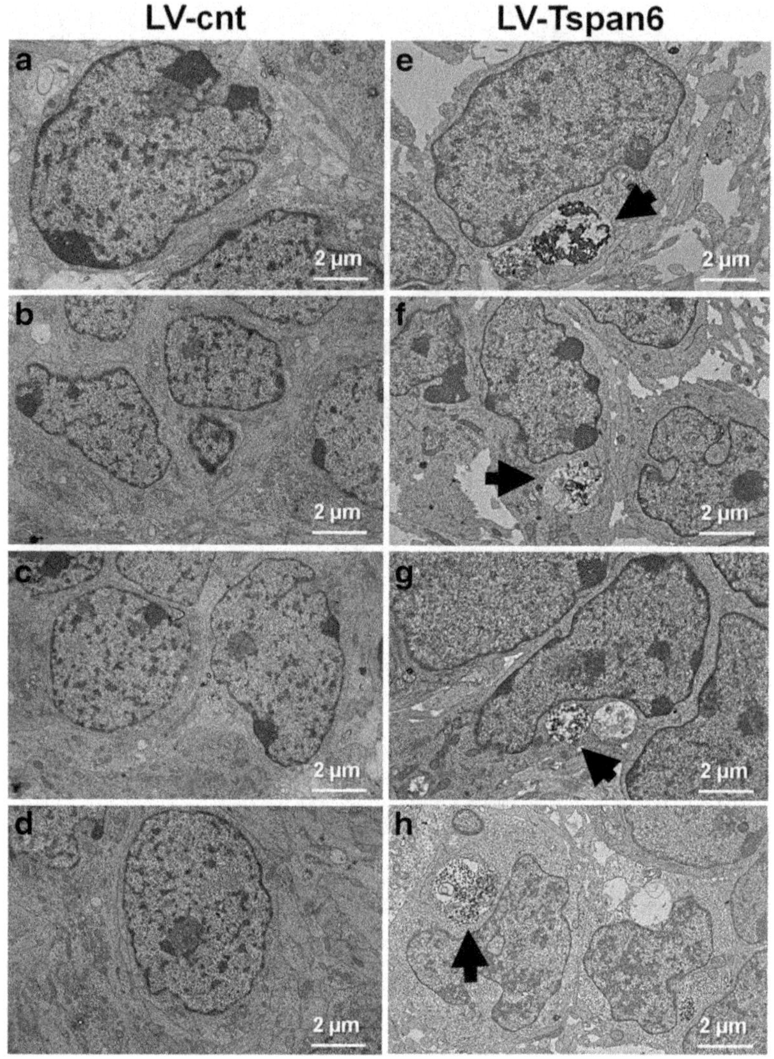

Fig. 10 6 DIV primary cortical neurons derived from *Tspan6 wt* (*Tspan6*$^{+/Y}$) E14.5 embryos were infected with an empty lentiviral vector (LV-cnt) or a lentiviral vector overexpressing Tspan6 (LV-Tspan6). At 9 DIV neurons were washed and processed for EM analysis. *Tspan6 wt* neurons that overexpressed Tspan6 (**e-h**) show alterations by EM consisting of accumulation of electron dense material inside large vesicles (arrow) in the soma compared to control neurons (**a-d**)

accumulation of APP-CTF fragments, indicating the existence of a TSPAN6-independent role of syntenin in stabilizing APP-CTF.

The enhancement of ESCRT-independent mechanisms impairs autophagy by affecting the fusion between autophagosomes and lysosomes, as illustrated by the accumulation of autophagosomes in ESCRT-depleted cells. Interestingly, TSPAN6 appears in a recently published list of newly identified modulators of autophagy [28]. Here, we find decreased fusion between autophagosomes and lysosomes in cells overexpressing TSPAN6, accompanied by the accumulation of the autophagic marker p62 in HEK293 cells. The impairment of autophagy provides a mechanistic explanation for the accumulation of APP-CTF in cells overexpressing TSPAN6. In agreement with a pivotal role for TSPAN6 at this critical junction, a reduction in the levels of TSPAN6 triggers the opposite effect of overexpression: a decrease in the levels of APP-CTF in HEK cells and in neurons. However, further work is needed to support an impairment of the ESCRT-pathway by TSPAN6.

Interestingly, alterations in the endolysosomal–autophagic system are well-recognized early pathological features of AD, which is marked by prominent enlargement of endosomal compartments and progressive accumulation of autophagic vacuoles [50]. In addition, neuronal deficiency of *presenilin 1*, whose mutations trigger the dominant form of the disease [51], causes accumulation of autophagosomes and MVBs [52, 53], while conditional knockout mice for *presenilin 1* accumulate autophagosomes in the brain [54], indicating a link between abnormal processing of presenilin substrates and abnormalities in those pathways. By co-expressing the $Rab5^{Q79L}$ mutant with TSPAN6 in HEK293 cells, we observe exacerbated enlarged Rab5-positive vesicles similar to those seen in neurons generated from induced pluripotent stem cells from AD patients and Down syndrome fibroblasts [55, 56]. Elevated levels of the APP-βCTF fragment generated by BACE1 are sufficient to trigger the accumulation of swollen endosomes by recruiting APPL1 [57]. Since BACE1 protein levels and the APP-βCTF fragment are increased in TSPAN6-overexpressing cells, it is plausible that the formation and accumulation of enlarged endosomes are the consequence of APP-βCTF accumulation. Further work should address to what extent the accumulating APP-CTF may contribute to some of these alterations. Further work is also needed to explain the effects of TSPAN6 on the processivity of γ-secretase processing reflected in increased $A\beta_{40}$. As the effect is not observed in cell free γ-secretase assays, it is likely indirect and possibly caused by redistribution of APP-CTF processing over different subcellular compartments or even different γ-secretase complexes [58] after TSPAN6 overexpression, however, this needs further investigation. On the other hand, the fact that the decreased expression levels of soluble Aβ and proteins involved in the amyloidogenic pathway observed in $App^{NL/F}$ x *Tspan6 KO* mice do not translate into a lower number of plaques in these animals, suggests that Tspan6 may be involved in other biological processes controlling Aβ accumulation in the brain such as glial-dependent Aβ uptake or clearance of the peptide from the brain through the blood brain barrier. Further studies should clarify these other potential roles.

Conclusions

In conclusion, our study identifies TSPAN6, a moderately up-regulated gene in the prefrontal cortex of AD patients, as a new modulator of APP-CTF proteostasis preventing its degradation by the impairment of the autolysosomal pathway, leading to consequent enhanced Aβ production, and turning the balance towards the formation of ILVs destined to form exosomes (Fig. 8 h). Human neurodegenerative diseases including Alzheimer's (AD), Huntington's, and Parkinson's diseases are associated with aberrant protein aggregation [59, 60], and loss of proteostatic mechanisms are likely very central in these diseases. Altogether, our work describes here the biological role of TSPAN6 in the MVB pathway and reinforces the idea that altered proteostasis in neurons may contribute to sporadic AD.

Additional files

Additional file 1: Figure S1. a TSPAN6 was transfected in HEK293 cells stably expressing human wtAPP (HEK-APPwt; 3 independent experiments per condition) and analyzed by western blot using antibodies against ADAM10, BACE1 and components of the γ-secretase complex. BACE1 levels were increased while γ-secretase components are not affected. A representative actin blot of the samples (run on a separate gel) is shown. b The activity of α- and β-secretase was determined by measuring the sAPPα and sAPPβ levels by western blot, respectively, in the 24 h-conditioned medium of the HEK293-APPwt cells from panel a. c The quantification of the intensity of the bands in panel a and b shows that BACE1 and sAPPβ levels are enhanced by TSPAN6 overexpression ($n = 3$ per condition) without any observable effect on sAPPα. d Same samples used in Fig. 1d were analyzed by western blot as in panel a. Briefly, HEK-APPwt cells were treated with a scrambled siRNA (*siRNA-cnt*) or a siRNA against *TSPAN6* (*siRNA-TSPAN6*). A polyclonal TSPAN6 antibody was used to corroborate the decrease of TSPAN6 in siRNA-*TSPAN6* treated cells. BACE1 levels were strongly reduced in *siRNA-TSPAN6*-treated cells. A representative actin blot of the samples (run on a separate gel) is shown. e sAPPα and sAPPβ levels present in the 24 h-conditioned medium of cells of panel d were determined by western blot. f Quantification of the intensity of the bands in panel d and e shows that BACE1 and sAPPβ levels are decreased by TSPAN6 downregulation without any observable effect on sAPPα. Statistical significance was determined by *t* test (*$p < 0.05$, **$p < 0.01$, ***$p < 0.001$).

Additional file 2: Figure S2. a Microsomal fractions from HEK293 cells downregulating (*siRNA-TSPAN6*; *siRNA-cnt* used as control; $n = 3$ technical repeats per condition) or overexpressing TSPAN6 (TSPAN6; empty vector used as control; $n = 3$ technical repeats per condition) were prepared for in vitro γ-secretase assay. The γ-secretase inhibitor DAPT (1 μM) was added as a negative control of the reaction. Analysis by western blot of the in vitro assays shows no effects on the production of AICD by downregulating or overexpressing TSPAN6. b In vitro γ-secretase assays were carried out by adding exogenous substrate (3xFlagAPP-C99) to microsomal fractions obtained from HEK293 cells overexpressing TSPAN6 or an empty vector (control) and analyzed by western blot. The γ-secretase inhibitor DAPT (1 μM) was added as a negative control. AICD production (detected with a monoclonal anti-Flag antibody) was not changed by overexpression of TSPAN6. The generation of different Aβ species during the in vitro reactions was determined by ELISA. No statistical differences in the different Aβ species produced were observed. c HEK293 cells treated with *siRNA-TSPAN6* or *siRNA-cnt* were transfected with the γ-secretase substrate myc-NΔE and analyzed by western blot (3 independent experiments). The blot was probed with a monoclonal anti-myc antibody to detect myc-NΔE, a monoclonal antibody against cleaved Notch1 (Val1744), a polyclonal antibody against TSPAN6 and a monoclonal antibody against actin. No effects on the myc-NΔE levels were observed when TSPAN6 is downregulated. d Plot of the ratio calculated from the bands in panel **c** between the γ-secretase-dependent generation of NICD and its substrate myc-NΔE. Cells down regulating TSPAN6 do not change the production of NICD. e Determination of *APP* mRNA levels of HEK293 cells transfected with an empty vector (control) or TSPAN6 by qPCR. No significant differences in the *APP* mRNA levels were observed between control or TSPAN6-overexpressing cells ($n = 3$ technical repeats per condition). f Determination of *BACE1* mRNA levels of HEK293 cells transfected with an empty vector (control) or TSPAN6 by qPCR. No significant differences in the *BACE1* mRNA levels were observed between control or TSPAN6-overexpressing cells ($n = 3$ technical repeats per condition).

Additional file 3: Figure S3. HEK293 cells transfected with myc-tagged TSPAN6 (myc-TSPAN6) were fixed and studied by immunofluorescence. Myc-TSPAN6, APP-CTF and APP-NTF were detected with a rat monoclonal antibody against myc, a rabbit monoclonal antibody against APP-CTF and a mouse monoclonal antibody against APP-NTF, respectively. Only APP-CTF shows a strong colocalization with myc-TSPAN6. Scale bar = 10 μM.

Additional file 4: Figure S4. a HEK293 cells were solubilized in 1% CHAPSO and fractionated by continuous sucrose gradient centrifugation. Fractions were collected and analyzed by western blot and probed with antibodies against markers for detergent-resistant (caveolin) or detergent-solubilized (calnexin) membranes, as well as APP, BACE1, γ-secretase components and TSPAN6. In the transfected cells APP-CTF showed a strong shift to the TSPAN6 positive fraction. The profile of the percentage of the intensity of the bands per each fraction versus the total intensity of APP-CTF and caveolin was plotted for control or TSPAN6-overexpressing cells. b Representative experiment of a proximity ligation assay (PLA) between APP-CTF and TSPAN6 on HEK293 cells transfected with an empty vector (control) or myc-tagged TSPAN6. Rabbit monoclonal antibody against APP-CTF (y188) and rat monoclonal antibody against myc were used as primary antibodies. Positive red dots indicating interaction events between APP-CTF and TSPAN6 were visualized by confocal microscopy, while cells expressing an empty vector were negative.

Additional file 5: Figure S5. Negative control of autophagosomes formation. HEK293 cells co-transfected with LC3-GFP-RFP and myc-tagged TSPAN6 (myc-TSPAN6) were left with culture medium containing 10% FBS. LC3-GFP-RFP was distributed over the cytosol in contrast to cells submitted to starvation (see Fig. 8e). Scale bars = 10 μm.

Additional file 6: Figure S6. Tspan6 immunoreactivity was present both in regions of high glutamatergic neuronal content (upper panels: GAD67, dentate gyrus) and high GABAergic neuronal content (lower panel: vGlut1, thalamic reticular nucleus). Scale bars = 18 μm.

Additional file 7: Figure S7. a Western blots of lysates of *Tspan6 wt* (*Tspan6 +/+* or *Tspan6 Y/+*) and *Tspan6 KO* (*Tspan6 -/-* or *Tspan6 Y/-*) primary neuronal cultures from different E14.5 embryos transduced with an empty lentiviral vector (LV-cnt) or a lentiviral vector overexpressing Tspan6 (LV-Tspan6). Overexpression of Tspan6 increases the levels of App and the autophagosomal marker p62, indicating a deficit in the autophagic pathway, but not of App-CTF and Bace1. Ponceau staining shows similar loading per well. b Increased levels of $A\beta_{40}$ (upper panel) and $A\beta_{42}$ (lower panel) determined by ELISA in the 12 h conditioned medium of *Tspan6 wt* (*Tspan6 +/+* or *Tspan6 Y/+*) and *Tspan6 KO* (*Tspan6 -/-* or *Tspan6 Y/-*) primary cortical neurons transduced with LV-Tspan6 ($n = 12$ different E14.5 embryos for *wt*, $n = 9$ different E14.5 embryos for *KO*) compared to neurons transduced with LV-cnt ($n = 13$ different E14.5 embryos for *wt*, $n = 10$ different E14.5 embryos for *KO*). Statistical significance was determined by *t* test (**p* <0.05, ***p* <0.01 and ****p* <0.001 for comparison between LV-cnt and LV-Tspan6 conditions, *ǂp* <0.05 for comparison between *Tspan6 wt* and *Tspan6 KO*).

Additional file 8: Figure S8. a Western blot analysis of lysates from the cerebral cortex of 12 months old $App^{NL/F}$ x *Tspan6 wt* ($n = 5$) and $App^{NL/F}$ x *Tspan6 KO* ($n = 6$) mice. The membranes were blotted with antibodies against sAppβ, App, Aβ peptide, Bace1, p62 and actin. b Plot showing the quantification of the bands on the western blot of panel a. The levels of App-CTF, Bace1, Aβ and p62 are decreased in $App^{NL/F}$ x *Tspan6 KO* mice ($n = 6$) compared to $App^{NL/F}$ x *Tspan6 wt* mice ($n = 5$). c Thioflavin staining of cleared brains was performed from 1 year old $App^{NL/F}$ x *Tspan6 wt* ($n = 5$) and $App^{NL/F}$ x *Tspan6 KO* mice ($n = 5$) mice to visualize and quantify the 3D content of amyloid plaques. No differences in the number or the volume occupied by amyloid plaques was detected in $App^{NL/F}$ x *Tspan6 KO* mice versus $App^{NL/F}$ x *Tspan6 wt* mice. Statistical significance was determined by *t*-test (**p* <0.05, ***p* <0.01).

Additional file 9: Figure S9. a 6 DIV *Tspan6 wt* (*Tspan6 +/+* or *Tspan6 Y/+*), *Tspan6 het* (*Tspan6 -/+*) and *Tspan6 KO* (*Tspan6 -/- or Tspan6 Y/-*) primary neuronal cultures were transduced with an adenoviral vector expressing the human APP-C99 triple tagged with a Flag peptide (AV-3xFlagAPP-C99) at a MOI of 100. After 48 h, 4 independent cultures of each condition were lysed and analyzed by western blot using a monoclonal antibody against Flag in order to detect the FlagAPP-C99 expression; Actin is used as a loading control. b Quantification of bands shown in panel a. *Tspan6 KO* neurons accumulate less FlagAPP-C99 after transduction in comparison to *Tspan6 wt* neurons. Statistical significance was determined by *t*-test (**p* <0.05, ****p* <0.001).

Abbreviations

AD: Alzheimer's disease; APP: Amyloid precursor protein; APP-CTF: APP-C-terminal fragments; EBSS: Earle's balanced salt solution; EE: Early endosomes; HEK293: Human embryonic kidney; ILVs: Intraluminal vesicles; MVBs: Multivesicular bodies; NICD: Notch intracelular domain; TSPAN6: Tetraspanin-6

Acknowledgements

We would like to thank Prof. Dr. Carlos Dotti for helpful discussion and critical reading of the manuscript. We also thank Dr. Ruzica Bago for providing us with some of the TSPAN6 constructs. We are grateful to Inframouse and Veronique Hendrickx and Jonas Verwaeren for animal husbandry. We thank the VIB Bio Imaging Core (LiMoNe and EMoNe facilities) where Confocal and Electron microscopy were performed.

Funding

The current work was supported by the Fonds Wetenschappelijk Onderzoek (FWO) Research Foundation (Postdoctoral Fellowship 95508 and Research Grant G094414N), a Methusalem grant from KU Leuven and the Flemish Government. BDS is the Bax-Vanluffelen Chair for Alzheimer's Disease and is supported directly by the Opening the Future campaign of the Leuven Universiteit Fonds (LUF). Confocal microscope equipment was acquired through a Hercules Type 1 A KUL/09/037 to Wim Annaert.

Authors' contributions

BSD designed the overall approach, coordinated the study and drafted the manuscript. FXG did most of the biochemical studies, statistical analysis of the data and wrote the relevant sections of the manuscript. RS did the co-localization studies in vitro, the statistical analysis for the confocal experiments and revised the manuscript. FB, SR and MO characterized the interaction of syntenin with TSPAN6 in vitro and revised the manuscript. AMA prepared the samples and took the images for the analysis by electron microscopy and revised the manuscript. KH provided technical and experimental assistance with the biochemical experiments and revised the manuscript. AS prepared neuronal primary cultures and revised the manuscript. AT did the fractionation of cell lysates by buoyant density gradient centrifugation, provided intellectual inputs and revised the manuscript. ER dissected and fixed the brains of mice for the histological studies and helped to revise the manuscript. SKS studied the expression of TSPAN6 in the corresponding histological slices and helped to revise the manuscript. IHS prepared *Tspan6 KO* primary neural cultures and helped to revise the manuscript. TS and TS provided the knock-in mice and provided input to the paper. JC developed the lightsheet Macroscope system and acquired volume images of amyloid plaques in cleared brains and ST created an ImageJ-based analysis workflow script to analyze the data generated from the images, both authors provided input to the paper. NC and SM performed a complete analysis of the data generated by the script developed by ST and provided input to the paper. WA provided critical analysis of the experiments and the results and helped to draft and revise the manuscript. All authors read and approved the final manuscript.

Competing interests

The authors declare that they have no conflict of interest with the context of this study BDS is consultant for Janssen pharmaceutica and Remynd. He receives research funding from Janssen pharmaceutica, but not for the work presented in the current manuscript.

Notes

Ragna Sannerud and Fedor Berditchevski contributed equally to the publication.

Author details

[1]VIB Center for Brain and Disease research – VIB, Leuven, Belgium. [2]Center of Human Genetics and Leuven Institute for Neurodegenerative Diseases (LIND), KULeuven, Leuven, Gasthuisberg O&N, Belgium. [3]School of Cancer Sciences, University of Birmingham, Edgbaston, Birmingham B15 2TT, UK. [4]Department of Neurobiology, University of Pittsburgh Brain Institute, Pittsburgh Institute for Neurodegenerative Disease, University of Pittsburgh School of Medicine, Biomedical Science Tower 3, Room 6062, 3501 Fifth Avenue, Pittsburgh, PA

15213-3301, USA. [5]Laboratory for Proteolytic Neuroscience, RIKEN Brain Science Institute, Wako-shi, 351-0198 Saitama, Japan. [6]Department of Biochemistry, Faculty of Medicine & Dentistry, University of Alberta, Edmonton, Canada. [7]Molecular Pathology Group, Cell Biology & Histology, Faculty of Medicine, University of Antwerp, Antwerp, Belgium. [8]Institute for Research in Biomedicine (IRB Barcelona), The Barcelona Institute of Science and Technology, c. Baldiri Reixac 10, 08028 Barcelona, Spain. [9]Dementia Research Institute (DRI-UK), University College London, Queen Square, WC1N 3BG London, UK.

References

1. Scheltens P, Blennow K, Breteler MM, de Strooper B, Frisoni GB, Salloway S, et al. Alzheimer's disease. Lancet. 2016. doi:10.1016/S0140-6736(15)01124-1.
2. De Strooper B, Karran E. The cellular phase of Alzheimer's disease. Cell. 2016;164:603–15.
3. De Strooper B. Proteases and proteolysis in Alzheimer disease: a multifactorial view on the disease process. Physiol Rev. 2010;90:465–94.
4. Chávez-Gutiérrez L, Bammens L, Benilova I, Vandersteen A, Benurwar M, Borgers M, et al. The mechanism of γ-secretase dysfunction in familial Alzheimer disease. EMBO J. 2012;31:2261–74.
5. Guix FX, Wahle T, Vennekens K, Snellinx A, Chávez-Gutiérrez L, Ill-Raga G, et al. Modification of γ-secretase by nitrosative stress links neuronal ageing to sporadic Alzheimer's disease. EMBO Mol Med. 2012;4:660–73.
6. Verghese PB, Castellano JM, Garai K, Wang Y, Jiang H, Shah A, et al. ApoE influences amyloid-β (Aβ) clearance despite minimalapoE/Aβ association in physiological conditions. Proc Natl Acad Sci U S A. 2013;110:1807–16.
7. Tarasoff-Conway JM, Carare RO, Osorio RS, Glodzik L, Butler T, Fieremans E, et al. Clearance systems in the brain implications for Alzheimer disease. Nat Rev Neurol. 2015;11:457–70.
8. Zhao Z, Sagare AP, Ma Q, Halliday MR, Kong P, Kisler K, et al. Central role for PICALM in amyloid-β blood-brain barrier transcytosis and clearance. Nat Neurosci. 2015;18:978–87.
9. Roh JH, Jiang H, Finn MB, Stewart FR, Mahan TE, Cirrito JR, et al. Potential role of orexin and sleep modulation in the pathogenesis of Alzheimer's disease. J Exp Med. 2014;211:2487–96.
10. Sagare AP, Bell RD, Zlokovic BV. Neurovascular defects and faulty amyloid-beta vascular clearance in Alzheimer's disease. Adv Alzheimer's Dis. 2012;3:87–100.
11. Szaruga M, Veugelen S, Benurwar M, Lismont S, Sepulveda-Falla D, Lleo A, et al. Qualitative changes in human γ-secretase underlie familial Alzheimer's disease. J Exp Med. 2015;212:2003–13.
12. Marquer C, Laine J, Dauphinot L, Hanbouch L, Lemercier-Neuillet C, Pierrot N, et al. Increasing membrane cholesterol of neurons in culture recapitulates Alzheimer's disease early phenotypes. Mol Neurodegener. 2014;9:60.
13. Vetrivel KS, Cheng H, Kim SH, Chen Y, Barnes NY, Parent AT, et al. Spatial segregation of gamma-secretase and substrates in distinct membrane domains. J Biol Chem. 2005;280:25892–900.
14. Rajendran L, Schneider A, Schlechtingen G, Weidlich S, Ries J, Braxmeier T, et al. Efficient inhibition of the Alzheimer's disease beta-secretase by membrane targeting. Science. 2008;320:520–3.
15. Holmes O, Paturi S, Ye W, Wolfe MS, Selkoe DJ. Effects of membrane lipids on the activity and processivity of purified γ-secretase. Biochemistry. 2012;51:3565–75.
16. Thathiah A, Horré K, Snellinx A, Vandewyer E, Huang Y, Ciesielska M, et al. β-arrestin 2 regulates Aβ generation and γ-secretase activity in Alzheimer's disease. Nat Med. 2013;19:43–9.
17. Chen AC, Kim S, Shepardson N, Patel S, Hong S, Selkoe DJ. Physical and functional interaction between the α- and γ-secretases : a new model of regulated intramembrane proteolysis. J Cell Biol. 2015;211:1157–76.
18. Odintsova E, Berditchevski F. Tetraspanins as regulators of protein trafficking. Traffic. 2007;8:89–96.
19. Hemler ME. Tetraspanin functions and associated microdomains. Nat Rev Mol Cell Biol. 2005;6:801–11.
20. Wakabayashi T, Craessaerts K, Bammens L, Bentahir M, Borgions F, Herdewijn P, et al. Analysis of the gamma-secretase interactome and validation of its association with tetraspanin-enriched microdomains. Nat Cell Biol. 2009;11:1340–6.
21. Dunn CD, Sulis ML, Ferrando AA, Greenwald I. A conserved tetraspanin subfamily promotes notch signaling in Caenorhabditis elegans and in human cells. Proc Natl Acad Sci U S A. 2010;107:5907–12.
22. Dornier E, Coumailleau F, Ottavi JF, Moretti J, Boucheix C, Mauduit P, et al. TspanC8 tetraspanins regulate ADAM10/kuzbanian trafficking and promote notch activation in flies and mammals. J Cell Biol. 2012;199:481–96.
23. Haining EJ, Yang J, Bailey RL, Khan K, Collier R, Tsai S, et al. The TspanC8 subgroup of tetraspanins interacts with a disintegrin and metalloprotease 10 (ADAM10) and regulates its maturation and cell surface expression. J Biol Chem. 2012;287:39753–65.
24. Jouannet S, Saint-Pol J, Fernandez L, Nguyen V, Charrin S, Boucheix C, et al. TspanC8 tetraspanins differentially regulate the cleavage of ADAM10 substrates, notch activation and ADAM10 membrane compartmentalization. Cell Mol Life Sci. 2015;73:1895–915.
25. Bassani S, Cingolani LA, Valnegri P, Folci A, Zapata J, Gianfelice A, et al. The X-linked intellectual disability protein TSPAN7 regulates excitatory synapse development and AMPAR trafficking. Neuron. 2012;73:1143–58.
26. Charrin S, Le Naour F, Silvie O, Milhiet PE, Boucheix C, Rubinstein E. Lateral organization of membrane proteins: tetraspanins spin their web. Biochem J. 2009;420:133–54.
27. Hemler ME. Targeting of tetraspanin proteins–potential benefits and strategies. Nat Rev Drug Discov. 2008;7:747–58.
28. Strohecker AM, Joshi S, Possemato R, Abraham RT, Sabatini DM, White E. Identification of 6-phosphofructo-2-kinase/fructose-2,6-bisphosphatase as a novel autophagy regulator by high content shRNA screening. Oncogene. 2015;34:5662–76.
29. Bossers K, Wirz KT, Meerhoff GF, Essing AH, Van Dongen JW, Houba P, et al. Concerted changes in transcripts in the prefrontal cortex precede neuropathology in Alzheimer's disease. Brain. 2010;133:3699–723.
30. Blalock EM, Geddes JW, Chen KC, Porter NM, Markesbery WR, Landfield PW. Incipient Alzheimer's disease: microarray correlation analyses reveal major transcriptional and tumor suppressor responses. Proc Natl Acad Sci U S A. 2004;101:2173–8.
31. Miller JA, Woltjer RL, Goodenbour JM, Horvath S, Geschwind DH. Genes and pathways underlying regional and cell type changes in Alzheimer's disease. Genome Med. 2013;5(5):48.
32. Kumar-Singh S, Pirici D, McGowan E, Serneels S, Ceuterick C, Hardy J, Duff K, Dickson D, Van Broeckhoven C. Dense-core plaques in Tg2576 and PSAPP mouse models of Alzheimer's disease are centered on vessel walls. Am J Pathol. 2005;167:527–43.
33. Zoncu R, Bar-Peled L, Efeyan A, Wang S, Sancak Y, Sabatini DM. mTORC1 senses lysosomal amino acids through an inside-out mechanism that requires the vacuolar H-ATPase. Science. 2011;334:678–83.
34. Kakuda N, Funamoto S, Yagishita S, Takami M, Osawa S, Dohmae N, Ihara Y. Equimolar production of amyloid beta-protein and amyloid precursor protein intracellular domain from beta-carboxyl-terminal fragment by gamma-secretase. J Biol Chem. 2006;281:14776–86.
35. Sannerud R, Declerck I, Peric A, Raemaekers T, Menendez G, Zhou L, et al. ADP ribosylation factor 6 (ARF6) controls amyloid precursor protein (APP) processing by mediating the endosomal sorting of BACE1. Proc Natl Acad Sci U S A. 2011;108:E559–68.
36. Bolte S, Cordelières FP. A guided tour into subcellular colocalization analysis in light microscopy. J Microsc. 2006;224:213–32.
37. Kang BS, Cooper DR, Jelen F, Devedjiev Y, Derewenda U, Dauter Z, et al. PDZ tandem of human syntenin: crystal structure and functional properties. Structure. 2003;11:459–68.
38. Kraulis PJ, Domaille PJ, Campbell-Burk SL, Van Aken T, Laue ED. Solution structure and dynamics of ras p21. GDP determined by heteronuclear three- and four-dimensional NMR spectroscopy. Biochemistry. 1994;33:3515–31.
39. Latysheva N, Muratov G, Rajesh S, Padgett M, Hotchin NA, Overduin M, et al. Syntenin-1 is a new component of tetraspanin-enriched microdomains: mechanisms and consequences of the interaction of syntenin-1 with CD63. Mol Cell Biol. 2006;26:7707–18.
40. Cierpicki T, Bushweller JH, Derewenda ZS. Probing the supramodular architecture of a multidomain protein: the structure of syntenin in solution. Structure. 2005;13:319–27.
41. Saito T, Matsuba Y, Mihira N, Takano J, Nilsson P, Itohara S, et al. Single App knock-in mouse models of Alzheimer's disease. Nat Neurosci. 2014;17:661–3.
42. Stenmark H, Parton RG, Steele-Mortimer O, Lütcke A, Gruenberg J, Zerial M. Inhibition of rab5 GTPase activity stimulates membrane fusion in endocytosis. EMBO J. 1994;13:1287–96.

43. Marsh M, Van Meer G. No ESCRTs for exosomes. Science. 2008;319:1191–2.
44. Stuffers S, Sem Wegner C, Stenmark H, Brech A. Multivesicular endosome biogenesis in the absence of ESCRTs. Traffic. 2009;10:925–37.
45. Baietti MF, Zhang Z, Mortier E, Melchior A, Degeest G, Geeraerts A, et al. Syndecan-syntenin-ALIX regulates the biogenesis of exosomes. Nat Cell Biol. 2012;14:677–85.
46. Doyle DA, Lee A, Lewis J, Kim E, Sheng M, MacKinnon R. Crystal structures of a complexed and peptide-free membrane protein-binding domain: molecular basis of peptide recognition by PDZ. Cell. 1996;85:1067–76.
47. Chen X, Li M, Chen D, Gao W, Guan JL, Komatsu M, et al. Autophagy induced by calcium phosphate precipitates involves endoplasmic reticulum membranes in autophagosome biogenesis. PLoS One. 2012;7:e52347.
48. Orsi A, Razi M, Dooley HC, Robinson D, Weston AE, Collinson LM, et al. Dynamic and transient interactions of Atg9 with autophagosomes, but not membrane integration, are required for autophagy. Mol Biol Cell. 2012;23:1860–73.
49. Bruno P, Calastretti A, Priulla M, Asnaghi L, Scarlatti F, Nicolin A, et al. Cell survival under nutrient stress is dependent on metabolic conditions regulated by Akt and not by autophagic vacuoles. Cell Signal. 2007;19:2118–26.
50. Nixon RA, Yang DS. Autophagy failure in Alzheimer's disease—locating the primary defect. Neurobiol Dis. 2011;43:38–45.
51. Sherrington R, Rogaev EI, Liang Y, Rogaeva EA, Levesque G, Ikeda M, et al. Cloning of a gene bearing missense mutations in early-onset familial Alzheimer's disease. Nature. 1995;375:754–60.
52. Dobrowolski R, Vick P, Ploper D, Gumper I, Snitkin H, Sabatini DD, et al. Presenilin deficiency or lysosomal inhibition enhances Wnt signaling through relocalization of GSK3 to the late-endosomal compartment. Cell Rep. 2012;2:1316–28.
53. Esselens C, Oorschot V, Baert V, Raemaekers T, Spittaels K, Serneels L, et al. Presenilin 1 mediates the turnover of telencephalin in hippocampal neurons via an autophagic degradative pathway. J Cell Biol. 2004;166:1041–54.
54. Lee JH, Yu WH, Kumar A, Lee S, Mohan PS, Peterhoff CM, et al. Lysosomal proteolysis and autophagy require presenilin 1 and are disrupted by Alzheimer-related PS1 mutations. Cell. 2010;141:1146–58.
55. Jiang Y, Mullaney KA, Peterhoff CM, Che S, Schmidt SD, Boyer-Boiteau A, et al. Alzheimer's-related endosome dysfunction in down syndrome is Aβ-independent but requires APP and is reversed by BACE-1 inhibition. Proc Natl Acad Sci U S A. 2010;107:1630–5.
56. Israel MA, Yuan Bardy SHC, Reyna SM, Mu Y, Herrera C, Hefferan MP, et al. Probing sporadic and familial Alzheimer's disease using induced pluripotent stem cells. Nature. 2012;482:216–20.
57. Kim S, Sato Y, Mohan PS, Peterhoff C, Pensalfini A, Rigoglioso A, et al. Evidence that the rab5 effector APPL1 mediates APP-βCTF-induced dysfunction of endosomes in down syndrome and Alzheimer's disease. Mol Psychiatry. 2015;21:707–16.
58. Sannerud R, Esselens C, Ejsmont P, Mattera R, Rochin L, Tharkeshwar AK, et al. Restricted location of PSEN2 γ-secretase determines substrate specificity and generates an intracellular Aβ pool. Cell. 2016;8674:30568–2.
59. Selkoe DJ. Folding proteins in fatal ways. Nature. 2003;426:900–4.
60. Kopito RR, Ron D. Conformational disease. Nat Cell Biol. 2000;2:E207–9.

3

Increased acetylation of Peroxiredoxin1 by HDAC6 inhibition leads to recovery of Aβ-induced impaired axonal transport

Heesun Choi[1], Haeng Jun Kim[1], Jisoo Kim[1], Soohyun Kim[2,3], Jinhee Yang[1], Wonik Lee[1], Yeonju Park[4], Seung Jae Hyeon[6], Dong-Sup Lee[4], Hoon Ryu[5,6], Junho Chung[2,3] and Inhee Mook-Jung[1*]

Abstract

Background: Reduction or inhibition of histone deacetylase 6 (HDAC6) has been shown to rescue memory in mouse models of Alzheimer's disease (AD) and is recently being considered a possible therapeutic strategy. However, the restoring mechanism of HDAC6 inhibition has not been fully understood.

Methods and results: Here, we found that an anti-oxidant protein Peroxdiredoxin1 (Prx1), a substrate of HDAC6, malfunctions in Aβ treated cells, the brains of 5xFAD AD model mice and AD patients. Malfunctioning Prx1, caused by reduced Prx1 acetylation levels, was recovered by HDAC6 inhibition. Increasing acetylation levels of Prx1 by HDAC6 inhibition recovered elevated reactive oxygen species (ROS) levels, elevated Ca^{2+} levels and impaired mitochondrial axonal transport, sequentially, even in the presence of Aβ. Prx1 mutant studies on the K197 site for an acetylation mimic or silencing mutation support the results showing that HDAC6 inhibitor restores Aβ-induced disruption of ROS, Ca^{2+} and axonal transport.

Conclusions: Taken together, increasing acetylation of Prx1 by HDAC6 inhibition has several beneficial effects in AD pathology. Here, we present the novel mechanism by which elevated acetylation of Prx1 rescues mitochondrial axonal transport impaired by Aβ. Therefore, our results suggest that modulation of Prx1 acetylation by HDAC6 inhibition has great therapeutic potential for AD and has further therapeutic possibilities for other neurodegenerative diseases as well.

Keywords: Alzheimer's disease, Histone deacetylase 6, Peroxiredoxin1, Axonal transport, Oxidative stress, Reactive oxygen species

Background

Alzheimer's disease (AD) is the most common neurodegenerative disease that leads to cognitive impairment. The major pathological features of AD are extracellular accumulation of beta-amyloid (Aβ), called senile plaque, and intracellular neurofibrillary tangles which are composed of hyperphosphorylated tau [1, 2]. There are several well-known cytotoxic effects and molecular changes of Aβ. Aβ disrupts axonal transport by dysregulating microtubule stability and affinity between motor or adaptor proteins and microtubule or cargos [3, 4]. Axonal transport is important for neuronal function and cell viability [5–7]. Oxidative stress, which is caused by increased reactive oxygen species (ROS), and excessive cytosolic Ca^{2+} are induced by Aβ [1]. ROS oxidize lipids, proteins and nucleic acids which are essential for normal cellular function, which leads to increased membrane permeability to Ca^{2+}, mitochondrial damage and apoptosis [8–11]. Excessive Ca^{2+} is involved in excitotoxicity which also contributes to neuronal cell death [12, 13]. In addition, ROS and Ca^{2+} damage to mitochondrial axonal transport is mediated by reduced affinity between Miro and kinesin [14, 15].

One of the molecular changes in AD include increased levels and activity of histone deacetylase 6 (HDAC6) in the brains of AD patients [16, 17]. HDAC6 is localized

* Correspondence: inhee@snu.ac.kr
[1]Department of Biochemistry and Biomedical Sciences, Seoul National University, College of Medicine, Seoul, Korea
Full list of author information is available at the end of the article

in the cytoplasm and deacetylates cytosolic proteins such as α-tubulin and Peroxiredoxin1 (Prx1) [18–20]. Some researchers have shown that reducing or inhibiting HDAC6 in AD model mice resulted in improved memory [21–23]. In addition, Aβ-induced impairment of mitochondrial axonal transport was rescued by HDAC6 inhibitor in primary neurons [24]. Even though HDAC6 has great possibility as an AD therapeutic target, the restoring mechanisms of HDAC6 inhibition are not fully understood.

Here we found one possible mechanism which is mediated by Prx1. A previous report has shown that increasing Prx1 acetylation elevates its reducing activity [19]. Since Prx1 is an HDAC6 substrate, increased HDAC6 activity may cause poor reducing activity of Prx1. Therefore, we studied whether HDAC6 inhibition can regulate ROS level through acetylation of Prx1. Furthermore, we tried to elucidate whether restored axonal transport by HDAC6 inhibitor is mediated by Prx1. Together, we propose that increased acetylation of Prx1 by HDAC6 inhibition leads to recovery of Aβ-induced pathology such as elevation of ROS and Ca^{2+} and impaired axonal transport, making HDAC6 a possible therapeutic target for AD.

Methods

Human brain samples

Neuropathological processing of normal and AD human brain samples followed the procedures previously established for the Boston University Alzheimer's Disease Center (BUADC). Entorhinal cortex and hippocampal regions were used for experiments. Detailed information of brain tissues is described in Additional file 1. In all cases where AD was diagnosed at autopsy, AD was stated as the cause of death. AD subjects had no evidence of other neurological disease based on neuropathological examination. Next of kin provided informed consent for participation and brain donation. The study was performed in accordance with principles of human subject protection in the Declaration of Helsinki. This study was reviewed by the Boston University School of Medicine Institutional Review Board and was approved as exempt because the study involves only tissue collected from post-mortem, and consequently not classified as human subjects.

Animals and intraperitoneal (i.p.) injection

Six-month-old 5xFAD mice (Tg6799; B6SJL-Tg (APPSwFlLon, PSEN* M146L*L286V) 6799Vas/J, stock number 006554, Jackson Labs, Bar Harbor, ME, USA) overexpressing human amyloid precursor protein 695 with three mutations (Swedish, Florida and London) and human presenilin 1 with two mutations (M146L and L286V) under transcriptional control of the murine Thy-1 promoter and wild type littermate (B6/SJL) were used for brain tissue analysis after Tubastatin A (TBA) injection. TBA (100 mg/kg) or saline was administrated daily by i.p. injection for 4 weeks. Animals were treated and maintained in accordance with the Animal Care and Use Guidelines of Seoul National University, Seoul, Korea.

Cell culture and transfection

HT22 cells were cultured in Dulbecco's modified Eagles medium (DMEM; HyClone, USA) supplemented with 10% fetal bovine serum (Hyclone, USA) and 1% penicillin/streptomycin (Sigma, USA) at 37 °C under 5% CO_2. Primary neuronal were previously described [25]. Briefly, primary hippocampal neurons were obtained from the brain tissue of Sprague–Dawley rat embryos (E18) (KOATECH, Korea). Brains were incubated in Hank's Balanced Salt Solution (HBSS; WelGENE, Korea) with 0.05% trypsin (Gibco, USA) for 20 min at 37 °C. Neurons dissociated in NeuroBasal medium (Gibco, USA) supplemented with B27 (Gibco, USA) and penicillin/streptomycin were plated on poly-D-lysine (Sigma, USA) coated dishes or microfluidic chambers for immunoprecipitation or mitochondrial axonal transport analysis, respectively. Half of the culture medium was replaced with fresh medium every 3 days for plates and every day for microfluidic chambers. For transfection, constructs were mixed with Lipofectamine LTX (Invitrogen, USA) in Opti-MEM (Gibco, USA) for HT22 cells and Lipofectamine 2000 (Invitrogen, USA) in fresh neuronal culture medium for primary neurons.

DNA constructs, reagents and antibodies

Three Flag-tagged Prx1 constructs – Prx1-WT-Flag, Prx1-K197Q-Flag and Prx1-K197R-Flag – and another three non-tagged vectors that express GFP separately – Prx1-WT, Prx1-K197Q and Prx1-K197R - were used. Prx1-WT-Flag construct based on pCR3.1 vector was kindly gifted by Dr. Sang Won Kang (Ewha Womans University, Seoul, Korea). Prx1-K197Q-Flag and Prx1-K197R-Flag vectors were generated by point mutation from Prx1-WT-Flag vector using site-directed mutagenesis kit (Enzynomics, Korea) according to manufacturer's instructions. Three non-tagged, separately GFP-expressing Prx1 vectors were constructed from Flag-tagged Prx1 vectors by BamHI and NotI restriction and insertion into pBI-CMV2 vector (Clontech, USA) which has two identical independently expressed promoters, one of which expresses AcGFP. For mitochondrial labeling, pDsRed2-Mito (Clontech, USA) were used. Tubastatin A (TBA) was purchased from Sigma (USA) and U-chem (Korea). N-acetyl cysteine (NAC), Trolox (Sigma, USA) and BAPTA-AM (ThermoFisher Scientific, USA), $A\beta_{1-42}$ peptide (American peptide, USA and Bachem, Switzerland) were used. Anti-Flag, acetyl-tubulin and β-actin antibodies were purchased from

Sigma (USA). Antibodies against Prx1 (CST, USA), 4-HNE, 8-OHdG (Abcam, UK) and Tom2 (SantaCruz, USA) were also used. Acetyl-Prx1 antibodies were generated from chicken using BSA-conjugated synthetic peptide (Peptron Inc., Korea) with a sequence of SKEYFS-K(Ac)QK, C-terminal of Prx1. For antibody selection, four rounds of bio-panning were performed as described previously using magnetic bead conjugated with BSA-acetylated Prx1 peptide after removing non-acetylated Prx1 binders using BSA-non-acetylated Prx1 peptide (BSA-CGGGSSKEYFSKQK) [26]. Affinity chromatography using Protein A agarose beads (Repligen 16 Corp., USA) was then used to purify acetyl-Prx1 antibodies (clone name: R2-31) [27].

Preparation of Aβ

$A\beta_{1-42}$ peptide (American peptide, USA and Bachem, Switzerland) was prepared as previously described [25]. In brief, $A\beta_{1-42}$ peptide was dissolved in 1,1,1,3,3,3-hexafluoro-2-propanol (Sigma, USA) and lyophilized in a Speedvac (Labconco, USA). The dry peptide was dissolved in anhydrous dimethyl sulfoxide (Sigma, USA) at a final concentration of 1 mM and diluted in DMEM or cell culture medium. During treating to cells, most of Aβ consisted predominantly of oligomers and some monomers [24].

Immunoprecipitation and western blotting

Cells were lysed in 1% Triton X-100 in TBS buffer (50 mM Tris HCl, 150 mM NaCl, pH 7.4) containing protease inhibitor cocktail, phenyl-methylsulfonyl fluoride (PMSF) (Sigma, USA) and TBA for HDAC6 inhibition. Flag-tagged Prx1 was immunoprecipitated using anti-Flag M2 magnetic beads (Sigma, USA) and eluted by competition with 3xFlag peptide (Sigma, USA) according to manufacturer's instructions. Elutes were mixed with SDS-PAGE sample buffer, and boiled at 95 °C for 3 min. For immunoprecipitation of endogenous Prx1, anti-Prx1 antibodies and protein A/G agarose beads (SantaCruz, USA) were crosslinked by BS3 (ThermoFisher Scientific, USA) according to manufacturer's instructions and then incubated with cell lysates overnight at 4 °C. Precipitates were eluted with SDS-PAGE sample buffer by boiling at 95 °C for 3 min. Both boiled elutes and equal amounts of input samples were separated via SDS-PAGE and transferred to polyvinylidene difluoride (PVDF) membranes. Membranes were blocked with 5% skim milk (Bioworld, USA) and probe with antibodies against indicated proteins. Western blotting process has been also described in a previous report [24].

DCFDA assay

For ROS measurement, cells were treated with 1 μM of cell-permeant 2′, 7′-dichlorodihydrofluorescein diacetate (H_2DCFDA, mentioned DCFDA in this paper) (Invitrogen, USA) in DMEM. After 1 h incubation at 37 °C, DCFDA was changed with DMEM. Fluorescent signals were captured using fluorescence microscope (Olympus, Japan) or CellInsight (Thermo Scientific, USA). Images obtained from fluorescence microscope were analyzed using Image J (NIH) and images from CellInsight using its software.

Fluo-4 assay

For measuring Ca^{2+} concentration, cells were incubated with fluo-4 (Invitrogen, USA) for 1 h at 37 °C. After changing medium to DMEM, fluorescent signals were captured using fluorescence microscope or CellInsight. Images obtained from fluorescence microscope were analyzed using Image J (NIH) and from CellInsight using its software.

Mitochondrial axonal transport analysis

Fabrication of microfluidic chambers and analysis of mitochondrial axonal transport were described in the reference [24]. In brief, neurons cultured in microfluidic chambers were transfected with pDsRed2-Mito at day in vitro (DIV) 7 or 8 to visualize mitochondria. Prx1 constructs, which express AcGFP, were simultaneously transfected with pDsRed2-Mito. After treatment with indicated compounds, live cells were time-lapse imaged using Olympus IX81 microscope (Japan) equipped with a Cool SNAP HQ2 CCD camera (Photometrics, USA), controlled by MetaMorph Software (Universal Imaging, USA), for 2 min, with a 1 s interval in an incubating equipment (Live cell instrument, Korea) which maintains 37 °C and 5% CO_2. Movies were processed using MetaMorph. Mitochondrial movement in axons were analyzed by using Image J installed with multiple kymograph plugins (by J. Rietdorf and A. Seitz).

Immunohistochemistry

Mice were anesthetized with a mixture of Zoletil 50 (Virbac, France) and Rompun (Bayer, USA) solution (3:1 ratio, 1 ml/kg, i.p.) and were transcardially perfused with phosphate buffered-saline (PBS). The hemisphere of the brain was dissected and incubated in 4% paraformaldehyde (PFA) for 36 h, followed by 30% sucrose for 72 h at 4 °C. Serial 30-μm-thick coronal tissue sections were made using freezing microtome (Leica, USA). For 4-HNE and 8-OHdG immunostaining using 3, 3′-diaminobenzidine (DAB), free-floating sections were incubated overnight at 4 °C with anti-4-HNE (1:200) and 8-OHdG (1:400) antibodies diluted in PBS containing 0.3% Triton X-100, 0.05% bovine serum albumin (BSA) and normal horse serum. Sections were then treated with 3% H_2O_2 in PBS for 30 min at room temperature (RT) to quench the activity of endogenous peroxidase, followed by incubation with biotinylated secondary antibodies (1:200; Vector Laboratories, USA) for 2 h at RT and then with an avidin-biotin complex (Vector Laboratories, USA) for 1 h at RT. Immunoreactivity was visualized by DAB in 0.05 M Tris-buffered saline (pH 7.6). Finally, sections were mounted on poly-L-lysine (Sigma, USA) coated Histobond glass slides (Marienfeld, Germany), air-dried overnight, serial ethanol dehydrated and coverslipped with Permount (Fisher Scientific, USA). For fluorescent staining with anti-acetyl-Prx1 (1:50) and Tom20 (1:200), sections were incubated overnight at 4 °C with indicated antibodies diluted in PBS containing 1% Triton X-100 and normal horse serum, followed by incubation with Alexa Fluor 488 and 594 secondary antibodies (Thermo-Fisher Scientific, USA) for 1 h at RT. Sections were washed with PBS every incubation step. For acetyl-Prx1 staining of human brain tissues using DAB, paraffin-embedded tissue sections were deparaffinized in 55 °C dry-oven for overnight. Rehydrated and endogenous peroxidase quenched tissue sections were incubated with anti-acetyl-Prx1 antibody (1:100) at 4 °C for overnight and the rest of procedures were equal to be described above. The images were acquired using Olympus FSX 100 (Olympus, Japan) or confocal microscope (Carl Zeiss, Germany) for DAB stained sections or fluorescent labeling sections, respectively. Image J was used for quantifying immunoreactivity.

Statistical analysis

Data were analyzed by two-way analysis of variance (ANOVA) or one-way ANOVA with Bonferroni post-hoc tests. All data were shown as mean ± SEM.

Results

Acetylation level of Prx1 was decreased in the brains of AD patients and acetylation of Prx1 is regulated by both Aβ and HDAC6

Since it was reported that the level and activity of HDAC6 were increased in AD [16, 17] and Prx1 is one of substrates of HDAC6 [19], we hypothesized that acetylation of Prx1 is reduced in AD conditions. First, we confirmed this hypothesis in human brain samples (Fig. 1a). As expected, Prx1 acetylation was decreased in the hippocampus and entorhinal cortex of AD patients compared to age- and sex-matched normal controls. This result suggests that upregulated HDAC6 in AD brains could affect Prx1 acetylation level, and reduced acetylation level of Prx1 is one of pathological features of AD brains. To determine whether acetylation of Prx1 is affected by Aβ and HDAC6, we used primary hippocampal neurons and HT22 cell line. Endogenous Prx1 in primary hippocampal neurons showed that acetylation of Prx1 was reduced by Aβ and recovered by Tubastatin A (TBA), an HDAC6 inhibitor (Fig. 1b). Similar results were shown in HT22 cells. In HT22 cells, Aβ decreased the level of Prx1 acetylation, however, TBA treatment increased the level of Prx1 acetylation even in the presence of Aβ (Fig. 1c). These results suggest that acetylation of Prx1 might be one of the crucial factors that modulate AD pathology and that HDAC6 is involved in these processes. To confirm the deacetylation site on Prx1 by HDAC6, antibodies against acetyl Prx1 at lysine (K) 197 residue were developed and validated by immunoprecipitation of a Prx1-WT-Flag and a Prx1-K197R-Flag which was not acetylated at K197 by substituting K to arginine (R) (see Additional file 2). To increase acetylation at K197 of Prx1, the Prx1-WT-Flag transfected HT22 cells were treated with TBA. It can be confirmed that the acetyl Prx1 antibody (R2-31) specifically detects acetylation of Prx1 at K197 because there was no signal in the Prx1-K197R-Flag, but there was in the Prx1-WT-Flag. In addition, a stronger signal appeared in the TBA-treated Prx1-WT-Flag than the non-treated one. These findings show that acetylation of Prx1 is regulated by both Aβ and HDAC6.

ROS and Ca^{2+} are regulated by HDAC6 inhibitor

Since increased acetylation of Prx1 shows more effective antioxidant activity [19], we tested whether acetylated Prx1 reduces ROS levels in HT22 cells. To prove it, we performed a DCFDA assay to measure ROS level in HT22 cells which were treated with Aβ with or without TBA. The fluorescence signal of DCFDA was increased in the Aβ treated group compared to veh. However, in the Aβ and TBA co-treatment group, the signal was decreased compared to the Aβ treated group (Fig. 2a). This indicates that the HDAC6 inhibitor can reduce the Aβ-induced elevated ROS level. Several reports showed that excessive ROS elevates cytoplasmic Ca^{2+} level through IP3R or RyR [28–30]. Since Aβ is also known to increase intracellular Ca^{2+} level, we measured Ca^{2+} level using Fluo-4 assay at the same condition as above. Similar with ROS level, Ca^{2+} level was increased by Aβ and rescued by TBA in the presence of Aβ (Fig. 2b). In addition, the results of TBA pretreatment before Aβ were also showed recovered Aβ-induced ROS and Ca^{2+} levels by TBA, which were similar to those of Fig. 2 - posttreatment of TBA (Additional file 3). These results provide evidence that increased acetylation of Prx1 by HDAC6 inhibitor might regulate ROS as well as Ca^{2+} levels in the presence of Aβ.

Aβ-induced ROS regulates intracellular Ca^{2+} level

To explore whether ROS can regulate Ca^{2+} level in the presence of Aβ, we treated trolox and N-acetyl cysteine (NAC) with Aβ to HT22 cells. Both trolox and NAC, which is an analog of vitamin E and a precursor to glutathione, respectively, were ROS inhibitors. 200 μM

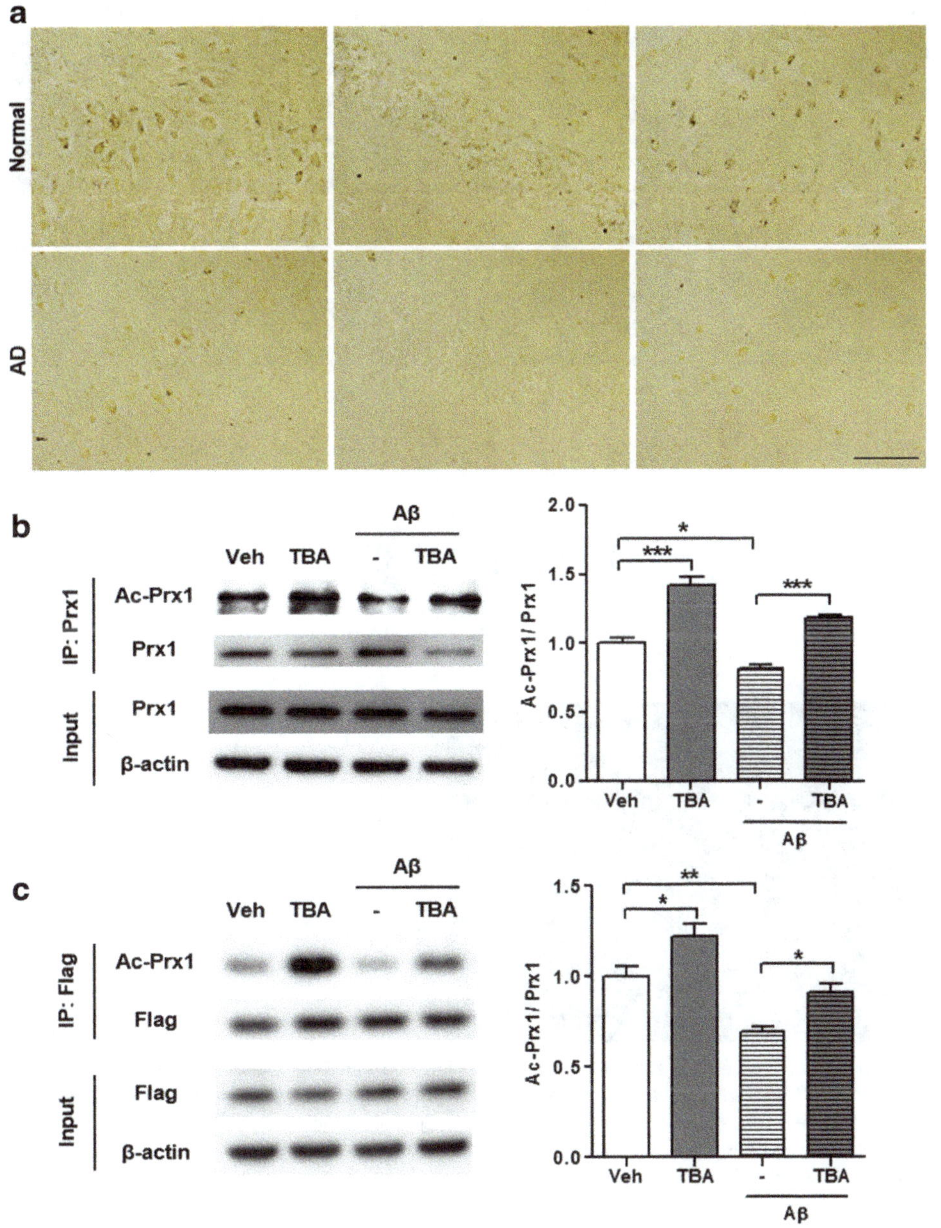

Fig. 1 Acetyl-Prx1 is decreased in AD patients' brains, and Aβ and HDAC6 inhibitor modulate Prx1 acetylation. **a** Representative images of acetyl-Prx1 level in human brain samples. *Top* row shows representative images of age- and sex-matched normal control brains and *bottom* row shows AD brains. Scale bar: 100 μm. **b** Acetylation level of Prx1 in primary hippocampal neurons. Primary hippocampal neurons were treated with Aβ (2 μM, 24 h) and then co-treated with TBA (1 μM, 3 h). Endogenous Prx1 was immunoprecipitated by anti-Prx1 antibody which was cross-linked to protein A/G coated agarose beads and probed by indicated antibodies. *Left* panel shows immunoblot images and *right* panel shows quantification of acetylation level of Prx1 which normalized by immunoprecipitated total Prx1 ($n = 4$, independent experiments). **c** Acetylation level of Prx1 in HT22 cells. Prx1-WT-Flag transfected HT22 cells were treated with Aβ (2 μM, 24 h) and then co-treated with TBA (0.5 μM, 3 h). Prx1-Flag was immunoprecipitated by anti-Flag M2 magnetic beads and probed by indicated antibodies. *Left* panel shows immunoblot images and right panel shows quantification of acetylation level of Prx1 which normalized by immunoprecipitated total Prx1 ($n = 4$, independent experiments). Data are presented as mean ± SEM. *$P < 0.05$, **$P < 0.01$, ***$P < 0.001$ (two-way ANOVA, Bonferroni post-hoc test)

of trolox was enough to suppress ROS when co-treated with Aβ in HT22 cells (Fig. 3a). Under this condition (200 μM trolox), where the ROS level is similar to veh even in the presence of Aβ, the Ca^{2+} level measured by Fluo-4 assay was also decreased compared to the Aβ-treated group (Fig. 3b). NAC, which is a different species of ROS inhibitor, had similar effects on Aβ-induced ROS and Ca^{2+} levels (Additional file 4). These results suggested that ROS could regulate Ca^{2+} level. In addition, the reverse direction, in which Ca^{2+} induces ROS, was

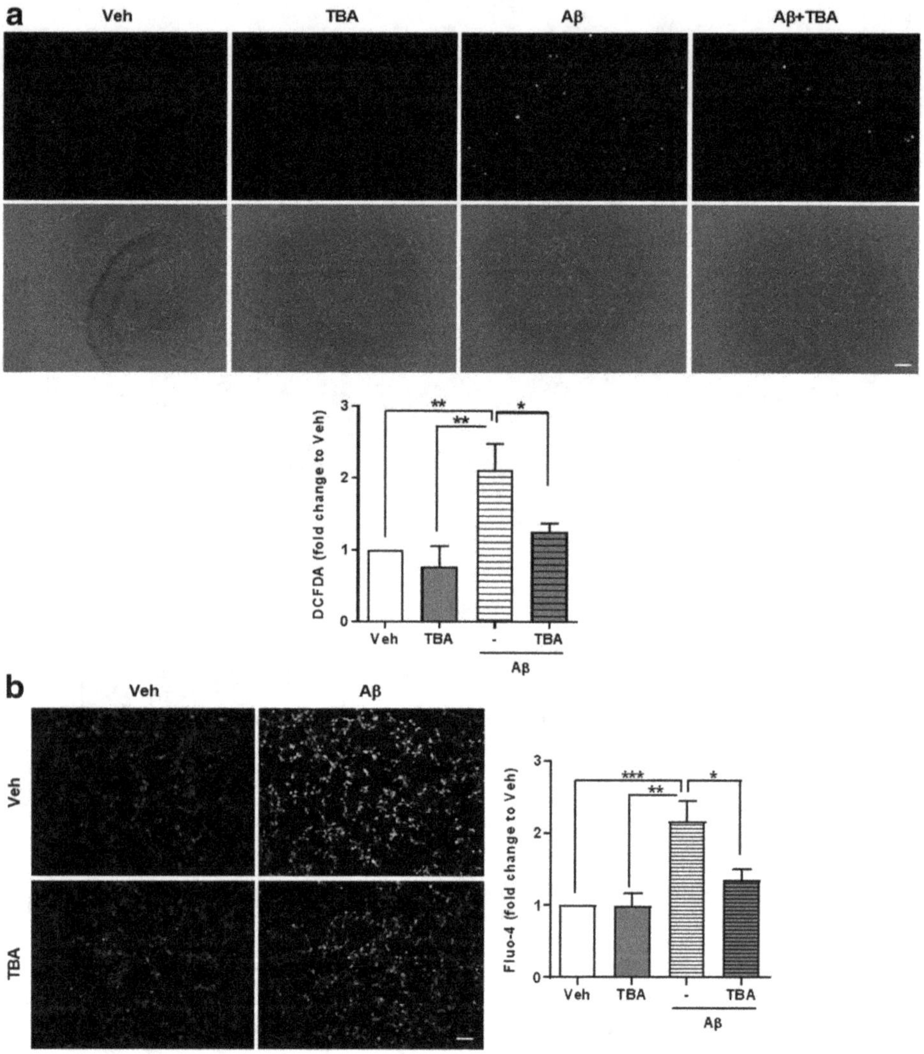

Fig. 2 HDAC6 inhibition decreases Aβ-induced ROS and Ca^{2+}. HT22 cells were treated with TBA (0.5 μM, 3 h) after being treated with Aβ (2 μM, 24 h). **a** ROS level was measured by DCFDA assay in HT22 cells. *Upper* panel shows representative DCFDA signals (*top* row) and bright field images (*bottom* row). *Lower* panel shows quantitative graph of fluorescent intensity ($n = 5$, independent experiments). **b** Ca^{2+} level was measured by Fluo-4 assay in HT22 cells. *Left* panel is representative images and *right* panel is quantification of fluorescent intensity ($n = 5$, independent experiments). Data are presented as mean ± SEM. $^{*}P < 0.05$, $^{**}P < 0.01$, $^{***}P < 0.001$ (two-way ANOVA, Bonferroni post-hoc test). Scale bar: 100 μm

examined in the presence of Aβ. HT22 cells were treated with BAPTA-AM, which is an intracellular Ca^{2+} chelator, and Aβ. The BAPTA-AM and Aβ co-treated group showed lower Ca^{2+} level, followed by reduced ROS level compared to Aβ only treated group (Additional file 5). These results suggest that ROS and Ca^{2+} regulate each other, and this leads to a vicious cycle, which accelerates AD pathology.

Recovery of Aβ-induced ROS and Ca^{2+} elevation by HDAC6 inhibitor is mediated by acetylation of Prx1

To determine the role of acetylated Prx1 in the recovery of Aβ-induced ROS and Ca^{2+}, we constructed acetyl mimic and silencing mutants, K197Q and K197R respectively, by substituting glutamine (Q) or R for K. The expression level is similar among constructs (Fig. 4a). Previous study shows that acetyl mimic mutant has stronger reducing activity compared to WT [19]. Indeed, acetyl mimic mutant transfected HT22 cells are partially resistant to Aβ-induced ROS elevation, while acetyl silencing mutant shows results similar to WT by Aβ. Moreover, even though TBA was co-treated with Aβ in acetyl silencing mutant transfected HT22 cells, increased ROS level by Aβ was not restored unlike in WT which showed restored ROS levels (Fig. 4b). In terms of Ca^{2+} level, it shows similar patterns to ROS level results (Fig. 4c). Acetyl mimic mutant groups showed protective effects against Aβ-induced increased Ca^{2+} level, and acetyl silencing mutant groups lost their function compared to WT. It provides evidence that increased Ca^{2+} by Aβ could be regulated by ROS level which is modulated

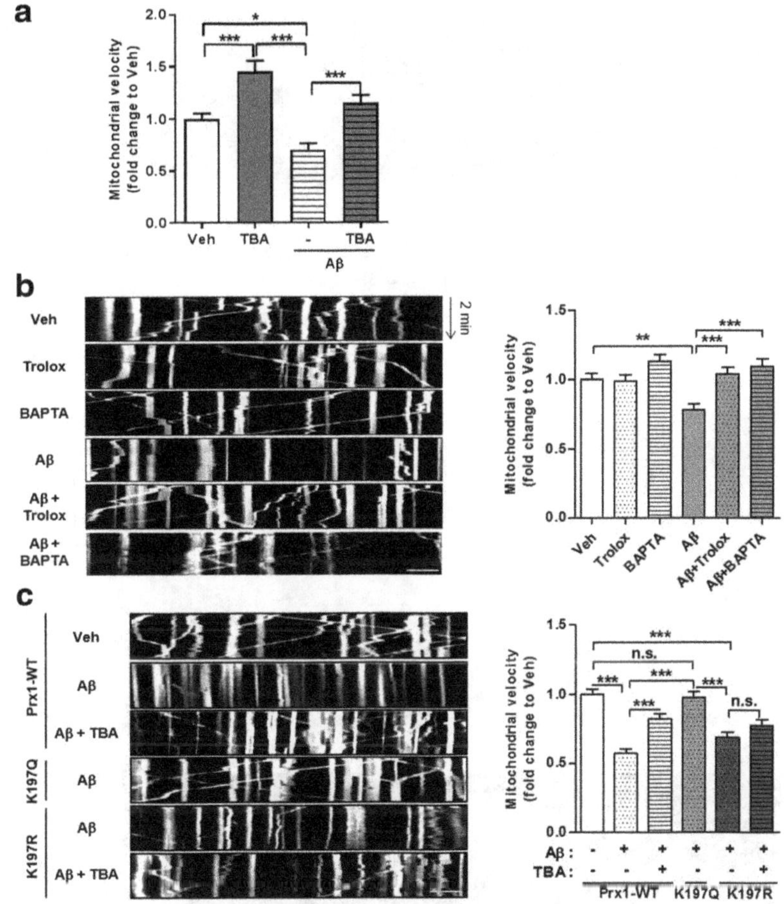

Fig. 5 Aβ-induced ROS disrupts mitochondrial axonal transport by elevating Ca^{2+} level. **a** Mitochondrial absolute velocity in axons of primary hippocampal neurons showing TBA recover impaired mitochondrial axonal transport by Aβ. Mito-dsRed2 transfected primary hippocampal neurons were treated with Aβ (2 μM, 24 h) followed by incubated with TBA (0.5 μM, 3 h). Data were obtained from 3 independent experiments ($n = 30$ cells per group). The results were shown as mean ± SEM. $^{*}P < 0.05$, $^{***}P < 0.001$ (two-way ANOVA, Bonferroni post-hoc test) (**b**) Disrupted mitochondrial axonal transport by Aβ is recovered by ROS inhibitor or Ca^{2+} chelator. Mito-dsRed2 transfected primary hippocampal neurons were pretreated with trolox (200 μM) or BAPTA (2 μM) for 1 h before incubation with 2 μM Aβ (24 h). *Left* panel shows kymograph and *right* panel shows quantitative graph of mitochondrial absolute velocity. Data were acquired from 4 independent experiments ($n = 40$ cells per group). The results were shown as mean ± SEM. $^{**}P < 0.01$, $^{***}P < 0.001$ (two-way ANOVA, Bonferroni post-hoc test) **c** Acetylation of Prx1 regulate mitochondrial axonal transport in the presence of Aβ. Prx1-WT or K197Q or K197R and mito-dsRed2 co-transfected primary hippocampal neurons were treated with Aβ (2 μM, 24 h) followed by incubated with TBA (0.5 μM, 3 h). *Left* panel shows kymograph and *right* panel shows quantitative graph of mitochondrial absolute velocity. Data were obtained from 5 independent experiments ($n = 40$ cells per group). The results were shown as mean ± SEM. $^{***}P < 0.001$, n.s.: non-significant (one-way ANOVA, Bonferroni post-hoc test), scale bar: 10 μm

in vivo using 5xFAD mice, an AD model mice. Six-month-old 5xFAD mice were injected TBA (100 mg/kg) for 4 weeks intraperitoneally. Consistent with the data from cultured cells, acetylation of Prx1 was reduced in the brains of 5xFAD mice compared to wild type. However, this reduction was recovered in TBA-injected 5xFAD by showing immunohistochemistry (Fig. 6a). There are reports showing that, in the brains of AD patients, some oxidative stress markers were elevated such as 8-hydroxydeoxyguanosine (8-OHdG), a marker of oxidative damage to DNA and RNA, and 4-hydroxynonenal (4-HNE), a product of lipid peroxidation [31–33]. We observed that 4-HNE and 8-OHdG were also increased in 5xFAD brains by western blotting and immunohistochemistry. However, increased acetylation of Prx1 by TBA recovered 4-HNE and 8-OHdG (Fig. 6b,c). These data suggest that reduced acetylation of Prx1 by Aβ might be involved in increased oxidative stress in 5xFAD. Since we identified that reduced ROS level recovers mitochondrial axonal transport in the presence of Aβ, mitochondrial axonal transport was analyzed with immunohistochemistry using Tom20, a mitochondrial marker protein, in mouse brains as previously described [21] (Fig. 6d). Mitochondrial localization presented by Tom20 immunoreactivity showed more mitochondria

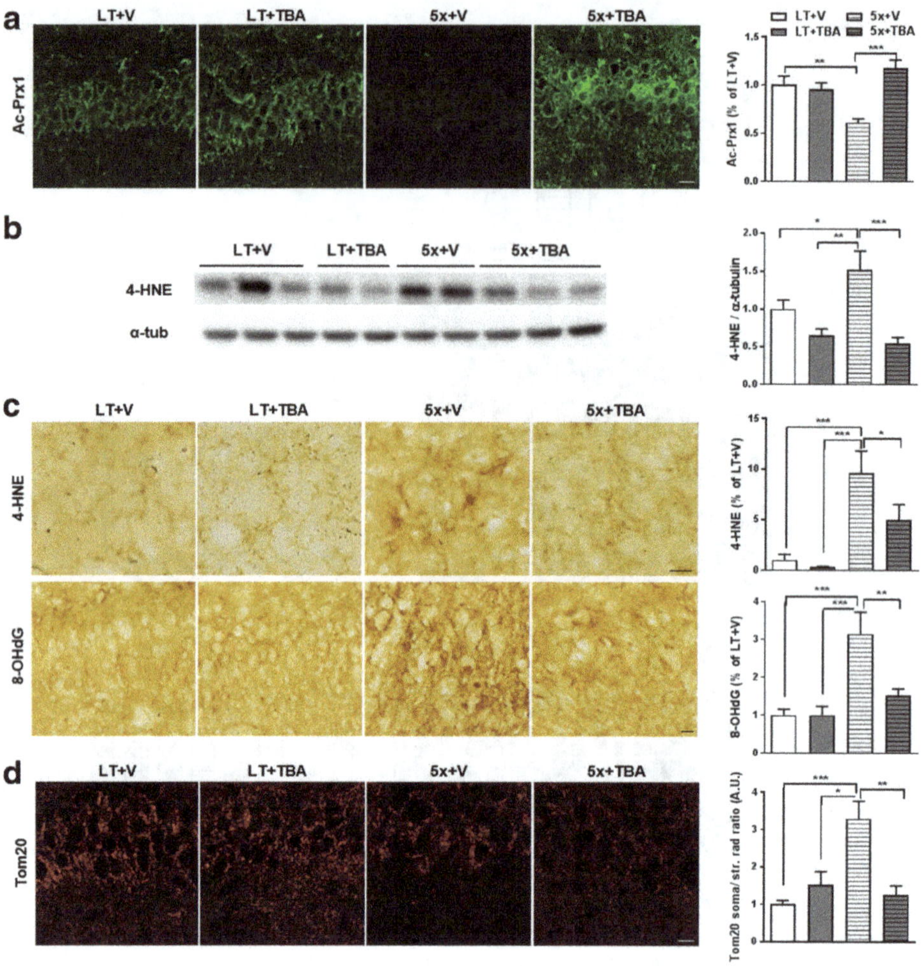

Fig. 6 HDAC6 inhibitor rescues oxidative stress and mitochondrial transport by elevating Prx1 acetylation in 5xFAD mice. TBA (100 mg/kg) was i.p. injected to 6-month-old 5xFAD female mice for 4 weeks. Five mice were used in each group. Cryosectioned brain slice were used in (**a**, **c** and **d**). Brain lysates were used in (**b**). **a** Reduced acetylation of Prx1 is recovered by TBA in 5xFAD mice. Representative images of Ac-Prx1 immunoreactivity in CA1 are shown in *left* panel and quantitative graph are in *right* panel. **b**, **c** Oxidative stress is recovered by TBA in 5xFAD mice. Representative immunoblot (*left*) and quantitative analysis (*right*) of 4-HNE are shown in **b**. Representative DAB stained images (*left*) against indicated antibodies and quantitative analysis (*right*) are shown in **c**. Immunoreactivity of 4-HNE and 8-OHdG was quantified in cortex and CA1, respectively. **d** Mitochondrial transport is rescued by TBA in 5xFAD mice. Anti-Tom20 shows mitochondrial distribution in CA1. Representative images are shown in *left* panel. Tom20 immunoreactivity in *right* panel was quantified as the ratio of intensity in soma to that in stratum radiatum. Data are presented as mean ± SEM ($n = 5$ per group). $^{*}P < 0.05$, $^{**}P < 0.01$, $^{***}P < 0.001$ (two-way ANOVA, Bonferroni post-hoc test), LT: wild-type littermate, 5x: 5xFAD, V: vehicle, TBA: Tubastatin A, scale bar: 10 μm

accumulation in the somata of neurons in the CA1 region of 5xFAD compared to wild type. However, mitochondria were distributed equally from the somata to the stratum radiatum in CA1 of TBA-injected 5xFAD, indicating that HDAC6 inhibition restores mitochondrial axonal transport *in vivo*. It is suggested that oxidative stress might be involved in the disruption of mitochondrial axonal transport in 5xFAD. Taken together, it is supposed that elevating acetylation of Prx1 by HDAC6 inhibitor plays an important role in recovering oxidative stress, followed by recovering mitochondrial axonal transport *in vivo*. Thus, regulating acetylation of Prx1 using HDAC6 inhibitor could be a new therapeutic strategy in AD.

Discussion

In the present study, we determine the new role of acetylation of Prx1 by HDAC6 modulation in AD pathogenesis related to Aβ. When acetylation of Prx1 at K197 was reduced, mitochondrial axonal transport was disrupted following the elevation of ROS and Ca^{2+} in the presence of Aβ. These pathologic features caused by Aβ were recovered by modulating acetylation of Prx1 through HDAC6 inhibition (Fig. 7). Given that Prx1 is a substrate of HDAC6, which is increased in level and activity in the brains of AD patients [16], reduced acetylation of Prx1 by Aβ might result from HDAC6 overactivation. Since deacetylated Prx1 has decreased anti-oxidant activity [19], excessive ROS and Ca^{2+}

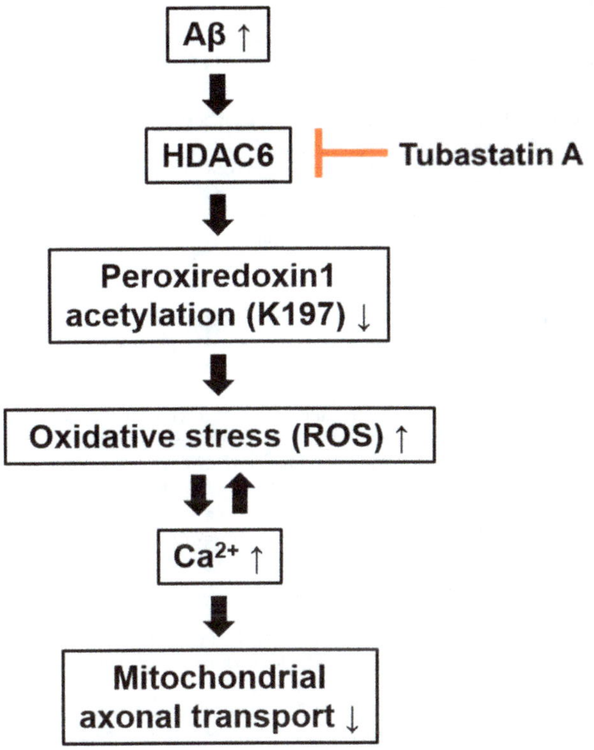

Fig. 7 Schematic diagram of the role of HDAC6 inhibitor and acetylation of Prx1 in AD. Increased acetylation of Prx1 by HDAC6 inhibitor rescues impaired mitochondrial axonal transport by restoring oxidative stress followed by reducing Ca^{2+} level in AD

caused by Aβ may also be downstream of HDAC6. It is reported that ROS and excessive Ca^{2+} impair mitochondrial axonal transport [14, 15]. Therefore, disrupted mitochondrial axonal transport in the presence of Aβ might be a result of reduced Prx1 acetylation caused by overactivated HDAC6. Previous studies have shown that HDAC6 inhibition rescues the Aβ-induced impairment of mitochondrial axonal transport by increasing acetylation of α-tubulin, resulting in increased microtubule stability and the recruitment of motor proteins to microtubules [3, 24, 34, 35]. Alpha-tubulin is a well-known substrate of HDAC6, and many researches have reported the relationship between acetylated α-tubulin and axonal transport [3, 24, 36, 37]. Here, we additively elucidated a novel mechanism of regulating mitochondrial axonal transport by HDAC6 inhibition, which modulates acetylation of Prx1 thereby regulating ROS and Ca^{2+} levels. This novel mechanism is more important, because it reveals that HDAC6 inhibitor can rescue excessive ROS and Ca^{2+} which are other major cellular pathogenic factors in AD.

In addition, modulation of Prx1 acetylation, not Prx1 itself, is more important for treatment of AD, because Prx1 is already increased in AD patients' brains [38, 39]. Although researchers consider that this may be the result of a cellular protective mechanism [38, 39], oxidative stress still remain in AD brains. Therefore, increasing acetylation of Prx1 is important to elevate antioxidant activity of Prx1. In this study, we demonstrated that elevating acetylation of Prx1 by HDAC6 inhibition in AD condition could recovered Aβ-induced oxidative stress followed by restoring excessive Ca^{2+} and mitochondrial axonal transport. Thus, modulating acetylation of Prx1 could be one of therapeutic targets for AD.

Several researchers showed that reduction or inhibition of HDAC6 ameliorated memory impairment in AD mice model [21–23, 40]. They proposed that the mechanism of memory rescue works by restoring axonal transport by increasing microtubule stability or recovering autophagy. In addition, the novel mechanism presented in this study could explain memory rescue through HDAC6 inhibition. Well-known pathogenic features of Aβ include elevated ROS and disrupted Ca^{2+} homeostasis and axonal transport [1, 41]. Excessive ROS in AD trigger oxidative stress, which leads to neuronal dysfunction and cell death by Aβ production, lipid peroxidation, enhancement of protein oxidation, and disruption of gene regulation through DNA oxidation [8, 31, 42, 43]. Lipid peroxidation causes ion imbalance and impairs metabolism by weakening cell membranes [44]. Moreover, Torres et al. suggested that the severity of cognitive impairment is directly related to the level of oxidative stress [45]. Elevated Ca^{2+} activates several enzymes such as calcineurin and calpain, which leads to neurite atrophy, disruption in synaptic plasticity and apoptotic cell death [12, 13, 46, 47]. A report also shows that the onset of cognitive symptoms in AD is tightly correlated with reduction of Ca^{2+}-binding proteins [48, 49]. Since neurons have unique polarized shapes such as long axons, axonal transport is important for communication between cell bodies and axon terminals. Therefore, axonal transport deficit leads to several deleterious effects in neurons. Clearance of misfolded proteins in axons and response to neurotrophic signals or stress insults require axonal transport [3, 5, 7]. Specifically, mitochondrial axonal transport is important for supplying energy to the distal axon to maintain synaptic function [6]. Amyloid precursor protein processing, from which Aβ is generated, is stimulated by axonal blockade [50]. In addition, it is reported that excessive ROS and Ca^{2+} damage axonal transport of mitochondria and synaptic vesicles [14, 15]. These findings suggest that disrupted ROS, Ca^{2+} homeostasis and axonal transport, assumed to be early pathologic events, are crucial for neuronal cell death and cognitive impairment in AD. Therefore, HDAC6 inhibitor could recover memory impairment in AD mice models. Moreover, since disrupted ROS, Ca^{2+} homeostasis and axonal transport are common pathologies of neurodegenerative diseases [3, 13, 51], it is expected that HDAC6 inhibitor could also have therapeutic effects in other neurodegenerative diseases.

To explore potential use for clinical treatment of HDAC6 inhibitor, we tested both posttreatment and pretreatment of TBA (Fig. 2 and Additional file 3). The results were similar in both treatment conditions, in which TBA could recover Aβ-induced ROS and Ca^{2+} levels. This indicates that TBA has both preventive and restorative ability for pathology of AD. However, we observed a little increasing of Ca^{2+} in TBA-alone-pretreatment group unlike in posttreatment group, although it wasn't severe increase as much as Aβ-alone-treated group.

We showed that ROS can regulate mitochondrial axonal transport mediated by Ca^{2+}. There are reports that excessive ROS or Ca^{2+} disrupts mitochondrial axonal transport [14, 15]. However, how ROS alter mitochondrial axonal transport is unclear. Our results show that when Aβ-induced ROS was blocked by ROS inhibitors or increased acetylation of Prx1 by HDAC6 inhibitor, Ca^{2+} level decreased, and rescue of mitochondrial axonal transport followed. It is reported that Ca^{2+} regulates mitochondrial axonal transport by modulating the interaction between mitochondria and motor proteins through Miro, which undergoes conformational changes as Ca^{2+} binds to it [15, 52]. Thus, we revealed for the first time that Ca^{2+} is a key mediator of ROS-induced mitochondrial axonal transport deficit.

Although ROS increase Ca^{2+} level by facilitating Ca^{2+} release from the ER or mitochondria, it is well-known that excessive Ca^{2+} can also elevate ROS by causing mitochondrial dysfunction [13, 31, 53, 54]. Consistent with previous reports, we showed that reduction of Aβ-induced Ca^{2+} by BAPTA decreased ROS levels (Additional file 5). Considering that Aβ-induced ROS elevate Ca^{2+}, and that Ca^{2+} also elevates ROS, a vicious cycle is formed. This cyclic nature suggests that mitochondrial axonal transport might be very susceptible to AD.

In this study, we investigated that the elevation of acetylation of Prx1 by HDAC6 inhibitor partially rescues increased ROS level in the presence of Aβ. Only partial recovery was achieved possibly due to other redox regulatory systems, which remain disrupted by Aβ, such as superoxide dismutase-2, glutaredoxin 1 and thioredoxin 1 [55]. The precise mechanism needs to be further studied.

Conclusions

We demonstrated a novel mechanism: mediated by restoring ROS and Ca^{2+} level in the presence of Aβ, increased acetylation of Prx1 by HDAC6 inhibitor rescues impaired mitochondrial axonal transport. This indicates the new role of Prx1 in regulating mitochondrial axonal transport which is downstream of HDAC6 and the new role of HDAC6 in restoring Aβ-induced oxidative stress and disrupted Ca^{2+} homeostasis. Therefore, HDAC6 inhibition might be a strong therapeutic strategy for AD.

Additional files

Additional file 1: Human brain samples that were used in the study. F: Female.

Additional file 2: Anti-acetyl Prx1 (R2-31) antibody specifically detects acetylated Prx1 at K197. R2-31 antibody specificity was validated by immunoprecipitation of Flag tagged Prx1-WT or Prx1-K197R using anti-Flag M2 magnetic beads and probed by R2-31 antibody. Expression and immunoprecipitation of exogenous Prx1-WT-Flag or Prx1-K197R-Flag was confirmed by anti-Flag antibody. Immunoblot of Ac-tub in Input shows TBA works well. N.C.: Negative Control, TBA: Tubastatin A.

Additional file 3: Pretreatment of TBA also decreases Aβ-induced ROS and Ca^{2+}. HT22 cells were pretreated with TBA (0.5 μM) for 1 h before incubation with Aβ (2 μM, 24 h). **a** ROS level was measured by DCFDA assay in HT22 cells. Upper panel is representative images of DCFDA signals (top row) and bright field images (bottom row) and lower panel is quantification of fluorescent intensity ($n = 6$, independent experiments). **b** Ca^{2+} level was measured by Fluo-4 assay in HT22 cells. Left panel is representative images and right panel is quantification of fluorescent intensity ($n = 4$, independent experiments). Data are presented as mean ± SEM. $*P < 0.05$, $**P < 0.01$, $***P < 0.001$ (two-way ANOVA, Bonferroni post-hoc test). Scale bar: 100 μm.

Additional file 4: NAC, an ROS inhibitor, also can regulate Aβ-induced intracellular calcium level. **a** Aβ-induced ROS was decreased by 2 mM NAC. HT22 cells were pretreated with indicated concentration of NAC for 1 h before incubation with 2 μM Aβ (24 h). Upper panel is representative images of DCFDA signals (top row) and bright field (bottom row) to measure ROS level in HT22 cells and lower penal is quantitative graph ($n = 5$, independent experiments). The results were shown as mean ± SEM. $**P < 0.01$ (one-way ANOVA, Bonferroni post-hoc test) **b** Reduction of Aβ-induced ROS level by NAC can decrease Ca^{2+} level. HT22 cells were pretreated with 2 mM NAC for 1 h before incubation with 2 μM Aβ (24 h). Left panel is representative images of Fluo-4 assay to measure Ca^{2+} level in HT22 cells and right panel is quantitative graph ($n = 7$, independent experiments). The results were shown as mean ± SEM. $**P < 0.01$, $***P < 0.001$ (two-way ANOVA, Bonferroni post-hoc test). Scale bar: 100 μm.

Additional file 5: Disrupted Ca^{2+} homeostasis induced by Aβ affects ROS level. **a** Increased Ca^{2+} level induced by Aβ was reduced by 2 μM BAPTA. HT22 cells were pretreated with indicated concentration of BAPTA for 1 h before incubation with 2 μM Aβ (24 h). Left panel is representative images of Fluo-4 assay to measure Ca^{2+} level and quantification is shown in right panel ($n = 6$, independent experiments). The results were shown as mean ± SEM. $*P < 0.05$, $**P < 0.01$ (one-way ANOVA, Bonferroni post-hoc test). **b** Reduction of Ca^{2+} by BAPTA can decrease ROS level in the presence of Aβ. HT22 cells were pretreated with 2 μM BAPTA for 1 h before incubation with 2 μM Aβ (24 h). In upper panel, representative DCFDA signals and bright field images were shown in top row and bottom row, respectively. Quantification graph was shown in lower panel ($n = 6$, independent experiments). The results were shown as mean ± SEM. $*P < 0.05$, $**P < 0.01$, $***P < 0.001$ (two-way ANOVA, Bonferroni post-hoc test). Scale bar: 100 μm.

Additional file 6: Disrupted mitochondrial axonal transport by Aβ is recovered by ROS inhibitor or Ca^{2+} chelator. Representative mitochondrial movements in axons of primary hippocampal neurons which are related to Fig. 5b. Scale bar: 10 μm.

Additional file 7: Acetylation of Prx1 regulate mitochondrial axonal transport in the presence of Aβ. Representative mitochondrial movements in axons of primary hippocampal neurons which are related to Fig. 5c. Scale bar: 10 μm.

Abbreviations

4-HNE: 4-hydroxynonenal; 8-OHdG: 8-hydroxydeoxyguanosine; AD: Alzheimer's disease; Aβ: Beta-amyloid; DAB: 3, 3'-diaminobenzidine; DCFDA: 2', 7'-dichlorodihydrofluorescein diacetate; DIV: Day in vitro; HDAC6: Histone deacetylase 6; i.p.: Intraperitoneal; NAC: N-acetyl cysteine; PFA: Paraformaldehyde; PMSF: Phenyl-methylsulfonyl fluoride;

Prx1: Peroxiredoxin1; PVDF: Polyvinylidene difluoride; ROS: Reactive oxygen species; RT: Room temperature; TBA: Tubastatin A; WT: Wild type

Acknowledgements
We thank Dr. Sang Won Kang for a generous gift of Prx1-Flag vector.

Funding
This research was supported by grants from NRF (2015R1A2A1A05001794, 2014M3C7A1046047, 2015M3C7A1028790 and MRC (2012R1A5A2A44671346)) for I.M-J.

Authors' contributions
HC designed the research, performed cloning, primary neuronal culture, cell culture, western blot analyses, DCFDA and Fluo-4 assays and immunohistochemical analyses, and drafted the manuscript. HJK contributed to develop antibodies and carried out mitochondrial transport analyses, primary neuronal culture, genotyping, TBA injection to mice, and immunohistochemical analyses. JK designed the research, performed cloning, DCFDA and Fluo-4 analyses, mitochondrial transport analyses, and primary neuronal culture. SK and JC carried out developing antibodies. JY served intellectual contribution about experiments. WL performed genotyping, and TBA injection to mice. YP and D-SL contributed to immunohistochemical analysis of human brain samples. SJH and HR gifted human brain samples and contributed to immunohistochemical analysis of human brain samples. IM-J designed the research, brought intellectual feedback, participated in interpretation of data and drafted manuscript. All authors have read and approved the final manuscript.

Competing interests
The authors declare that they have no competing interests.

Consent for publication
Not applicable.

Ethics approval and consent to participate
Neuropathological processing of normal and AD human brain samples followed the procedures previously established for the Boston University Alzheimer's Disease Center (BUADC). Next of kin provided informed consent for participation and brain donation. The study was performed in accordance with principles of human subject protection in the Declaration of Helsinki. This study was reviewed by the Boston University School of Medicine Institutional Review Board and was approved as exempt because the study involves only tissue collected from post-mortem, and consequently not classified as human subjects. Animals were treated and maintained as per the Helsinki Treaty, the Principles of Laboratory Animal Care (NIH publication No. 85–23, revised 1985), and the Animal Care and Use Guidelines of Seoul National University, Seoul, Korea. All experimental procedures were reviewed and approved by the Institutional Animal Care and Use Committee (IACUC) of Seoul National University.

Author details
[1]Department of Biochemistry and Biomedical Sciences, Seoul National University, College of Medicine, Seoul, Korea. [2]Department of Biochemistry and Molecular Biology, Seoul National University, College of Medicine, Seoul, Korea. [3]Cancer Research Institute, Seoul National University College of Medicine, Seoul, Korea. [4]Department of Biomedical Sciences, Laboratory of Immunology and Cancer Biology, Seoul National University College of Medicine, Seoul, Korea. [5]VA Boston Healthcare System, Boston University Alzheimer's Disease Center, and Department of Neurology, Boston University School of Medicine, Boston MA02130, USA. [6]Center for Neuromedicine, Brain Science Institute, Korea Institute of Science and Technology, Seoul, Korea.

References

1. Querfurth HW, LaFerla FM. Alzheimer's disease. N Engl J Med. 2010;362:329–44.
2. Kumar A, Singh A, Ekavali. A review on Alzheimer's disease pathophysiology and its management: an update. Pharmacol Rep. 2015;67:195–203.
3. Millecamps S, Julien JP. Axonal transport deficits and neurodegenerative diseases. Nat Rev Neurosci. 2013;14:161–76.
4. Rui Y, Tiwari P, Xie Z, Zheng JQ. Acute impairment of mitochondrial trafficking by beta-amyloid peptides in hippocampal neurons. J Neurosci. 2006;26:10480–7.
5. Perlson E, Maday S, Fu MM, Moughamian AJ, Holzbaur EL. Retrograde axonal transport: pathways to cell death? Trends Neurosci. 2010;33:335–44.
6. Calkins MJ, Reddy PH. Amyloid beta impairs mitochondrial anterograde transport and degenerates synapses in Alzheimer's disease neurons. Biochim Biophys Acta. 2011;1812:507–13.
7. Maday S, Twelvetrees AE, Moughamian AJ, Holzbaur EL. Axonal transport: cargo-specific mechanisms of motility and regulation. Neuron. 2014;84:292–309.
8. Huang WJ, Zhang X, Chen WW. Role of oxidative stress in Alzheimer's disease. Biomed Rep. 2016;4:519–22.
9. Jomova K, Vondrakova D, Lawson M, Valko M. Metals, oxidative stress and neurodegenerative disorders. Mol Cell Biochem. 2010;345:91–104.
10. Fleming JL, Phiel CJ, Toland AE. The role for oxidative stress in aberrant DNA methylation in Alzheimer's disease. Curr Alzheimer Res. 2012;9:1077–96.
11. Jin SM, Cho HJ, Jung ES, Shim MY, Mook-Jung I. DNA damage-inducing agents elicit gamma-secretase activation mediated by oxidative stress. Cell Death Differ. 2008;15:1375–84.
12. Kuchibhotla KV, Goldman ST, Lattarulo CR, Wu HY, Hyman BT, Bacskai BJ. Abeta plaques lead to aberrant regulation of calcium homeostasis in vivo resulting in structural and functional disruption of neuronal networks. Neuron. 2008;59:214–25.
13. Bezprozvanny I. Calcium signaling and neurodegenerative diseases. Trends Mol Med. 2009;15:89–100.
14. Fang C, Bourdette D, Banker G. Oxidative stress inhibits axonal transport: implications for neurodegenerative diseases. Mol Neurodegener. 2012;7:29.
15. Wang X, Schwarz TL. The mechanism of Ca2+ – dependent regulation of kinesin-mediated mitochondrial motility. Cell. 2009;136:163–74.
16. Ding H, Dolan PJ, Johnson GV. Histone deacetylase 6 interacts with the microtubule-associated protein tau. J Neurochem. 2008;106:2119–30.
17. Hempen B, Brion JP. Reduction of acetylated alpha-tubulin immunoreactivity in neurofibrillary tangle-bearing neurons in Alzheimer's disease. J Neuropathol Exp Neurol. 1996;55:964–72.
18. Hubbert C, Guardiola A, Shao R, Kawaguchi Y, Ito A, Nixon A, Yoshida M, Wang XF, Yao TP. HDAC6 is a microtubule-associated deacetylase. Nature. 2002;417:455–8.
19. Parmigiani RB, Xu WS, Venta-Perez G, Erdjument-Bromage H, Yaneva M, Tempst P, Marks PA. HDAC6 is a specific deacetylase of peroxiredoxins and is involved in redox regulation. Proc Natl Acad Sci U S A. 2008;105:9633–8.
20. d'Ydewalle C, Bogaert E, Van Den Bosch L. HDAC6 at the intersection of neuroprotection and neurodegeneration. Traffic. 2012;13:771–9.
21. Govindarajan N, Rao P, Burkhardt S, Sananbenesi F, Schluter OM, Bradke F, Lu J, Fischer A. Reducing HDAC6 ameliorates cognitive deficits in a mouse model for Alzheimer's disease. EMBO Mol Med. 2013;5:52–63.
22. Majid T, Griffin D, Criss Z, Jarpe M, Pautler RG. Pharmocologic treatment with histone deacetylase 6 inhibitor (ACY-738) recovers Alzheimer's disease phenotype in amyloid precursor protein/presenilin 1 (APP/PS1) mice. Alzheimers Dement. 2015;1:170–81.
23. Zhang L, Liu C, Wu J, Tao JJ, Sui XL, Yao ZG, Xu YF, Huang L, Zhu H, Sheng SL, Qin C. Tubastatin A/ACY-1215 improves cognition in Alzheimer's disease transgenic mice. J Alzheimers Dis. 2014;41:1193–205.
24. Kim C, Choi H, Jung ES, Lee W, Oh S, Jeon NL, Mook-Jung I. HDAC6 inhibitor blocks amyloid beta-induced impairment of mitochondrial transport in hippocampal neurons. PLoS One. 2012;7:e42983.
25. Cha MY, Cho HJ, Kim C, Jung YO, Kang MJ, Murray ME, Hong HS, Choi YJ, Choi H, Kim DK, et al. Mitochondrial ATP synthase activity is impaired by suppressed O-GlcNAcylation in Alzheimer's disease. Hum Mol Genet. 2015; 24:6492–504.
26. Barbas CF, Burton DR, Scott JK, Silverman GJ. Phage display. New York: CSHL Press; 2004.

27. Park S, Lee DH, Park JG, Lee YT, Chung J. A sensitive enzyme immunoassay for measuring cotinine in passive smokers. Clin Chim Acta. 2010;411:1238–42.
28. Camara AK, Bienengraeber M, Stowe DF. Mitochondrial approaches to protect against cardiac ischemia and reperfusion injury. Front Physiol. 2011;2:13.
29. Hidalgo C, Bull R, Behrens MI, Donoso P. Redox regulation of RyR-mediated Ca2+ release in muscle and neurons. Biol Res. 2004;37:539–52.
30. Gorlach A, Bertram K, Hudecova S, Krizanova O. Calcium and ROS: a mutual interplay. Redox Biol. 2015;6:260–71.
31. Zhao Y, Zhao B. Oxidative stress and the pathogenesis of Alzheimer's disease. Oxid Med Cell Longev. 2013;2013:316523.
32. Nunomura A, Perry G, Pappolla MA, Wade R, Hirai K, Chiba S, Smith MA. RNA oxidation is a prominent feature of vulnerable neurons in Alzheimer's disease. J Neurosci. 1999;19:1959–64.
33. Markesbery WR, Lovell MA. Four-hydroxynonenal, a product of lipid peroxidation, is increased in the brain in Alzheimer's disease. Neurobiol Aging. 1998;19:33–6.
34. Dompierre JP, Godin JD, Charrin BC, Cordelieres FP, King SJ, Humbert S, Saudou F. Histone deacetylase 6 inhibition compensates for the transport deficit in Huntington's disease by increasing tubulin acetylation. J Neurosci. 2007;27:3571–83.
35. Reed NA, Cai D, Blasius TL, Jih GT, Meyhofer E, Gaertig J, Verhey KJ. Microtubule acetylation promotes kinesin-1 binding and transport. Curr Biol. 2006;16:2166–72.
36. Li G, Jiang H, Chang M, Xie H, Hu L. HDAC6 alpha-tubulin deacetylase: a potential therapeutic target in neurodegenerative diseases. J Neurol Sci. 2011;304:1–8.
37. Matsuyama A, Shimazu T, Sumida Y, Saito A, Yoshimatsu Y, Seigneurin-Berny D, Osada H, Komatsu Y, Nishino N, Khochbin S, et al. In vivo destabilization of dynamic microtubules by HDAC6-mediated deacetylation. EMBO J. 2002;21:6820–31.
38. Kim SH, Fountoulakis M, Cairns N, Lubec G. Protein levels of human peroxiredoxin subtypes in brains of patients with Alzheimer's disease and Down syndrome. J Neural Transm Suppl. 2001;(61):223–235.
39. Chang RY, Etheridge N, Dodd PR, Nouwens AS. Targeted quantitative analysis of synaptic proteins in Alzheimer's disease brain. Neurochem Int. 2014;75:66–75.
40. Selenica ML, Benner L, Housley SB, Manchec B, Lee DC, Nash KR, Kalin J, Bergman JA, Kozikowski A, Gordon MN, Morgan D. Histone deacetylase 6 inhibition improves memory and reduces total tau levels in a mouse model of tau deposition. Alzheimers Res Ther. 2014;6:12.
41. Vicario-Orri E, Opazo CM, Munoz FJ. The pathophysiology of axonal transport in Alzheimer's disease. J Alzheimers Dis. 2015;43:1097–113.
42. Murakami K, Murata N, Noda Y, Tahara S, Kaneko T, Kinoshita N, Hatsuta H, Murayama S, Barnham KJ, Irie K, et al. SOD1 (copper/zinc superoxide dismutase) deficiency drives amyloid beta protein oligomerization and memory loss in mouse model of Alzheimer disease. J Biol Chem. 2011;286:44557–68.
43. Oda A, Tamaoka A, Araki W. Oxidative stress up-regulates presenilin 1 in lipid rafts in neuronal cells. J Neurosci Res. 2010;88:1137–45.
44. Madeo J. The Role of Oxidative Stress in Alzheimer 's Disease. J Alzheimers Dis Parkinsonism. 2013;03:116.
45. Torres LL, Quaglio NB, de Souza GT, Garcia RT, Dati LM, Moreira WL, Loureiro AP, de Souza-Talarico JN, Smid J, Porto CS, et al. Peripheral oxidative stress biomarkers in mild cognitive impairment and Alzheimer's disease. J Alzheimers Dis. 2011;26:59–68.
46. Trinchese F, Fa M, Liu S, Zhang H, Hidalgo A, Schmidt SD, Yamaguchi H, Yoshii N, Mathews PM, Nixon RA, Arancio O. Inhibition of calpains improves memory and synaptic transmission in a mouse model of Alzheimer disease. J Clin Invest. 2008;118:2796–807.
47. Son SM, Byun J, Roh SE, Kim SJ, Mook-Jung I. Reduced IRE1alpha mediates apoptotic cell death by disrupting calcium homeostasis via the InsP3 receptor. Cell Death Dis. 2014;5:e1188.
48. Palop JJ, Jones B, Kekonius L, Chin J, Yu GQ, Raber J, Masliah E, Mucke L. Neuronal depletion of calcium-dependent proteins in the dentate gyrus is tightly linked to Alzheimer's disease-related cognitive deficits. Proc Natl Acad Sci U S A. 2003;100:9572–7.
49. Kook SY, Jeong H, Kang MJ, Park R, Shin HJ, Han SH, Son SM, Song H, Baik SH, Moon M, et al. Crucial role of calbindin-D28k in the pathogenesis of Alzheimer's disease mouse model. Cell Death Differ. 2014;21:1575–87.
50. Kamal A, Almenar-Queralt A, LeBlanc JF, Roberts EA, Goldstein LS. Kinesin-mediated axonal transport of a membrane compartment containing beta-secretase and presenilin-1 requires APP. Nature. 2001;414:643–8.
51. Kim GH, Kim JE, Rhie SJ, Yoon S. The role of oxidative stress in neurodegenerative diseases. Exp Neurobiol. 2015;24:325–40.
52. Stephen TL, Gupta-Agarwal S, Kittler JT. Mitochondrial dynamics in astrocytes. Biochem Soc Trans. 2014;42:1302–10.
53. Hidalgo C, Carrasco MA, Munoz P, Nunez MT. A role for reactive oxygen/nitrogen species and iron on neuronal synaptic plasticity. Antioxid Redox Signal. 2007;9:245–55.
54. Sanmartin CD, Paula-Lima AC, Garcia A, Barattini P, Hartel S, Nunez MT, Hidalgo C. Ryanodine receptor-mediated Ca(2+) release underlies iron-induced mitochondrial fission and stimulates mitochondrial Ca(2+) uptake in primary hippocampal neurons. Front Mol Neurosci. 2014;7:13.
55. Massaad CA, Klann E. Reactive oxygen species in the regulation of synaptic plasticity and memory. Antioxid Redox Signal. 2011;14:2013–54.

4

Diurnal oscillation of CSF Aβ and other AD biomarkers

Brendan P. Lucey*, Anne M. Fagan, David M. Holtzman, John C. Morris and Randall J. Bateman

Abstract

To assess stages of Alzheimer's disease (AD) pathogenesis and the efficacy of drugs during clinical trials, there has been immense interest in the field to establish baseline cerebrospinal fluid (CSF) concentrations for potential AD biomarkers such as amyloid-β (Aβ) and tau. Significant within-person variations in CSF Aβ concentrations over time found that this variation followed the sleep-wake cycle. A recent paper in Molecular Neurodegeneration reported the absence of diurnal variations in multiple classical and candidate AD biomarkers, such as soluble APP, Aβ, tau, p-tau, YKL-40, VILIP-1, or apolipoprotein E. This commentary addresses these apparently discordant results regarding the diurnal variability of APP and Aβ compared with the literature. Despite our concerns, we appreciate the authors' interest in this important topic and contribution to improve our knowledge about the factors influencing Aβ diurnal variation.

Keywords: Alzheimer's disease, Amyloid-β, Biomarkers

Background

To assess stages of Alzheimer's disease (AD) pathogenesis and the efficacy of drugs during clinical trials, there has been immense interest in the field to establish baseline cerebrospinal fluid (CSF) concentrations for potential AD biomarkers such as amyloid-β (Aβ) and tau. For instance, lumbar punctures performed in individuals demonstrate low levels of Aβ42 in individuals cerebral with amyloid deposition [1]. Large fluctuations in Aβ levels also were noted in individuals over years when sampled by lumbar puncture [2]. Indwelling lumbar catheters have also been used to obtain more frequent CSF sampling over 24–48 h to understand Aβ metabolism for pharmacological modeling during drug trials. These catheter studies found significant within-person variability in CSF Aβ concentrations over the sampled time [3].

After Aβ release was demonstrated to be driven by neuronal activity in vivo [4], further investigations in rodents and humans found that the central nervous system concentration of Aβ fluctuated with the sleep-wake cycle. The amplitude of Aβ oscillation was decreased by both amyloid deposition in the brains of AD mouse models and humans, and in individuals with autosomal dominant AD mutations [5–7]. Soluble amyloid precursor protein (APP) and plasma Aβ also oscillate with sleep-wake activity [8, 9]. An analysis of serial Aβ concentrations from 178 participants who underwent CSF sampling via indwelling lumbar catheters in multiple academic and industry studies found an Aβ diurnal pattern in 16 of 17 studies [10]. The only study without a diurnal oscillation was confounded by a bacterial filter placed on the catheter during collection that removed Aβ from the CSF samples [11]. The Aβ diurnal pattern has also been replicated using different assays (enzyme-linked immunosorbent assay and mass spectrometry) [12].

Main text

Recently, Cicognola et al. [13] reported the absence of diurnal variations in multiple classical and candidate AD biomarkers, such as soluble APP, Aβ, tau, p-tau, YKL-40, VILIP-1, or apolipoprotein E. The authors sampled from 13 neurosurgical patients by either ventricular or lumbar CSF drainage at six time points over a 24-h period: 08:00, 12:00, 16:00, 20:00, 00:00, and 08:00. Four ml of CSF was collected at each time point.

* Correspondence: luceyb@wustl.edu
Department of Neurology, Washington University School of Medicine, 660 South Euclid Avenue, Campus Box 8111, St Louis, MO 63110, USA

Several factors may have led to the apparently discordant results regarding the diurnal variability of APP and Aβ, compared with the literature, in the Cicognola et al. study. First, it is possible that neurosurgical patients may have disrupted sleep-wake cycles that might alter diurnal patterns, particularly if the patients were sampled while in intensive care units where sleep would be fragmented due to frequent interruptions for clinical care. Further, brain tumors, hydrocephalus, and other intracranial pathologies could independently disturb sleep-wake activity and CSF flow.

Second, a longer sampling period may be necessary to observe fluctuations of Aβ in this population. For example, sampling periods up to 168 h were required to correlate Aβ fluctuations with changes in neurological status in patients with brain injury [14].

Third, the authors collected CSF from two different types of drains. Presumably, CSF was collected during the patients' routine clinical care between the research sampling time points. Previous reports have found that more frequent sampling will increase the rate of linear rise in Aβ [10, 15]. The authors do not record how much CSF was drained between these time points for clinical purposes to control for this effect.

Fourth, we expect that CSF sampling was not frequent enough to detect an Aβ oscillation over 24 h and that the study is underpowered to detect any oscillation that may be present in this patient population.

Fifth, a repeated measures ANOVA may not be the correct test to determine if there is a diurnal oscillation as we would predict Aβ concentrations to oscillate together over the 24 h day.

Conclusion

Understanding how Aβ concentrations change over short periods of time (e.g. hours) in the human central nervous system is critical to the design and implementation of anti-Aβ AD treatment trials. Despite our concerns, we appreciate the authors' interest in this important topic and contribution to improve our knowledge about the factors influencing Aβ diurnal variation.

Author's response: Is there an association of diurnal variation with cerebrospinal fluid biomarkers for Alzheimer's disease?

Claudia Cicognola[1,2], Davide Chiasserini[3], Paolo Eusebi[3], Ulf Andreasson[1,2], Hugo Vanderstichele[4], Henrik Zetterberg[1,2,5], Lucilla Parnetti[3], Kaj Blennow[1,2]

[1]Institute of Neuroscience and Physiology, Department of Psychiatry and Neurochemistry, The Sahlgrenska Academy at University of Gothenburg, Mölndal, Sweden
[2]Clinical Neurochemistry Laboratory, Sahlgrenska University Hospital Mölndal, SE-431 80 Mölndal, Sweden
[3]Section of Neurology, Department of Medicine, Center for Memory Disturbances, University of Perugia Sant' Andrea delle Fratte, 06132 Perugia, Italy
[4]ADx NeuroSciences, Gent, Belgium
[5]UCL Institute of Neurology, Queen Square, London, UK

We thank Lucey and co-workers [16] for their interest in our paper [13]. The authors point out some potential confounders that may influence sleep-wake cycles and variability of biomarkers for Alzheimer's disease pathophysiology, thereby affecting the possibility to identify diurnal patterns of variation in biomarker concentrations [16]. As acknowledged in the discussion section of our paper, these types of potential confounders may underlie the inconsistencies in outcomes between studies, as also recently reviewed [17]. For example, acute brain trauma [18] and other possible disease- or drug-related effects on brain functioning and Aβ metabolism in neurosurgical patients [13, 14], may give different results than studies in healthy controls [10, 19]. Further, sampling procedures, e.g., the use of lumbar or ventricular catheters [10, 13, 19] or intracerebral microdialysis catheters [14], or even plasma [9], reflect different compartments that will impact the results.

Undoubtedly, we need to perform more studies using highly standardized protocols, controlling for clinical confounder as well possible artefacts due to variable sampling time-points and volume-related disturbances in CSF dynamics [15], to resolve whether Aβ and other biomarkers reflecting AD pathophysiology vary with the normal sleep-wake cycle, and show a true diurnal variation.

Abbreviations
AD: Alzheimer's disease; ANOVA: Analysis of variance; APP: Amyloid precursor protein; Aβ: Amyloid-β; CSF: Cerebrospinal fluid

Acknowledgements
None.

Funding
Dr. Brendan Lucey's is supported by a career development award funded by the National Institute on Aging (1K76AG054863-01). The funding source had no role in the writing of this manuscript.

Authors' contributions
BPL drafted this commentary. AMF, DMH, JCM, and RJB revised and edited this commentary. CC drafted the Author's response. DC, PE, UA, HV, HZ, LP and KB revised and edited the Author's response. All authors read and approved the final manuscript.

Competing interests
The authors declare that they have no competing interests.

References
1. Fagan AM, Mintun MA, Mach RH, Lee S-Y, Dence CS, Shah AR, et al. Inverse relation between in vivo amyloid imaging load and cerebrospinal fluid Amyloid-beta-42 in humans. Ann Neurol. 2006;59(3):512–9.
2. Kanai M, Matsubara E, Isoe K, Urakami K, Nakashima K, Arai H, et al. Longitudinal study of cerebrospinal fluid levels of tau, Aβ1-40, and Aβ1-42(43) in Alzheimer's disease: a study in Japan. Ann Neurol. 1998;44:17–26.
3. Bateman RJ, Wen G, Morris JC, Holtzman DM. Fluctuations of CSF amyloid-β levels: implications for a diagnostic and therapeutic biomarker. Neurology. 2007;68:666–9.
4. Cirrito JR, Yamada KA, Finn MB, Sloviter RS, Bales KR, May PC, et al. Synaptic activity regulates interstitial fluid amyloid-β levels in vivo. Neuron. 2005;48: 913–22.
5. Kang J-E, Lim MM, Bateman RJ, Lee JJ, Smyth LP, Cirrito JR, et al. Amyloid-β dynamics are regulated by orexin and the sleep-wake cycle. Science. 2009; 326(5955):1005–7. Pubmed Central PMCID: PMC2789838.
6. Huang Y, Potter R, Sigurdson W, Santacruz A, Shih S, Ju Y-E, et al. Effects of age and amyloid deposition on Aβ dynamics in the human central nervous system. Arch Neurol. 2012;69(1):51–8. Pubmed Central PMCID: PMC3254706.
7. Roh JH, Huang Y, Bero AW, Kasten T, Stewart FR, Bateman RJ, et al. Disruption of the sleep-wake cycle and diurnal fluctuation of amyloid-β in mice with Alzheimer's disease pathology. Sci Transl Med. 2012;4(15):150ra22. Pubmed Central PMCID: PMC3654377.
8. Dobrowolska JA, Kasten T, Huang Y, Benzinger TL, Sigurdson W, Ovod V, et al. Diurnal patterns of soluble amyloid precursor protein metabolites in the human central nervous system. PLoS One. 2014;9(3):e89998. Pubmed Central PMCID: PMC3960093.
9. Huang Y, Potter R, Sigurdson W, Kasten T, Connors R, Morris JC, et al. Beta-amyloid dynamics in human plasma. Arch Neurol. 2012;69(12):1591–7. Pubmed Central PMCID: PMC3808092.
10. Lucey BP, Gonzales C, Das U, Li J, Siemers ER, Slemmon JR, et al. An integrated multi-study analysis of intra-subject variability in cerebrospinal fluid amyloid-β concentrations collected by lumbar puncture and indwelling lumbar catheter. Alzheimers Res Ther. 2015;7(1):53. Pubmed Central PMCID: PMC4518529.
11. Slats D, Claassen JA, Spies PE, Borm G, Besse KT, Aalst W, et al. Hourly variability of cerebrospinal fluid biomarkers in Alzheimer's disease subjects and healthy older volunteers. Neurobiol Aging. 2012;33(4):831.e1–9.
12. Lucey BP, Mawuenyega KG, Patterson BW, Elbert DL, Ovod V, Kasten T, et al. Associations Between β-Amyloid Kinetics and the β-Amyloid Diurnal Pattern in the Central Nervous System. JAMA Neurol. 2017;74(2):207–20.
13. Cicognola C, Chiasserini D, Eusebi P, Andreasson U, Vanderstichele H, Zetterberg H, et al. No diurnal variation of classical and candidate biomarkers of Alzheimer's disease in CSF. Mol Neurodegener. 2016;11(1):65. Pubmed Central PMCID: PMC5013624.
14. Brody DL, Magnoni S, Schwetye KE, Spinner ML, Esparza TJ, Stocchetti N, et al. Amyloid-β dynamics correlate with neurological status in the injured human brain. Science. 2008;321(5893):1221–4.
15. Li J, Llano DA, Ellis T, LeBlond D, Bhathena A, Jhee SS, et al. Effect of human cerebrospinal fluid sampling frequency on amyloid-β levels. Alzheimers Dement. 2012;8(4):295–303.
16. Lucey BP, Fagan AM, Holtzman DM, Morris JC, Bateman RJ. Diurnal oscillation of CSF Aβ and other AD biomarkers. Mol Neurodeg. 2016. doi:10.1186/s13024-017-0161-4.
17. Cicognola C, Chiasserini D, Parnetti L. Preanalytical confounding factors in the analysis of cerebrospinal fluid biomarkers for Alzheimer's disease: the issue of diurnal variation. Front Neurol. 2015;6:143.
18. Olsson A, Csajbok L, Öst M, Höglund K, Nylén K, Rosengren L, Nellgård B, Blennow K. Marked increase of β-amyloid (1–42) and amyloid precursor protein in ventricular cerebrospinal fluid after severe traumatic brain injury. J Neurol. 2004;251:870–6.
19. Bjerke M, Portelius E, Minthon L, Wallin A, Anckarsäter H, Anckarsäter R, Andreasen N, Zetterberg H, Andreasson U, Blennow K. Confounding factors influencing amyloid Beta concentration in cerebrospinal fluid. Int J Alzheimers Dis. 2010. doi:10.4061/2010/986310.

5

The novel RAGE interactor PRAK is associated with autophagy signaling in Alzheimer's disease pathogenesis

Yoonhee Kim[†], Chaeyoung Kim[†], Sung Min Son, Hyundong Song, Hyun Seok Hong, Sun-ho Han and Inhee Mook-Jung[*]

Abstract

Background: The receptor for advanced glycation end products (RAGE) has been found to interact with amyloid β (Aβ). Although RAGE does not have any kinase motifs in its cytosolic domain, the interaction between RAGE and Aβ triggers multiple cellular signaling involved in Alzheimer's disease (AD). However, the mechanism of signal transduction by RAGE remains still unknown. Therefore, identifying binding proteins of RAGE may provide novel therapeutic targets for AD.

Results: In this study, we identified p38-regulated/activated protein kinase (PRAK) as a novel RAGE interacting molecule. To investigate the effect of Aβ on PRAK mediated RAGE signaling pathway, we treated SH-SY5Y cells with monomeric form of Aβ. We demonstrated that Aβ significantly increased the phosphorylation of PRAK as well as the interaction between PRAK and RAGE. We showed that knockdown of PRAK rescued mTORC1 inactivation induced by Aβ treatment and decreased the formation of Aβ-induced autophagosome.

Conclusions: We provide evidence that PRAK plays a critical role in AD pathology as a key interactor of RAGE. Thus, our data suggest that PRAK might be a potential therapeutic target of AD involved in RAGE-mediated cell signaling induced by Aβ.

Keywords: PRAK, RAGE, Alzheimer's disease, Autophagy, Aβ

Background

Alzheimer's disease (AD), a progressive neurodegenerative disorder, is the most common type of dementia [1]. Notably, Amyloid β (Aβ) is a major pathological characteristic of AD [2]. Along with neurofibrillary tangles and neuronal loss, Aβ influences AD pathogenesis, including oxidative injury, synaptic degeneration, inflammatory response and neuronal death. Unfortunately, the intermediate mechanism underlying toxic Aβ interactions and AD pathogenesis remains unelucidated. As a result, current treatments can merely alleviate AD symptoms and delay deterioration [3].

The receptor for advanced glycation end-products (RAGE) is a multi-ligand receptor that belongs to the immunoglobulin superfamily [4, 5]. RAGE ligands are comprised of advanced glycation end-products [4], high mobility group box 1 (HMGB1, also known as amphoterin) [6], S100/calgranulins [7, 8], Mac-1 [9], phosphatidylserine [10] and Aβ [11]. Interactions of ligand-RAGE activate multiple intracellular signaling pathways involving MAPKs such as ERK1/2, p38, JNK, PI3K, Src kinase, JAK/STAT, TGFβ/Smad, and members of the Rho GTPase signaling pathway [12]. Moreover, ligand-RAGE interactions cause the generation of reactive oxygen species [13], influence cellular homeostasis and inflammatory response, and lead to diseases such as cancer, diabetes and AD [14].

Multiple lines of evidence underscore the importance of the 42 amino acids of the RAGE cytoplasmic domain in intracellular signal transduction. For example, deletion in this RAGE cytoplasmic domain (DN-RAGE) renders RAGE incapable of facilitating signal transduction following ligand-RAGE interaction [15]. Furthermore, the

* Correspondence: inhee@snu.ac.kr
[†]Equal contributors
Department of Biochemistry and Biomedical Sciences, Seoul National University College of Medicine, 103 Daehak-ro, Jongro-gu, Seoul 110-799, Korea

absence of any known signal transduction motifs in the RAGE cytoplasmic domain has limited our understanding of AD pathogenesis through Aβ-RAGE interaction-mediated signaling. mDia-1 is known to interact with the RAGE cytoplasmic domain and requires RAGE-mediated cellular migration, Rho GTPases (particularly cdc42 and rac-1) activation for this interaction [16]. However, RAGE cytoplasmic domain binding proteins responsible for triggering other RAGE-mediated signaling pathways remain unknown.

p38-regulated/activated protein kinase (PRAK), also known as the mitogen-activated protein kinase (MAPK) activated protein kinase-5 (MK5), is a Ser/Thr protein kinase and a member of the MAPKs [17]. PRAK can be activated by cellular stress and inflammatory cytokines [18]. PRAK is known to phosphorylate Heat shock protein 27 (HSP27) [17], cytosolic phospholipase A2 (cPLA2) [19], tyrosine hydroxylase [20], FOXO3a [21], FAK [22], septin8 [23] and p53 [24]. Thus, PRAK plays a crucial role in cellular signaling phenomena such as the cell cycle, angiogenesis, and neuronal plasticity [25]. Moreover, PRAK regulates the phosphorylation of Ras homologue enriched in brain (Rheb), a main component of mammalian target of rapamycin complex 1 (mTORC1), leading to decreased cell growth [26].

In this study, we found PRAK as a novel interactor of the RAGE cytoplasmic domain using the yeast two-hybrid approach. The interaction between PRAK and RAGE was further verified by immunoprecipitation (IP), surface plasmon resonance (SPR). We identified that Aβ treatment induced phosphorylation of PRAK and increased interaction between PRAK and RAGE. More interestingly, the interaction between PRAK and RAGE was also increased in the brains of Tg6799 mouse, AD animal model. Furthermore, knockdown of PRAK reduced RAGE-mediated formation of autophagosome via mTORC1 signaling pathway. Our results indicate that PRAK binds to the RAGE cytoplasmic domain and regulates Aβ-RAGE-mediated autophagy.

Results

Identification of PRAK as a binding partner of RAGE

To identify proteins that interact with the RAGE cytoplasmic domain, we carried out the yeast two-hybrid screening between the human brain cDNA library and RAGE cytoplasmic domain, the latter was used as the bait. We identified interaction between PRAK and the RAGE cytoplasmic domain through the expression of three reporter genes, *lacZ*, *ura3*, and *ade2*, each being under the control of different GAL4 promoters. To ensure the reliability of the results, both the positive and negative controls were incorporated on the same filter (Fig. 1a). To validate the interaction between PRAK and RAGE, we transfected PRAK-GFP and RAGE into cells and performed immunoprecipitation with anti-GFP antibodies (Fig. 1b). We also confirmed the interaction between PRAK and RAGE at endogenous levels in SH-SY5Y cells by antibodies against both PRAK and RAGE (Additional file 1: Figure S1). We investigated the binding kinetics between PRAK and RAGE using surface plasmon resonance (SPR) by immobilizing PRAK protein on the chip surface. The response unit (RU) was gradually increased by the RAGE concentration from 2.5 μM to 40 μM (Fig. 1c). The K_d value of the binding strength of the RAGE cytoplasmic domain to PRAK is 0.5086 nM. This SPR data supported that the PRAK is a specific binding protein to the RAGE cytosolic domain.

Aβ increases PRAK-RAGE interaction

The binding of RAGE to its ligands triggers various signaling pathways and this process is dependent on the RAGE cytoplasmic domain. In AD, RAGE expression is increased in the brain [11]. Aβ-RAGE interaction induces the cellular effects associated with AD pathology [27–29]. To investigate the effect of Aβ on interaction between PRAK and RAGE, we performed in situ proximity ligation assay on cells overexpressing both RAGE and PRAK after 2 μM monomeric Aβ treatment. The red dots suggest closely apposed binding of the two proteins (~40 nm). The red dot signals increased substantially in treatment of cells with Aβ compared to treatment of cell with vehicle (Fig. 2a). Furthermore, to see the colocalization between PRAK and RAGE, we used the structure illumination microscopy (SIM) with high resolution. After treatment of monomeric Aβ for 6 h, we stained using anti-PRAK antibody (green) and anti-RAGE antibodies (red). Compared to vehicle treatment, Aβ treatment increased the colocalization between PRAK and RAGE (Fig. 2b). These data indicate that Aβ treatment increases the interaction between PRAK and RAGE. In addition, we confirmed the interaction between PRAK and RAGE in vivo using the brains of Tg6799 mice as AD animal model. Consistent with cell data using Aβ, the binding of PRAK to RAGE was increased in the brains of Tg6799 compared to litter mate (Fig. 2c, 19.2 % ± 1.684, * $p < 0.05$, n = 4 independent experiments). Taken together, these data implicate that the interaction between PRAK and RAGE was increased under Aβ abundant conditions in cells as well as in vivo.

Aβ induces phosphorylation of PRAK via RAGE-intracellular domain

Since PRAK is a protein kinase activated through phosphorylation in response to cellular stress and proinflammatory cytokine [17]. We examined whether 2 μM monomeric Aβ treatment can induce phosphorylation of PRAK. As expected, Aβ treatment increased the level

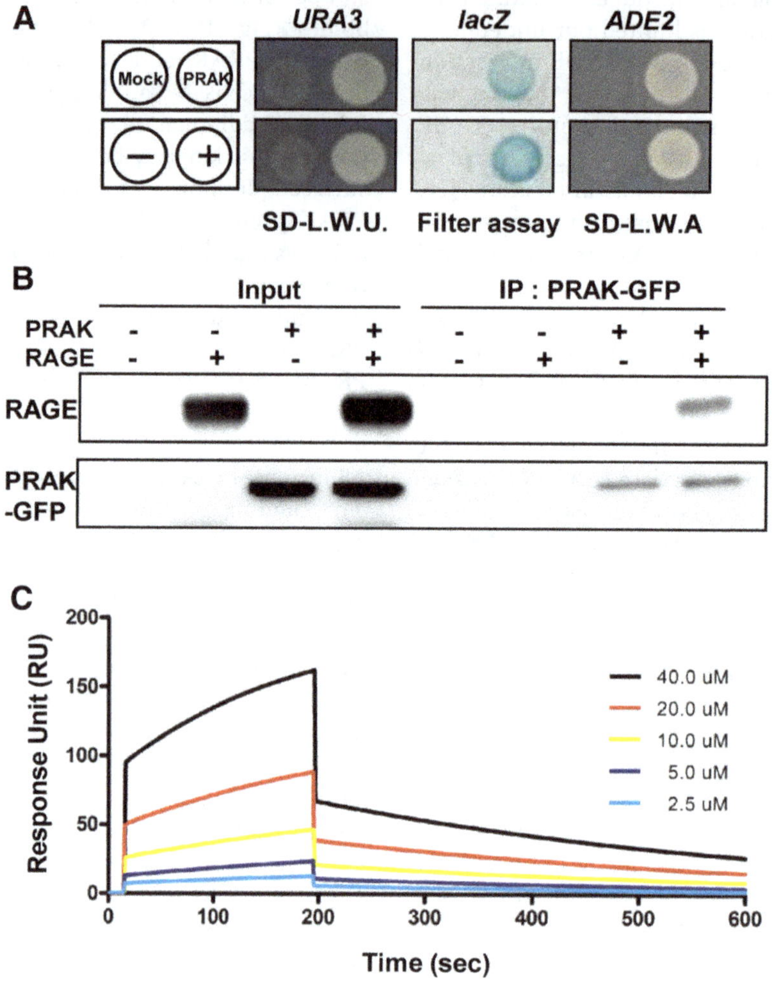

Fig. 1 PRAK interacts with the RAGE. **a** Yeast two-hybrid screening to identify RAGE interacting proteins in a human brain cDNA library. Yeast transformants of the RAGE bait and human brain cDNA library were spread on selection medium SD-LWU (SD without leucine, tryptophan and uracil), SD-LWA (SD without leucine, tryptophan and adenosine) and filter assay. pGBKT- PTB and pACT2-PTB served as the positive control (+). pGBKT and pACT2 were used as negative control (−). **b** PRAK and RAGE binding in vitro. Immunoprecipitation (IP) with anti-GFP antibody was accomplished using lysates from CHO cells transfected with RAGE and GFP-tagged PRAK, followed by western blotting with anti-RAGE antibody. **c** Binding kinetics of the RAGE C-term to PRAK protein. GST-fused PRAK protein was immobilized onto a CM5 sensor chip as the ligand. The RAGE C-term was used as the analyte from 0 to 40 μM to measure the kinetics of binding. Curves corresponding to multiple analyte concentrations were generated to ensure the precision of the calculation of the kinetics. The binding kinetics were analyzed using BIAevaluation 3.1 software

of phosphorylated PRAK at Thr-142 compared to vehicle. The mean change was about 18 % ± 3.3 (*** $p < 0.001$, n = 4 independent experiments, Fig. 3a). To test whether the RAGE cytoplasmic domain, the PRAK binding site, is critical for phosphorylation of PRAK after Aβ stimulation, we used cells overexpressing RAGE or the RAGE cytoplasmic domain deletion mutant (DN-RAGE). Full length of RAGE induced PRAK phosphorylation by Aβ stimulation compared with the vehicle (19.4 % ± 4.38, ** $p < 0.01$, n = 3 independent experiments). However, phosphorylation of PRAK was not altered by Aβ treatment in cells overexpressing DN-RAGE (Fig. 3b). This result suggests that phosphorylation of PRAK induced by Aβ treatment is dependent on RAGE-cytoplasmic domain.

Aβ induces mTORC1 inactivation via PRAK and RAGE

mTORC1/p70S6K signaling associated with autophagy formation is one of Aβ induced downstream signaling pathways [29]. In addition, Rheb, the main component of the mTORC1 complex, is a downstream substrate of PRAK [26]. We investigated the status of Rheb and mTORC1/p70S6K activation as a downstream signaling pathway of Aβ induced PRAK-RAGE interaction. To see if alteration of phosphorylation on Rheb or mTORC1/p70S6k induced by Aβ is dependent on both PRAK and RAGE, we used SH-SY5Y cells overexpressing DN-RAGE or siPRAK. 2 μM monomeric Aβ treatment increased phosphorylation of Rheb, compared with the vehicle (13.1 % ± 2.55, ** $p < 0.01$, n = 4 independent experiments,

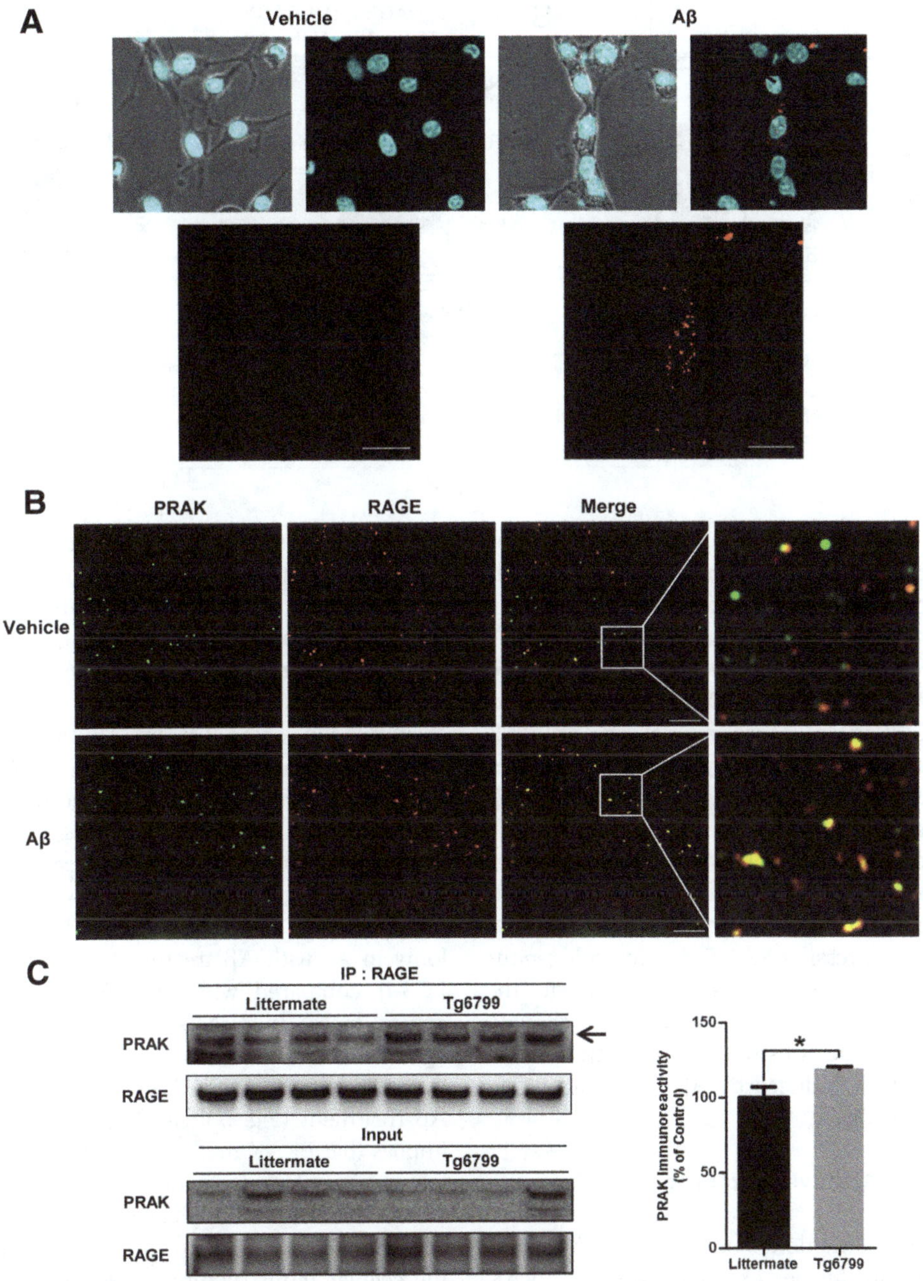

Fig. 2 Aβ treatment increases the interaction between PRAK and RAGE. **a** Aβ treatment increases RAGE-PRAK binding. Overexpression of RAGE and PRAK in SH-SY5Y cells were treated with either DMSO or monomeric Aβ 2 μM for 6 h and co-localization was detected using in situ proximity ligation assay kit. Probes in close proximity (<40 nm) are indicated by fluorescent dot signals. Scale bars represent 20 μm. **b** Aβ enhances the co-localization between RAGE and PRAK. SH-SY5Y cells was induced by a 6 h treatment of DMSO or monomeric 2 μM Aβ. Immunofluorescence analysis using anti-PRAK (green) and anti-RAGE (red) antibodies. SIM was used for image analysis. Scale bars represent 5 μm. **c** PRAK and RAGE binding in vivo. Immunoprecipitation (IP) with anti-RAGE antibody was accomplished using total brain lysates from 3 months wild-type litter mates and Tg6799, followed by western blotting with anti-PRAK antibody. Quantification of protein level was performed by densitometric analysis. Data are mean ± SEM. n = 4. *$P < 0.05$

Fig. 4a in RAGE overexpressed cells). In contrast, Aβ treatment did not alter phosphorylation of Rheb in cells overexpressing DN-RAGE (n = 4 independent experiments, Fig. 4a). Consistent with the results of Fig. 4a, knockdown of PRAK using siRNA against PRAK did not significantly increase phosphorylation of Rheb even in the presence of Aβ (in the case of control si-RNA treated group: 19.8 % ±9.06 increase in Aβ treated cells compared to vehicle treated cells, ** $p < 0.01$, n = 4 independent experiments, Fig. 4b). Since phosphorylation of Rheb inhibits

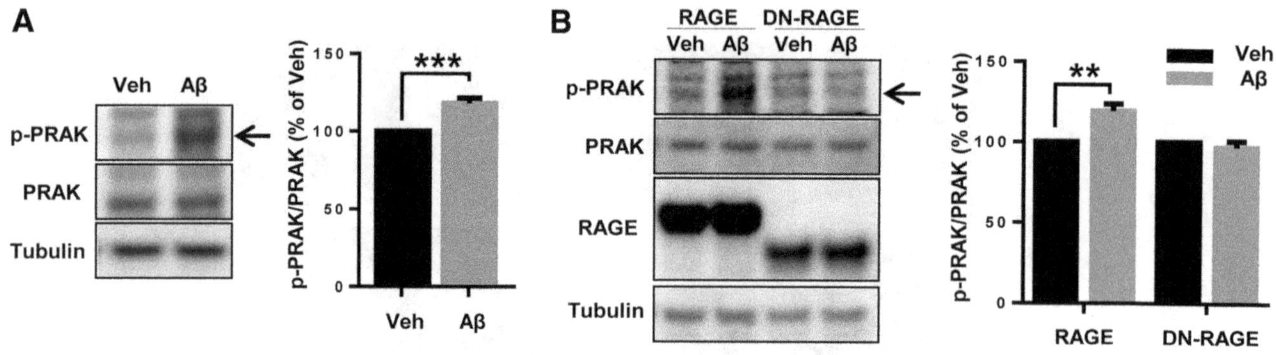

Fig. 3 Aβ treatment induces phosphorylation of PRAK via RAGE. **a** SH-SY5Y cells were treated with either DMSO or 2 μM monomeric Aβ for 6 h. **b** SH-SY5Y cells were transfected with full length RAGE and DN-RAGE and subsequently treated with either DMSO or 2 μM monomeric Aβ for 6 h. Western blot was performed with the indicated antibodies. Quantification of protein level was performed by densitometric analysis. Data are mean ± SEM of at least 3 independent experiments. $^{**}P < 0.01$, $^{***}P < 0.001$

the mTORC1/p70S6K pathway [30], we examined the p70s6k phosphorylation levels. Compared with vehicle treatment, phosphorylation of p70s6k was significantly decreased by Aβ treatment (24.1 % ± 5.34, ** $p < 0.01$, n = 4 independent experiments, Fig. 4c). However, Aβ treatment did not significantly decrease p-p70s6k in cells overexpressing DN-RAGE (Fig. 4c). Moreover, deletion of PRAK by si-PRAK did not alter p-p70s6k by Aβ treatment compared with vehicle treated group, while si-control cells decreased p-p70s6k by Aβ treatment compared with vehicle treated group (21.7 % ±2.95, ** $p < 0.01$, n = 4 independent experiments, Fig. 4d). Mock-transfected cells showed similar trends on phosphorylation of Rheb and p70s6k as cells overexpressing RAGE due to endogenous RAGE effects when Aβ was treated even though the degree of phosphorylation is much less (data not shown). Therefore, these results demonstrate that the activation of Rheb-mTORC1/p70S6K induced by Aβ is dependent on PRAK-RAGE interaction.

PRAK mediates RAGE-Aβ-driven autophagosome formation

Since autophagosome formation is one of the Rheb-mTOR downstream effects, we further examined whether PRAK involves formation of autophagosome induced by Aβ. Since activation of mTOR suppresses autophagy induction by phosphorylation of serine/threonine kinases, UNC-51-like kinase 1 (ULK1) [31], we measured phosphorylation of mTOR and ULK1 as an early marker of autophagy induction. ULK1, a mammalian autophagy initiating kinase, plays a critical role in the early stage of autophagy [31]. 2 μM monomeric Aβ treatment significantly decreased the phosphorylation of mTOR and ULK1 compared with vehicle (mTOR: 21.4 % ±4.96, ULK1: 17.8 % ±5.21 ** $p < 0.01$, n = 5 independent experiments). However, the levels of p-mTOR and p-ULK were not changed by Aβ treatment in cells transfected with siRNA against PRAK (Fig 5a). Because microtubule-associated protein 1A/1B-light chain 3-II (LC3-II) is increased during formation of autophagosome [32] and Aβ is known to induce autophagosome formation [33], we measured the level of LC3-II by Western blot. 2 μM monomeric Aβ treatment induced accumulation of LC3-II, but siRNA against PRAK transfected cells reduced accumulation of LC3-II by Aβ treatment compared to vehicle (Fig. 5b). The accumulation of LC3-II could be due to either formation of autophagosome or blockage of downstream in autophagy (autophagic flux) [32]. To distinguish these two possibilities, we used bafilomycin A_1 that blocks fusion of autophagosome with lysosomes to make autolysosome, resulting in accumulation of LC3-II. Bafilomycin A_1 with Aβ treatment increased accumulation of LC3-II compared with only Aβ treatment (Fig. 5b, si-control lanes). In contrast, knockdown of PRAK by siRNA against PRAK did not induce accumulation of LC3-II level by Bafilomycin A_1 with Aβ treatment compared with only Aβ treatment (Fig. 5b, si-PRAK lanes). Taken together, it implies that PRAK mediated accumulation of LC3-II is due to autophagy formation, not by blockage of autophagic flux. To evaluate actual autophagosome formation via PRAK, we used transmission electron microscopy (TEM) to examine the cellular ultrastructure. As shown in Fig. 5c and d, Aβ treatment increased the accumulation of autophagosomes (red arrows), compared with vehicle. In contrast, deletion of PRAK did not induce accumulation of autophagosomes by Aβ treatment. Taken together, these results demonstrate that the Aβ-RAGE-induced autophagosome formation is mediated by PRAK.

Discussion

RAGE mediates diverse cellular signaling pathways triggered by specific ligands [34]. In this study, we provide evidence that alteration of Rheb-mTOR/p70S6K by interaction of Aβ-RAGE is mediated by PRAK. Since Aβ-RAGE interaction also leads to the activation of an

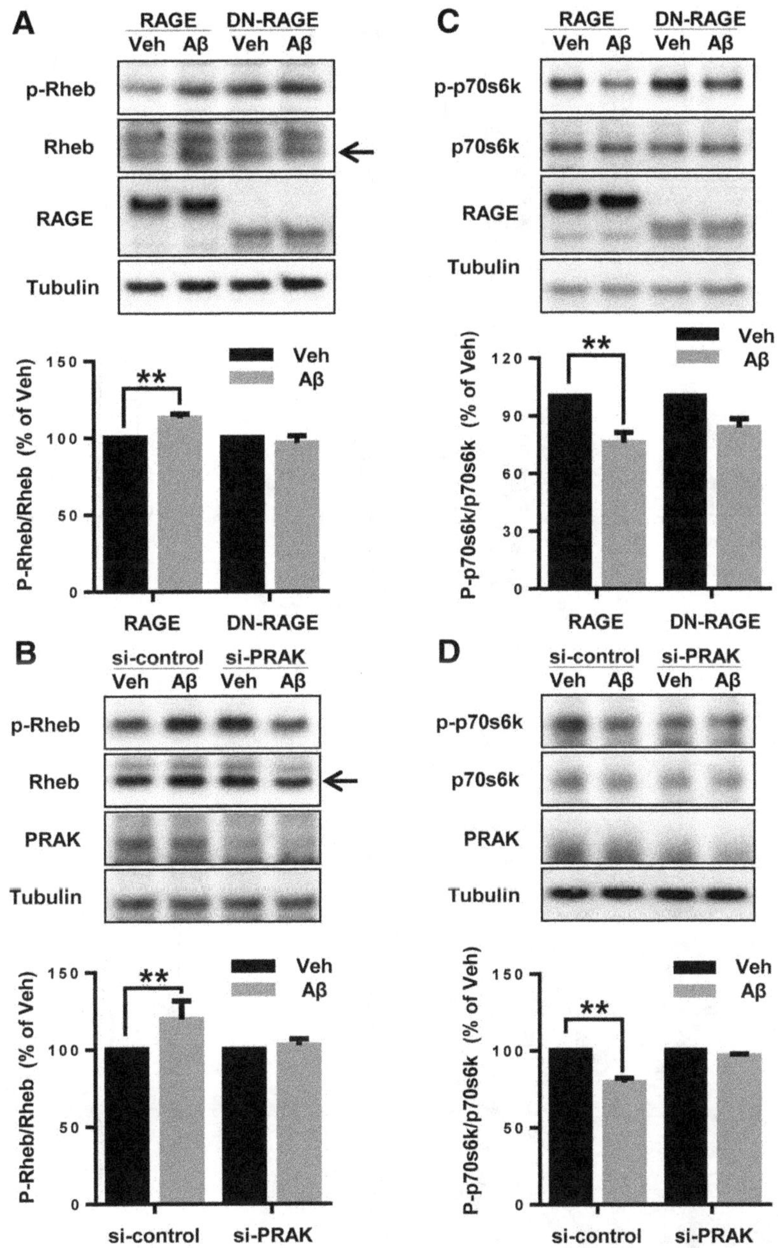

Fig. 4 RAGE and PRAK mediate mTORC1 inactivation by Aβ treatment. **a** RAGE and DN-RAGE-overexpressing SH-SY5Y cells were treated with either DMSO or 2 μM monomeric Aβ for 6 h. **b** SH-SY5Y cells were transfected with plasmids expressing RAGE and then transiently re-transfected with PRAK siRNA or scrambled control siRNA. Cells were treated with either DMSO or 2 μM monomeric Aβ for 6 h. **c** RAGE and DN-RAGE-overexpressing SH-SY5Y cells were treated with either DMSO or 2 μM monomeric Aβ for 6 h. **d** SH-SY5Y cells were transfected with plasmids expressing RAGE and then transiently re-transfected with PRAK siRNA or scrambled control siRNA. Cells were treated with either DMSO or 2 μM monomeric Aβ for 6 h. Western blot was performed with the indicated antibodies. Quantification of protein level was performed by densitometric analysis. Data are mean ± SEM of 4 separate experiments. $^{**}P < 0.01$

NF-κB dependent signaling pathway [11], we investigated if PRAK can modulate activation of NF-κB induced by Aβ-RAGE interaction. As expected, Aβ treatment increased p-IκB compared with vehicle treatment. However, knockdown of PRAK did not change the level of p-IκB by Aβ treatment (Additional file 2: Figure S2). Therefore, our data support that PRAK specifically mediates Rheb-mTORC1/p70S6K signaling pathway among various downstream signaling pathways of Aβ-RAGE interaction.

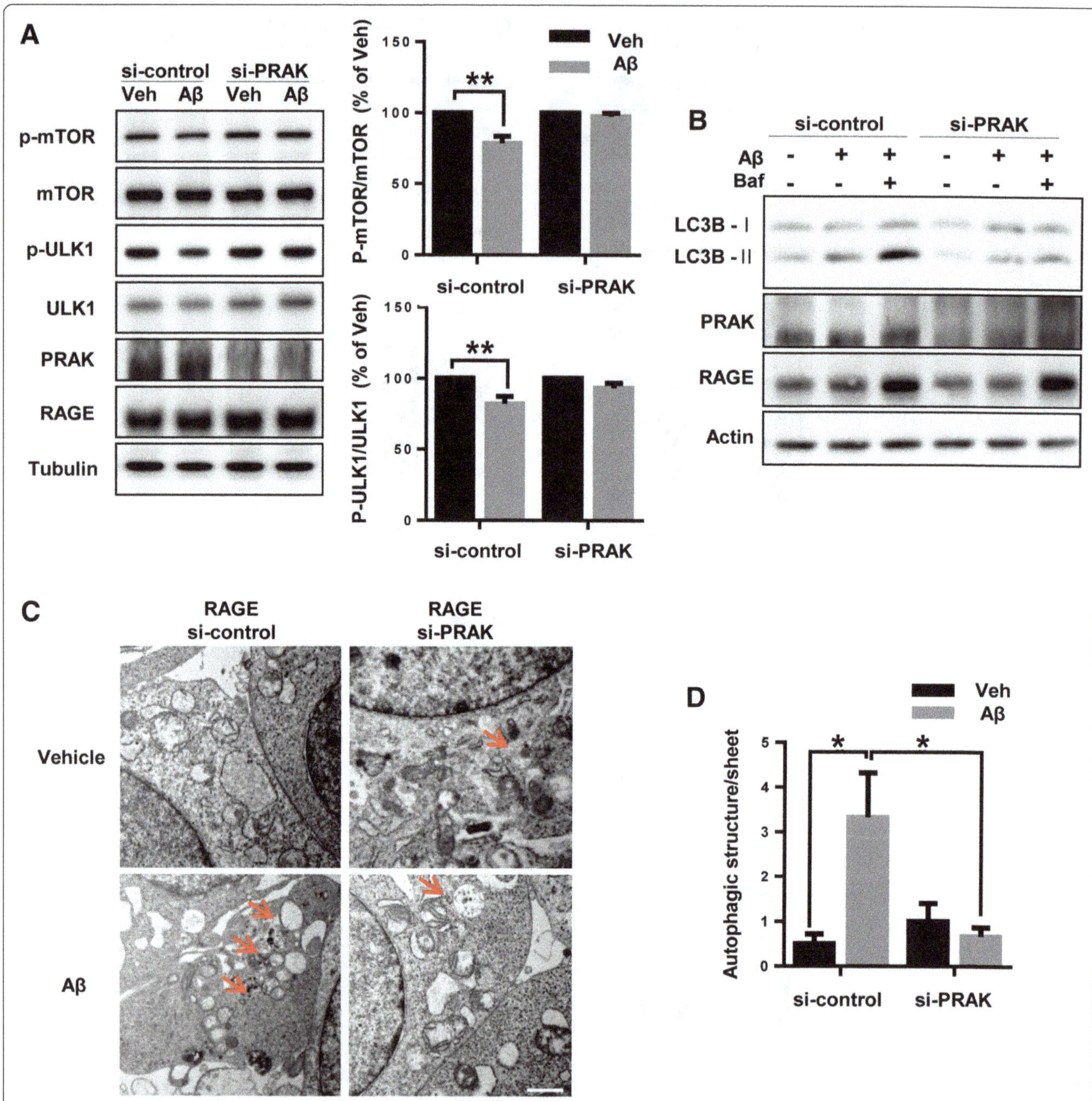

Fig. 5 PRAK mediates Aβ-induced autophagy signaling pathway. **a** SH-SY5Y cells were transfected with plasmids expressing RAGE and then transiently re-transfected with PRAK siRNA or scrambled control siRNA. After 24 h, cells were treated with either DMSO or 2 μM monomeric Aβ for 6 h. **b** SH-SY5Y cells were transfected with plasmids expressing RAGE and transiently retransfected with PRAK siRNA or scrambled control siRNA. After 24 h, cells were pretreatment with 10 nM Bafilomycin A_1 for 1 h and treated with either DMSO or 2 μM monomeric Aβ for 6 h. Western blot analysis was performed with the indicated antibodies. Quantification of protein level was performed by densitometric analysis. Data are mean ± SEM of 5 separate experiments. $^{**}P < 0.01$. **c** Cells were co-transfected with RAGE plasmid DNA and PRAK siRNA or scrambled control siRNA. After 24 h, cells were treated with either DMSO or 2 μM monomeric Aβ for 6 h, fixed, and stained for TEM as described in the methods section. EM images indicate PRAK-mediated changes in the number of autophagosomes (arrows). Quantification of autophagosomes is shown in (**d**). Scale bars represent 1 μm. $^{*}P < 0.05$

Although ligands of RAGE and their associated signaling pathways are well known, there are few studies of RAGE cytoplasmic domain-interacting proteins [28]. In this study, we identified that PRAK as an interactor of the RAGE is recruited and phosphorylated by Aβ treatment and interact with RAGE cytoplasmic domain. Previous studies reported that PRAK, a substrate for atypical and conventional MAPKs, is phosphorylated and activated by p38 and ERK3/4 [17, 35]. In addition, it is well known that p38 is phosphorylated by Aβ mediated-RAGE activation [12, 36]. To investigate if p38 phosphorylates PRAK by Aβ-RAGE interaction, we measured the level of phosphorylated p38 using western blot. Consistent with previous studies, the interaction between Aβ-RAGE activates p38 (Additional file 3: Figure S3). However, p38 is also phosphorylated by Aβ treatment in DN-RAGE overexpressing cells. This data suggests that PRAK might be phosphorylated by the other MAPK, but not p38, because PRAK is not phosphorylated by Aβ treatment in DN-RAGE overexpressing cell (Fig 3b).

Zheng et al., reported that PRAK regulates mTORC1 by phosphorylation of Rheb. They also showed that alteration of mTORC1 by PRAK is independent of AMP-activated protein kinase (AMPK) and Tuberous Sclerosis Complex 2 (TSC2) [26]. Our data also suggest that interaction between RAGE and PRAK by Aβ treatment regulate mTORC1, leading to autophagosome formation. The mTOR forms two catalytic distinct complexes: mTOR complex 1 (mTORC1) and mTOR complex 2 (mTORC2). mTORC1 and mTORC2 are regulated by different upstream and downstream components. mTORC1 is regulated by various upstream effects, such as PI3K/Akt, GSK-3β, AMPK, LKB1, IRS-1 and MAPK [37–41]. There are a number of downstream components of mTORC1, including STAT3, 4EBPs and p70S6Ks [42]. mTORC1 is highly expressed in brain and regulates multiple signaling pathways related with protein synthesis, autophagy, cell growth and mitochondrial function [43]. Accumulating evidences suggest that mTORC1 plays a critical role in AD pathology [44, 45]. In a previous study, we demonstrated that interaction between Aβ and RAGE induces autophagic vacuoles via the Ca^{2+}/calmodulin-dependent protein kinase kinase-AMPK pathway [29]. In this study, we focused our efforts on autophagy among several PRAK downstream signals and found that Aβ treatment increases the interaction between RAGE and PRAK, inducing autophagosome formation via Rheb-mTORC1/p70s6k. Therefore, we further provided evidence that Aβ-RAGE-mediated autophagosome formation is regulated not only by CaMKKβ-AMPK signaling through calcium, but also by Rheb-mTORC1 signaling through PRAK. Inhibition of mTOR can induce autophagosome formation [46] and many autophagic vacuoles can be seen in the brains of AD patients [33, 47]. When beclin 1, one of autophagy initiating molecules, was knocked down in neurons and transgenic mice in AD mouse model, less autophagosome were shown and more Aβ depositions were examined [48, 49], suggesting autophagy has a beneficial role to remove Aβ accumulation. However, since the disruption of lysosomal function has been reported in the brains of AD patients and animal models [50, 51], autophagic flux, fusion between autophagosome and lysosome, might be impaired, resulting in less autolysosomes. It causes the inhibition of abnormal protein degradation [52, 53]. Many autophagic vacuoles in the brains of AD patients might be resulted in accumulation of autophagosomes due to blockade of autophagic flux with lysosomal dysfunction. Out data showed that Aβ-RAGE-PRAK axis stimulates autophagic formation via inhibiting mTORC1/p70s6k to make autophagosome. If the function of lysosome is intact in the brains, Aβ-RAGE-PRAK axis-induced autophagosomes might be beneficial. Since the exact status of lysosomes in each stages of AD is still unknown, the role of autophagy in AD pathogenesis is controversial. The detailed mechanism regarding autophagic flux in AD should be clarified as a further study.

Conclusions

In summary, we identified that PRAK is a novel RAGE interactor, and mediates downstream signaling by direct binding to the cytoplasmic domain of RAGE. Specifically, PRAK mediates the Rheb-mTORC1/p70s6k pathway by Aβ-RAGE interaction. Our data suggest that PRAK is a critical regulating factor that modulates RAGE downstream signaling and RAGE-induced AD pathology.

Methods

Yeast two-hybrid screening

Yeast two-hybrid screening was performed by Panbionet, (http://www.panbionet.com/), with the RAGE carboxyl terminal (C-terminal) region (BD, binding domain) and the human brain cDNA domain (AD, activation domain) library. RAGE C-terminal region (361-end amino acids of RAGE) was amplified by PCR using the following primers pair: F primer, 5′-GGC GAA TTC ATC TTG TGG CAA AGG CGG–3′; R primer, 5′-GGC AGA TCT TCA AGG CCC TCC AGT ACT–3′. The RAGE bait (135 nt) was cloned into the BamHI/EcoRI sites of the pGBKT vector, which contain the GAL4 DNA binding domain (GAL4DB). The AD library inserts were cloned into pACT2 vector containing a GAL4 activation domain. These two-hybrid plasmids were co-transformed into yeast strain PBN204, containing 3 reporters (*URA3, lacZ, and ADE2*) under the control of dissimilar GAL4 promoters. In order to confirm the interaction, positive clones were amplified by *Escherichia coli* transformation or PCR. The amplified clones were reintroduced into yeast PBN204 strain with the RAGE bait plasmid or with a negative control plasmid expressing GAL4-binding domain without the bait. pACT2-polypyrimidine tract-binding protein (PTB) and pGBKT-PTB served were used as positive controls for the protein-protein interactions. pACT2 and pGBKT served were used as the negative controls. The identity of the interactors was determined by sequencing.

Cell culture and animals

SH-SY5Y human neuroblastoma and Chinese hamster ovary (CHO) cell lines were maintained in Dulbecco's modified Eagle's medium (DMEM, HyClone) then added to 10 % FBS (HyClone), 0.1 mg/mL penicillin and streptomycin (Sigma) at 37 °C in a 5 % CO_2 incubator. Tg6799 (B6SJL-Tg [APPSwFlLon, PSEN*M146L*L286V] 6799Vas/J, Jackson Lab, stock no. 006554) and B6SJL wild-type (littermate) mice were used for the experiments. All animal use was performed according to the Principles of Laboratory Animal Care (NIH publication no. 85–23, revised 1985) and use guidelines of Seoul National University, Seoul, Korea.

Transfection

Approximately 100×10^3 cells were seeded in tissue culture plates and plated at 70 % confluence after 24 h. Cells were transfected with full-length human RAGE or DN-RAGE or PRAK constructs by using Lipofectamine LTX (Invitrogen) according to the manufacturer's protocol. PRAK siRNA (three to five target-specific 19–25 nt siRNAs designed to knockdown gene expression) or scrambled cotrol siRNA (Santa Cruz Biotechnology) by using RNAiMAX (Invitrogen) according to the manufacturer's protocol.

Reagents

$A\beta_{42}$ peptide (AP62-0-80; American Peptide;2 μM) was dissolved in hexafluoroisopropanol for 4 days at room temperature. The lyophilized peptide was then dissolved in DMSO (Sigma) [54]. For this experiments, an monomeric preparation of $A\beta_{42}$ peptide was utilized, that was characterized by atomic force microscopy (AFM). Bafilomycin A_1 (Sigma; 10nM) was dissolved in DMSO and pretreatment 1 h before Aβ treatment.

Immunoprecipitation

CHO cells transfected with RAGE and GFP-tagged PRAK were washed with PBS and lysed with 1 % CHAPS buffer (Sigma). To reduce non-specific binding, pre-clearing with protein A/G agarose (Santa Cruz Biotechnology) was performed for 1 h at 4 °C with gentle rotating. After bicinchoninic acid assay, equal protein lysates were immunoprecipitated with anti-GFP antibodies (1 μg/mL; Santa Cruz Biotechnology), incubated overnight at 4 °C with gentle rotating, and added to the beads for 1 h. The samples were washed in the lysis buffer and elution protein complex with the SDS-PAGE sample loading buffer and analyzed by western blotting as described above. Brain tissue or SH-SY5Y cells were lysed with RIPA and using ImmunoCruz™ IP/WB Optima E System (Santa Cruz Biotechnology) according to the manufacturer's protocol with anti-RAGE antibodies (1 μg/mL; Millipore).

Western blot

Cells were washed with PBS and lysed in RIPA buffer supplemented with a proteinase and phosphatase inhibitor cocktail (Sigma). For whole cell lysates, cells were sonicated and centrifuged for 20 min at 17,950 g at 4 °C. Cell lysates were run on SDS-PAGE gels, and then transferred to PVDF membrane. After overnight incubation at 4 °C with the primary antibody in 3 % BSA, the signal was enhanced using Enhanced chemiluminescence (ECL, GE Healthcare Biosciences) followed by image analysis with Bioimaging analyzer (LAS-3000, Fuji Film, Inc.) and Multi-Gauge (Fuji). Primary antibodies were used against RAGE (Millipore), LC3B, p-ULK1 (S757), ULK1, p-mTOR (S2481), mTOR, p-p70s6k, p70s6k, p-p38, p38, p-IkB, IkB, tubulin (Cell Signaling Technology), PRAK, GFP (Santa Cruz Biotechnology), and actin (Sigma). Anti-p-PRAK (T182) and anti-p-Rheb (S130) antibodies were obtained from Jiahuai Han's Lab (Xiamen University).

Surface plasmon resonance spectroscopy (SPR)

The sensor chip CM5 with pre-immobilized anti-GST antibodies in one flow cell was first saturated with GST-fused PRAK protein. To analyze the binding kinetics, multiple concentrations of RAGE C-terminal region were diluted in HBS-EP buffer (0.01 M HEPES, pH 7.4; 0.15 M NaCl; 3 mM EDTA; 0.005 % Surfactant P20) and infused onto the sensor chip at a flow rate of 30 μL/min for 180 s. The response unit (RU) was recorded in real time by Biacore (Biacore X-100 plus, Biacore, Inc.). After the analyte infusion was stopped, the HBS-EP buffer was poured over the chip for 420 s at a flow rate of 30 μL/min. In order to dissociate the bounded analytes from the immobilized PRAK and for acquisition of the dissociation curves. Injection of 1 % PBS, including the HBS-EP buffer was performed as the vehicle control. The Biacore control software was used to measure the changes in plot, the binding curve, and RU. The curves obtained from the SPR experiments were analyzed and the dissociation equilibrium constant for RAGE C-terminus to immobilized PRAK was calculated using kinetic evaluation software. The dissociation constant KD (M) was derived from the equation, KD = kd/ka, where kd and ka are dissociation-and association-rate constants, respectively.

In Situ Proximity Ligation Assay

SH-SY5Y cells were co-transfected with RAGE and PRAK, stimulated with 2 μM of Aβ for 6 h, and stained according to the manufacturer's instructions (Duolink; 92008, Olink Bioscience).

Immunofluorescence assay

For immunocytochemistry, cells were fixed with 4 % PFA for 20 min at RT. Incubation was performed with 5 % BSA in PBS containing 1 % Triton X-100 for 30 min for blocking and permeabilization. The cells were then incubated with primary antibodies against human RAGE (1:200; R&D Systems) and PRAK (1:500; Santa Cruz Biotechnology) at 4 °C overnight. Finally, the cells were incubated with anti-rabbit Alexa 488 and anti-goat Alexa 594 (Invitrogen) at RT for 1 h, followed by DAPI staining and rinsing. The fluorescence was visualized by a super resolution structured illumination microscopy (Nikon N-SIM, Nikon Instruments Inc.).

Transmission electron microscopy (TEM)

Cells were fixed with 2 % PFA in 0.1 M phosphate or cacodylate buffer (pH 7.2) and 2.5 % glutaraldehyde in 0.1 M phosphate buffer (pH 7.2) at 4 °C for 24 h. Cells were then embedded with epoxy resin and polymerized at 38 °C for 12 h and then at 60 °C for 48 h. Thin sections, cut on an ultramicrotome (MT-XL, RMC Products), were collected on a copper grid. Samples were thin sectioned at 65 nm. Sections were then stained with 4 % lead citrate and saturated 4 % uranyl acetate, and examined under an electron microscope (JEM-1400, JEOL) at 80 kV [55]. Counting the number of autophagic structure per sheet (n = 6), using photographs taken at 20,000x magnification.

Statistical analysis

For statistical analysis, the unpaired *t*-test or the One-Way/Two-Way ANOVA was performed using Graphpad Instat 5.1 (GraphPad Software Inc.). Data in figures represent mean ± SEM.

Additional files

Additional file 1: Figure S1. Interaction between endogenous PRAK and RAGE. SH-SY5Y cell lysates were immunoprecipitated with RAGE antibody or normal IgG antibody. Western blot analysis performed with the indicated antibodies.

Additional file 2: Figure S2. PRAK does not mediate NF-κB activation through Aβ-RAGE interaction. SH-SY5Y cells were transfected with plasmids expressing RAGE and then transiently re-transfected with PRAK siRNA or scrambled control siRNA. After 24 h, cells were treated with DMSO or 2 μM monomeric Aβ for 30 min and western blot analysis performed with the indicated antibodies.

Additional file 3: Figure S3. RAGE-independent pathway activates p38 via Aβ. RAGE and DN-RAGE-overexpressing SH-SY5Y cells were treated with either DMSO or 2 μM monomeric Aβ for 6 h. Western blot analysis performed with the indicated antibodies.

Abbreviations

AD: Alzheimer's disease; Aβ: Amyloid beta; DN-RAGE: dominant negative RAGE; GFP: green fluorescent protein; IP: immunoprecipitation; LC3: microtubule-associated protein 1 light chain 3; mTORC1: mammalian target of rapamycin complex 1; NF-κB: nuclear factor of kappa light polypeptide gene enhancer in B-cells; PRAK: p38-regulated/activated protein kinase; RAGE: receptor for advanced glycation endproducts; Rheb: ras homologue enriched in brain; SPR: surface plasmon resonance; TEM: transmission electron microscopy; ULK1: UNC-51-like kinase 1.

Competing interest

The authors have no potential conflicts of interest to declare.

Authors' contributions

Y.K., C.K., S.M.S., I. M-J. conceived the study. Y.K., C.K., H.S.H. and S.H. designed the research. Y.K., C.K. performed and analyzed experiments. H.S. performed SPR analysis. The manuscript was written by Y.K., C.K. and I. M-J with assistance from other authors. All authors read and approved the final manuscript.

Acknowledgements

This work was supported by grants from the National Research Foundation [2015R1A2A1A05001794, 2014M3C7A1046047, 2015M3C7A1028790 and the Medical Research Center (2012R1A5A2A44671346)] and Protein metabolism medical research center through Seoul National University Nobel Laureates Invitation program for I. M-J.

References

1. Blennow K, De Leon MJ, Zetterberg H. Alzheimer's disease. Lancet. 2006;368:387–403.
2. Skaper SD. Alzheimer's disease and amyloid: culprit or coincidence? Int Rev Neurobiol. 2012;102:277–316.
3. Querfurth HW, LaFerla FM. Alzheimer's disease. N Engl J Med. 2010;362:329–44.
4. Neeper M, Schmidt AM, Brett J, Yan SD, Wang F, Pan YC, et al. Cloning and expression of a cell surface receptor for advanced glycosylation end products of proteins. J Biol Chem. 1992;267:14998–5004.
5. Schmidt AM, Vianna M, Gerlach M, Brett J, Ryan J, Kao J, et al. Isolation and characterization of two binding proteins for advanced glycosylation end products from bovine lung which are present on the endothelial cell surface. J Biol Chem. 1992;267:14987–97.
6. Hori O, Brett J, Slattery T, Cao R, Zhang J, Chen JX, et al. The receptor for advanced glycation end products (RAGE) is a cellular binding site for amphoterin. Mediation of neurite outgrowth and co-expression of rage and amphoterin in the developing nervous system. J Biol Chem. 1995;270:25752–61.
7. Hofmann MA, Drury S, Fu C, Qu W, Taguchi A, Lu Y, et al. RAGE mediates a novel proinflammatory axis: a central cell surface receptor for S100/calgranulin polypeptides. Cell. 1999;97:889–901.
8. Donato R. RAGE: a single receptor for several ligands and different cellular responses: the case of certain S100 proteins. Curr Mol Med. 2007;7:711–24.
9. Chavakis T, Bierhaus A, Al-Fakhri N, Schneider D, Witte S, Linn T, et al. The pattern recognition receptor (RAGE) is a counterreceptor for leukocyte integrins: a novel pathway for inflammatory cell recruitment. J Exp Med. 2003;198:1507–15.
10. He M, Kubo H, Morimoto K, Fujino N, Suzuki T, Takahasi T, et al. Receptor for advanced glycation end products binds to phosphatidylserine and assists in the clearance of apoptotic cells. EMBO Rep. 2011;12:358–64.
11. Yan SD, Chen X, Fu J, Chen M, Zhu H, Roher A, et al. RAGE and amyloid-beta peptide neurotoxicity in Alzheimer's disease. Nature. 1996;382:685–91.
12. Ramasamy R, Yan SF, Schmidt AM. RAGE: therapeutic target and biomarker of the inflammatory response–the evidence mounts. J Leukoc Biol. 2009;86:505–12.
13. Wautier MP, Chappey O, Corda S, Stern DM, Schmidt AM, Wautier JL. Activation of NADPH oxidase by AGE links oxidant stress to altered gene expression via RAGE. Am J Physiol Endocrinol Metab. 2001;280:E685–94.
14. Ramasamy R, Vannucci SJ, Yan SS, Herold K, Yan SF, Schmidt AM. Advanced glycation end products and RAGE: a common thread in aging, diabetes, neurodegeneration, and inflammation. Glycobiology. 2005;15:16R–28R.
15. Rai V, Maldonado AY, Burz DS, Reverdatto S, Yan SF, Schmidt AM, et al. Signal transduction in receptor for advanced glycation end products (RAGE): solution structure of C-terminal rage (ctRAGE) and its binding to mDia1. J Biol Chem. 2012;287:5133–44.
16. Hudson BI, Kalea AZ, Del Mar AM, Harja E, Boulanger E, D'Agati V, et al. Interaction of the RAGE cytoplasmic domain with diaphanous-1 is required for ligand-stimulated cellular migration through activation of Rac1 and Cdc42. J Biol Chem. 2008;283:34457–68.
17. New L, Jiang Y, Zhao M, Liu K, Zhu W, Flood LJ, et al. PRAK, a novel protein kinase regulated by the p38 MAP kinase. EMBO J. 1998;17:3372–84.
18. New L, Jiang Y, Han J. Regulation of PRAK subcellular location by p38 MAP kinases. Mol Biol Cell. 2003;14:2603–16.
19. Hefner Y, Borsch-Haubold AG, Murakami M, Wilde JI, Pasquet S, Schieltz D, et al. Serine 727 phosphorylation and activation of cytosolic phospholipase A2 by MNK1-related protein kinases. J Biol Chem. 2000;275:37542–51.
20. Toska K, Kleppe R, Armstrong CG, Morrice NA, Cohen P, Haavik J. Regulation of tyrosine hydroxylase by stress-activated protein kinases. J Neurochem. 2002;83:775–83.

21. Kress TR, Cannell IG, Brenkman AB, Samans B, Gaestel M, Roepman P, et al. The MK5/PRAK kinase and Myc form a negative feedback loop that is disrupted during colorectal tumorigenesis. Mol Cell. 2011;41:445–57.
22. Zhao X, Guan JL. Focal adhesion kinase and its signaling pathways in cell migration and angiogenesis. Adv Drug Deliv Rev. 2011;63:610–5.
23. Shiryaev A, Kostenko S, Dumitriu G, Moens U. Septin 8 is an interaction partner and in vitro substrate of MK5. World J Biol Chem. 2012;3:98–109.
24. Sun P, Yoshizuka N, New L, Moser BA, Li Y, Liao R, et al. PRAK is essential for ras-induced senescence and tumor suppression. Cell. 2007;128:295–308.
25. Moens U, Kostenko S. Structure and function of MK5/PRAK: the loner among the mitogen-activated protein kinase-activated protein kinases. Biol Chem. 2013;394:1115–32.
26. Zheng M, Wang YH, Wu XN, Wu SQ, Lu BJ, Dong MQ, et al. Inactivation of Rheb by PRAK-mediated phosphorylation is essential for energy-depletion-induced suppression of mTORC1. Nat Cell Biol. 2011;13:263–72.
27. Arancio O, Zhang HP, Chen X, Lin C, Trinchese F, Puzzo D, et al. RAGE potentiates Abeta-induced perturbation of neuronal function in transgenic mice. EMBO J. 2004;23:4096–105.
28. Ding Q, Keller JN. Evaluation of rage isoforms, ligands, and signaling in the brain. Biochim Biophys Acta. 2005;1746:18–27.
29. Son SM, Jung ES, Shin HJ, Byun J, Mook-Jung I. Abeta-induced formation of autophagosomes is mediated by RAGE-CaMKKbeta-AMPK signaling. Neurobiol Aging. 2012;33:1006 e1011–1023.
30. Long X, Lin Y, Ortiz-Vega S, Yonezawa K, Avruch J. Rheb binds and regulates the mTOR kinase. Curr Biol. 2005;15:702–13.
31. Kim J, Kundu M, Viollet B, Guan KL. AMPK and mTOR regulate autophagy through direct phosphorylation of Ulk1. Nat Cell Biol. 2011;13:132–41.
32. Klionsky DJ, Abeliovich H, Agostinis P, Agrawal DK, Aliev G, Askew DS, et al. Guidelines for the use and interpretation of assays for monitoring autophagy in higher eukaryotes. Autophagy. 2008;4:151–75.
33. Nixon RA. Autophagy, amyloidogenesis and Alzheimer disease. J Cell Sci. 2007;120:4081–91.
34. Han SH, Kim YH, Mook-Jung I. RAGE: the beneficial and deleterious effects by diverse mechanisms of actions. Mol Cell. 2011;31:91–7.
35. Seternes OM, Mikalsen T, Johansen B, Michaelsen E, Armstrong CG, Morrice NA, et al. Activation of MK5/PRAK by the atypical MAP kinase ERK3 defines a novel signal transduction pathway. EMBO J. 2004;23:4780–91.
36. Origlia N, Righi M, Capsoni S, Cattaneo A, Fang F, Stern DM, et al. Receptor for advanced glycation end product-dependent activation of p38 mitogen-activated protein kinase contributes to amyloid-beta-mediated cortical synaptic dysfunction. J Neurosci. 2008;28:3521–30.
37. Bertrand FE, Spengemen JD, Shelton JG, McCubrey JA. Inhibition of PI3K, mTOR and MEK signaling pathways promotes rapid apoptosis in B-lineage ALL in the presence of stromal cell support. Leukemia. 2005;19:98–102.
38. Woiwode A, Johnson SA, Zhong S, Zhang C, Roeder RG, Teichmann M, et al. PTEN represses RNA polymerase III-dependent transcription by targeting the TFIIIB complex. Mol Cell Biol. 2008;28:4204–14.
39. Narayanan SP, Flores AI, Wang F, Macklin WB. Akt signals through the mammalian target of rapamycin pathway to regulate CNS myelination. J Neurosci. 2009;29:6860–70.
40. Feldman ME, Apsel B, Uotila A, Loewith R, Knight ZA, Ruggero D, et al. Active-site inhibitors of mTOR target rapamycin-resistant outputs of mTORC1 and mTORC2. PLoS Biol. 2009;7, e38.
41. Cleveland-Donovan K, Maile LA, Tsiaras WG, Tchkonia T, Kirkland JL, Boney CM. IGF-I activation of the AKT pathway is impaired in visceral but not subcutaneous preadipocytes from obese subjects. Endocrinology. 2010;151:3752–63.
42. Hoeffer CA, Klann E. mTOR signaling: at the crossroads of plasticity, memory and disease. Trends Neurosci. 2010;33:67–75.
43. Perluigi M, Di Domenico F, Butterfield DA. mTOR signaling in aging and neurodegeneration: At the crossroad between metabolism dysfunction and impairment of autophagy. Neurobiol Dis. 2015.
44. Ma T, Hoeffer CA, Capetillo-Zarate E, Yu F, Wong H, Lin MT, et al. Dysregulation of the mTOR pathway mediates impairment of synaptic plasticity in a mouse model of Alzheimer's disease. PLoS ONE. 2010;5.
45. Paccalin M, Pain-Barc S, Pluchon C, Paul C, Besson MN, Carret-Rebillat AS, et al. Activated mTOR and PKR kinases in lymphocytes correlate with memory and cognitive decline in Alzheimer's disease. Dement Geriatr Cogn Disord. 2006;22:320–6.
46. Kim YC, Guan KL. mTOR: a pharmacologic target for autophagy regulation. J Clin Invest. 2015;125:25–32.
47. Yu WH, Kumar A, Peterhoff C, Shapiro Kulnane L, Uchiyama Y, Lamb BT, et al. Autophagic vacuoles are enriched in amyloid precursor protein-secretase activities: implications for beta-amyloid peptide over-production and localization in Alzheimer's disease. Int J Biochem Cell Biol. 2004;36:2531–40.
48. Salminen A, Kaarniranta K, Kauppinen A, Ojala J, Haapasalo A, Soininen H, et al. Impaired autophagy and APP processing in Alzheimer's disease: The potential role of Beclin 1 interactome. Prog Neurobiol. 2013;106–107:33–54.
49. Pickford F, Masliah E, Britschgi M, Lucin K, Narasimhan R, Jaeger PA, et al. The autophagy-related protein beclin 1 shows reduced expression in early Alzheimer disease and regulates amyloid beta accumulation in mice. J Clin Invest. 2008;118:2190–9.
50. Nixon RA, Yang DS. Autophagy failure in Alzheimer's disease–locating the primary defect. Neurobiol Dis. 2011;43:38–45.
51. Nixon RA, Wegiel J, Kumar A, Yu WH, Peterhoff C, Cataldo A, et al. Extensive involvement of autophagy in Alzheimer disease: an immuno-electron microscopy study. J Neuropathol Exp Neurol. 2005;64:113–22.
52. Nixon RA. Autophagy in neurodegenerative disease: friend, foe or turncoat? Trends Neurosci. 2006;29:528–35.
53. Li L, Zhang X, Le W. Autophagy dysfunction in Alzheimer's disease. Neuro-degenerative diseases. 2010;7:265–71.
54. Dahlgren KN, Manelli AM, Stine Jr WB, Baker LK, Krafft GA, LaDu MJ. Oligomeric and fibrillar species of amyloid-beta peptides differentially affect neuronal viability. J Biol Chem. 2002;277:32046–53.
55. Eskelinen EL, Schmidt CK, Neu S, Willenborg M, Fuertes G, Salvador N, et al. Disturbed cholesterol traffic but normal proteolytic function in LAMP-1/LAMP-2 double-deficient fibroblasts. Mol Biol Cell. 2004;15:3132–45.

6

3D culture models of Alzheimer's disease: a road map to a "cure-in-a-dish"

Se Hoon Choi[1†], Young Hye Kim[2†], Luisa Quinti[1], Rudolph E. Tanzi[1*] and Doo Yeon Kim[1*]

Abstract

Alzheimer's disease (AD) transgenic mice have been used as a standard AD model for basic mechanistic studies and drug discovery. These mouse models showed symbolic AD pathologies including β-amyloid (Aβ) plaques, gliosis and memory deficits but failed to fully recapitulate AD pathogenic cascades including robust phospho tau (p-tau) accumulation, clear neurofibrillary tangles (NFTs) and neurodegeneration, solely driven by familial AD (FAD) mutation(s). Recent advances in human stem cell and three-dimensional (3D) culture technologies made it possible to generate novel 3D neural cell culture models that recapitulate AD pathologies including robust Aβ deposition and Aβ-driven NFT-like tau pathology. These new 3D human cell culture models of AD hold a promise for a novel platform that can be used for mechanism studies in human brain-like environment and high-throughput drug screening (HTS). In this review, we will summarize the current progress in recapitulating AD pathogenic cascades in human neural cell culture models using AD patient-derived induced pluripotent stem cells (iPSCs) or genetically modified human stem cell lines. We will also explain how new 3D culture technologies were applied to accelerate Aβ and p-tau pathologies in human neural cell cultures, as compared the standard two-dimensional (2D) culture conditions. Finally, we will discuss a potential impact of the human 3D human neural cell culture models on the AD drug-development process. These revolutionary 3D culture models of AD will contribute to accelerate the discovery of novel AD drugs.

Keywords: Alzheimer's disease, Three-dimensional culture, Amyloid plaques, Neurofibrillary tangles, Induced-pluripotent stem cell, High-throughput drug screening

Background

Alzheimer's disease (AD) is the most common neurodegenerative disease worldwide. AD begins with short-term memory impairments, gets worse over time, and culminates in total loss of cognition [1]. Familial, early-onset (<60 years), rare, autosomal-dominant forms of AD (FAD) is caused by fully penetrant mutations either in the amyloid precursor protein (APP), presenilin 1 (PSEN1), or presenilin 2 (PSEN2) genes. Sporadic AD (SAD) is the more common form of the disease, and usually involves late onset owing to multifactorial genetic and environmental risk factors [1–3]. Currently, AD affects 5.3 million people in the United States and the number of AD patients are predicted to increase dramatically over the next decade [4]. However, there is no clear therapeutic option for AD patients yet, except for some symptomatic reliefs [3, 5, 6].

Two key pathological hallmarks of AD are amyloid plaques (a.k.a. senile plaques), and neurofibrillary tangles (NFTs) [4]. The amyloid plaques are extracellular amyloid filaments, composed primarily of small ~4 kDa peptides called β-amyloid (Aβ), which are liberated from the amyloid precursor protein (APP) via sequential proteolytic cleavages by β- and γ-secretase [1, 7, 8]. NFTs are composed of highly phosphorylated forms of the microtubule-associated protein tau (p-tau) [9, 10]. In AD, p-tau dramatically accumulates in the unusual cellular compartments including soma and dendrites, possibly due to an imbalance between the activities of protein kinases and phosphatases [11–13].

For the past decade, AD transgenic mice overexpressing APP or APP/Presenilin (PSEN) with single or multiple familial AD mutations have been used as a

* Correspondence: tanzi@helix.mgh.harvard.edu; dkim@helix.mgh.harvard.edu
†Equal contributors
[1]Genetics and Aging Research Unit, MassGeneral Institute for Neurodegenerative Disease, Massachusetts General Hospital, Harvard Medical School, 02129 Charlestown, MA, USA
Full list of author information is available at the end of the article

standard AD model for basic mechanistic studies and drug discovery [9, 14, 15]. However, these AD transgenic mouse models do not develop clear NFTs nor robust neurodegeneration as observed in human AD patients, despite strong Aβ deposition, synaptic deficits and clear gliosis [9, 14–18]. According to the "amyloid hypothesis," the accumulation of pathogenic Aβ species, causing amyloid plaques, would trigger a pathogenic cascade that leads to hyperphosphorylation of tau causing NFTs, and ultimately, neuronal death [1, 19–22]. The failures of anti-Aβ therapies in humans, which were highly effective in mouse models, might be explained by the limitation of AD mouse models in comprehensively modeling human AD pathologies [23, 24].

Advances in stem cell technology made it possible to generate human neurons with FAD mutations. Induced-pluripotent stem cell (iPSC) technology can even provide human neurons harboring the identical genetic information of AD patients [1, 25–30]. These new exciting human neural cell culture models cast light on making new AD cellular models that can comprehensively recapitulate pathogenic cascades of AD in human brain-like environment. Indeed, we recently showed that the overexpression of APP and PSEN1 with multiple FAD mutations were enough to induce robust Aβ deposition (amyloid plaques), and detergent-resistant, fibrillary p-tau aggregates in human neural cells cultured in our unique Matrigel-based three-dimensional (3D) culture system (Fig. 1), which has not been feasible in AD transgenic mouse models [17, 18, 31, 32]. Our results clearly demonstrate the advantage of human neuronal cells in modeling pathogenic cascades of AD as compared to mouse models.

In this review, we will summarize the current progress in recapitulating AD pathogenic cascades, including Aβ and p-tau pathologies in human neural cell culture models. In addition to new human AD neuronal cell models, derived from fibroblasts, blood cells and CRISPR/CAS9-edited iPSCs, we will focus on how our and other 3D culture technologies were applied to accelerate Aβ and/or p-tau pathologies in human neural cell cultures. Finally, we will discuss a potential impact of these revolutionary human 3D culture models of neurodegenerative diseases on drug-development pipelines.

Main text

The identification of Aβ as the main component of amyloid plaques resulted in the original formation of the "amyloid hypothesis", by Drs. Glenner and Wong in 1984 [33], which was later renamed the "amyloid cascade hypothesis" by Drs. Hardy and Higgins [34]. This hypothesis posits that the accumulation of Aβ is the initial pathological trigger in the disease, subsequently leading to the formation of NFTs, neuronal cell death

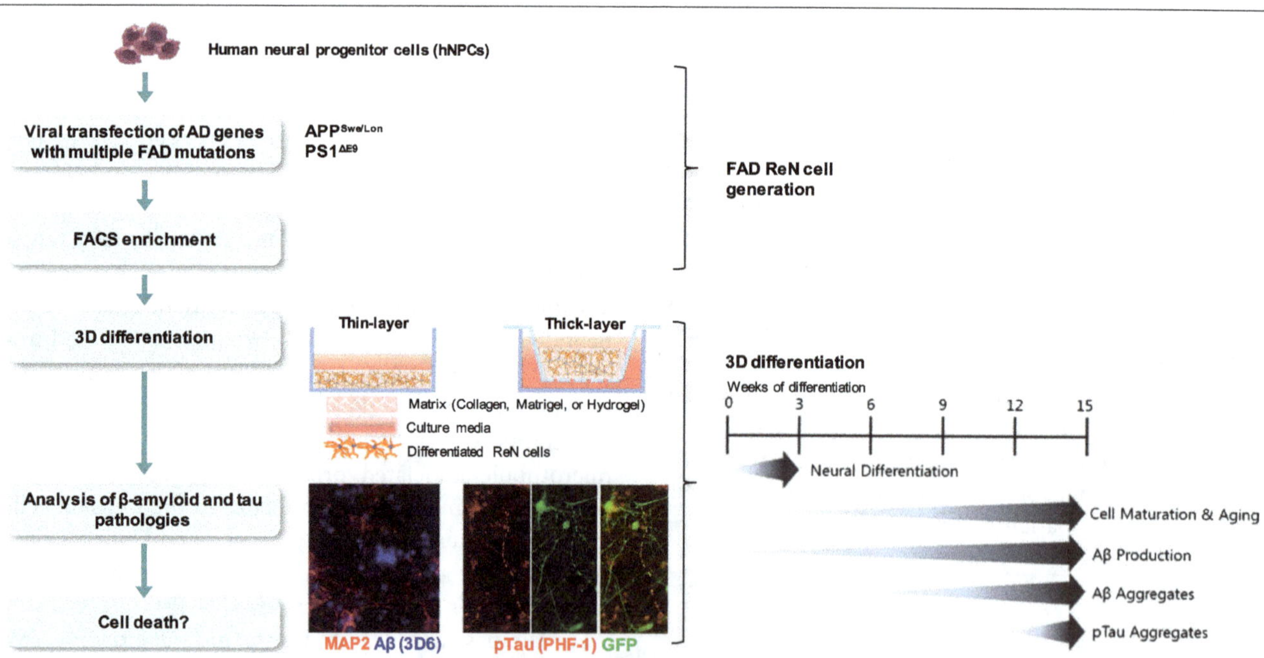

Fig. 1 Recapitulation of Aβ and Tau pathology in a 3D human neural cell culture model of AD. Human neural progenitor cells (hNPCs) are virally transfected with APP and/or PSEN1 FAD mutations with either GFP or mCherry as a reporter for viral infection. These cells are enriched based on GFP and/or mCherry signals by FACS, and then differentiated in 3D Matrigel culture systems. Thin-layer (~100–300 μm) culture format is suited for immunostaining analyses and thick-layer (~4 mm) culture format is used for biochemical analyses. In 3D-differentiated hNPCs with FAD mutations, extracellular Aβ aggregates develop ~6 weeks of differentiation and robust increase in tauopathy is evident from ~10–14 weeks of differentiation

and dementia [2]. However, it has not been easy to fully validate the hypothesis, partly due to the absence of appropriate experimental models. Researchers have taken advantage of FAD-linked APP and/or PSEN1 mutations by developing transgenic mice that express these mutated proteins. Various AD transgenic mouse models have been generated by overexpressing human APP and/or PSEN1 with single or multiple FAD mutations, in which accumulation of Aβ peptides is a common target [9, 14–18]. Since then, AD transgenic mouse models have become the standard model system in vivo for mechanistic studies and AD drug discovery.

It is beyond the scope of this review to discuss all the different AD mouse models, which has already been covered by many reviews including ours [17]. However, although most AD transgenic mouse models recapitulated amyloid plaques and β-amyloid-induced synaptic/memory deficits, none of the AD transgenic mouse models have successfully recapitulated clear Aβ-driven NFT formation nor neuronal death [17]. The limitation of AD mouse models in comprehensively modeling human AD pathologies have led to the failures of anti-Aβ therapies in humans, which were otherwise highly effective in mouse models [23, 24]. 3xTg mice, which express mutant forms of APP, PSEN1 and tau, have shown to develop both plaques and tangle-like pathology [35]. However, this model contains a tau mutation which is associated with frontotemporal dementia (FTD), not AD. It is crucial to note that no mutation has been located in the tau gene in AD and that normal human tau becomes pathological in the disease. Fundamental species-specific differences in genome and proteoforms between mice and humans may preclude the recapitulation of *bona fide* AD pathological events in mouse models. Indeed, adult mice do not express the six human isoforms of tau proteins and endogenous mouse tau seems to interfere with aggregation of human tau proteins [17, 31, 36].

Recapitulating Aβ pathology in human iPSC-derived neurons

Human neurons derived from AD patients by iPSC technology appear to be an ideal platform for modeling AD in human neuronal environment [25, 26, 29, 30, 37–51]. To date, several research groups have reported the usage of iPSCs in AD modeling, which provide a proof-of-principle for modeling patient-specific AD pathology in human brain-like environment [25–30, 37–42, 48, 49, 52, 53]. These patient-derived AD neurons were mainly generated from FAD patients but also a few from sAD patients. As summarized in our previous review, human iPSC-derived neurons could have successfully recapitulated several pathological features of AD [17]. Most of the FAD neurons carrying FAD mutations in PSEN1 and PSEN2 showed significant increase in the Aβ42/Aβ40 ratio as compared to the non-AD control neurons, confirming that PSEN1 FAD mutations increase pathogenic Aβ42 levels as predicted [1, 25–29]. The iPSC neurons carrying PSEN1 FAD mutations, ΔE9 and L166P were also used as model systems to explore if the PSEN FAD mutations induce "loss of function" of presenilin/γ-secretase in human physiological neurons, which contribute to resolve the controversy over the presenilin/γ-secretase impairment by PSEN FAD mutations [27, 28, 54, 55].

Similar to PSEN FAD neurons, iPSC-derived human neurons harboring APP FAD mutations also showed increases in pathogenic Aβ levels [25, 29, 40, 56]. APP^{V717I} FAD mutation (also termed as London mutation) significantly increased the Aβ42/40 ratio in human forebrain neurons as predicted in non-human model systems [25, 29]. APP E693Δ is a rare autosomal FAD mutation associated with early-onset AD symptoms without Aβ plaques. Consistent with the finding in a different system, AD leads to a reduction in extracellular Aβ levels while inducing the accumulation of intracellular Aβ oligomers in a human iPSC-derived neuronal model [39]. APP duplication (APP^{Dp}) is another early-onset FAD mutation, which has been tested in human iPSC-derived neurons [25, 40]. Due to the presence of two copies of the APP gene, these neurons produce high levels of Aβ40 and 42 as compared to other iPSC-derived FAD neurons. Down syndrome (DS) neurons also showed robust increases in total Aβ levels due to the APP gene duplication located on chromosome 21 [57].

In addition to FAD patient-derived neurons, Paquet et al., recently reported the generation of knock-in human neurons harboring heterozygous and homozygous APP or PSEN1 FAD mutations ($APP^{KM670/671NL}$ and $PSEN1^{M146V}$) using modified CRISPR/Cas9 gene editing technology [56]. As predicted, $APP^{KM670/671NL}$ knock-in neurons showed increase in total Aβ levels, while the neurons with $PSEN1^{M146V}$ showed ~2 fold increases in Aβ42/Aβ40 ratio [56]. Since these neurons were originated from non-AD patients, this is a clear demonstration that APP or PSEN1 FAD mutations are sufficient to increase pathogenic Aβ species in human neurons.

Human neurons derived from SAD patients showed variable results in Aβ levels. In general, only a handful of SAD patients showed the increased Aβ levels, which have not been replicable between patients [38–41, 49, 50]. It is not easy to determine whether these variabilities stem from the presence of multiple genetic variants or differential neuronal differentiation conditions due to the lack of isogenic control cell lines. Very limited amount of genetic information is available for these cell lines.

In addition to Aβ accumulation, select AD neurons showed various deficits, which might be triggered by the pathogenic Aβ species. Increased active/total glycogen synthase kinase-3β (GSK3β) levels and enlarged RAB5-positive early endosomes were observed in FAD neurons with APP mutations [29, 40]. $APP^{E693\Delta}$ neurons showed elevated endoplasmic reticulum (ER), oxidative stress and altered glycosylation, which can be blocked by Docosahexaenoic acid (DHA) treatments [39]. Abnormal Ca^{2+} influx and the increased susceptibility to cell death have been reported in SAD basal forebrain cholinergic neurons harboring APOε3/ε4alleles [38]. However, it not clear if these deficits are directly connected to the accumulation of pathogenic Aβ. The elevated GSK3β levels in AD neurons were reduced by β-secretase inhibitors, but not by β-secretase inhibitors, which suggest that the accumulation of pathogenic Aβ cannot fully explain the GSK3β changes [40].

Recapitulating tau pathology in human AD neurons: driven by Aβ or APP-C99?

As previously discussed, AD transgenic mouse model with single or multiple FAD mutations failed to show clear tau/NFT pathologies despite robust Aβ accumulation. As discussed earlier, adult mice do not express tau isoforms as the human brains and even knock in mouse study showed that the presence of endogenous mouse tau inhibit the aggregation of human tau proteins [17, 36].

Patient-derived human neurons can be an excellent alternative model to test if the accumulation of pathogenic Aβ species can induce tau pathology as predicted by the Aβ hypothesis. Indeed, iPSC-derived human neurons with frontotemporal dementia (FTD)-associated tau mutations showed pronounced tau pathology with increased fragmentation of neurites, elevated p-tau immunoreactivity and various cellular deficits including decreased neurite extension, increased cellular stress markers and altered vesicle trafficking [58–60]. Some of these deficits were not observed in parental fibroblast cells, suggesting that FTD tau mutation elicit neuron-specific pathology [59]. These results clearly demonstrate that iPSC-derived human neuronal cultures can be a valid model system for studying tau pathology in vitro.

In the case of AD neurons, not all, but select FAD neurons showed moderate but consistent alteration in p-tau, total tau and/or p-tau/total tau ratio [17]. Israel et al., reported increases tau phosphorylation (p-tau/total tau ratio) in neurons from APP^{Dp} FAD patients and one of the sAD patients, as well as other pathological markers Aβ, p-tau (Thr231) and active glycogen synthase kinase-3β (aGSK-3β), which suggest possible connections among elevated tau phosphorylation, Aβ and GSK-3β activities [40]. However, two Aβ blockers, β-secretase and γ-secretase inhibitors showed contradicting result in reducing tau phosphorylation, which suggests that p-tau increases in these neurons were not solely induced by Aβ species [17, 40]. Muratore et al., also observed the increases in both total tau and p-tau levels in APP^{V717I} FAD neurons [29]. Interestingly, the early treatments with Aβ-specific antibodies reduced the total and p-tau (T231) levels in these neurons, which is a strong evidence that the accumulation of pathogenic Aβ species is responsible for alteration in total and phospho tau levels in APP^{V717I} FAD neurons [29].

Moore et al., also reconfirmed that cortical neurons derived from iPSCs harboring APP^{V717I} or APP^{Dp} duplication mutation showed increases in both total and p-tau (S202/T205, S396 and S404) levels [25]. Interestingly, altered tau metabolism was not observed in neurons carrying PSEN1 FAD mutations (Y111C, M146I and Intron 4) [25]. β-secretase inhibitor or γ-secretase modulator treatments decreased the total and p-tau levels in APP^{V717I}, APP^{Dp}, DS neurons while the impact of γ-secretase modulator treatments was relatively moderate as compared to β-secretase inhibitor treatments [17, 25]. Interestingly, again, γ-secretase inhibitor treatments did not reduce these tau levels, rather dramatically increased in FAD and even in the control cells [25]. Based on these results, Moore et al., proposed an interesting hypothesis that the total and p-tau change (termed as "tau proteostasis) is regulated by APP metabolism, likely by one of the APP cleavage product, APP-C99, not by Aβ. This hypothesis suggest that BACE1 inhibition therapies can be more effective in reducing p-tau levels in human neurons derived from FAD patients, as compared to other anti-Aβ therapies. The current BACE1 inhibitor clinical trials may be an interesting test for this hypothesis in vivo [61–63]. Moreover, it is not still clear whether the tau proteostasis in these cells is directly relevant to advanced tau/NFT pathology since there is no evidence for tau aggregation nor tau-related pathologies. Also, γ-secretase inhibitor treatments may have also affected other physiological neuronal functions via regulating multiple neuronal substrate cleavages. Further studies will be needed to fully demonstrate the connection among tau proteostasis, APP-C99, and Aβ accumulation [17].

The limitation of human AD neurons in recapitulating robust AD pathologies

As aforementioned, the human iPSC-derived FAD neurons successfully recapitulated early features of AD including the increases in pathogenic Aβ species. However, these FAD neurons that were not able to fully recapitulate did not show robust extracellular Aβ plaques, Aβ-induced p-tau pathology, NFT pathologies such as aggregated with paired helical filaments (PHFs); neither did they display any signs of neurodegeneration, as predicted in the amyloid hypothesis and observed in AD patients.

Lack of robust AD hallmarks in the iPSC-derived neuronal models might be a result of the following reasons: 1) production of lower levels of pathogenic Aβ species, especially Aβ42, compared to AD patients; 2) insufficient maturation and aging of neuronal cells; 3) fundamental limitation of conventional 2D cell culture systems to mimic complex and dynamic 3D brain environment. The levels of pathogenic Aβ42 in FAD neurons are in the range from 4 to 80 fmol/mg [29, 40, 64]. However, the mean insoluble Aβ42 levels measured in AD brains were ~1,659 pmol/g [65], much higher than the levels observed in iPSC-derived FAD neuronal culture. Thus, the levels of Aβ species generated from FAD iPSC-derived neurons might not be sufficient to form Aβ plaques and other Aβ-triggered pathogenic events. Insufficient neuronal maturation and aging may also contribute to the inability of FAD neurons to reconstitute AD pathologies. As well known, aging is one of the major risk factors of AD and it is still technically challenging to reconstitute mature and possibly aged neuronal culture with human iPSCs. In the case of tau pathology, wild-type human iPSC-derived neurons seem to express low levels of adult 4-repeat (4R) tau isoforms even after 90-days of differentiation [58–60, 66]. 4R tau plays an important role in tau aggregation and NFT pathology in the adult brain, and therefore, low 4R tau levels might also explain why human FAD neurons could not show robust tauopathy with detergent-resistant helical filamentous aggregation [10, 67, 68].

Accelerating AD pathology using matrigel-based 3D culture system

To overcome the aforementioned limitations of animal models and AD iPSCs-derived neurons, we have recently developed a 3D human neuronal culture model of AD by combining genetically engineered human neuronal progenitor cells (hNPCs) and Matrigel-based 3D culture technology [31, 32]. In order to establish the system, we first generated hNPCs producing high levels of pathogenic Aβ species by overexpressing human APP and PSEN1 with multiple FAD mutations in the ReNcell VM cell line (ReN cells), an immortalized hNPC line that readily differentiates into neurons and glial cells [69]. For FAD mutations, we chose the $APP^{K670N/M671L}$ and APP^{V717I} and $PSEN1^{\Delta E9}$ mutation to produce high levels of Aβ species and elevate Aβ42/Aβ40 ratio. Using Fluorescence-activated cell sorting (FACS) enrichment protocols, we generated FAD ReN cell lines which produced ~1000 fold higher levels of Aβ as compared to iPSC-derived FAD neurons (Fig. 1).

In conventional 2D cell culture systems, the secreted Aβ might diffuse into the relatively large volume of cell culture media, and is likely to be removed during regular media changes preventing aggregation of Aβ [17, 31]. To provide the brain tissue-like closed 3D environment which provides a local niche that promotes aggregation of β-amyloid, which can trigger pathogenic cascades, including NFTs, our FAD ReN cells were grown in Matrigel. We chose Matrigel specifically as our 3D matrix because it contains high levels of brain ECM proteins (i.e., laminin, entactin, collagen, and heparin sulfate proteoglycans) and easily solidifies with cells upon moderate thermal change [70]. Cells that were mixed with Matrigel were grown in a thin-layer 3D format (~100–300 μm in thickness) on cell culture vessels with a cover-glass bottom for cellular imaging and in a thick-layer 3D format (up to 4 mm in thickness) using cell culture inserts for molecular and biochemical analyses, respectively (Fig. 1).

Besides the 3D neural cell culture systems being suitable for reconstituting extracellular aggregation of Aβ, they also have advantages in recapitulating in vivo brain environments and can accelerate neuronal differentiation and neural network formation [71–76]. Indeed, we found that our Matrigel-based 3D culture conditions dramatically increased neural differentiation of ReN hNPCs as compared to 2D cultures conditions [17, 32]. More importantly, we found the 3D culture conditions also dramatically elevated 4R adult tau isoforms, which are essential for reconstituting the tau aggregation and NFT pathology [32, 67]. RT-PCR analysis showed 4R/3R tau ratio in 3D-differentiated ReN cells is ~1, which is similar to the ratio in adult human brains [32]. Since we use the same BD Matrigel for 2D and 3D differentiation protocols (only difference is Matrigel concentration), these differences cannot be explained by differential Matrix composition. Together, our results showed that 3D culture conditions have advantages for both accelerating Aβ and NFT pathologies.

The differentiated FAD ReN cells revealed dramatic increases in Aβ40 (~9-fold) and Aβ42 (~17-fold) levels as compared to the control ReN cells, and the Aβ42:Aβ40 ratio was also increased (~5-fold) in ReN cells expressing PSEN ΔE9 mutation [32]. After 6 weeks of 3D-differentiation, not in 2D conditions, we were able to detect clear formation of amyloid plaque pathology: extracellular Aβ deposits were detected by Aβ immunostaining and Amylo-Glo, a Aβ dye and detergent sodium dodecyl sulfate (SDS)-resistant Aβ aggregates were confirmed by biochemical analysis [31, 32].

One of the most interesting aspects of our 3D human neuronal culture model is successful recapitulation of tauopathy without any FTD tau mutation. After ~10 weeks of differentiation, FAD ReN cells showed dramatic increases in phospho tau (pSer199/Ser202/Thr205, pSer396/Ser404) levels in detergent-insoluble fractions from FAD ReN cells without significantly affecting total tau levels. Intracellular accumulation of aggregated, hyperphosphorylated tau proteins was clear in the somatodendritic compartments of FAD neurons, and also we were able to observe the formation of filamentous structures of detergent-insoluble tau proteins [31, 32]. More importantly, inhibition of Aβ generation with β-secretase or γ-secretase inhibitors not only decreased the levels of pathogenic Aβ plaques but also attenuated tau pathology in our 3D cultures, which supports that tau pathology in our system is driven by Aβ accumulation.

Interestingly, we also observed that neurites with high levels of p-tau showed unusual dystrophic morphologies, implying that our 3D models possibly recapitulate dystrophic neurites which is another important pathological feature of AD [32] (*a manuscript under preparation*). The neurite dystrophy, which refer to neuritic sprouting, swollen dendrites and/or axons, has been shown to be the critical neuropathological correlate of dementia in AD [77–83]. Several molecular pathways have been proposed as underlying mechanisms of the neurite dystrophy in AD, based on the studies using AD mouse models and human AD brain samples [78–80, 84, 85]. For example, Hu et al. reported that overexpression of reticulon 3 (RTN3), of which levels were closely related with neurite dystrophy in the brains of AD patients and APP transgenic mice, led to cognitive deficits in mice without Aβ and tau pathologies [85]. In the future studies, it will be interesting to determine potential roles of these proposed pathways on the neurite dystrophy observed in our 3D human neural culture model of AD.

Accelerating AD pathology using 3D organoid cultures

The self-organizing structures such as cerebral organoids are another way to achieve 3D structures that can facilitate interstitial compartments for Aβ deposition [32]. As previously shown, these brain organoids/neuro-spheroids model can more closely mimic brain structures that are affected in the brains of AD patients [86]. Recently, two groups reported the generation of 3D brain organoid cultures using AD patient-derived iPSCs. Raja et al., used APP^{Dp}, $PSEN1^{M146L}$ and $PSEN1^{A246E}$ FAD iPSCs to generate 3D brain organoids/neuro-spheroids that recapitulated AD-like pathologies, including Aβ aggregation, p-tau accumulation at somatodendritic compartments, and endosome abnormalities. The incidence of AD pathology was more robust and consistent as compared to the same cell lines in 2D culture conditions [25, 40, 41]. More importantly, treatment of patient-derived organoids with β- and γ-secretase inhibitors significantly reduces Aβ deposition and tau pathology [32]. Instead of FAD iPSCs, Lee et al. used iPSCs that were derived from 5 different sAD patients' blood samples [49]. In agreement with Raja et al., they have reported the detection of Aβ and p-tau in brain organoids/neuro-spheroids from sAD iPSCs. They also reported that β- and γ-secretase inhibitors showed less potency in decreasing Aβ levels in neural cells differentiated under 3D culture conditions.

These results clearly demonstrate that 3D organoids culture conditions can accelerate AD pathogenesis in iPSC-derived AD neural cultures, possibly by promoting local Aβ eposition as we proposed in our 3D Matrigel culture models [17, 31, 32]. More importantly, β- and γ-secretase inhibitors significantly reduce p-tau pathology in these organoid cultures, which also support our conclusion that Aβ accumulation is mainly responsible for the robust tauopathy in 3D-cultured AD iPSC-derived neurons. Although it is not shown in these studies, the potential increases in 4R tau isoforms in 3D conditions may also contribute to achieve more robust tau pathology as we showed in our Matrigel-based 3D cultures.

Application of 3D culture models of AD for drug discovery: looking for a cure in a dish?

In the past decade, AD transgenic mice have been used as a standard preclinical model for testing candidate AD drug targets, which are pre-selected by basic mechanistic studies or by the chemical/peptide library screening using a simple biochemical or cellular model (i.e., APP processing, synthetic Aβ aggregation, tau phosphorylation and etc.) (Fig. 2). The candidate compounds are tested in AD transgenic mice with multiple doses to explore their potential toxicity and the impact on AD pathology, including pathogenic Aβ accumulation, p-tau accumulation and the behavioral and memory deficits. This process takes more than 2–3 years and is relatively expensive. Only small portions of primary candidate compounds can pass through this process. However, a majority of AD drug targets which showed favorable outcome in all the biochemical, cell culture and AD transgenic models, have failed to show efficacy in human clinical trials [23, 87]. A possible explanation for these failures is the limitation of AD transgenic mouse model to fully recapitulate human AD pathology including Aβ-driven NFT and clear neurodegeneration as we discussed earlier.

One of the interesting applications of 3D human neural cell culture models of AD is to use them as a drug-screening platform to accelerate AD drug discovery. 3D culture models of AD can suitably supplement the current drug-development pipeline by providing additional model systems to cross-check the impact of candidate drugs on AD pathogenesis in human brain-like environment (Fig. 2). 3D culture models of AD are also relatively cheaper and faster (6–10 weeks for our 3D culture model; 12 weeks for 3D organoid models) as compared to AD transgenic mouse model. Therefore, they can be easily added to the current drug-development process (Fig. 2). Cross-checking AD drug

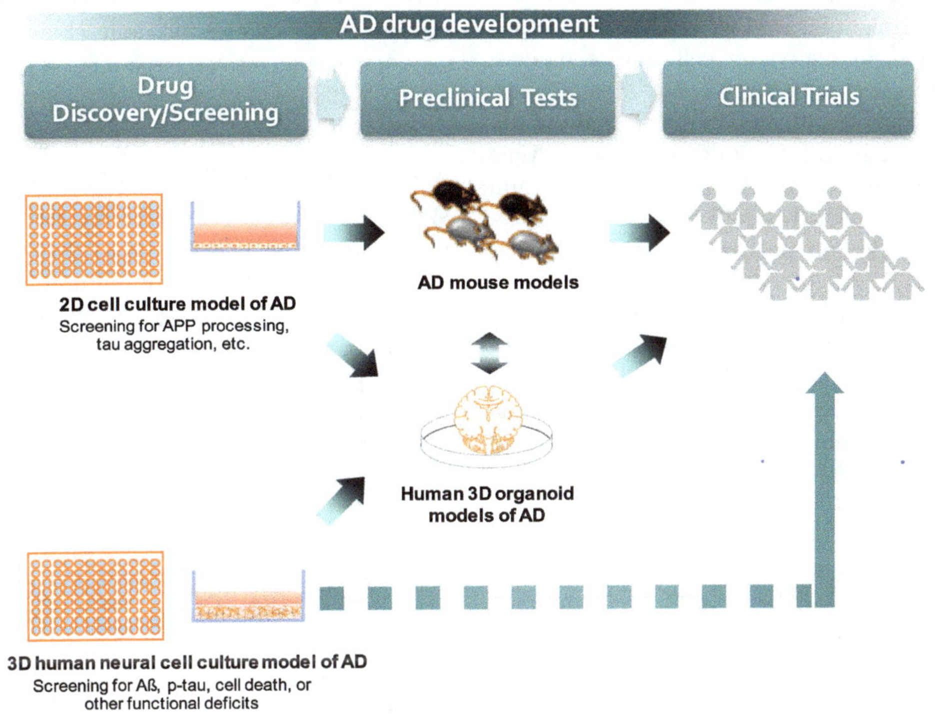

Fig. 2 Platform for AD drug screening in a 3D human neural cell culture model of AD. Typically, discovery of new AD drugs goes through three steps: Development and screening drugs in conventional 2D cell culture models of AD (Drug Discovery/Screening); followed by confirming the effects of drugs in AD transgenic mouse models (Preclinical Tests); and after their effects were confirmed both in cell culture and mouse models, drugs are further tested in humans (Clinical Trials). As compared to the conventional 2D cell cultures and animal models, 3D human cell culture models of AD can be more cost-effective and less time-consuming in developing novel AD drugs

targets in both human and mouse based models will be helpful to minimize chance of failure in human clinical trials [17, 23]. In addition to the impact on AD pathology, 3D human cellular models can also provide information regarding human-specific toxicity and/or potential side-effects. For some of the candidate drugs that are targeting Aβ driven tau pathology, 3D culture models can be the primary system to assess the efficacy of the drug (Fig. 2).

The most exciting application of the 3D culture models of AD is the unbiased, high-throughput screening (HTS) of new AD drugs in a human brain-like environment (Fig. 2). HTS allows rapid and parallel testing of thousands of compounds in a short time, which is not feasible with AD transgenic mouse models due to their high-maintenance, cost and time-consuming nature. We have previously shown that our Matrigel-based 3D culture model can be easily adapted to HTS formats including 96-well and even in 384-well culture systems [31]. The immortalized and single-clonal ReN cells in our 3D cultures also fit well for large-scale, HTS studies due to their rapid proliferation and stability over multiple passages [17]. Both ELISA and automated immunofluorescence microscopy can be used for measuring AD pathologies in HTS format [31]. Using validated drug libraries like FDA-approved drugs, we can dramatically save time by minimizing the new animal tests since they had already been validated for their toxicity in mouse and human models (Fig. 2). 3D organoids models of AD might be also used to cross-check AD drug targets screened from 3D HTS [53] (Fig. 2).

Challenges and perspectives

While many advances have been made, challenges still lie ahead to create comprehensive 3D human culture models for AD drug testing and screening. Although our current 3D culture models have successfully recapitulated the AD pathogenic cascades, the overexpression of FAD genes in our 3D culture system, may add additional artificial pathologies, as shown in AD transgenic mouse models [88]. Lack of functional tests such as behavior assessments, is another disadvantage of the current human 3D culture models. Therefore, immediate application of these culture models of AD may be limited to early stage drug development, possibly replacing in vitro cell culture models and conventional cell based HTS assays. The outcome from 3D neuronal HTS assays should provide better predictions of the pharmacokinetic-pharmacodynamic relationship in animal and human trials.

The limited protocols for differentiating forebrain neurons and glial cells might be another technical challenge for reconstituting brain regions in cell culture models, which were mostly affected in AD [17, 31]. Most 2D culture models could not recapitulate complex brain structures and inflammatory components, such as multiple neuronal layer systems, the blood-brain-barrier and microglial components, which would make it hard to assess pharmacodynamic and pharmacokinetic properties that animal models do. In particular, recent studies clearly showed that brain inflammatory components and blood-brain-barrier system play important roles in AD pathogenesis [89–92]. Adoption of advanced cell culture technology, including hydrogel-based 3D culture models, cerebral organoids and microfluidic systems (i.e., organ-on-chip) will be crucial to recapitulating functional brain structures with multiple cell types [17, 32, 76, 86, 93–96].

The 3D organoids models of AD do not rely on the overexpression of FAD genes and have advantages in recapitulating organized brain structures with multiple neural cell types. However, the 3D organoids models of AD might not be suitable for HTS in the current forms due to their well-known heterogeneity [86, 93] and the requirement for longer drug treatments (30–60 days). As we discussed, these 3D organoids models may successfully complement animal preclinical testing (Fig. 2).

The flexible scalability and the use of single-clonal human stem cell lines, which showed rapid and robust AD pathologies, made it easy to fit our Matrigel-based 3D culture model into HTS AD drug screening [17, 31]. However, the use of heterogeneous Matrigel with under-defined and complex protein components, may cause variability for drug testing [70, 97]. Natural hydrogels based on simple extracellular matrix protein components may be potential alternatives for Matrigel [76, 98, 99]. Synthetic hydrogels generally provide much better matrix uniformity and reproducibility than natural hydrogels [94, 100–102]. Further studies will be needed if these synthetic hydrogels can be applicable in 3D human neural cell culture models of AD and the drug testing.

Conclusions

Developing disease models that fully mirror all, at least key, aspects of the disease is important to understand the disease and ultimately to find cure for it. In AD research, various in vitro 2D cell cultures and animal models, mostly transgenic mouse models, have been widely used. Although they have enormously contributed to AD research, unfortunately, none of these models have successfully reproduced the disease progression found in human AD patients. Recently, we have developed a 3D human neural cell culture model of AD, in which human neural progenitors expressing FAD mutations are grown and differentiated in 3D culture system, which mimics the brain environment [31, 32]. In our 3D culture system, but not in 2D, these neurons successfully generated extracellular aggregation of Aβ and tauopathy driven by the Aβ accumulation, which was not feasible in AD transgenic mouse models. Recently studies also showed that 3D organoids cultures were successfully adapted to accelerate AD pathogenesis in iPSC-derived AD neural cultures. These exciting 3D human cell culture models of AD will serve to facilitate the development of more precise human cellular models of AD for basic mechanistic studies and contribute to the discovery of novel AD drugs.

Abbreviations

2D: Two-dimensional; 3D: Three-dimensional; AD: Alzheimer's disease; APP: Amyloid precursor protein; Aβ: β-Amyloid; FAD: Familial Alzheimer's disease; hNPCs: Human neural progenitor cells; HTS: High-throughput screening; NFT: Neurofibrillary tangle; PSEN: Presenilin; ReN: ReNcell VM; SAD: Sporadic Alzheimer's disease

Acknowledgements

We would also like to thank Drs. Weiming Xia (BU), Daniel Irimia (MGH) and Stephan Wong (Texas Methodist Hospital) for the helpful discussion regarding the human iPSC technology and 3D organoid models.

Funding

This work is supported by the grants from the Cure Alzheimer's fund to D. Y. K., S. H. C. and R. E. T., National Institute of Health (1RF1AG048080-01, D.Y.K. and R.E.T.; 5P01AG15379, D.Y.K. and R.E.T.; 2R01AG014713, D.Y.K.; 5R37MH060009, R.E.T.), BrightFocus Foundation (D.Y.K.) and National Research Foundation of Korea (NRF) grant funded by the Korea government (MSIP) (2016R1A2B4015694, 2015M3A9C7030151, and 2016R1A5A2921654, Y.H.K.) and by the KBSI research grant (T36416, Y.H.K.).

Authors' contributions

SHC, YHK, and DYK mainly contributed to writing the manuscript. LQ partially contribute to "drug discovery section" and DYK and RET supervised the manuscript. All authors read and approved the final manuscript.

Authors' information

Information for all the co-authors are listed in the title page.

Competing interests

The authors declare that they have no competing interests.

Author details

[1]Genetics and Aging Research Unit, MassGeneral Institute for Neurodegenerative Disease, Massachusetts General Hospital, Harvard Medical School, 02129 Charlestown, MA, USA. [2]Biomedical Omics Group, Korea Basic Science Institute, Cheongju-si, Chungbuk 363-883, Republic of Korea.

References

1. Tanzi RE, Bertram L. Twenty years of the Alzheimer's disease amyloid hypothesis: a genetic perspective. Cell. 2005;120:545–55.

2. Tanzi RE. A brief history of Alzheimer's disease gene discovery. J Alzheimers Dis. 2013;33 Suppl 1:S5–13.
3. Bertram L, Tanzi RE. Thirty years of Alzheimer's disease genetics: the implications of systematic meta-analyses. Nat Rev Neurosci. 2008;9:768–78.
4. Alzheimer's Association. 2015 Alzheimer's disease facts and figures. Alzheimers Dement. 2015;11:332–84.
5. Karran E, De Strooper B. The amyloid cascade hypothesis: are we poised for success or failure?. J Neurochem. 2016;139(Suppl 2):237–52.
6. Cutler N, Sramek J. Review of the next generation of Alzheimer's disease therapeutics: challenges for drug development. Prog Neuropsychopharmacol Biol Psychiatry. 2001;25:27–57.
7. Selkoe D. Alzheimer's disease: genes, proteins, and therapy. Physiol Rev. 2001;81:741–66.
8. Selkoe DJ, Hardy J. The amyloid hypothesis of Alzheimer's disease at 25 years. EMBO Mol Med EMBO Press. 2016;8:595–608.
9. Götz J, Ittner LM. Animal models of Alzheimer's disease and frontotemporal dementia. Nat Rev Neurosci. 2008;9:532–44.
10. Iqbal K, Liu F, Gong C-X, Grundke-Iqbal I. Tau in Alzheimer disease and related tauopathies. Curr Alzheimer Res NIH Public Access. 2010;7:656–64.
11. Trojanowski JQ, Lee VM-Y. The role of tau in Alzheimer's disease. Med Clin North Am. 2002;86:615–27.
12. Lee VMY, Lee VM-Y, Brunden KR, Brunden KR, Hutton M, Hutton M, et al. Developing therapeutic approaches to tau, selected kinases, and related neuronal protein targets. Cold Spring Harb Perspect Med. 2011;1:a006437–7.
13. Ballatore C, Lee VM-Y, Trojanowski JQ. Tau-mediated neurodegeneration in Alzheimer's disease and related disorders. Nat Rev Neurosci. 2007;8:663–72.
14. Chin J. Selecting a mouse model of Alzheimer's disease. Methods Mol Biol. 2011;670:169–89.
15. Armstrong RA. A critical analysis of the "amyloid cascade hypothesis". Folia Neuropathol. 2014;52(3):211–25.
16. Duff K, Rao MV. Progress in the modeling of neurodegenerative diseases in transgenic mice. Curr Opin Neurol. 2001;14:441–7.
17. D'Avanzo C, Aronson J, Kim YH, Choi SH, Tanzi RE, Kim DY. Alzheimer's in 3D culture: challenges and perspectives. Bioessays. 2015;37:1139–48.
18. Choi SH, Kim YH, D'Avanzo C, Aronson J, Tanzi RE, Kim DY. Recapitulating amyloid β and tau pathology in human neural cell culture models: clinical implications. US Neurology. 2015;11:102–5.
19. Hardy J. The amyloid hypothesis of Alzheimer's disease: progress and problems on the road to therapeutics. Science. 2002;297:353–6.
20. Selkoe D. Alzheimer's disease is a synaptic failure. Science. 2002;298:789–91.
21. Benilova I, Karran E, De Strooper B. The toxic Aβ oligomer and Alzheimer's disease: an emperor in need of clothes. Nat Neurosci. 2012;15:349–57.
22. Karran E, Mercken M, Strooper BD, De Strooper B. The amyloid cascade hypothesis for Alzheimer's disease: an appraisal for the development of therapeutics. Nat Rev Drug Discov. 2011;10:698–712.
23. De Strooper B. Lessons from a failed γ-secretase Alzheimer trial. Cell. 2014; 159:721–6.
24. Henley DB, Sundell KL, Sethuraman G, Dowsett SA, May PC. Safety profile of semagacestat, a gamma-secretase inhibitor: IDENTITY trial findings. Curr Med Res Opin. 2014;30:2021–32.
25. Moore S, Evans LDB, Andersson T, Portelius E, Smith J, Dias TB, et al. APP metabolism regulates tau proteostasis in human cerebral cortex neurons. Cell Rep. 2015;11:689–96.
26. Sproul AA, Sproul AA, Jacob S, Jacob S, Pre D, Pre D, et al. Characterization and molecular profiling of PSEN1 familial Alzheimer's disease iPSC-derived neural progenitors. PLoS ONE. 2014;9:e84547. Borchelt DR.
27. Woodruff G, Young JE, Martinez FJ, Buen F, Gore A, Kinaga J, et al. The presenilin-1 ΔE9 mutation results in reduced γ-secretase activity, but not total loss of PS1 function, in isogenic human stem cells. Cell Rep. 2013;5:974–85.
28. Koch P, Tamboli IY, Mertens J, Wunderlich P, Ladewig J, Stüber K, et al. Presenilin-1 L166P mutant human pluripotent stem cell–derived neurons exhibit partial loss of γ-secretase activity in endogenous amyloid-β generation. Am J Pathol. 2012;180:2404–16.
29. Muratore CR, Rice HC, Srikanth P, Callahan DG, Shin T, Benjamin LNP, et al. The familial Alzheimer's disease APPV717I mutation alters APP processing and Tau expression in iPSC-derived neurons. Hum Mol Genet. 2014;23:3523–36.
30. Hu W, Hu W, Qiu B, Qiu B, Guan W, Guan W, et al. Direct conversion of normal and alzheimer's disease human fibroblasts into neuronal cells by small molecules. Cell Stem Cell. 2015;17:204–12.
31. Kim YH, Bylykbashi E, Washicosky KJ. A 3D human neural cell culture system for modeling Alzheimer's disease. Nat Protoc. 2015;10:985–1006.
32. Choi SH, Kim YH, Hebisch M, Sliwinski C, Lee S, D'Avanzo C, et al. A three-dimensional human neural cell culture model of Alzheimer's disease. Nature. 2014;515:274–8.
33. Glenner GG, Wong CW. Alzheimer's disease: initial report of the purification and characterization of a novel cerebrovascular amyloid protein. Biochem Biophys Res Commun. 1984;120:885–90.
34. Hardy JA, Higgins GA. Alzheimer's disease: the amyloid cascade hypothesis. Science. 1992;256:184–5.
35. Oddo S, Caccamo A, Shepherd JD, Murphy MP, Golde TE, Kayed R, et al. Triple-transgenic model of Alzheimer's disease with plaques and tangles: intracellular Abeta and synaptic dysfunction. Neuron. 2003;39:409–21. 2003rd ed.
36. Ando K, Leroy K, Héraud C, Yilmaz Z, Authelet M, Suain V, et al. Accelerated human mutant tau aggregation by knocking out murine tau in a transgenic mouse model. Am J Pathol. 2011;178:803–16.
37. Mohamet L, Miazga NJ, Ward CM. Familial Alzheimer's disease modelling using induced pluripotent stem cell technology. WJSC. 2014;6:239–47.
38. Duan L, Bhattacharyya BJ, Belmadani A, Pan L, Miller RJ, Kessler JA. Stem cell derived basal forebrain cholinergic neurons from Alzheimer's disease patients are more susceptible to cell death. Mol Neurodegener. 2014;9:3. BioMed Central Ltd.
39. Kondo T, Asai M, Tsukita K, Kutoku Y, Ohsawa Y, Sunada Y, et al. Modeling Alzheimer's disease with iPSCs reveals stress phenotypes associated with intracellular aβ and differential drug responsiveness. Cell Stem Cell. 2013;12:487–96.
40. Israel MA, Israel MA, Yuan SH, Yuan SH, Bardy C, Bardy C, et al. Probing sporadic and familial Alzheimer's disease using induced pluripotent stem cells. Nature. 2012;482:216–20.
41. Yagi T, Ito D, Okada Y, Akamatsu W, Nihei Y, Yoshizaki T, et al. Modeling familial Alzheimer's disease with induced pluripotent stem cells. Hum Mol Genet. 2011;20:4530–9.
42. Li T, Pires C, Nielsen TT, Waldemar G, Hjermind LE, Nielsen JE, et al. Generation of induced pluripotent stem cells (iPSCs) from an Alzheimer's disease patient carrying an A79V mutation in PSEN1. Stem Cell Res. 2016;16:229–32.
43. Ochalek A, Nemes C, Varga E, Táncos Z, Kobolák J, Dinnyés A. Establishment of induced pluripotent stem cell (iPSC) line from a 57-year old patient with sporadic Alzheimer's disease. Stem Cell Res. 2016;17:72–4.
44. Chandrasekaran A, Varga E, Nemes C, Táncos Z, Kobolák J, Dinnyés A. Establishment of induced pluripotent stem cell (iPSC) line from a 63-year old patient with late onset Alzheimer's disease (LOAD). Stem Cell Res. 2016; 17:78–80.
45. Táncos Z, Varga E, Kovács E, Dinnyés A, Kobolák J. Establishment of induced pluripotent stem cell (iPSC) line from a 75-year old patient with late onset Alzheimer's disease (LOAD). Stem Cell Res. 2016;17:81–3.
46. Táncos Z, Varga E, Kovács E, Dinnyés A, Kobolák J. Establishment of induced pluripotent stem cell (iPSC) line from an 84-year old patient with late onset Alzheimer's disease (LOAD). Stem Cell Res. 2016;17:75–7.
47. Nemes C, Varga E, Táncos Z, Bock I, Francz B, Kobolák J, et al. Establishment of PSEN1 mutant induced pluripotent stem cell (iPSC) line from an Alzheimer's disease (AD) female patient. Stem Cell Res. 2016;17:69–71.
48. Liu Q, Waltz S, Woodruff G, Ouyang J, Israel MA, Herrera C, et al. Effect of potent γ-secretase modulator in human neurons derived from multiple presenilin 1–induced pluripotent stem cell mutant carriers. NIH Public Access. 2014;71:1481–9.
49. Lee H-K, Velazquez Sanchez C, Chen M, Morin PJ, Wells JM, Hanlon EB, et al. Three dimensional human neuro-spheroid model of Alzheimer's disease based on differentiated induced pluripotent stem cells. PLoS ONE. 2016;11: e0163072. Yan R.
50. Hossini AM, Megges M, Prigione A, Lichtner B, Toliat MR, Wruck W, et al. Induced pluripotent stem cell-derived neuronal cells from a sporadic Alzheimer's disease donor as a model for investigating AD-associated gene regulatory networks. BMC Genomics. 2015;16:84. BioMed Central Ltd.
51. Lee H-K, Morin P, Xia W. Peripheral blood mononuclear cell-converted induced pluripotent stem cells (iPSCs) from an early onset Alzheimer's patient. Stem Cell Res. 2016;16:213–5.
52. Liao M-C, Muratore CR, Gierahn TM, Sullivan SE, Srikanth P, De Jager PL, et al. Single-cell detection of secreted Aβ and sAPPα from human IPSC-derived neurons and astrocytes. J Neurosci. 2016;36:1730–46.
53. Raja WK, Mungenast AE, Lin Y-T, Ko T, Abdurrob F, Seo J, et al. Self-Organizing 3D human neural tissue derived from induced pluripotent stem cells recapitulate Alzheimer's disease phenotypes. PLoS ONE. 2016;11: e0161969. Padmanabhan J.

54. De Strooper B. Loss-of-function presenilin mutations in Alzheimer disease. Talking point on the role of presenilin mutations in Alzheimer disease. EMBO Rep. 2007;8:141–6.
55. Shen J, Kelleher RJ. The presenilin hypothesis of Alzheimer's disease: evidence for a loss-of-function pathogenic mechanism. Proc Natl Acad Sci U S A. 2007;104:403–9.
56. Paquet D, Kwart D, Chen A, Sproul A, Jacob S, Teo S, et al. Efficient introduction of specific homozygous and heterozygous mutations using CRISPR/Cas9. Nature. 2016;533:125–9.
57. Shi Y, Kirwan P, Smith J, MacLean G, Orkin SH, Livesey FJ. A human stem cell model of early alzheimer's disease pathology in down syndrome. Sci Transl Med. 2012;4:124ra29–9.
58. Iovino M, Agathou S, González-Rueda A, Del Castillo Velasco-Herrera M, Borroni B, Alberici A, et al. Early maturation and distinct tau pathology in induced pluripotent stem cell-derived neurons from patients with MAPT mutations. Brain. 2015;138:3345–59.
59. Ehrlich M, Hallmann A-L, Reinhardt P, Araúzo-Bravo MJ, Korr S, Röpke A, et al. Distinct neurodegenerative changes in an induced pluripotent stem cell model of frontotemporal dementia linked to mutant TAU protein. Stem Cell Reports. 2015;5:83–96.
60. Wren MC, Zhao J, Liu C-C, Murray ME, Atagi Y, Davis MD, et al. Frontotemporal dementia-associated N279K tau mutant disrupts subcellular vesicle trafficking and induces cellular stress in iPSC-derived neural stem cells. Mol Neurodegener. 2015;10:46.
61. Vassar R. BACE1 inhibitor drugs in clinical trials for Alzheimer's disease. Alzheimers Res Ther. 2014;6:89.
62. Yan R. Stepping closer to treating Alzheimer's disease patients with BACE1 inhibitor drugs. Transl Neurodegener. 2016;5:13.
63. Yan R, Fan Q, Zhou J, Vassar R. Inhibiting BACE1 to reverse synaptic dysfunctions in Alzheimer's disease. Neurosci Biobehav Rev. 2016;65: 326–40.
64. Falk A, Koch P, Kesavan J, Takashima Y, Ladewig J, Alexander M, et al. Capture of neuroepithelial-like stem cells from pluripotent stem cells provides a versatile system for in vitro production of human neurons. PLoS ONE. 2012;7:e29597. Pera M.
65. Wang J, Dickson DW, Trojanowski JQ, Lee VM. The levels of soluble versus insoluble brain Abeta distinguish Alzheimer's disease from normal and pathologic aging. Exp Neurol. 1999;158:328–37.
66. Sposito T, Preza E, Mahoney CJ, Setó-Salvia N, Ryan NS, Morris HR, et al. Developmental regulation of tau splicing is disrupted in stem cell-derived neurons from frontotemporal dementia patients with the 10 + 16 splice-site mutation in MAPT. Hum Mol Genet. 2015;24:5260–9. Oxford University Press.
67. D'Souza I, Schellenberg GD. Regulation of tau isoform expression and dementia. Biochim Biophys Acta. 2005;1739:104–15.
68. Gasparini L, Terni B, Spillantini MG. Frontotemporal dementia with tau pathology. Neurodegener Dis. 2007;4:236–53. Karger Publishers.
69. Donato R, Miljan EA, Hines SJ, Aouabdi S, Pollock K, Patel S, et al. Differential development of neuronal physiological responsiveness in two human neural stem cell lines. BMC Neurosci. 2007;8:36.
70. Hughes CS, Postovit LM, Lajoie GA. Matrigel: a complex protein mixture required for optimal growth of cell culture. Proteomics. 2010;10:1886–90.
71. Ortinau S, Ortinau S, Schmich J, Schmich J, Block S, Block S, et al. Effect of 3D-scaffold formation on differentiation and survival in human neural progenitor cells. BioMed Eng OnLine. 2010;9:70.
72. LaPlaca MC, Vernekar VN, Shoemaker JT, Cullen DK. Three-Dimensional Neuronal Cultures. In: Morgan JR, Berthiaume F, editors. Methods in bioengineering: 3D tissue engineering. methods in bioengineering: 3D tissue engineering. 2010. p. 187–204.
73. Suga H, Suga H, Kadoshima T, Kadoshima T, Minaguchi M, Minaguchi M, et al. Self-formation of functional adenohypophysis in three-dimensional culture. Nature. 2011;480:57–62.
74. Li H, Li H, Wijekoon A, Wijekoon A, Leipzig ND, Leipzig ND. 3D differentiation of neural stem cells in macroporous photopolymerizable hydrogel scaffolds. PLoS ONE. 2012;7:e48824. Gelain F.
75. Liedmann A, Liedmann A, Frech S, Frech S, Morgan PJ, Morgan PJ, et al. Differentiation of human neural progenitor cells in functionalized hydrogel matrices. BioResearch Open Access. 2012;1:16–24.
76. Tang-Schomer MD, White JD, Tien LW, Schmitt LI, Valentin TM, Graziano DJ, et al. Bioengineered functional brain-like cortical tissue. Proc Natl Acad Sci U S A. 2014;111:13811–6.
77. Onorato M, Mulvihill P, Connolly J, Galloway P, Whitehouse P, Perry G. Alteration of neuritic cytoarchitecture in Alzheimer disease. Prog Clin Biol Res. 1989;317:781–9.
78. Sharoar MG, Shi Q, Ge Y, He W, Hu X, Perry G, et al. Dysfunctional tubular endoplasmic reticulum constitutes a pathological feature of Alzheimer's disease. Molecular Psychiatry. 2016;21:1263–71. Nature Publishing Group.
79. Sadleir KR, Kandalepas PC, Buggia-Prévot V, Nicholson DA, Thinakaran G, Vassar R. Presynaptic dystrophic neurites surrounding amyloid plaques are sites of microtubule disruption, BACE1 elevation, and increased Aβ generation in Alzheimer's disease. Acta Neuropathologica. 2016;132:235–56. Springer Berlin Heidelberg.
80. Sanchez-Varo R, Trujillo-Estrada L, Sanchez-Mejias E, Torres M, Baglietto-Vargas D, Moreno-Gonzalez I, et al. Abnormal accumulation of autophagic vesicles correlates with axonal and synaptic pathology in young Alzheimer's mice hippocampus. Acta Neuropathologica. 2012;123:53–70. Springer-Verlag.
81. Woodhouse A, Vickers JC, Adlard PA, Dickson TC. Dystrophic neurites in TgCRND8 and Tg2576 mice mimic human pathological brain aging. Neurobiol Aging. 2009;30:864–74.
82. Bell KFS, de Kort GJL, Steggerda S, Shigemoto R, Ribeiro-da-Silva A, Cuello AC. Structural involvement of the glutamatergic presynaptic boutons in a transgenic mouse model expressing early onset amyloid pathology. Neurosci Lett. 2003;353:143–7.
83. Blanchard V, Moussaoui S, Czech C, Touchet N, Bonici B, Planche M, et al. Time sequence of maturation of dystrophic neurites associated with Abeta deposits in APP/PS1 transgenic mice. Exp Neurol. 2003;184:247–63.
84. Uchida Y, Gomi F. The role of calsyntenin-3 in dystrophic neurite formation in Alzheimer's disease brain. Geriatr Gerontol Int. 2016;16 Suppl 1:43–50.
85. Hu X, Shi Q, Zhou X, He W, Yi H, Yin X, et al. Transgenic mice overexpressing reticulon 3 develop neuritic abnormalities. EMBO J. 2007;26: 2755–67.
86. Lancaster MA, Renner M, Martin C-A, Wenzel D, Bicknell LS, Hurles ME, et al. Cerebral organoids model human brain development and microcephaly. Nature. 2013;501:373–9.
87. Orgogozo J-M, Gilman S, Dartigues J-F, Laurent B, Puel M, Kirby LC, et al. Subacute meningoencephalitis in a subset of patients with AD after Abeta42 immunization. Neurology. 2003;61:46–54.
88. Saito T, Matsuba Y, Mihira N, Takano J, Nilsson P, Itohara S, et al. Single App knock-in mouse models of Alzheimer's disease. Nat Neurosci. 2014;17:661–3.
89. Hong S, Beja-Glasser VF, Nfonoyim BM, Frouin A, Li S, Ramakrishnan S, et al. Complement and microglia mediate early synapse loss in Alzheimer mouse models. Science. 2016;352:712–6.
90. Chung W-S, Verghese PB, Chakraborty C, Joung J, Hyman BT, Ulrich JD, et al. Novel allele-dependent role for APOE in controlling the rate of synapse pruning by astrocytes. Proc Natl Acad Sci U S A. 2016;113:10186–91.
91. Montagne A, Barnes SR, Sweeney MD, Halliday MR, Sagare AP, Zhao Z, et al. Blood-brain barrier breakdown in the aging human hippocampus. Neuron. 2015;85:296–302.
92. Zhao Z, Sagare AP, Ma Q, Halliday MR, Kong P, Kisler K, et al. Central role for PICALM in amyloid-β blood-brain barrier transcytosis and clearance. Nat Neurosci. 2015;18:978–87.
93. Bershteyn M, Kriegstein AR. Cerebral organoids in a dish: progress and prospects. Cell. 2013;155:19–20.
94. Verhulsel M, Vignes M, Descroix S, Malaquin L, Vignjevic DM, Viovy J-L. A review of microfabrication and hydrogel engineering for micro-organs on chips. Biomaterials. 2014;35:1816–32.
95. Moreno EL, Hachi S, Hemmer K, Trietsch SJ, Baumuratov AS, Hankemeier T, et al. Differentiation of neuroepithelial stem cells into functional dopaminergic neurons in 3D microfluidic cell culture. Lab Chip. 2015;15:2419–28.
96. Adriani G, Ma D, Pavesi A, Goh ELK, Kamm RD. Modeling the blood-brain barrier in a 3D triple co-culture microfluidic system. Conf Proc IEEE Eng Med Biol Soc IEEE. 2015;2015:338–41.
97. Kleinman HK, McGarvey ML, Liotta LA, Robey PG, Tryggvason K, Martin GR. Isolation and characterization of type IV procollagen, laminin, and heparan sulfate proteoglycan from the EHS sarcoma. Biochemistry. 1982;21:6188–93.
98. Bozza A, Coates EE, Incitti T, Ferlin KM, Messina A, Menna E, et al. Neural differentiation of pluripotent cells in 3D alginate-based cultures. Biomaterials. 2014;35:4636–45.
99. Pellett S, Schwartz MP, Tepp WH, Josephson R, Scherf JM, Pier CL, et al. Human induced pluripotent stem cell derived neuronal cells cultured on chemically-defined hydrogels for sensitive in vitro detection of botulinum neurotoxin. Sci Rep. 2015;5:14566. Nature Publishing Group.

100. Shao Y, Sang J, Fu J. On human pluripotent stem cell control: the rise of 3D bioengineering and mechanobiology. Biomaterials. 2015;52:26–43.
101. Krutty JD, Schmitt SK, Gopalan P, Murphy WL. Surface functionalization and dynamics of polymeric cell culture substrates. Curr Opin Biotechnol. 2016;40:164–9.
102. Lee J, Cuddihy MJ, Kotov NA. Three-dimensional cell culture matrices: state of the art. Tissue Eng Part B Rev. 2008;14:61–86. Mary Ann Liebert, Inc. 140 Huguenot Street, 3rd Floor New Rochelle, NY 10801 USA.

7

Vitamin D interacts with Esr1 and Igf1 to regulate molecular pathways relevant to Alzheimer's disease

Véréna Landel[1], Pascal Millet[1,2], Kévin Baranger[1], Béatrice Loriod[3] and François Féron[1*]

Abstract

Background: Increasing evidence suggests a potential therapeutic benefit of vitamin D supplementation against Alzheimer's disease (AD). Although studies have shown improvements in cognitive performance and decreases in markers of the pathology after chronic treatment, the mechanisms by which vitamin D acts on brain cells are multiple and remain to be thoroughly studied. We analyzed the molecular changes observed after 5 months of vitamin D3 supplementation in the brains of transgenic 5xFAD (Tg) mice, a recognized mouse model of AD, and their wild type (Wt) littermates. We first performed a kinematic behavioural examination at 4, 6 and 8 months of age (M4, M6 and M8) followed by a histologic assessment of AD markers. We then performed a comparative transcriptomic analysis of mRNA regulation in the neocortex and hippocampus of 9 months old (M9) female mice.

Results: Transcriptomic analysis of the hippocampus and neocortex of both Wt and Tg mice at M9, following 5 months of vitamin D3 treatment, reveals a large panel of dysregulated pathways related to i) immune and inflammatory response, ii) neurotransmitter activity, iii) endothelial and vascular processes and iv) hormonal alterations. The differentially expressed genes are not all direct targets of the vitamin D-VDR pathway and it appears that vitamin D action engages in the crosstalk with estrogen and insulin signaling. The misexpression of the large number of genes observed in this study translates into improved learning and memory performance and a decrease in amyloid plaques and astrogliosis in Tg animals.

Conclusions: This study underlies the multiplicity of action of this potent neurosteroid in an aging and AD-like brain. The classical and non-classical actions of vitamin D3 can act in an additive and possibly synergistic manner to induce neuroprotective activities in a context-specific way.

Keywords: Vitamin D, Alzheimer's disease, Transcriptome, Nervous system, Inflammatory response, Hormonal activity

Background

The world is currently facing a global Alzheimer's disease (AD) pandemic and there is an urgent necessity to find drugs that can halt, or even better, cure this pathology. Clinicians and researchers are actively looking for molecules with neuro-protective, regenerative and immunomodulatory properties [1]. Preferably, to speed up their delivery to AD patients, the selected compounds should be FDA-approved with a well-known toxicity range.

With the intention of unveiling new molecular candidates, we elected a recognized animal model for this disease, namely the 5XFAD transgenic mice [2], that exhibit mnesic deficits, increased Amyloid Precursor Protein (APP) processing and an early onset for inflammation and plaque formation [3]. We timely assessed gene misexpression in the hippocampus and neocortex of 5XFAD female mice at presymptomatic, prodromal-like and symptomatic stages of the pathology. As expected, we observed a dysregulated expression of genes involved in inflammation, NADPH oxidase complex, phagocytic processes and interferon-γ-related pathways [4]. Remarkably, we also found a modulated expression of 784 vitamin D-associated transcripts (Additional file 1).

Vitamin D3 is a fat-soluble and seco-steroid hormone. Unlike other vitamins, vitamin D3 is mainly produced after adequate exposure to sunlight. Where this exposure

* Correspondence: francois.feron@univ-amu.fr
[1]Aix Marseille Université, CNRS, NICN UMR 7259, Marseille 13916, France
Full list of author information is available at the end of the article

is lacking, dietary intake of vitamin D (vitamin D2 or vitamin D3) is required. The epidermis contains a cholesterol metabolite that under ultraviolet light produces a precursor, previtamin D3. After isomerization and two separate hydroxylations, the active 1,25-dihydroxyvitamin D3 (1,25(OH)2D3 or calcitriol) is produced. 1,25(OH)2D3 operates *via* both nuclear receptors named Vitamin D Receptor (VDR) (part of the superfamily of steroid hormone receptors) and non-genomic systems. The 1,25(OH)2D3/VDR complex interacts with specific genomic sequences named Vitamin D Responsive Elements (VDRE) found in promoter regions and has been shown to regulate the transcription of a large number (up to 1000) of target genes [5, 6].

Epidemiological and clinical data have shown that i) high serum levels of 25-hydroxyvitamin D (25(OH)D) associate with better cognitive test performance [7, 8] and ii) vitamin D deficiency is found in patients with Alzheimer's disease [9–13]. Other studies reported i) associations between VDR polymorphisms and cognitive function in Alzheimer's disease patients [14–19] and ii) decreased VDR mRNA levels in the hippocampus of AD patients [20].

1,25(OH)2D3 has also been shown to i) enhance cerebral clearance of human Amyloid Beta (Aβ) peptide from mouse brain across the blood–brain barrier [21], ii) prevent Aβ-induced alterations in cortical neurons through upregulation of the VDR and downregulation of L-type voltage sensitive calcium channels [22, 23]. Experimental observations confirmed that i) vitamin D deficiency increases spatial learning deficits in a rat model of AD [24] likely by enhancing Aβ deposition through modulation of amyloid processing [25] and ii) vitamin D3 supplementation decreases pathological markers of the disease, such as Aβ deposition, in a transgenic mouse model [26]. However, relatively little is known about the mechanisms of action of this steroid hormone in demented brains.

Purposely, we assessed the therapeutic benefit of vitamin D3 in 5XFAD mice, supplemented after the onset of the symptoms, from month 4 (M4) to month 9 (M9). Along the course of the disease, we measured memory abilities and, at the end of the experiment, we quantified amyloid plaque load. In addition, using pangenomic cDNA microarrays and bioinformatic tools, we identified the genes that were regulated, directly or indirectly, by a vitamin D3 intervention. This study is the first to provide insight into the molecular mechanisms at play after chronic treatment with vitamin D3 in both healthy aging and AD-like brains.

Results

Vitamin D3 supplementation induces an extensive gene dysregulation

To reveal the potential molecular targets of vitamin D3 in specific brain regions, we conducted a series of transcriptomic experiments. The study allowed a comparison of dysregulated genes and associated molecular pathways affected by vitamin D3 supplementation in both a non-AD and AD context, *i.e.* Wild-type (Wt) versus Transgenic (Tg) animals. Figure 1 reveals the total number of transcripts affected in Wt or Tg animals after 5 months of vitamin D3 supplementation. A total of 2211 genes are dysregulated in Wt animals in both the hippocampus and cortex combined, compared to a total of 1277 Differentially Expressed Genes (DEGs) in Tg mice after vitamin D3 treatment (Fig. 1a). Vitamin D3 supplementation induces a dysregulation of nearly twice as many genes in Wt animals as compared to Tg. Details about these DEGs are given in Additional file 2. There is no significant difference in terms of the number of upregulated or downregulated genes in both genotypes and brain regions (Fig. 1a). When considering each brain area analyzed, there is little difference in the number of dysregulated genes for a given genotype (Fig. 1b). In Wt mice, about 10 % of DEGs are common to both tissues while 13 % shared DEGs can be observed in Tg animals (Fig. 1b). Interestingly, a number of DEGs are common to both genotypes in both brain areas (Fig. 1c). Up to 366 genes are commonly dysregulated after vitamin D3 treatment in both Wt and Tg mice (Fig. 1d). Using Ingenuity Pathway Analysis (IPA) software, the clustering of the 366 genes indicates that among the top canonical pathways, the ones displaying the largest number of DEGs are: Axon guidance signaling (13 genes), Protein kinase A signaling (13), ILK signaling (9), Huntington's disease signaling (9), Glioblastoma Multiform signaling (8), Cdc42 signaling (8), IL8 signaling (8), Agranulocyte adhesion and diapedesis (8), Tight junction signaling (7), Embryonic stem cell pluripotency (6), Corticotropin Releasing Hormone signaling (6), Communication between innate and adaptive immune cells (5), Glutamate receptor signaling (5) and Dopamine receptor signaling (5). Furthermore, 39 out of 366 genes are associated to inflammatory response, 26 to cognition and 25 to Alzheimer's disease (Fig. 1e).

An intriguing expression of hormone transcripts in the cortex and hippocampus

One of the aims of this transcriptomic analysis was to extract information about genes whose expression is modified in the nervous system after 5 months of vitamin D3 supplementation, regardless of the pathological context. One way to obtain such information is to refine the working dataset to include only genes that are commonly dysregulated in all tested conditions. Table 1 shows the list of genes found to be dysregulated in Wt and Tg mice, in both the hippocampus and cortex. In these four conditions, we found 28 DEGs, with varying fold changes according to the genotype and brain region

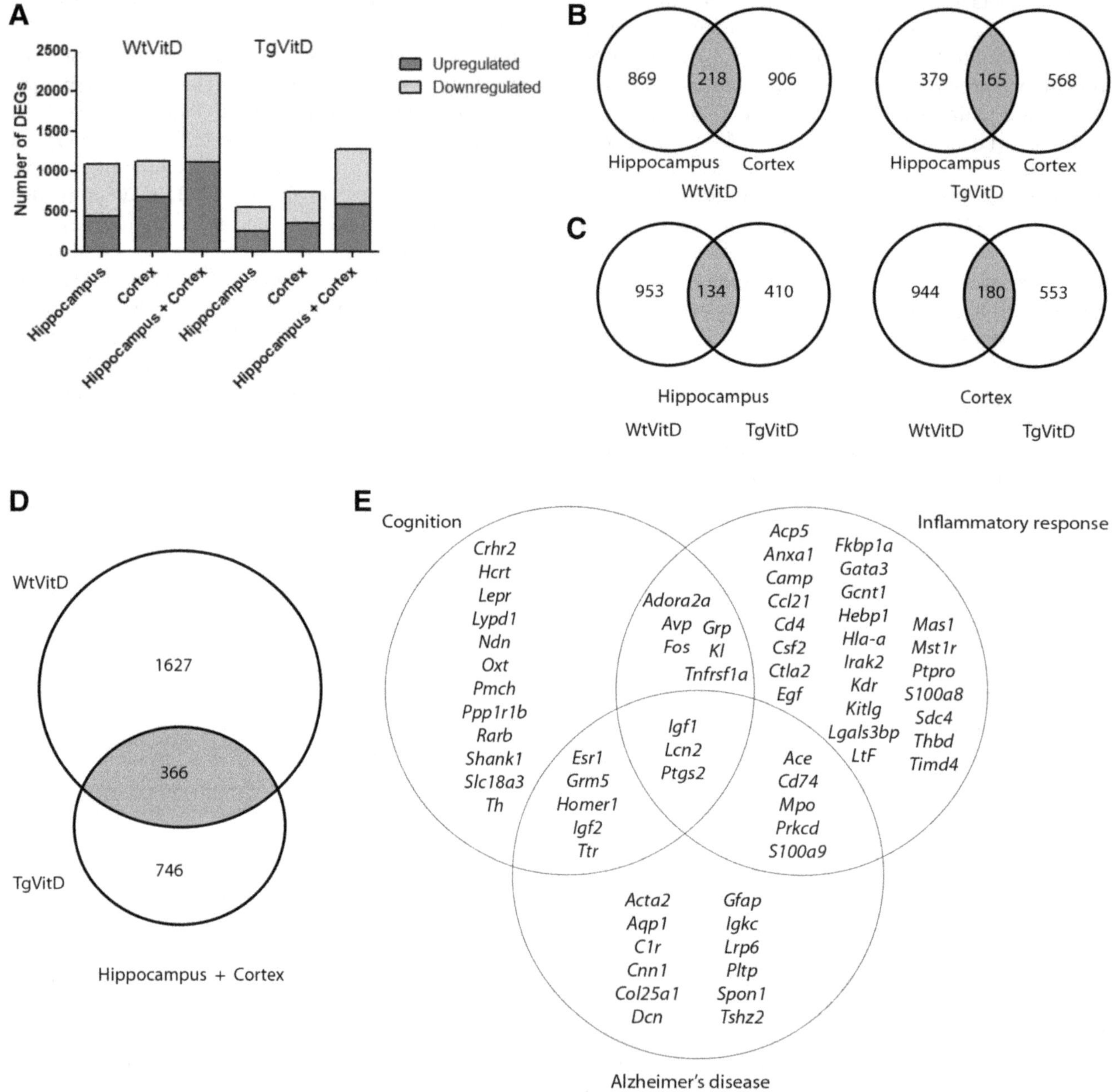

Fig. 1 Schematic overview of gene expression in cortex and hippocampus of 9 month-old wild type and transgenic mice reveals that a 5 month vitamin D3 supplementation induces an extensive transcript dysregulation. **a** Graphical representation of the number of upregulated (*dark grey*) and downregulated (*light grey*) DEGs in either the hippocampus, cortex or combined regions in both Wt and Tg animals having been fed a vitamin D3 diet for 5 months. The number of genes specifically dysregulated in wild type mice is twice as large as in transgenic mice. **b-c** Venn diagrams indicating the number of overlapping (*grey*) and non overlapping DEGs when the two brain areas are compared in wild type and transgenic mice (**b**) and when the two strains are compared at the hippocampal or cortex level (**c**). **d** Venn diagram showing that, when hippocampal and cortical data are combined, vitamin D3 supplementation triggers the dysregulation of 366 genes in both strains. **e** List and top associated biological functions of the 366 DEGs common to both strains. Overall, 39 are associated to inflammatory response, 26 to cognition and 25 to Alzheimer's disease. Fold change (FC) cutoff used for above analyses was -1.5> FC <1.5

studied, that are consistently regulated after 5 months of vitamin D3 supplementation. To gain better sense of the biological functions represented by the differentially expressed genes, we performed a Functional Annotation Clustering using the NIH David tool. This analysis revealed that the genes in this dataset are related to five different biological clusters: regulation of phosphorylation, hormone activity, membrane trafficking, nucleotide binding and metal ion binding. A less restrictive additional analysis was performed on DEGs found in at

Table 1 List of commonly dysregulated genes in the cortex and hippocampus of transgenic and wild type mice

		Fold change			
		Hipocampus		Cortex	
Gene symbol	Entrez gene name	WtVitD/Wt	TgVitD/Tg	WtVitD/Wt	TgVitD/Tg
Ahcy	adenosylhomocysteinase	−1,73	−2,07	1,79	2,07
Atg4c	autophagy related 4C, cysteine peptidase	−2,72	−2,75	4,49	4,82
Avp	arginine vasopressin	−1,59	2,21	1,73	3,96
C130078n14	uncharacterized protein C130078N14	−2,13	−2,17	3,92	2,77
Cdk5rap1	CDK5 regulatory subunit associated protein 1	−1,78	−2,14	2,66	2,92
Cpne1	copine I	−1,56	−1,82	1,6	1,71
Dnajb8	DnaJ (Hsp40) homolog, subfamily B, member 8	−1,85	1,98	−1,92	−1,73
Fam205a	family with sequence similarity 205, member A	2,34	2,78	1,61	−1,55
Fkbp1a	FK506 binding protein 1A, 12kDa	1,97	1,62	−1,72	−1,52
Gbp6	guanylate binding protein family, member 6	2,19	2,21	−2,65	−3,23
Gm4924	predicted gene 4924	1,68	1,94	2,14	1,53
Hla-drb5	major histocompatibility complex, class II, DR beta 5	1,86	1,53	−2,53	−2,34
Iqcf4	IQ motif containing F4	2,74	2,22	−1,54	−1,73
Iqsec3	IQ motif and Sec7 domain 3	−5,23	4,49	−3,3	1,58
Kcnj6	potassium channel, inwardly rectifying subfamily J, member 6	1,61	1,93	−1,79	−1,67
Kdr	kinase insert domain receptor	−1,6	1,68	1,53	−1,64
Mirg	miRNA containing gene	−1,91	1,88	−3,41	−1,68
Nanog	Nanog homeobox	−2,91	1,53	−1,52	−1,66
Ocel1	occludin/ELL domain containing 1	−3,07	−3,98	3,52	3,21
Omp	olfactory marker protein	−1,54	−10,41	3,18	1,66
Oxt	oxytocin/neurophysin I prepropeptide	−2,75	4,04	2,03	4,74
Ppp1r16b	protein phosphatase 1, regulatory subunit 16B	2,29	2,39	−1,78	−1,78
Prkcd	protein kinase C, delta	−2,18	−2,52	1,84	1,65
Prl	prolactin	1,93	−1,88	10,07	10,54
Rnase4	ribonuclease, RNase A family, 4	1,61	2,12	−2,14	−2,07
Sdc4	syndecan 4	2,38	1,95	−1,91	−1,81
Serpina3g	serine (or cysteine) peptidase inhibitor, clade A, member 3G	2,78	1,94	−1,8	−2,42
Znf669	zinc finger protein 669	−2,08	−1,9	1,84	2,2

Dysregulated transcripts in the hippocampus and cortex of vitamin D3 supplemented wild type and transgenic mice in comparison with unsupplemented littermates. The gene symbol, the full name and the fold change of each gene are indicated

least three out of the four conditions. Table 2 represents the top ten biological clusters associated with this dataset. One hundred thirty-six genes were differentially expressed (Additional file 3) and when performing functional annotation clustering of these DEGs, the number one biological function is hormone activity (Table 2). Eight genes fall into this ontological category: *Avp, Igf1, Igf2, Nppa, Oxt, Pmch, Prl, Trh.* Bearing in mind that several of these neuropeptides are largely found in the pituitary axis, it is extremely intriguing to find them differentially expressed in the cortex or hippocampus of 5XFAD mice.

Among the top ten biological pathways affected by vitamin D3 treatment, two of them concern synaptic processes and neurotransmission with dysregulation of genes such as *Syn3, Syt10* and *Sv2c,* while two others are related to immune responses including genes such as *C1qb, Cd4* and *Cd74* (Table 2). A literature search was then performed to determine whether some of these genes contain a putative VDRE in their sequence. Among the 136 genes commonly dysregulated, only four, *Fos, Gcnt1, Irak2, St6galnac1,* were found to present a known functional VDRE in their promoter region [6].

The effects of vitamin D3 supplementation vary according to the health status of the animal

To move further and comprehensively assess the effect of vitamin D on brain functioning, we analyzed the

Table 2 Top ten biological clusters associated with transcripts dysregulated in at least 3 out of 4 conditions: misexpression in the hippocampus and/or cortex of transgenic and/or wild type mice

Annotation term	Number of genes	Genes
Hormone activity	8	*Avp, Igf1, Igf2, Nppa, Oxt, Pmch, Prl, Trh*
Synaptic vesicle	5	*Doc2g, Slc17a6, Syn3, Sv2c, Syt10*
Regulation of phosphorylation	6	*Cd4, Cd74, Cdk5rap1, Fkbp1a, Irak2, Prkcd*
Membrane-bounded vesicle	8	*Capn11, Doc2g, Gpnmb, Prl, Slc17a6, Syn3, Sv2c, Syt10*
Striated muscle tissue development	4	*Fkbp1a, Foxp1, Rxrg, Tnnt2*
Blood circulation	4	*Acta2, Ace, Avp, Nppa*
Lymphocyte activation	4	*Cd4, Cd74, Fkbp1a, Foxp1*
C2 calcium-dependent membrane targeting	4	*Cpne1, Doc2g, Prkcd, Syt10*
Immune effector process	4	*Cd74, C1qb, Foxp1, Prkcd*
Synapse	5	*Shc4, Slc17a6, Syn3, Sv2c, Syt10*

Cluster name, number of genes within each cluster and acronym of each gene are indicated

record of dysregulated genes, in accordance with their role in well-described metabolic pathways. For each strain, we combined transcriptomic data from the hippocampus and the neocortex at M9 and, using Ingenuity software, we listed the main canonical pathways that were modified by the vitamin D3-enriched diet. We then compared the two strains of animals (Wt *vs* Tg). All perturbed pathways and the names of their associated DEGs are recorded in Additional file 4. Out of the 90 major modified canonical pathways, 42 were common to both strains. As shown in Fig. 2, 16 of them are related to either the nervous or the immune system.

In regard to the brain (Fig. 2a), the largest number of dysregulated genes – 53 and 38 for the Wt and Tg animals, respectively – is associated to Axon guidance signaling. Within both strains, we observe a modified expression of growth factors (e.g. *Bdnf, Bmp1, Bmp6, Egf, Igf1, Figf, Ntf3, Vegfc*), chemo-attractive/repulsive agents (e.g. *Sema3b, Sema3c, Sema4g, Sema6b, Sema6c*), proteases (e.g. *Ace, Adam11, Adamts2, Adamts8, Adamts9, Mmp9*) and TGF/WNT/β-catenin-associated molecules (e.g. *Tgfb1, Tgfbr1, Tgfbr2, Wnt1, Wnt3, Wnt6, Wnt9a, Wnt9b, Wnt16*). Two other metabolic pathways - the signaling of the corticotropin releasing hormone and the multiform glioblastoma – include large subsets of dysregulated genes. However, the highest ratio (number of dysregulated genes/number of genes involved in the pathway) is found for the neuroprotective role of THOP1 in Alzheimer's disease.

With respect to the immune system (Fig. 2b), three canonical pathways – Role of macrophages, fibroblasts and endothelial cells in rheumatoid arthritis, Agranulocyte adhesion and diapedesis and Dendritic cell maturation - emerge as primarily affected by vitamin D3 supplementation, in both strains. Other modified metabolic pathways include Communication between innate and adaptive immune cells, Complement system and MIF regulation of innate immunity. Nonetheless, the peak ratios are observed for the Role of Il17F in inflammatory diseases and the role of Il17A in psoriasis.

In addition to this strain independent response to vitamin D3 supplementation, the brains display specific modifications in line with the health status of the animal. For example, vitamin D3-enriched diet modify the expression of glucocorticoid and glutamate receptors in wild type animals and GABA, dopamine and serotonin receptors in transgenic animals (Fig. 2a). Similarly, vitamin D3 alters interleukin signaling in a strain-dependent manner. IL-12 and IL-8 pathways are adjusted in Wt and Tg brains, respectively (Fig. 2b). Other examples of discrepancies can be listed. The non pathological brain responds to vitamin D3 treatment by modifying the expression of i) nitric oxide in macrophages, ii) neurotrophins and iii) molecules related to Huntington disease whereas the pathological brain reacts by altering the expression of iv) nitric oxide in endothelial cells, v) cathecholamines and vi) molecules associated to Multiple Sclerosis.

Vitamin D3, a potent upstream regulator altering the expression of Alzheimer's disease-associated genes

To further decipher the detailed role of vitamin D in brain functioning, we narrowed our analysis to the genes that are directly or indirectly regulated by vitamin D or its related-metabolites. Using Ingenuity software, we listed all dysregulated molecules whose expression has been associated, in the literature, to this steroid.

As summarized in Fig. 3, we observed 290 and 249 vitamin D-related DEGs respectively, when comparing vitamin D3-supplemented Wt and Tg mice with their unsupplemented littermates. Within these two pools, 188 and 151 genes are part of the initial list of 784 vitamin D-associated transcripts whose expression is altered in the brain of transgenic animals (Additional file 5).

Furthermore, when assessing the presence of a VDRE in the promoter region of these DEGs [6], we found 25 (13 %) and 18 (12 %) transcripts in the two above-mentioned populations (highlighted in grey in Additional file 5). As a comparison, 68 (9 %) out of the 784 genes listed in Additional file 1 harbor a VDRE. We then clustered the two populations of vitamin D-related DEGs and, as shown on Fig. 3, we highlighted three sub-populations, composed of transcripts involved in inflammatory response, Alzheimer's disease and cognition.

At this point, we decided to validate the observed expression of certain DEGs of our dataset, using quantitative PCR (qPCR). We chose two hormones, *Oxt* and *Avp*, which are, according to the microarray results, dysregulated in the hippocampus and cortex of both Wt and Tg animals. We also focused on four vitamin D-related genes involved in AD commonly dysregulated in the neocortex and hippocampus of Tg animals, namely *Lcn2, Ptgs2, Esr1* and *Igf1*. An overexpression of the transcripts *Oxt* and *Avp* is confirmed in the cortex as well as an upregulation of *Esr1* in the hippocampus. The gene coding for *Lcn2* is overexpressed in both the hippocampus and the cortex. However, the downregulation of *Igf1* is not confirmed by qPCR analysis (Fig. 3b).

Vitamin D3 supplementation alters the expression of many Alzheimer's disease-associated genes, even in Wt brains. However, major differences can be observed. As reported on Fig. 4, 29 and 27 transcripts are uniquely misexpressed in Wt and Tg animals, respectively. In addition, 13 out of the 16 vitamin D-related DEGs emerging at the intersection of both strains are inversely expressed. The three transcripts that are similarly misexpressed are *Ace, Igf1* and *Gfap*, strongly related to Alzheimer's disease. All three are underexpressed when compared to unsupplemented animals (Fig. 4).

The consequences of this discordant response to vitamin D3 treatment are unknown since the Wt mice display no AD symptoms and features. Nevertheless, it allowed us to envision the putative mechanism of action of vitamin D3 or its related metabolites (Fig. 4). Vitamin D3 or 1,25(OH)2D3 and its receptor likely act *via* four regulators, namely IGF1, ESR1, ERK and NF-κB. *Igf1* is underexpressed in both strains while *Esr1* is overexpressed in Tg brains and underexpressed in Wt brains. The expression of *Erk* and *Nf-κb* is unchanged in both strains but many transcripts under their control are misexpressed in Tg and Wt animals. Downstream gene regulators include *Fos, Stat1 and Stat3*. The former is overexpressed in Tg and underexpressed in Wt animals.

Vitamin D3 treatment impacts amyloid plaque load and gliosis in transgenic animals

In order to examine whether a 5-month therapeutic intervention with vitamin D3 translated into a positive functional outcome, animals were analyzed at the histological and behavioral levels for known markers of AD pathogenesis. At the histological level, vitamin D3 supplementation decreased the quantity of plaques in three different brain regions of Tg mice: frontal cortex, hippocampus and neocortex (Fig. 5a). Astrogliosis, assessed through GFAP-immunostaining, is greatly increased in Tg animals compared to Wt. Vitamin D3 treatment of Tg animals during 5 months significantly decreases GFAP reactivity. However, this significant decrease is only observed in the frontal cortex (Fig. 5b). Microglial activation was assessed through immunostaining with IBA1 antibody and although there is an increase in this microglial marker between Wt and Tg control mice, vitamin D3 supplementation increases IBA1 immunoreactivity only in the frontal cortex of Tg animals when compared to their unsupplemented littermates (Fig. 5c).

Four months of vitamin D3-enriched diet is sufficient to rescue cognitive deficits in the 5XFAD model

After 4 months of vitamin D3-supplemented diet, cognitive performance was evaluated using two different paradigms: the Y-maze and the 6-radial arm water maze. A longitudinal study was first performed from M4 to M8 using the Y-maze. This study shows that Tg animals display a decreased percent of alternation with time whereas aging Tg animals on a high vitamin D3 diet do not show any cognitive decline between M4 and M8 (Fig. 5d). At M8, we observed a significant decrease in percent alternation performance in Tg mice. This effect is rescued by treatment with vitamin D3 during 4 months with no significant difference in the number of arms entered (Fig. 5e and f). However, a high vitamin D3 diet does not improve working memory in wild-type animals, even at M8 (Fig. 5e). The RAWM was used in addition to the Y-maze to assess hippocampal-dependent spatial working memory and reference memory. At the end of the learning process (end of day 3), results show a significant decrease in the total number of errors for Tg animals having been fed a vitamin D3 supplemented diet compared to Tg animals on a control diet (Fig. 5g).

Discussion

Despite growing evidence that vitamin D deficiency is a risk factor for cognitive decline and possibly Alzheimer's disease, very few studies have investigated the effect of vitamin D supplementation in AD mouse models. To our knowledge, this is the first transcriptomic study to assess the effect of long-term vitamin D3 supplementation in the nervous system of an AD mouse model. This work allowed us to examine the effects of chronic vitamin D3 treatment in both normal aging and AD-like brains, at the transcriptomic, histological and behavioral levels. We observed a very large number of dysregulated

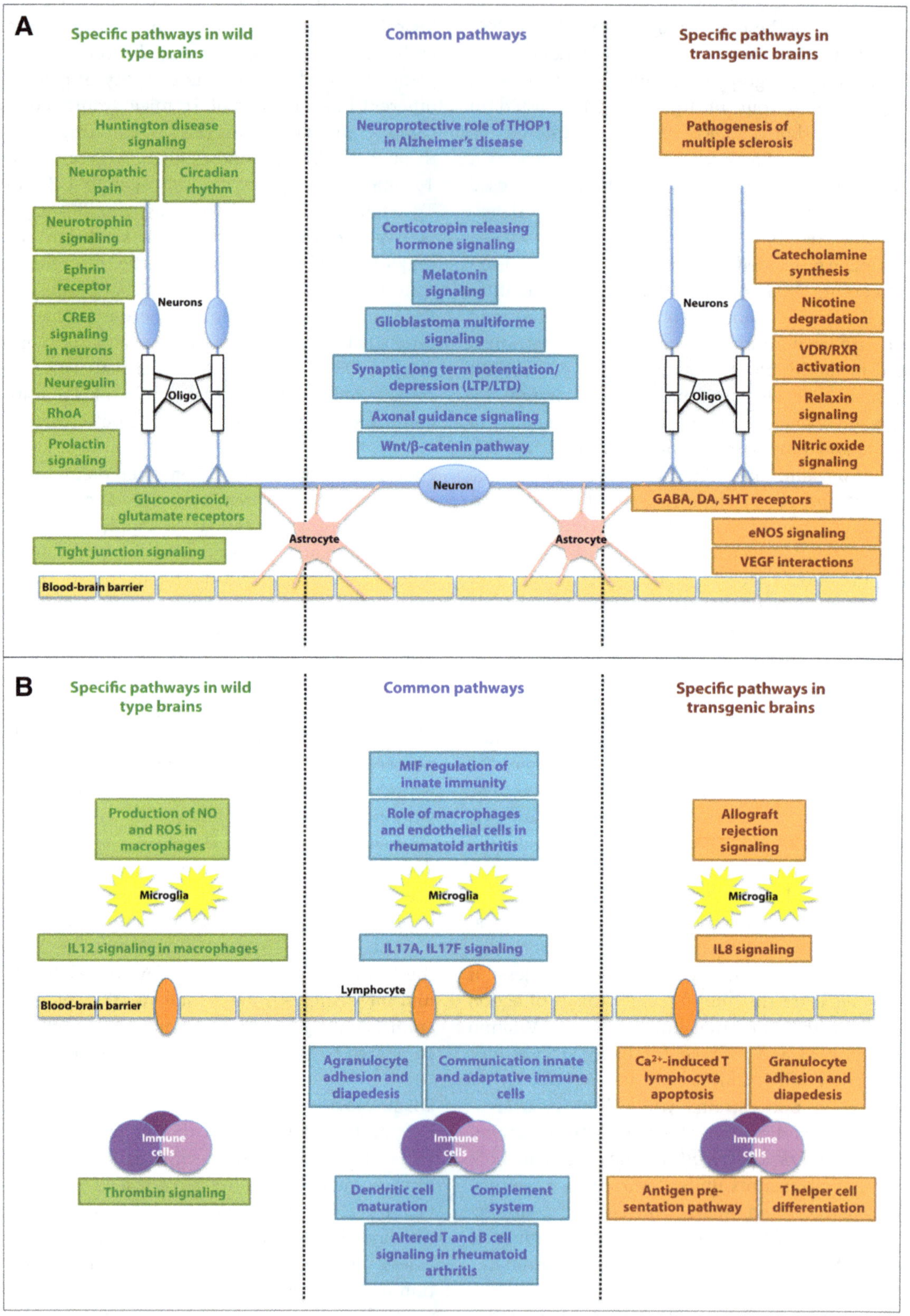

Fig. 2 (See legend on next page.)

(See figure on previous page.)
Fig. 2 Top canonical metabolic pathways associated to gene dysregulation in the cortex and hippocampus of mice after 5 months of vitamin D3 supplementation: common versus strain-specific processes. Metabolic pathways associated to gene expression dysregulation were identified using Ingenuity Pathway Analysis (IPA). Data from both the cortex and hippocampus were analyzed as one dataset and the main metabolic pathways affected were clustered according to their association to the nervous (**a**) or the immune (**b**) system

genes in both the pathological and non AD-like cortex and hippocampus of these animals at M9. On the one hand, our results point out that, although there are nearly double the number of DEGs in Wt animals compared to Tg, a high number of genes misexpressed after vitamin D3 supplementation are common to both genotypes. On the other hand, when considering the biological pathways affected by these DEGs, the common pathways between Wt and Tg often include different subsets of genes for a given pathway or an inversed expression for the same gene. Our study underlines some well-known actions of vitamin D and related metabolites, namely its impact on immune and inflammatory processes and cell cycle, along with previously shown effects on nervous system molecules such as neurotrophins and nitric oxide. However, our results also comprise unexpected effects on the expression of hormonal transcripts and reveal regulation of genes involved in synaptic function, axon guidance, endothelial and vascular processes and stem cell pluripotency. A reassuring result is that among the 784 genes predicted to be related to vitamin D action in Tg animals, almost a third of them are indeed regulated after 5 months of supplementation. On top of that, the majority of the

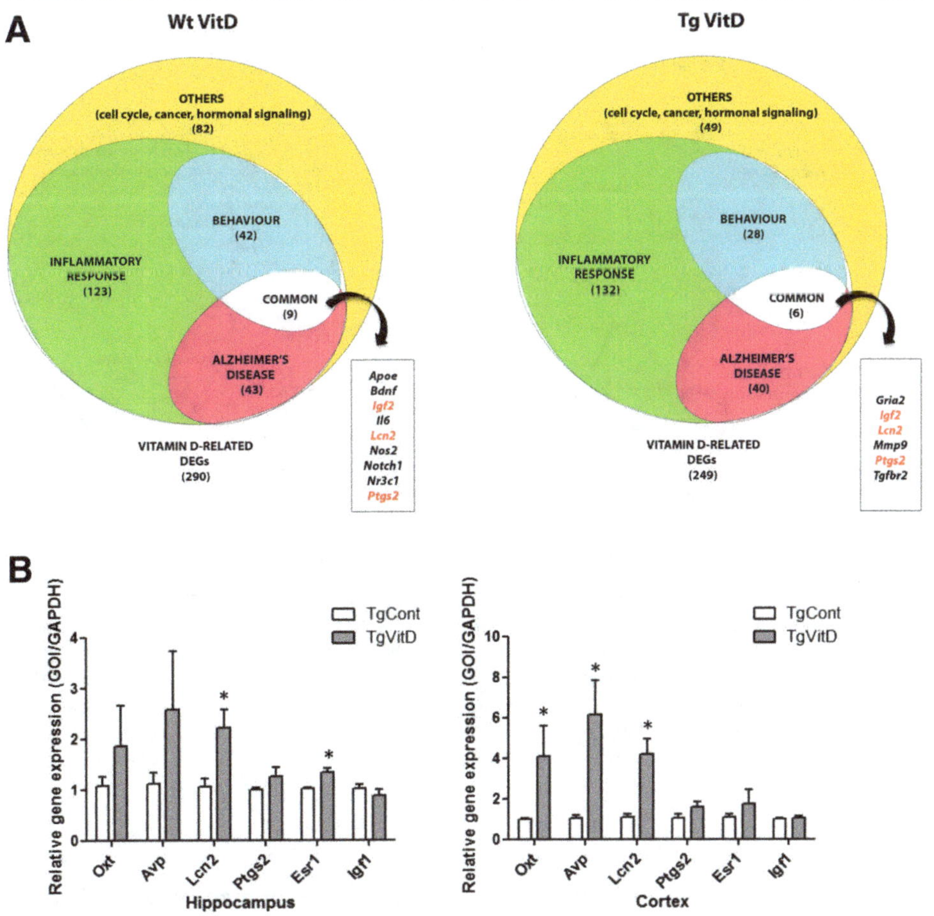

Fig. 3 Analysis of vitamin D3-related dysregulated genes indicates an association with inflammatory response, Alzheimer's disease and behavior. **a** Overall, 290 and 249 vitamin D-related DEGs are found misexpressed when comparing vitamin D3-supplemented wild type and transgenic mice with their unsupplemented littermates, respectively. Functional classification of these DEGs show importance of inflammatory, behavioural and Alzheimer's disease related processes. **b** qPCR validation of several dysregulated transcripts ($n = 6$ per group). An overexpression of the transcripts oxytocin (*Oxt*) and arginine vasopressin (*Avp*) is confirmed in the cortex as well as an upregulation of estrogen receptor 1 (*Esr1*) in the hippocampus. The gene coding for lipocalin 2 (*Lcn2*) is overexpressed in both the hippocampus and the cortex. * = $p < 0.05$

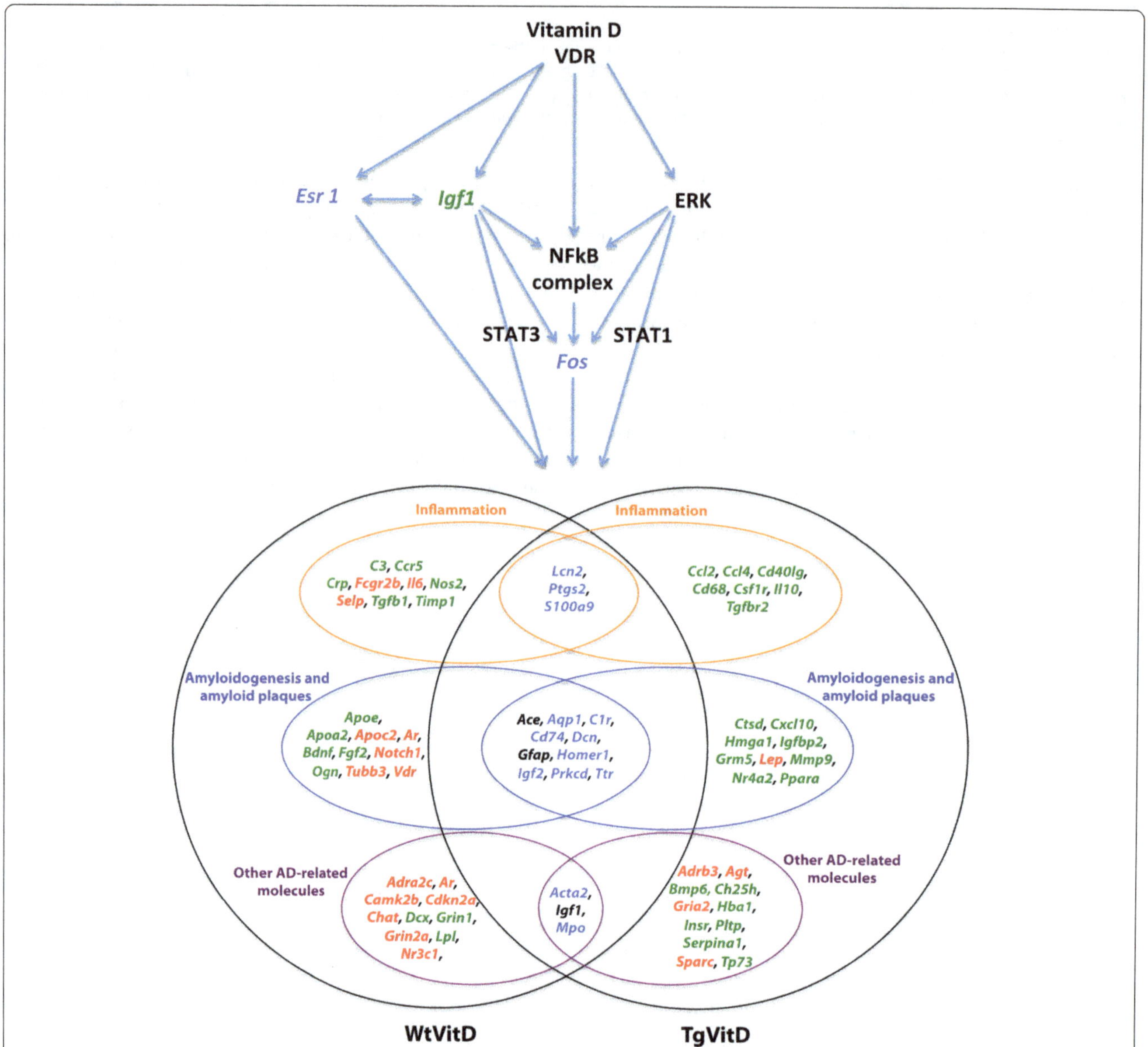

Fig. 4 Schematic view of the putative mechanisms of vitamin D3 action in the brain. Vitamin D3 or its related metabolites and their receptors act via four main regulators: IGF1, ESR1, ERK and NF-κB. *Igf1* is underexpressed (*green*) in both strains while *Esr1* is overexpressed in transgenic brains and underexpressed in wild type brains (*blue*). The expression of *Erk* and *NF-κB* is unchanged in both strains but many transcripts under their control are misexpressed in transgenic and wild type animals. Downstream gene regulators include *Fos*, *Stat1* and *Stat3*. *Fos* is overexpressed in transgenic animals and underexpressed in wild type animals (*blue*). Overall, 72 vitamin D-related transcripts are associated to either inflammation (19 genes) or amyloidogenesis and amyloid plaques (29) or AD-related features (24). Sixteen genes are dysregulated in both strains (*center areas*). However, only three of them - *Ace*, *Igf1* and *Gfap* - are similarly misexpressed (*black colour*). Specific up- (*red*) and down-regulated (*green*) are indicated for each strain

vitamin D-related genes are associated to Alzheimer's disease, in both the Wt and Tg brains. We show that vitamin D action in the brain of this AD mouse model likely involves signaling through ESR1 and IGF1 and that a 5-month therapeutic intervention reduces the histological markers of the disease and restores learning and memory capacities.

A common set of brain-associated genes regulated by vitamin D

As mentioned earlier, no pangenomic study previously assessed the effect of vitamin D3 supplementation in a mouse model of Alzheimer's disease. As a result, no direct comparison can be performed. However, three teams performed a thorough transcriptomic analysis on

i) brains from adult rats that were vitamin D-deprived during gestation [27] ii) 1,25(OH)2D3-supplemented cultures of neurons and glia [28] or pericytes [29] and iii) hippocampus from middle aged rats after chronic treatment with increasing doses of vitamin D3 [30]. A cross examination of our data with those reported in these studies reveals that the dysregulated expression of 46 genes – *Aaas, Aldoa, Atp2b4, Bcam, Bmp1, C3, Cat, Ccl2, Cntn4, Col16a1, Dpp6, Epas1, Fam120c, Fam70a, Fbln1, Fkbp1a, Foxc1, Gfap, Grp, Hspa12a, Htr2c, Igf1, Kdr, Kif1a, Lcat, Lpl, Ndst4, Nmbr, Nr4a2, Pde3b, Pmch, Polr1b, Ppp2r2b, Rab33b, Sdc4, Senp7, Serinc2, Slc17a6, Syt2, Thbd, Tia1, Trhr, Ttc39c, Vcam1, Vdr and Vps13c* – was formerly observed. The newly generated list may appear relatively restricted when compared to our initial dataset of 3488 dysregulated genes. However, given the variety of scientific paradigms (depletion *vs* supplementation), the nature of the samples (cells vs different brain regions), the molecular diversity of the administered molecule (vitamin D3 *vs* 1,25(OH)2D3) and the heterogeneous size of the datasets, it is not of minor importance to be able to establish an inventory of commonly misexpressed genes in nervous cells or brain areas after vitamin D3 treatment. Moreover, some studies have performed targeted analysis of specific gene expression in nervous system cells or tissues. For instance, Kaneko and collaborators demonstrated that calcitriol regulates the expression of two human brain-related genes containing VDREs, tryptophan hydroxylase (Tph) and leptin (Lep) [31]. These genes are also modulated in the brains of either Wt or Tg mice in our study. In a set of experiments examining the effect of maternal vitamin D deficiency on fetal brain development, Hawes and colleagues found that the pups from deficient mothers display a modulated expression of *Bdnf, Foxp2, Tgfb1* and *Th,* which are also affected in certain conditions of our study [32]. Altogether, these results underline the necessity for additional work to be performed on the genomic effects of vitamin D3 or 1,25(OH)2D3 in nervous system cells, as there are clearly multiple targets relevant to brain function and these could potentially explain a causal relationship between vitamin D status and brain aging or AD.

We chose to perform a literature-based analysis of possible VDRE-containing DEGs in our datasets. To avoid discrepancies between study designs, we initially based our search on a large *in silico* and microarray-based study by Wang and colleagues [6]. This revealed the presence of a very limited number of putative VDREs in our dataset. However, although ChiP-seq and genome-wide studies have found that the most frequent sequence located in VDR binding regions is the classic consensus VDRE motif, these data also suggest the presence of other motifs whose configuration diverge from the classic one and that might or might not interact directly with the VDR [33]. Moreover, there appears to be 1000–10,000 possible chromatin VDR binding sites, according to the cell-type considered. In contrast the number of primary 1,25(OH)2D3 target genes is thought to be around 100–1000 per tissue, suggesting that some genes are controlled by more than one VDR binding site [33]. It is therefore difficult to conclude on the complete list of VDR direct targets in our dataset. For instance, the study by Latimer and coworkers, reported putative VDRE sequences in three genes from our dataset – *Cntn4, Ppp2r2b and Syt2* - which were not previously identified by Wang and colleagues [6, 30]. These potential VDRE-containing DEGs are involved in synaptic vesicle trafficking and neurotransmission, indicating a possible direct modulation of these processes by 1,25(OH)2D3 in the 5XFAD animal model. Since the determination of true VDRE sequences would require further investigation and that vitamin D metabolites are also known to interact with various membrane-based signaling pathways, the search for indirect actions, for instance through modulation of immune processes, is not to be excluded.

A confirmed immuno-modulatory role, several mechanisms of action

The impact of vitamin D3 on inflammatory and immune processes is all but unexpected since it is now well established that vitamin D is a potent immune modulator [34]. 1,25(0H)2D3 adjusts the expression of inflammatory cytokines and prevents the proliferation of proinflammatory cells [35]. As a general rule, 1,25(OH)2D3-treated T-cells produce less proinflammatory Th1 (IL-2, interferon-γ, tumor necrosis factor-α), Th9 (IL-9) and Th22 (IL-22) cytokines and more anti-inflammatory Th2 (IL-3, IL-4, IL-5, IL-10) cytokines [36–39]. In addition, Th17 activity is affected by vitamin D. Activated T-cells treated with 1,25(OH)2D3 secrete reduced levels of IL-17, interferon-γ and IL-21 [40]. The overall picture remains slightly blurry. However, several key regulatory mechanisms begin to surface.

Characteristically, when calcitriol binds the VDR/RXR, the complex recognizes VDREs located in the promoter region of target genes and activates or inhibits their transcription. Concerning IL8 signaling, one of the top commonly affected processes in both Wt and Tg animals in our study, it is likely that IL8 is under the primary control of 1,25(OH)D and VDR as a study recently demonstrated the presence of VDR binding sites, in human monocytes, within the interleukin 8 (IL8) cluster [41]. However, direct activation/repression of gene expression is not the only mechanism by which the vitamin D system can act on immune processes [42]. As presented in Fig. 2, IL17A and IL17F signaling are affected by vitamin D3 supplementation in both strains. No known VDREs are present in the promoter regions of the TH17-

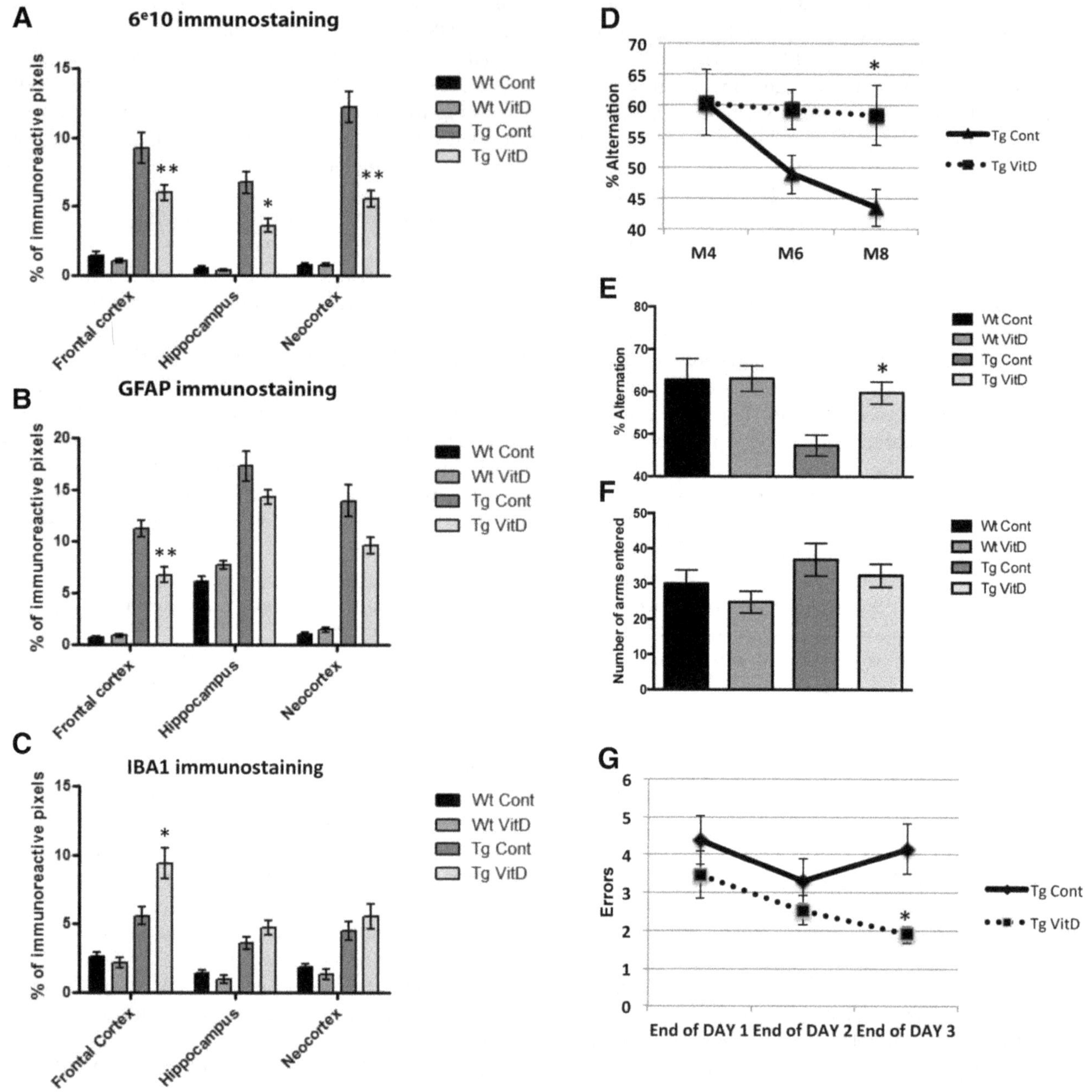

Fig. 5 Vitamin D3 supplementation reduces amyloid plaque load and cognitive deficits in transgenic animals. **a** In the three assessed brain regions - frontal cortex, hippocampus and neocortex – the number of amyloid plaques is reduced in transgenic supplemented brains. Vitamin D3 treatment limits astrogliosis (GFAP staining) in the frontal cortex and neocortex (**b**) and increases microglial activation (IBA1 staining) in the frontal cortex (**c**) of transgenic mice. Cognitive performance was assessed using the Y-maze and the radial arm water maze. **d** Vitamin D3 supplemented transgenic mice do not display the decreased percent of alternation (Y maze) observed in unsupplemented transgenic mice over time as measured at M4, M6 and M8. **e**, **f** At the end of the supplementation period (M8), a significant decrease in percent alternation performance is observed in transgenic mice. This effect is rescued by vitamin D3 supplementation with no significant difference in the number of arms entered. **g** Using the radial arm water maze, hippocampal-dependent spatial working memory was assessed. At the end of the learning process (Day 3), a significantly reduced number of errors is observed in supplemented transgenic mice. * = $p < 0.05$; ** = $p < 0.01$

signature cytokines that are *Il17a* and *Il17f*. Recently, it was reported that vitamin D inhibition of Th17 differentiation is obtained through modulation of Smads. More specifically, the presence of a negative VDRE in *Smad7* promoter leading to *Smad7* repression along with a VDR-dependent increase in *Smad3* explain the changes observed in Th17 cells during differentiation. In parallel, 1,25(OH)2D3 indirectly regulates the expression of

Th17-specific genes *Il17a* and *Il17f* through activation of ERK [43]. On top of direct transcriptomic action and indirect signaling through vitamin D receptors, it is also possible that epigenetic mechanisms are also at play. For example, 1,25(OH)2D3 regulates TLR-mediated inflammation signaling by downregulating miR-155 in macrophages [44]. In our study, the modulated expression of several members of the TLR family (*Tlr1, Tlr2* and *Tlr7*), with no known VDREs, could potentially involve such mechanisms [45].

In addition to these various mechanisms, 1,25(OH)2D3 interacts with other transcription factors, such as the glucocorticoid receptor, the nuclear factor of activated T-cells (NFAT) or NF-κB resulting in overall decreased inflammatory states [46]. It has been shown that, when activated by its ligand, the VDR dimerizes with the glucocorticoid receptor and together they bind to glucocorticoid responsive elements of genes, leading to an up-regulation of anti-inflammatory molecules and a down-regulation of pro-inflammatory genes [47]. Glucocorticoid receptor signaling is one of the top biological functions affected in our study, in both Wt and Tg brains. VDR is also able to bind to an NFAT binding site, inducing a diminished NFAT activity and downstream a repressed expression of IL-2, cyclooxygenase 2 [48] and IL-17 [49]. Similarly, 1,25(OH)2D3 has been shown to inhibit NF-κB activation and signaling through up-regulation of IκB expression [50], interference with DNA binding [51] and by enhancing FBW-7 dependent turnover of NF-κB subunits [52], leading to a reduced production of pro-inflammatory cytokines and pro-inflammatory enzymes such as cyclooxygenase 2 [53]. Deciphering the exact mode of action for 1,25(OH)2D3 modulation of immune and inflammatory pathways, whether it involves direct gene regulation, interactions and cross-talks between various signaling pathways, and epigenetic mechanisms is beyond the scope of this study. However, it is clear that in both the healthy and AD-like brain, vitamin D3 supplementation induces a strong effect on inflammatory and immune processes.

A background-specific action of vitamin D3

As established during the last 25 years, vitamin D and its metabolites play crucial roles in cell proliferation and differentiation, neuroprotection, neurotransmission and neuroplasticity [54]. However, as observed in the immune system, vitamin D3 action is space- and time-specific. For example, a hypervitaminosis D alters the synthesis of calcium binding proteins in the caudate/putamen but not in the hippocampus and the cerebral cortex [55]. Likewise, 3 weeks after the induction of an experimental allergic encephalomyelitis, vitamin D3 supplementation provokes a massive downregulation of inducible nitric oxide synthase (iNOS) only in the rat cerebellum and brainstem [56]. The time window for vitamin D depletion or supplementation can be essential as well. A transient developmental vitamin D deficiency induces persistent morphological and molecular changes in the adult rat brain [57–59] while an adult vitamin D deficiency is associated with less profound modifications [60].

An important finding from our transcriptomic analysis is the effect of the pathological context on gene response to vitamin D3 treatment. Indeed, our study provides evidence that vitamin D3 has distinct genomic effects in a non-pathologic and an AD-like brain. It is clear that, when given to healthy animals, vitamin D3 induces dysregulation of genes implicated in an important number of nervous system related pathways, whereas it appears to act preferentially on immune system processes in Tg mice, as illustrated in Fig. 2 and Additional file 4. When considering nervous system related pathways, distinct actions also appear. For instance, the non-pathologic brain expresses genes associated to neurological functions such as neurotrophins or tight junction modulation while the pathologic brain activates/represses genes related to catecholamine synthesis or nitric oxide signaling (Fig. 2). Another mean to demonstrate the effect of the pathological background on gene dysregulation is to observe the subtle strain-associated changes in a common canonical pathway. One of the most remarkable is the Wnt/β-catenin signaling. Out of seven genes whose expression is dysregulated in both strains – *Dsh, Frizzled, Lef/Tgf, Lrp1, Rar, Tgfbr, Wnt* – 5 are inversely misexpressed, indicating a putative opposite action of vitamin D3. In addition, 12 and 7 genes are exclusively dysregulated in the wild type and transgenic brains, respectively (Additional file 6).

Several studies have highlighted the importance of various factors, such as genetic settings, pathological backgrounds, organ areas, cell subtypes, delivery time windows, molecule concentrations, in determining the response to vitamin D treatment. We can list a few examples. Conversely to cells from healthy individuals, 1,25(OH)2D3 increases the production of IL-2 in peripheral blood mononuclear cells from hemodialysis patients [61]. 1,25(OH)2D3 addition in the culture medium of either monocytes or macrophages induces an up-regulation and a down-regulation of IL-1 and IL-6 mRNA, respectively. These results were abolished or modified when cells, before being stimulated with LPS or TNF-α, were pre-incubated with 1,25(OH)2D3 [62]. 1,25(OH)2D3 triggers a lessened expression of IL-10, followed by an increased production, at a later stage [46].

Such regulation variability may explain some observed discrepancies between the mouse strains used in the current study. Genetically similar mice from the same ages were fed with the same diet, during the same time window, and the same brain areas were analyzed. Yet, one strain differs from the other by carrying two mutated human genes – APP and PSEN1 - that induce molecular, morphological and behavioral changes. The 5XFAD mouse model is an inflammatory model [4, 63] and, as mentioned above, 1,25(OH)2D3 induces a different response when acting on an inflamed tissue. Interestingly, this may even apply to the canonical pathways that are dysregulated in both strains (Additional file 4). In most if not all cases, the two lists of misexpressed genes are not fully identical. This confirms that the pleiotropic action of vitamin D3 and its related metabolites strongly varies according to the health status of the animal.

In addition, the strain-associated differences may be related to the mechanism of action of vitamin D metabolites at play, whether it is a genomic response or the induction of membrane based signaling pathways. In a recent review, Michael Berridge develops the hypothesis that vitamin D acts as a guardian of phenotypic stability in a cell- and context-specific manner [64]. This stability is maintained through modulation of various intracellular signaling pathways that are linked to vitamin D action. For instance, vitamin D is capable of regulating the expression of many components of pathways activated by insulin, TGFB1, WNT and NOTCH [65], whose mRNA expression is affected in our study.

A strong link with Alzheimer's disease in both Wt and Tg

The 5XFAD model is based on the insertion of two human transgenes leading to a major increase of Aβ 1-42 that accumulates rapidly in the brains of transgenic animals. Overall, this model is both an inflammatory and amyloidogenic model of Alzheimer's disease [2, 4, 66]. As seen so far, the inflammatory component present in Tg animals is highly addressed by vitamin D3 treatment and, to a lesser extent, in Wt animals. Other effects of gene dysregulation in the brain of both Wt and Tg mice relate to Alzheimer's disease. For instance, one of the commonly dysregulated pathways, described in Additional file 4, concerns the neuroprotective role of THOP1. THOP1, an oligopeptidase whose levels increase upon Aβ exposure, is found overexpressed in human AD brains, and appears to engage in neuroprotective activities against toxic effects of Aβ at early stages of the disease [67]. This pathway is significantly affected in our study, however it is difficult to conclude about the outcome induced by such dysregulation at the functional level, especially since the expression of different genes in the pathway is modified according to the genotype.

Within the THOP1 pathway, the expression of angiotensin-converting enzyme (ACE), which converts angiotensin I to angiotensin II, a potent vasoconstrictor, is affected in both wild type and transgenic animals. No study has focused on the effect of vitamin D3 supplementation on ACE expression. However, it has been observed that VDR knockout mice display an increased production of ACE mRNA [68]. Interestingly, this metalloprotease is involved in Alzheimer's disease since human ACE increases degradation and cleavage of Aβ [69–72].

Another interesting result is the finding that a number of DEGs relate to vascular processes. Angiogenesis is a complex process that involves the activation and modification of several signaling pathways within endothelial cells. A key mediator of this process is VEGF. Pathological angiogenesis is now considered as a key contributor to the development of AD. Substantial evidence suggests that the neurodegenerative process can be caused by cerebral hypoperfusion which induces reduced oxygen, glucose and nutrient supply to the brain, and damages the parenchymal cells and the blood–brain barrier (BBB). BBB dysfunction promotes oxidative stress, inflammation, paracellular permeability and dysregulation of nitric oxide [73]. Several signaling pathways such as VEGF signaling, tight junction signaling, nitric oxide signaling in macrophages and eNos signaling are disturbed by vitamin D3 treatment, especially in Tg mice.

Conversely, we observed a misexpression of *Apoe* mRNA only in wild type supplemented animals. This protein is associated to cardiovascular diseases as well as Alzheimer's disease [74]. No direct interaction between vitamin D3 and ApoE has been unveiled so far. However, several studies indicate putative interplays. For example, the VDR mRNA regulates the phosphorylation and production of STAT1 [75] which in turn is involved in the expression of apoE mRNA [76]. Furthermore, the vitamin D system interacts with IGF1 and Esr1 (see below), the latter upregulating *Apoe* mRNA in rat primary culture of hippocampal neurons [77]. On the other hand, ApoE ε4 alleles have been associated with reduced memory function and higher serum 25(OH)D concentrations [78].

Overall, the fact that a large number of vitamin D-related genes are categorized as AD-related in both Wt and Tg animals is intriguing. This is suggestive of a close link between vitamin D signaling and AD-related signaling, as has been proposed by researchers [25, 79]. Although we observed a positive effect of vitamin D3 treatment on the amount of amyloid plaques, we never detected a misexpression of the endogenous *App* transcript in our transgenic or wild type animals. This comes as a relative surprise since it has been reported that either the cotransfection of VDR or a calcitriol treatment reduces, in a dose dependent manner, APP transcription in neuroblastoma cells [18]. It is hypothesized that VDR interacts with SMAD3 [80], a transcription factor known to regulate APP transcription through TGF beta signaling [81]. However, our data failed to confirm these findings. In wild type mice, vitamin D3 supplementation induces an under-expression of *Smad6, Tgfb1* and *Tgfbr1* transcripts without affecting *App* expression. In addition, no misexpression of these four mRNAs is observed in transgenic animals. It is therefore likely that other intermediate molecules, such as those described below, are involved in the reduction of amyloid burden.

An unexpected regulation of oxytocin and arginine vasopressin transcripts in the cortex

One very intriguing result is the mRNA regulation of a number of hormones classically known to be present in the pituitary axis. It is true that OXT and AVP, for instance, act as both hormones and central neurotransmitters. However, to our knowledge, the presence of local regulation of gene expression in the hippocampus or cortex for both these hormones has never been reported before. Binding sites for both hormones have been described in different central regions such as the amygdala, septum and olfactory region [82]. However, while AVP receptors have been reported within the hippocampus no OXT receptor has been found in this area [83]. Both neuropeptides regulate rodent, primate and human social behaviors and stress responses [84]. AVP influences memory processes in the brain by facilitating memory consolidation and retrieval [85, 86]. Regarding its role in AD pathology, a significant decrease in AVP concentration was found in the brain of AD patients while application of AVP improves learning and memory in aged people and in rats having received Aβ [87–90]. OXT regulates hippocampal synaptic plasticity and improves hippocampal-dependent cognitive functions [91–93]. The direct or indirect regulation of these neuropeptides by vitamin D3 could have important implications for a number of behavioral and cognitive processes in both the normal and pathological brain. Differential expression of these two genes (*Oxt* and *Avp*) was then measured by qPCR. A significant increase for both these genes was only confirmed in the cortex, although the same tendency is observed in the hippocampus. It appears that important inter-individual variations are present among the tested mice, further supporting the idea that vitamin D3 acts not only in a space- and time-specific manner, but also in an individual-specific way.

A putative role of insulin growth factor 1 and estrogen receptor 1 as downstream regulators

Four other gene expressions were assessed with qPCR and, once again, not all were validated in each brain area analyzed. *Lcn2* and *Ptgs2* are both involved in inflammatory signaling processes and have been found to contribute to amyloid response in AD [94, 95]. *Esr1* and *Igf1* induce signaling pathways known to be affected in AD. Several interactions between the estrogen and vitamin D endocrine system have been described so far. 1,25(OH)2D3 may play an important role in estrogen biosynthesis suggested by the fact that serum estrogen levels are decreased in VDR knock-out mice as compared with wild-type mice [96]. The direct action of vitamin D on estrogen signaling is also cell-specific as demonstrated by the fact that 1,25-(OH)2D3 increases estrogen receptor (ER) expression in osteoblast-like cells, while it exerts a negative effect on ER in MCF-7 human breast cancer cells [97, 98]. An alteration in ER distribution in AD hippocampal neurons has been described, and, more precisely, a shift in cellular localization of these receptors inhibits the development of AD pathology [99, 100]. Collectively, investigations suggest that levels of estrogen receptors play an important role in neuroprotection and against neuroinflammation-induced degeneration in AD [101, 102]. ESR1 has also been shown to interact directly with amyloid processing through non-genomic signaling via activation of MAPK/ERK pathway [103]. Recently, two potential negative VDREs have been identified in the promoter region of *Esr1* [104] suggesting a direct transcriptional action of vitamin D/VDR on ER leading to an altered estrogen signaling mechanism important to both Wt and AD-like brains. A possible mechanism by which ESR1 confers neuroprotective effects in AD is through interaction with IGF1R. Both in vivo and in vitro studies have revealed interaction between ERs and IGF1R in the promotion of neuronal survival, synaptic plasticity and against Aβ toxicity [105, 106]. Insulin signaling is emerging as an important event in neurodegenerative processes and aging in general. However, inconsistencies regarding the role of insulin-like signaling and its association to AD have appeared. In rodents, reduced insulin/IGF1 signaling slows aging and therefore prevents development of neurodegenerative diseases [107] but normal aging is associated with declining levels of IGF1 and administration of insulin can improve cognitive function in AD patients [108, 109]. Regardless, in vivo evidence shows that AD-like pathology is significantly delayed in IGF1R knock out mouse models of AD [110, 111]. Potential crosstalks between vitamin D and IGF1 signaling have been put forward. VDR knock-out mice display decreased expression of *Igf1, Igf1r* and *Nf- kb* [112]. 1,25(OH)2D3 also regulates the expression of a well-known anti-aging gene, Klotho (*Kl*), whose expression is modified in the hippocampus of both Wt and Tg mice in our study. *Kl* dysregulation is linked to modulation of Insulin/IGF1 signaling pathways [113]. Taken together, these results largely support both direct and indirect action of vitamin D/VDR on ESR1 and IGF1 signaling pathways in both Wt and 5XFAD mice, as a mechanism to reduce brain aging processes.

Convergent data on amyloid plaque load and divergent results on astrogliosis

The bulk of our study focuses on describing the similarities or differences induced by chronic vitamin D3 supplementation at the transcriptomic level in Wt and Tg animals at M9. Importantly, the altered gene expression translates into a modification of functional outcomes. We note a link between the action of vitamin D3 on gene regulation in our model and its effect at the histological and behavioral levels. We show here that 5 months of vitamin D3 treatment restores learning and memory performance in Tg animals in both the Y-maze and RAWM but does not affect cognitive outcome in Wt mice. This is accompanied by a decrease in the number of amyloid plaques, astrocytic reactivity and subtle changes in microglial activation for Tg animals having been fed a vitamin D3 diet. Several studies have shown an improvement in memory and cognitive function in different models of AD or aging following vitamin D2, vitamin D3 or 1,25(OH)2D3 treatment. In their work, Yu and colleagues used young AβPP transgenic mice and found an amelioration of performance in the Morris Water Maze (MWM) for animals under a high vitamin D3 diet. These behavioral changes were accompanied by a diminished Aβ load, along with an increase in astrocytic reactivity, NGF levels and decreased TNF-α in the brain of treated mice. This study focused on a preventive action of vitamin D3, which might explain some of the differences observed when comparing their data to ours. Specifically, the increase in astrocytic marker GFAP is inconsistent with the diminished GFAP staining observed in our study [26]. This discrepancy might reflect the balance by which vitamin D3 exerts its effects according to the pathological context and the time of delivery. An increase in GFAP expression is a hallmark of reactive gliosis and is found in many neuropathological conditions, including AD. The functional changes associated to this increased expression however are not fully understood. To study the functional outcomes of GFAP dysregulation on the surrounding brain tissue and cells, GFAP knock-outs (KO) have been generated and when combined to brain injury models, studies suggest that GFAP increase is associated to protective mechanisms [114, 115]. When GFAP KO mice were crossed with a mouse model for AD, the deposition of amyloid plaques was accelerated. Furthermore, neuritic dystrophy was exacerbated and the interaction of astrocytes with plaques was decreased [116]. These observations lead to the conclusion that astrogliosis can be considered as a brain defense mechanism attempting to prevent plaque formation and neuronal damage, and this would take place during the onset of the disease. However, we cannot rule out that, at the same time, gliosis affects the synaptic and metabolic support functions of astrocytes [116, 117]. It is then probable that with age and repeated insults, chronic astrocyte reactivity may become deleterious, engaging the opposite effect of vitamin D3 on GFAP expression when compared to a younger tissue. We and others have shown that genes involved in glial reactivity and inflammation are among the earliest affected during disease pathogenesis in the 5xFAD model and that these are correlated with cognitive impairment [4]. We show here that vitamin D3 is able to act specifically on both astrocytic and microglial activation at both the transcriptomic and histological levels. In the AD brain, microglial activation is the driving force for the elaboration of an inflammatory cascade [118] and reports show an upregulation of VDR mRNA in microglia stimulated by Aβ in vitro [119], indicating that microglia found around amyloid plaques could increase their responsiveness to vitamin D metabolites. Microglia, unlike the other cells of the nervous system, stems from the myeloid lineage and is considered the macrophages of the brain. As discussed thoroughly here and elsewhere, the vitamin D system displays potent anti-inflammatory roles in immune cells and the increase in microglial activity in the frontal cortex of 5xFAD mice reflects the capacity of vitamin D3 to balance the pro- and anti-inflammatory cytokine production regulated by microglia [118, 120]. In addition, this enhanced activation of microglia at the proteomic level could also reflect increased phagocytic activity of Aβ, a process demonstrated to be promoted by vitamin D3 in the macrophages of AD patients [121, 122]. Once again, it appears that vitamin D3 acts on both nervous system and the immune system pathways to reduce alteration in neuronal metabolism and further preserve cognitive outcomes.

An age- and concentration-dependent action on cognition

The study by Yu and colleagues does not present the effect of vitamin D3 on cognitive functions in the Wt counterpart, leaving no comparison possible [26]. Accordingly, an 8 week treatment with intraperitoneal injections of 1,25(OH)2D3 in a different mouse model of AD restored learning and memory deficits, assessed by the fear conditioning paradigm, compared to vehicle-treated Tg mice but did not affect cognitive performance in non-Tg animals [123]. Yet, another study, which tested a 7 months vitamin D2 supplementation in another AD mouse model, concluded that, in this case, vitamin D2 improved cognitive performance more reliably in Wt mice rather than Tg at M9 [124]. And when focusing solely on the implication of vitamin D in normal aging and memory disabilities, Latimer and colleagues showed that a high vitamin D3 diet (10,000 IU/Kg diet) lasting 5 to 6 months prevented cognitive decline in aging rats. The study demonstrates a causal relationship between enhanced learning and memory during aging with vitamin D3 status which is underlined by enhanced synaptic transmission due to gene expression changes in the brain [30]. At approximately the same time, Briones and Darwish performed subcutaneous injections of 1,25(OH)2D3, for 21 days, to both young and aged rats (6 and 20 months, respectively) and observed an attenuation of cognitive impairment accompanied by enhanced brain energy metabolism, modulation of inflammatory and redox state in aged rats after treatment compared to controls [125, 126]. Both these studies underlie a role for vitamin D metabolite supplementation in the preservation of cognitive function in "normal" aging animals. The middle-age period is characterized by the onset of subtle changes in cognitive performance that might not be detected by the straightforward tests that are the Y-maze and RAWM. It is probable that M9 is not old enough to detect memory decline in Wt animals or that tests aiming at detecting more subtle performance changes in executive function or processing speed would be required to allow analysis of vitamin D3 treatment on cognitive performance in Wt aging animals.

Conclusions

Classically, investigations into physiological processes and neurodegenerative disease pathogenesis have moved from the whole organism to the molecular level as the advent of genome-wide microarrays and large-scale genome sequencing have become powerful tools for probing physiological mechanisms. Vitamin D signaling is ideally suited for genomic analysis as its main receptor VDR is a direct regulator of gene transcription. However, although transcriptomic technologies have evolved greatly, there is still no consensus about an optimal way to analyze transcriptomic data. This renders comparison with other studies rather difficult, especially when platform and data analysis programs differ. The growing knowledge about epigenetic mechanisms at play in gene regulation and its relevance to vitamin D action in the brain could not be addressed in this study but needs further investigation in future experimental designs. The absence of a clear consensus motif for VDREs also impedes the pinpointing of direct vitamin D targets. Moreover, a 5-month supplementation entails that transcriptional activation is not the only mechanism at play, and that membrane-based actions of vitamin D and its related metabolites are to be considered. The interactions between the vitamin D system and other signaling pathways are clearly as important as direct transcriptional activation or repression of 1,25(OH)2D3 targets, as shown in this study.

The aim of this study was to i) assess the potential therapeutic benefit and the mechanisms of action of a chronic vitamin D3 supplementation in an AD model and ii) extract information about specific signaling pathways affected by vitamin D3 in the nervous system. Therefore, validating each DEG obtained by microarray assay using qPCR or proteomic approaches was largely beyond the scope of the study but this needs to be further addressed, especially for those genes put forward as key partners or downstream actors. It is important to note that the discordant results observed between microarray data and qPCR analysis might reflect the importance of inter-individual variability in response to vitamin D3 treatment but also the limitations for each method used. Indeed, transcriptomic data are normalized to global measures while qPCR results are obtained in reference to one housekeeping gene. Concerning *Igf1* mRNA quantification, it is also likely that putatively low levels followed by further reduction in gene expression is more error prone and reaches the limit of qPCR analysis. Moreover, as our study emphasizes the time-, background- and individual-specific action of vitamin D3 in the brain, it is obvious that differential activity at the transcriptomic level is operated between the cortex and hippocampus. Additional analysis of our data would allow for more precise deciphering of vitamin D3 impact in each brain area known to be affected in AD. The study was also designed using a female cohort, and it would seem extremely relevant to repeat such experiments in male animals. This could help contribute to the ongoing debate about the relevance of gender differences in the pathogenesis of the disease. Especially since estrogen signaling appears to play an important part in the events observed here, along with the mRNA dysregulation of a certain number of hormones, we cannot exclude a sex-impact to be considered in the way vitamin D3 acts on brain cells.

Lastly, animal studies using vitamin D treatment in AD models, including ours, show improvement in various markers of the disease but interventional clinical trials, to date, failed to show such effects. It is important to bear in mind that animal models of AD do not recapitulate fully the complex physiopathology of the disease and major differences in regulation by the vitamin D signaling system are observed, according to the species concerned [127], possibly further increasing the gap between the results obtained from animal and human studies. Moreover, we chose to place ourselves in a therapeutic context, however, reproducing such a study in a preventive manner would allow refining the analysis of vitamin D3 action in a time-dependent manner. Indeed, one major current problem concerning clinical trials, using vitamin D as a protective agent against cognitive decline and AD, is the time and dose for treatment. When comparing our study to others, we highlight the differences in functional outcomes depending on the time of treatment, the dose or metabolite used. As with clinical trials, there is a great need for additional work in rodents before deciphering the exact mechanisms of action of vitamin D in the nervous system. However, we feel confident that the present dataset is a useful public resource which reflects the variety and pleiotropy of vitamin D3 actions in the brain with particular emphasis on the crosstalk between vitamin D3 activated pathways and those affected in AD and should allow future studies to further validate the use of vitamin D3 as a potent therapeutic agent in AD.

Methods

Animals and experimental design

Female 5XFAD transgenic mice were used for this study. These mice overexpress two transgenes bearing five mutations linked to familial AD: human *APP* (Swedish mutation K670N, M671L; Florida mutation I716V; London mutation V717I) and human *presenilin 1* (*PSEN1* M146L, L286V), under transcriptional control of the mouse Thy1 promoter. 5XFAD lines from the B6/SJL genetic background were maintained by crossing hemizygous transgenic mice with B6/SJL F1 breeders. These mice exhibit AD-related symptoms earlier than other animal models and amyloid deposition starts in the cortex and subiculum at 2 months of age [2, 128]. Heterozygous 5XFAD transgenic animals and wild type (Wt) controls were obtained after breeding of progenitors purchased from the Jackson Laboratory. Newborn pups were genotyped by polymerase chain reaction (PCR) of tail DNA biopsies in order to detect the human *PSEN1* gene as previously described [128]. Animals were weaned at 4 weeks of age and fed an identical diet until M4. Mice were then allocated to different groups: Wt animals on a control diet (1000 IU/kg) ($n = 10$), Wt animals on a vitamin D3 enriched diet (7500 IU/kg) ($n = 11$), transgenic animals on a control diet ($n = 14$) and transgenic animals fed with the vitamin D3 enriched diet ($n = 16$) (INRA, France). Mice were tested at M4, M6 and M8 in the Y-maze, and at M8 in the 6-radial-arm water maze before euthanasia at M9. Animal experiments were approved by the Ethics Committee of the Medical Faculty of Marseille and were carried out in accordance with the guidelines published in the European Communities Council Directive of November 24, 1986 (86/609/EEC). All efforts were made to reduce animal suffering and the number of mice needed for the study.

Behavioural testing

Y-maze

Spontaneous alternation in the Y-maze was tested according to the following protocol: each mouse was placed in a random arm of the symmetrical Y-maze and was allowed to explore freely through the maze during an 8 min session. The sequence and total number of arms entered was recorded. Arm entry was considered complete when the hind paws were completely in the arm. Experiments were done blind with respect to the genotype and diet of the mice. Washing with water and ethanol was performed between each passage. Percentage of alternation was determined as follows: number of triads containing entries into all three arms/maximum possible alternations (total number of arms entered – 2) x 100.

6-Radial arm water maze

The 6-RAWM is a hybrid of the Morris water maze and a radial arm maze. The test allows assessment of spatial and reference memory. The mouse version of this maze uses a circular pool with six swim alleys (arms) radiating out from an open central area with a hidden escape platform submerged at the end of one goal arm. The overall design of the study was adapted from Alamed and collaborators [129], using a 3-day protocol containing 12 sessions per day. Visual cues were displayed around the room and the experimenter remained visible throughout the training sessions. For this procedure the goal arm differed between mice but was held constant for each mouse during all trials with a different start arm on successive trials. The first day of training comprised of alternating between hidden and visible platform. During the 12 trials of the second and third day, the platform remained hidden and the mice were required to use the visual cues to locate the goal arm. When a mouse entered a wrong arm, which did not contain the platform, an error was scored. At the end of the procedure, mice were tested in the circular pool using a visible platform, to ensure their visual abilities were satisfactory for inclusion in the study.

Tissue isolation

Brain tissues were collected at M9, from all groups. Mice were anesthetized with isoflurane before sacrifice and brains isolated from each animal. The hippocampus and neocortex from a half brain were dissected, snap-frozen in liquid nitrogen and stored at -80 °C until use. The other hemi-brain was placed in 4 % paraformaldehyde during 6 days at 4 °C, for further immunohistological processing.

Tissue processing and immunostaining

Coronal brain sections from hemi-brains previously collected and fixed in 4 % paraformaldehyde were serially generated using a cryostat and stored at -20 °C in six-well plates containing a cryoprotectant (30 % glycerol; 30 % ethylene glycol (Sigma Aldrich, Saint-Quentin Fallavier, France) diluted in 0,05 M PBS phosphate buffered saline (pH 7.4) until being processed for immunostaining.

After washing in PBS, floating sections were incubated, during 1 h at room temperature (RT), with a blocking buffer (3 % BSA, 0.1 % Triton X-100 in PBS pH 7.4) and, overnight at 4 °C, with the following primary antibodies diluted in the blocking solution: rabbit polyclonal anti-GFAP (1/500, Dako France, Trappes, France), mouse monoclonal anti-Aβ, 6E10 (1/300, Covance, Eurogentec, Angers, France) and rabbit polyclonal anti-IBA1 (1/200, Wako, Sobioda, Montbonnot-Saint-Martin, France). Then, slices were rinsed in PBS and incubated for 90 min at RT with cross-absorbed Alexafluor 488-conjugated anti-rabbit or 594-conjugated anti-mouse secondary antibodies (1/500, Life Technologies, Saint Aubin, France) along with Hoechst blue (1/1000, Sigma Aldrich) in dark conditions. After several washes in PBS, slides were mounted with ProLong Gold Antifade reagent (Life Technologies).

Microscopic analysis and quantification of gliosis and amyloid plaques

Quantification of gliosis and amyloid plaques were performed on 30 μm thick brain coronal sections co-stained with either GFAP and 6E10 or IBA1 and 6E10 antibodies, at the frontal cortex, hippocampal and sensory cortex levels. Images were acquired using an inverted Axio Observer microscope (Zeiss, Jena, Germany) equipped with DAPI, FITC and TRITC epifluorescence filters. Images of large brain sections were obtained using the mosaic mode of the Axiovision software (Zeiss). For 6E10, GFAP and IBA1 staining quantifications, ImageJ software was used. The pictures were binarized to 16 bit black and white images and a fixed intensity threshold was applied for all images. Percentage of covered area by the fluorescent staining was calculated. Eight mice per group and three sections per mouse at three different levels were used.

RNA isolation

Total RNA was isolated from the snap-frozen hippocampi and cortices using RNeasy Mini kit (Qiagen, Courtaboeuf, France), according to the manufacturer's instructions. RNA concentration was determined using a Nanodrop 2000 spectrophotometer (Life Technologies ThermoFisher Scientific, Villebon sur Yvette, France) and RNA integrity assessed on an Agilent 2100 Bioanalyzer (Agilent Technologies, Les Ulis, France).

Microarray assay

RNA samples from three animals in each group were pooled for microarray hybridization. Sample amplification, labeling, and hybridization were performed in line with the Agilent one-color microarray-base analysis (low input quick amp labeling) protocol (Agilent Technologies). Briefly, total RNA was reverse-transcribed into cDNA using the T7 promoter primer. The reaction intending to synthesize cyanine-3-labeled cRNA from cDNA was performed in a solution containing dNTP mix, T7 RNA polymerase and cyanine 3-dCTP and then incubated at 40 °C for 2 h. Labeled cRNA was purified and fragmented before hybridization on Agilent 8x60k Mouse Gene Expression Arrays (Agilent Technologies), containing 62,975 oligonucleotide probes, at 65 °C for 17 h. Raw microarray signals were scanned and extracted using Agilent Feature Extraction Software (Agilent Technologies). AgiND R package was used for quality control and normalization. Quantile methods and a background correction were applied for data normalization. Microarray data are available in the ArrayExpress database under accession number E-MTAB-1937.

Microarray data analysis

Biological interpretation of the data was performed using two different programs. The NIH DAVID tool was used to obtain functional annotation clusters related to the datasets of interest. Ingenuity Pathway Analysis (IPA, Ingenuity Systems) was also used to identify biological functions and upstream regulators relevant to the lists of DEGs analyzed. The main criterion to validate a differentially expressed gene was a fold change over 1.5 or under -1.5 when considering expression values in the group supplemented with vitamin D3 relative to the control diet group, whether considering wild type or transgenic animals. Upregulated and downregulated genes were analyzed in the same datasets to obtain the biologically relevant function categories. Right-tailed Fisher's exact test was used to calculate a *p*-value determining the top statistically significant biological functions assigned to the data set.

Real-time quantitative PCR (qPCR)

Total RNA (750 ng) was subjected to reverse transcription reaction to synthetize cDNA using oligo dT, RNase Out and M-MLV RT enzyme (Life Technologies, ThermoFisher Scientific) according to the manufacturer's instructions.

Real time qPCR experiments were carried out with the 7500 Fast real-Time PCR system (Applied Biosystems, ThermoFisher Scientific), using TaqMan® Fast Universal PCR Master Mix (2X) and the following TaqMan® Gene Expression Assays: *Oxt* (Mm00726655_s1), *Avp* (Mm00437761_g1), *Lcn2* (Mm01324470_m1), *Ptgs2* (Mm00478374_m1), *Esr1* (Mm00433149_m1), *Igf1* (Mm00439560_m1), *Gapdh* (Mm99999915_g1). Experiments used 7.5 ng of previously prepared cDNA and samples were run in triplicates on six different biological samples for each group. Relative expression levels were determined according to the ΔΔCt method where the expression level of the mRNA of interest is given by $2^{-\Delta\Delta CT}$ where $\Delta\Delta CT = \Delta CT$ target mRNA − ΔCT reference mRNA (*Gapdh*) in the same sample as previously described [4, 128].

Statistical analysis

Significant differences between groups were determined using the Kaleida Graph software. We used one-way ANOVA followed by a post-hoc Bonferroni test for multiple comparisons. Kruskal-Wallis test was used to compare two experimental groups. Values represent the mean ± SEM of the indicated number of independent experiments/animals, and the level of significance was set for $p < 0.05$ * or $p < 0{,}01$**.

Additional files

Additional file 1: Table S1. List of vitamin D-related transcripts dysregulated in transgenic 5XFAD mice. Dysregulated transcripts in the adult brain of 9 month-old 5XFAD transgenic female mice in comparison with wild type mice. The acronym and the full name of each gene are indicated. Genes with a VDRE are highlighted in grey.

Additional file 2: Comparative analysis of DEGs between different conditions. Table S2. Common DEGs between cortex and hippocampus in Wt mice supplemented with vitamin D3. Table S3. Specific DEGs in cortex of Wt mice supplemented with vitamin D3. Table S4. Specific DEGs in hippocampus of Wt mice supplemented with vitamin D3. Table S5. Common DEGs between cortex and hippocampus in Tg mice supplemented with vitamin D3. Table S6. Specific DEGs in cortex of Tg mice supplemented with vitamin D3. Table S7. Specific DEGs in hippocampus of Tg mice supplemented with vitamin D3. Table S8. Common DEGs between cortex and hippocampus of both Wt and Tg mice supplemented with vitamin D3.

Additional file 3: Table S9. Common DEGs in at least 3 out 4 conditions (cortex; hippocampus; WtVitD; TgVitD).

Additional file 4: List of canonical pathways modified by a vitamin D3-enriched diet in Wt and Tg animals. Table S10. Common canonical pathways between Wt and Tg mice supplemented with vitamin D3 and associated DEGs. Table S11. Canonical pathways specifically modified in Wt VitD animals. Table S12. Canonical pathways specifically modified in Tg VitD animals.

Additional file 5: List of DEGs known to be related to vitamin D action in the corertx and hippocampus of Wt and Tg mice. Genes containing a VDRE sequence are highlighted in grey. Table S13. Vitamin D related DEGs in Tg Cont, Tg VitD and Wt VitD mice. Table S14. Common vitamin D related DEGS between Tg Cont and TgVitD or between Tg Cont and Wt VitD. Table S15. Common vitamin D related DEGs between Tg Cont, Tg VitD and Wt VitD mice.

Additional file 6: Figure S1. Comparison of the different DEGs affected in the Wnt/β-catenin signaling pathway according to mouse genotype (Wt VitD versus Tg VitD).

Abbreviations

1,25(OH)2D3: 1,25-dihydroxycholecalciferol or calcitriol; 25(OH)D: 25-hydroxyvitamin D or calcidiol; 5XFAD: 5 mutations of familial Alzheimer's disease; AD: Alzheimer's disease; APP: amyloid precursor protein; Aβ: amyloid beta peptide; BBB: blood brain barrier; DEG: differentially expressed genes; ESR1: estrogen receptor 1; FC: fold change; IGF1: insulin growth factor 1; IPA: ingenuity pathway analysis; KO: knock-out; M4; M6; M9: month 4; month 6; month 9; MWM: Morris water maze; PSEN1: presenilin 1; RAWM: radial arm water maze; RXR: retinoid X receptor; TG: transgenic; VDR: vitamin D receptor; VDRE: vitamin D responsive element; VitD: vitamin D; WT: wild type.

Competing interests

The authors declare that they have no competing interests

Authors' contributions

VL performed the experiments and wrote the manuscript. PM participated in interpreting the data and helped draft the manuscript. KB bred and genotyped the mice and helped draft the manuscript. BL performed the microarray assay and helped draft the manuscript. FF designed, and coordinated the study, wrote the manuscript. All authors read and approved the final manuscript.

Acknowledgments

Aurélia Cès for her help with the behavioral experiments and Philippe Benech for his input in analyzing the transcriptomic data.
This work was supported by public [*Aix-Marseille Université* (AMU), *Centrel National de la Recherche Scientifique* (CNRS)] and private grants [*Fondation de 'Avenir, Demain Debout, Combattre la Paralysie*]. KB was granted a research associate fellowship by the French "Fondation Plan Alzheimer" and A*MIDEX (Management of talents).

Author details

Aix Marseille Université, CNRS, NICN UMR 7259, Marseille 13916, France. [2]APHP, Groupe hospitalier universitaire Saint Louis-Lariboisière-Fernand Widal, Centre Mémoire de Ressources et de Recherche, Hôpital Fernand Widal, Paris, France. [3]Aix Marseille Université, INSERM UMR 1090, TAGC, Marseille, France, Marseille 13288, France.

References

1. Bateman R. Alzheimer's disease and other dementias: advances in 2014. Lancet Neurol. 2015;14:4–6.
2. Oakley H, Cole SL, Logan S, Maus E, Shao P, Craft J, Guillozet-Bongaarts A, Ohno M, Disterhoft J, Van Eldik L, Berry R, Vassar R. Intraneuronal beta-amyloid aggregates, neurodegeneration, and neuron loss in transgenic mice with five familial Alzheimer's disease mutations: potential factors in amyloid plaque formation. J Neurosci Off J Soc Neurosci. 2006;26:10129–40.
3. Webster SJ, Bachstetter AD, Nelson PT, Schmitt FA, Van Eldik LJ. Using mice to model Alzheimer's dementia: an overview of the clinical disease and the preclinical behavioral changes in 10 mouse models. Front Genet. 2014;5:88.
4. Landel V, Baranger K, Virard I, Loriod B, Khrestchatisky M, Rivera S, Benech P, Féron F. Temporal gene profiling of the 5XFAD transgenic mouse model highlights the importance of microglial activation in Alzheimer's disease. Mol Neurodegener. 2014;9:33.
5. Christakos S, Dhawan P, Liu Y, Peng X, Porta A. New insights into the mechanisms of vitamin D action. J Cell Biochem. 2003;88:695–705.
6. Wang T-T, Tavera-Mendoza LE, Laperriere D, Libby E, MacLeod NB, Nagai Y, Bourdeau V, Konstorum A, Lallemant B, Zhang R, Mader S, White JH. Large-scale in silico and microarray-based identification of direct 1,25-dihydroxyvitamin D3 target genes. Mol Endocrinol. 2005;19:2685–95.
7. Przybelski R, Agrawal S, Krueger D, Engelke JA, Walbrun F, Binkley N. Rapid correction of low vitamin D status in nursing home residents. Osteoporos Int. 2008;19:1621–8.
8. Anastasiou CA, Yannakoulia M, Scarmeas N. Vitamin D and cognition: an update of the current evidence. J Alzheimers Dis. 2014;42 Suppl 3:S71–80.
9. Sato Y, Asoh T, Oizumi K. High prevalence of vitamin D deficiency and reduced bone mass in elderly women with Alzheimer's disease. Bone. 1998;23:555–7.
10. Evatt ML, Delong MR, Khazai N, Rosen A, Triche S, Tangpricha V. Prevalence of vitamin d insufficiency in patients with Parkinson disease and Alzheimer disease. Arch Neurol. 2008;65:1348–52.
11. Annweiler C, Maby E, Meyerber M, Beauchet O. Hypovitaminosis D and executive dysfunction in older adults with memory complaint: a memory clinic-based study. Dement Geriatr Cogn Disord. 2014;37:286–93.
12. Annweiler C, Rolland Y, Schott AM, Blain H, Vellas B, Beauchet O. Serum vitamin D deficiency as a predictor of incident non-Alzheimer dementias: a 7-year longitudinal study. Dement Geriatr Cogn Disord. 2011;32:273–8.
13. Littlejohns TJ, Henley WE, Lang IA, Annweiler C, Beauchet O, Chaves PHM, Fried L, Kestenbaum BR, Kuller LH, Langa KM, Lopez OL, Kos K, Soni M, Llewellyn DJ. Vitamin D and the risk of dementia and Alzheimer disease. Neurology. 2014;83:920–8.
14. Gezen-Ak D, Dursun E, Ertan T, Hanagasi H, Gurvit H, Emre M, Eker E, Ozturk M, Engin F, Yilmazer S. Association between vitamin D receptor gene polymorphism and Alzheimer's disease. Tohoku J Exp Med. 2007;212:275–82.
15. Kuningas M, Mooijaart SP, Jolles J, Slagboom PE, Westendorp RG, van Heemst D. VDR gene variants associate with cognitive function and depressive symptoms in old age. Neurobiol Aging. 2009;30:466–73.

16. Lehmann DJ, Refsum H, Warden DR, Medway C, Wilcock GK, Smith AD. The vitamin D receptor gene is associated with Alzheimer's disease. Neurosci Lett. 2011;504:79–82.
17. Gezen-Ak D, Dursun E, Bilgic B, Hanagasi H, Ertan T, Gurvit H, Emre M, Eker E, Ulutin T, Uysal O, Yilmazer S. Vitamin D receptor gene haplotype is associated with late-onset Alzheimer's disease. Tohoku J Exp Med. 2012;228:189–96.
18. Wang L, Hara K, Van Baaren JM, Price JC, Beecham GW, Gallins PJ, Whitehead PL, Wang G, Lu C, Slifer MA, Zuchner S, Martin ER, Mash D, Haines JL, Pericak-Vance MA, Gilbert JR. Vitamin D receptor and Alzheimer's disease: a genetic and functional study. Neurobiol Aging. 2012;1844(33):e1–9.
19. Laczmanski L, Jakubik M, Bednarek-Tupikowska G, Rymaszewska J, Sloka N, Lwow F. Vitamin D receptor gene polymorphisms in Alzheimer's disease patients. Exp Gerontol. 2015;69:142–7.
20. Sutherland MK, Somerville MJ, Yoong LK, Bergeron C, Haussler MR, McLachlan DR. Reduction of vitamin D hormone receptor mRNA levels in Alzheimer as compared to Huntington hippocampus: correlation with calbindin-28k mRNA levels. Brain Res Mol Brain Res. 1992;13:239–50.
21. Ito S, Ohtsuki S, Nezu Y, Koitabashi Y, Murata S, Terasaki T. 1alpha,25-Dihydroxyvitamin D3 enhances cerebral clearance of human amyloid-beta peptide(1-40) from mouse brain across the blood–brain barrier. Fluids Barriers CNS. 2011;8:20.
22. Dursun E, Gezen-Ak D, Yilmazer S. A novel perspective for Alzheimer's disease: vitamin D receptor suppression by amyloid-beta and preventing the amyloid-beta induced alterations by vitamin D in cortical neurons. J Alzheimers Dis. 2011;23:207–19.
23. Gezen-Ak D, Dursun E, Yilmazer S. The effects of vitamin D receptor silencing on the expression of LVSCC-A1C and LVSCC-A1D and the release of NGF in cortical neurons. PLoS One. 2011;6:e17553.
24. Taghizadeh M, Djazayery A, Salami M, Eshraghian MR, Zavareh SA. Vitamin-D-free regimen intensifies the spatial learning deficit in Alzheimer's disease. Int J Neurosci. 2011;121:16–24.
25. Grimm MO, Lehmann J, Mett J, Zimmer VC, Grosgen S, Stahlmann CP, Hundsdorfer B, Haupenthal VJ, Rothhaar TL, Herr C, Bals R, Grimm HS, Hartmann T. Impact of Vitamin D on amyloid precursor protein processing and amyloid-beta peptide degradation in Alzheimer's disease. Neurodegener Dis. 2014;13:75–81.
26. Yu J, Gattoni-Celli M, Zhu H, Bhat NR, Sambamurti K, Gattoni-Celli S, Kindy MS. Vitamin D3-enriched diet correlates with a decrease of amyloid plaques in the brain of AbetaPP transgenic mice. J Alzheimers Dis. 2011;25:295–307.
27. Eyles D, Almeras L, Benech P, Patatian A, Mackay-Sim A, McGrath J, Feron F. Developmental vitamin D deficiency alters the expression of genes encoding mitochondrial, cytoskeletal and synaptic proteins in the adult rat brain. J Steroid Biochem Mol Biol. 2007;103:538–45.
28. Nissou MF, Brocard J, El Atifi M, Guttin A, Andrieux A, Berger F, Issartel JP, Wion D. The transcriptomic response of mixed neuron-glial cell cultures to 1,25-dihydroxyvitamin d3 includes genes limiting the progression of neurodegenerative diseases. J Alzheimers Dis. 2013;35:553–64.
29. Nissou MF, Guttin A, Zenga C, Berger F, Issartel JP, Wion D. Additional clues for a protective role of vitamin D in neurodegenerative diseases: 1,25-dihydroxyvitamin D3 triggers an anti-inflammatory response in brain pericytes. J Alzheimers Dis. 2014;42:789–99.
30. Latimer CS, Brewer LD, Searcy JL, Chen KC, Popovic J, Kraner SD, Thibault O, Blalock EM, Landfield PW, Porter NM. Vitamin D prevents cognitive decline and enhances hippocampal synaptic function in aging rats. Proc Natl Acad Sci U S A. 2014;111:E4359–66.
31. Kaneko I, Sabir MS, Dussik CM, Whitfield GK, Karrys A, Hsieh J-C, Haussler MR, Meyer MB, Pike JW, Jurutka PW. 1,25-Dihydroxyvitamin D regulates expression of the tryptophan hydroxylase 2 and leptin genes: implication for behavioral influences of vitamin D. FASEB J Off Publ Fed Am Soc Exp Biol. 2015;29:4023–35.
32. Hawes JE, Tesic D, Whitehouse AJ, Zosky GR, Smith JT, Wyrwoll CS. Maternal vitamin D deficiency alters fetal brain development in the BALB/c mouse. Behav Brain Res. 2015;286:192–200.
33. Carlberg C. Genome-wide (over)view on the actions of vitamin D. Front Physiol. 2014;5:167.
34. de Abreu Fernandes DA, Eyles D, Feron F. Vitamin D, a neuro-immunomodulator: implications for neurodegenerative and autoimmune diseases. Psychoneuroendocrinology. 2009;34 Suppl 1:S265–77.
35. Yin K, Agrawal DK. Vitamin D and inflammatory diseases. J Inflamm Res. 2014;7:69–87.
36. Lemire JM, Archer DC, Beck L, Spiegelberg HL. Immunosuppressive actions of 1,25-dihydroxyvitamin D3: preferential inhibition of Th1 functions. J Nutr. 1995;125(6 Suppl):1704S–8S.
37. Boonstra A, Barrat FJ, Crain C, Heath VL, Savelkoul HF, O'Garra A. 1alpha,25-Dihydroxyvitamin d3 has a direct effect on naive CD4(+) T cells to enhance the development of Th2 cells. J Immunol. 2001;167:4974–80.
38. Cantorna MT, Waddell A. The vitamin D receptor turns off chronically activated T cells. Ann N Y Acad Sci. 2014;1317:70–5.
39. Hewison M. Vitamin D and the immune system: new perspectives on an old theme. Rheum Dis Clin North Am. 2012;38:125–39.
40. Jeffery LE, Burke F, Mura M, Zheng Y, Qureshi OS, Hewison M, Walker LSK, Lammas DA, Raza K, Sansom DM. 1,25-Dihydroxyvitamin D3 and IL-2 combine to inhibit T cell production of inflammatory cytokines and promote development of regulatory T cells expressing CTLA-4 and FoxP3. J Immunol. 2009;183:5458–67.
41. Ryynänen J, Carlberg C. Primary 1,25-dihydroxyvitamin D3 response of the interleukin 8 gene cluster in human monocyte- and macrophage-like cells. PLoS One. 2013;8:e78170.
42. Campbell MJ. Vitamin D and the RNA transcriptome: more than mRNA regulation. Front Physiol. 2014;5:181.
43. Nanduri R, Mahajan S, Bhagyaraj E, Sethi K, Kalra R, Chandra V, Gupta P. The Active Form of Vitamin D Transcriptionally Represses Smad7 Signaling and Activates Extracellular Signal-regulated Kinase (ERK) to Inhibit the Differentiation of a Inflammatory T Helper Cell Subset and Suppress Experimental Autoimmune Encephalomyelitis. J Biol Chem. 2015;290:12222–36.
44. Chen Y, Liu W, Sun T, Huang Y, Wang Y, Deb DK, Yoon D, Kong J, Thadhani R, Li YC 1,25-Dihydroxyvitamin D Promotes Negative Feedback Regulation of Toll-Like Receptor Signaling via Targeting MicroRNA-155-SOCS1 in Macrophages. J Immunol. 2013;190:3687–95.
45. Li YC, Chen Y, Liu W, Thadhani R. MicroRNA-mediated mechanism of vitamin D regulation of innate immune response. J Steroid Biochem Mol Biol. 2014;144(Pt A):81–6.
46. Wöbke TK, Sorg BL, Steinhilber D. Vitamin D in inflammatory diseases. Front Physiol. 2014;5:244.
47. Barnes PJ. Anti-inflammatory actions of glucocorticoids: molecular mechanisms. Clin Sci (Lond). 1998;94:557–72.
48. Müller MR, Rao A. NFAT, immunity and cancer: a transcription factor comes of age. Nat Rev Immunol. 2010;10:645–56.
49. Joshi S, Pantalena L-C, Liu XK, Gaffen SL, Liu H, Rohowsky-Kochan C, Ichiyama K, Yoshimura A, Steinman L, Christakos S, Youssef S. 1,25-dihydroxyvitamin D(3) ameliorates Th17 autoimmunity via transcriptional modulation of interleukin-17A. Mol Cell Biol. 2011;31:3653–69.
50. Cohen-Lahav M, Shany S, Tobvin D, Chaimovitz C, Douvdevani A. Vitamin D decreases NFκB activity by increasing IκBα levels. Nephrol Dial Transplant. 2006;21:889–97.
51. Harant H, Wolff B, Lindley IJD. 1α,25-Dihydroxyvitamin D3 decreases DNA binding of nuclear factor-κB in human fibroblasts. FEBS Lett. 1998;436:329–34.
52. Fekrmandi F, Wang T-T, White JH. The hormone-bound vitamin D receptor enhances the FBW7-dependent turnover of NF-κB subunits. Sci Rep. 2015;5:13002.
53. Tsatsanis C, Androulidaki A, Venihaki M, Margioris AN. Signalling networks regulating cyclooxygenase-2. Int J Biochem Cell Biol. 2006;38:1654–61.
54. DeLuca GC, Kimball SM, Kolasinski J, Ramagopalan SV, Ebers GC. Review: the role of vitamin D in nervous system health and disease. Neuropathol Appl Neurobiol. 2013;39:458–84.
55. de Viragh PA, Haglid KG, Celio MR. Parvalbumin increases in the caudate putamen of rats with vitamin D hypervitaminosis. Proc Natl Acad Sci U S A. 1989;86:3887–90.
56. Garcion E, Nataf S, Berod A, Darcy F, Brachet P. 1,25-Dihydroxyvitamin D3 inhibits the expression of inducible nitric oxide synthase in rat central nervous system during experimental allergic encephalomyelitis. Brain Res Mol Brain Res. 1997;45:255–67.
57. Féron F, Burne THJ, Brown J, Smith E, McGrath JJ, Mackay-Sim A, Eyles DW. Developmental Vitamin D3 deficiency alters the adult rat brain. Brain Res Bull. 2005;65:141–8.
58. Almeras L, Eyles D, Benech P, Laffite D, Villard C, Patatian A, Boucraut J, Mackay-Sim A, McGrath J, Feron F. Developmental vitamin D deficiency alters brain protein expression in the adult rat: implications for neuropsychiatric disorders. Proteomics. 2007;7:769–80.

59. McGrath JJ, Féron FP, Burne TH, Mackay-Sim A, Eyles DW. Vitamin D3-implications for brain development. J Steroid Biochem Mol Biol. 2004;89-90(1-5):557–60.
60. Cui X, Gooch H, Groves NJ, Sah P, Burne TH, Eyles DW, McGrath JJ. Vitamin D and the brain: key questions for future research. J Steroid Biochem Mol Biol. 2015;148:305–9.
61. Tabata T, Shoji T, Kikunami K, Matsushita Y, Inoue T, Tanaka S, Hino M, Miki T, Nishizawa Y, Morii H. In vivo effect of 1 alpha-hydroxyvitamin D3 on interleukin-2 production in hemodialysis patients. Nephron. 1988;50:295–8.
62. Di Rosa M, Malaguarnera G, De Gregorio C, Palumbo M, Nunnari G, Malaguarnera L. Immuno-modulatory effects of vitamin D3 in human monocyte and macrophages. Cell Immunol. 2012;280:36–43.
63. Bouter Y, Kacprowski T, Weissmann R, Dietrich K, Borgers H, Brauß A, Sperling C, Wirths O, Albrecht M, Jensen LR, Kuss AW, Bayer TA. Deciphering the molecular profile of plaques, memory decline and neuron loss in two mouse models for Alzheimer's disease by deep sequencing. Front Aging Neurosci. 2014;6:75.
64. Berridge MJ. Vitamin D: a custodian of cell signalling stability in health and disease. Biochem Soc Trans. 2015;43:349–58.
65. Larriba MJ, González-Sancho JM, Bonilla F, Muñoz A. Interaction of vitamin D with membrane-based signaling pathways. Front Physiol. 2014;5:60.
66. Bilkei-Gorzo A. Genetic mouse models of brain ageing and Alzheimer's disease. Pharmacol Ther. 2014;142:244–57.
67. Pollio G, Hoozemans JJM, Andersen CA, Roncarati R, Rosi MC, van Haastert ES, Seredenina T, Diamanti D, Gotta S, Fiorentini A, Magnoni L, Raggiaschi R, Rozemuller AJM, Casamenti F, Caricasole A, Terstappen GC. Increased expression of the oligopeptidase THOP1 is a neuroprotective response to Abeta toxicity. Neurobiol Dis. 2008;31:145–58.
68. Dougherty U, Mustafi R, Sadiq F, Almoghrabi A, Mustafi D, Kreisheh M, Sundaramurthy S, Liu W, Konda VJ, Pekow J, Khare S, Hart J, Joseph L, Wyrwicz A, Karczmar GS, Li YC, Bissonnette M. The renin-angiotensin system mediates EGF receptor-vitamin d receptor cross-talk in colitis-associated colon cancer. Clin Cancer Res. 2014;20:5848–59.
69. Carson JA, Turner AJ. Beta-amyloid catabolism: roles for neprilysin (NEP) and other metallopeptidases? J Neurochem. 2002;81:1–8.
70. Hemming ML, Selkoe DJ. Amyloid beta-protein is degraded by cellular angiotensin-converting enzyme (ACE) and elevated by an ACE inhibitor. J Biol Chem. 2005;280:37644–50.
71. Zou K, Yamaguchi H, Akatsu H, Sakamoto T, Ko M, Mizoguchi K, Gong J-S, Yu W, Yamamoto T, Kosaka K, Yanagisawa K, Michikawa M. Angiotensin-converting enzyme converts amyloid beta-protein 1-42 (Abeta(1-42)) to Abeta(1-40), and its inhibition enhances brain Abeta deposition. J Neurosci Off J Soc Neurosci. 2007;27:8628–35.
72. Carter CJ. Convergence of genes implicated in Alzheimer's disease on the cerebral cholesterol shuttle: APP, cholesterol, lipoproteins, and atherosclerosis. Neurochem Int. 2007;50:12–38.
73. Di Marco LY, Venneri A, Farkas E, Evans PC, Marzo A, Frangi AF. Vascular dysfunction in the pathogenesis of Alzheimer's disease - A review of endothelium-mediated mechanisms and ensuing vicious circles. Neurobiol Dis. 2015;82:593–606.
74. Giau VV, Bagyinszky E, An SSA, Kim SY. Role of apolipoprotein E in neurodegenerative diseases. Neuropsychiatr Dis Treat. 2015;11:1723–37.
75. Lange CM, Gouttenoire J, Duong FHT, Morikawa K, Heim MH, Moradpour D. Vitamin D receptor and Jak-STAT signaling crosstalk results in calcitriol-mediated increase of hepatocellular response to IFN-α. J Immunol. 2014;192:6037–44.
76. Trusca VG, Fuior EV, Florea IC, Kardassis D, Simionescu M, Gafencu AV. Macrophage-specific up-regulation of apolipoprotein E gene expression by STAT1 is achieved via long range genomic interactions. J Biol Chem. 2011;286:13891–904.
77. Wang JM, Irwin RW, Brinton RD. Activation of estrogen receptor alpha increases and estrogen receptor beta decreases apolipoprotein E expression in hippocampus in vitro and in vivo. Proc Natl Acad Sci U S A. 2006;103:16983–8.
78. Maddock J, Cavadino A, Power C, Hyppönen E. 25-hydroxyvitamin D, APOE ε4 genotype and cognitive function: findings from the 1958 British birth cohort. Eur J Clin Nutr. 2015;69:505–8.
79. Gezen-Ak D, Yilmazer S, Dursun E. Why vitamin D in Alzheimer's disease? The hypothesis. J Alzheimers Dis. 2014;40:257–69.
80. Yanagisawa J, Yanagi Y, Masuhiro Y, Suzawa M, Watanabe M, Kashiwagi K, Toriyabe T, Kawabata M, Miyazono K, Kato S. Convergence of transforming growth factor-beta and vitamin D signaling pathways on SMAD transcriptional coactivators. Science. 1999;283:1317–21.
81. Lesné S, Docagne F, Gabriel C, Liot G, Lahiri DK, Buée L, Plawinski L, Delacourte A, MacKenzie ET, Buisson A, Vivien D. Transforming growth factor-beta 1 potentiates amyloid-beta generation in astrocytes and in transgenic mice. J Biol Chem. 2003;278:18408–18.
82. Biegon A, Terlou M, Voorhuis TD, de Kloet ER. Arginine-vasopressin binding sites in rat brain: a quantitative autoradiographic study. Neurosci Lett. 1984;44:229–34.
83. Boccia ML, Petrusz P, Suzuki K, Marson L, Pedersen CA. Immunohistochemical localization of oxytocin receptors in human brain. Neuroscience. 2013;253:155–64.
84. Kim T-K, Lee J-E, Kim J-E, Park J-Y, Choi J, Kim H, Lee E-H, Han P-L: G9a-Mediated Regulation of OXT and AVP Expression in the Basolateral Amygdala Mediates Stress-Induced Lasting Behavioral Depression and Its Reversal by Exercise. Mol Neurobiol 2015. Epub ahead of print.
85. Metzger D, Alescio-Lautier B, Soumireu-Mourat B. Facilitation of retention performance in mice by pretest microinjection of AVP into dorsal or ventral hippocampus: differential influence of the peptide on appetitive task. Neurosci Lett. 1989;101:77–82.
86. Sato T, Tanaka K, Teramoto T, Ohnishi Y, Hirate K, Irifune M, Nishikawa T. Facilitative effect of a novel AVP fragment analog, NC-1900, on memory retention and recall in mice. Peptides. 2004;25:1139–46.
87. Fujiyoshi K, Suga H, Okamoto K, Nakamura S, Kameyama M. Reduction of arginine-vasopressin in the cerebral cortex in Alzheimer type senile dementia. J Neurol Neurosurg Psychiatry. 1987;50:929–32.
88. Perras B, Wagner U, Born J, Fehm HL. Improvement of sleep and pituitary-adrenal inhibition after subchronic intranasal vasopressin treatment in elderly humans. J Clin Psychopharmacol. 2003;23:35–44.
89. Jing W, Guo F, Cheng L, Zhang J-F, Qi J-S. Arginine vasopressin prevents amyloid beta protein-induced impairment of long-term potentiation in rat hippocampus in vivo. Neurosci Lett. 2009;450:306–10.
90. Pan Y-F, Chen X-R, Wu M-N, Ma C-G, Qi J-S. Arginine vasopressin prevents against Abeta(25-35)-induced impairment of spatial learning and memory in rats. Horm Behav. 2010;57:448–54.
91. Lin Y-T, Huang C-C, Hsu K-S. Oxytocin promotes long-term potentiation by enhancing epidermal growth factor receptor-mediated local translation of protein kinase Mζ. J Neurosci Off J Soc Neurosci. 2012;32:15476–88.
92. Hu J, Qi S, Becker B, Luo L, Gao S, Gong Q, Hurlemann R, Kendrick KM. Oxytocin selectively facilitates learning with social feedback and increases activity and functional connectivity in emotional memory and reward processing regions. Hum Brain Mapp. 2015;36:2132–46.
93. Wang Y, Zhao S, Wu Z, Feng Y, Zhao C, Zhang C. Oxytocin in the regulation of social behaviours in medial amygdala-lesioned mice via the inhibition of the extracellular signal-regulated kinase signalling pathway. Clin Exp Pharmacol Physiol. 2015;42:465–74.
94. Naudé PJW, Nyakas C, Eiden LE, Ait-Ali D, van der Heide R, Engelborghs S, Luiten PGM, De Deyn PP, Boer JA den, Eisel ULM. Lipocalin 2: novel component of proinflammatory signaling in Alzheimer's disease. FASEB J. 2012;26:2811–23.
95. Mesquita SD, Ferreira AC, Falcao AM, Sousa JC, Oliveira TG, Correia-Neves M, Sousa N, Marques F, Palha JA. Lipocalin 2 modulates the cellular response to amyloid beta. Cell Death Differ. 2014;21:1588–99.
96. Kinuta K, Tanaka H, Moriwake T, Aya K, Kato S, Seino Y. Vitamin D is an important factor in estrogen biosynthesis of both female and male gonads. Endocrinology. 2000;141:1317–24.
97. Swami S, Krishnan AV, Wang JY, Jensen K, Peng L, Albertelli MA, Feldman D. Inhibitory effects of calcitriol on the growth of MCF-7 breast cancer xenografts in nude mice: selective modulation of aromatase expression in vivo. Horm Cancer. 2011;2:190–202.
98. Katzburg S, Hendel D, Waisman A, Posner GH, Kaye AM, Somjen D. Treatment with non-hypercalcemic analogs of 1,25-dihydroxyvitamin D3 increases responsiveness to 17beta-estradiol, dihydrotestosterone or raloxifene in primary human osteoblasts. J Steroid Biochem Mol Biol. 2004;88:213–9.
99. Jorm AF, Korten AE, Henderson AS. The prevalence of dementia: a quantitative integration of the literature. Acta Psychiatr Scand. 1987;76:465–79.
100. Henderson VW, Paganini-Hill A, Emanuel CK, Dunn ME, Buckwalter JG. Estrogen replacement therapy in older women. Comparisons between Alzheimer's disease cases and nondemented control subjects. Arch Neurol. 1994;51:896–900.
101. Liu S, Zhao M. Neuroprotective effect of estrogen: role of nonsynaptic NR2B-containing NMDA receptors. Brain Res Bull. 2013;93:27–31.

102. Lan Y-L, Zhao J, Li S. Update on the neuroprotective effect of estrogen receptor alpha against Alzheimer's disease. J Alzheimers Dis. 2015;43:1137–48.
103. Shi C, Zhu X, Wang J, Long D. Estrogen receptor α promotes non-amyloidogenic processing of platelet amyloid precursor protein via the MAPK/ERK pathway. J Steroid Biochem Mol Biol. 2014;144(Pt B):280–5.
104. Swami S, Krishnan AV, Peng L, Lundqvist J, Feldman D. Transrepression of the estrogen receptor promoter by calcitriol in human breast cancer cells via two negative vitamin D response elements. Endocr Relat Cancer. 2013;20:565–77.
105. Mendez P, Azcoitia I, Garcia-Segura LM. Estrogen receptor alpha forms estrogen-dependent multimolecular complexes with insulin-like growth factor receptor and phosphatidylinositol 3-kinase in the adult rat brain. Brain Res Mol Brain Res. 2003;112:170–6.
106. Chen W-F, Zhou L-P, Chen L, Wu L, Gao Q-G, Wong M-S. Involvement of IGF-I receptor and estrogen receptor pathways in the protective effects of ginsenoside Rg1 against A $\beta_{25\text{-}35}$-induced toxicity in PC12 cells. Neurochem Int. 2013;62:1065–71.
107. Taguchi A, White MF. Insulin-like signaling, nutrient homeostasis, and life span. Annu Rev Physiol. 2008;70:191–212.
108. Rozing MP, Westendorp RGJ, Frölich M, de Craen AJM, Beekman M, Heijmans BT, Mooijaart SP, Blauw G-J, Slagboom PE, van Heemst D, Leiden Longevity Study (LLS) Group. Human insulin/IGF-1 and familial longevity at middle age. Aging. 2009;1:714–22.
109. Moloney AM, Griffin RJ, Timmons S, O'Connor R, Ravid R, O'Neill C. Defects in IGF-1 receptor, insulin receptor and IRS-1/2 in Alzheimer's disease indicate possible resistance to IGF-1 and insulin signalling. Neurobiol Aging. 2010;31:224–43.
110. Freude S, Schilbach K, Schubert M. The role of IGF-1 receptor and insulin receptor signaling for the pathogenesis of Alzheimer's disease: from model organisms to human disease. Curr Alzheimer Res. 2009;6:213–23.
111. Gontier G, George C, Chaker Z, Holzenberger M, Aïd S. Blocking IGF Signaling in Adult Neurons Alleviates Alzheimer's Disease Pathology through Amyloid-β Clearance. J Neurosci Off J Soc Neurosci. 2015;35:11500–13.
112. Keisala T, Minasyan A, Lou YR, Zou J, Kalueff AV, Pyykko I, Tuohimaa P. Premature aging in vitamin D receptor mutant mice. J Steroid Biochem Mol Biol. 2009;115:91–7.
113. Wang Y, Sun Z. Current understanding of klotho. Ageing Res Rev. 2009;8:43–51.
114. Nawashiro H, Messing A, Azzam N, Brenner M. Mice lacking GFAP are hypersensitive to traumatic cerebrospinal injury. Neuroreport. 1998;9:1691–6.
115. Otani N, Nawashiro H, Fukui S, Ooigawa H, Ohsumi A, Toyooka T, Shima K, Gomi H, Brenner M. Enhanced hippocampal neurodegeneration after traumatic or kainate excitotoxicity in GFAP-null mice. J Clin Neurosci. 2006;13:934–8.
116. Kraft AW, Hu X, Yoon H, Yan P, Xiao Q, Wang Y, Gil SC, Brown J, Wilhelmsson U, Restivo JL, Cirrito JR, Holtzman DM, Kim J, Pekny M, Lee J-M. Attenuating astrocyte activation accelerates plaque pathogenesis in APP/PS1 mice. FASEB J. 2013;27:187–98.
117. Orre M, Kamphuis W, Osborn LM, Jansen AHP, Kooijman L, Bossers K, Hol EM. Isolation of glia from Alzheimer's mice reveals inflammation and dysfunction. Neurobiol Aging. 2014;35:2746–60.
118. Lue LF, Kuo YM, Beach T, Walker DG. Microglia activation and anti-inflammatory regulation in Alzheimer's disease. Mol Neurobiol. 2010;41:115–28.
119. Walker DG, Link J, Lue L-F, Dalsing-Hernandez JE, Boyes BE. Gene expression changes by amyloid beta peptide-stimulated human postmortem brain microglia identify activation of multiple inflammatory processes. J Leukoc Biol. 2006;79:596–610.
120. Qiao D-L, Zhang S-Q, Giunta B. Is Vitamin D Beneficial to Alzheimer Disease? A Surprising Dilemma. CNS Neurosci Ther. 2012;18:601–3.
121. Mizwicki MT, Menegaz D, Zhang J, Barrientos-Duran A, Tse S, Cashman JR, Griffin PR, Fiala M. Genomic and nongenomic signaling induced by 1alpha,25(OH)2-vitamin D3 promotes the recovery of amyloid-beta phagocytosis by Alzheimer's disease macrophages. J Alzheimers Dis. 2012;29:51–62.
122. Mizwicki MT, Liu G, Fiala M, Magpantay L, Sayre J, Siani A, Mahanian M, Weitzman R, Hayden EY, Rosenthal MJ, Nemere I, Ringman J, Teplow DB. 1alpha,25-dihydroxyvitamin D3 and resolvin D1 retune the balance between amyloid-beta phagocytosis and inflammation in Alzheimer's disease patients. J Alzheimers Dis. 2013;34:155–70.
123. Durk MR, Han K, Chow EC, Ahrens R, Henderson JT, Fraser PE, Pang KS. 1alpha,25-Dihydroxyvitamin D3 reduces cerebral amyloid-beta accumulation and improves cognition in mouse models of Alzheimer's disease. J Neurosci. 2014;34:7091–101.
124. Bennett L, Kersaitis C, Macaulay SL, Munch G, Niedermayer G, Nigro J, Payne M, Sheean P, Vallotton P, Zabaras D, Bird M. Vitamin D2-enriched button mushroom (Agaricus bisporus) improves memory in both wild type and APPswe/PS1dE9 transgenic mice. PLoS One. 2013;8:e76362.
125. Briones TL, Darwish H. Vitamin D mitigates age-related cognitive decline through the modulation of pro-inflammatory state and decrease in amyloid burden. J Neuroinflammation. 2012;9:244.
126. Briones TL, Darwish H. Decrease in age-related tau hyperphosphorylation and cognitive improvement following vitamin D supplementation are associated with modulation of brain energy metabolism and redox state. Neuroscience. 2014;262:143–55.
127. Dimitrov V, White JH: Species-specific regulation of innate immunity by vitamin D signaling. J Steroid Biochem Mol Biol. 2015. Epub ahead of print.
128. Py NA, Bonnet AE, Bernard A, Marchalant Y, Charrat E, Checler F, Khrestchatisky M, Baranger K, Rivera S. Differential spatio-temporal regulation of MMPs in the 5xFAD mouse model of Alzheimer's disease: evidence for a pro-amyloidogenic role of MT1-MMP. Front Aging Neurosci. 2014;6:247.
129. Alamed J, Wilcock DM, Diamond DM, Gordon MN, Morgan D. Two-day radial-arm water maze learning and memory task; robust resolution of amyloid-related memory deficits in transgenic mice. Nat Protoc. 2006;1:1671–9.

8

Neurotrophic factor small-molecule mimetics mediated neuroregeneration and synaptic repair: emerging therapeutic modality for Alzheimer's disease

Syed Faraz Kazim[1,2] and Khalid Iqbal[1*]

Abstract

Alzheimer's disease (AD) is an incurable and debilitating chronic progressive neurodegenerative disorder which is the leading cause of dementia worldwide. AD is a heterogeneous and multifactorial disorder, histopathologically characterized by the presence of amyloid β (Aβ) plaques and neurofibrillary tangles composed of Aβ peptides and abnormally hyperphosphorylated tau protein, respectively. Independent of the various etiopathogenic mechanisms, neurodegeneration is a final common outcome of AD neuropathology. Synaptic loss is a better correlate of cognitive impairment in AD than Aβ or tau pathologies. Thus a highly promising therapeutic strategy for AD is to shift the balance from neurodegeneration to neuroregeneration and synaptic repair. Neurotrophic factors, by virtue of their neurogenic and neurotrophic activities, have potential for the treatment of AD. However, the clinical therapeutic usage of recombinant neurotrophic factors is limited because of the insurmountable hurdles of unfavorable pharmacokinetic properties, poor blood–brain barrier (BBB) permeability, and severe adverse effects. Neurotrophic factor small-molecule mimetics, in this context, represent a potential strategy to overcome these short comings, and have shown promise in preclinical studies. Neurotrophic factor small-molecule mimetics have been the focus of intense research in recent years for AD drug development. Here, we review the relevant literature regarding the therapeutic beneficial effect of neurotrophic factors in AD, and then discuss the recent status of research regarding the neurotrophic factor small-molecule mimetics as therapeutic candidates for AD. Lastly, we summarize the preclinical studies with a ciliary neurotrophic factor (CNTF) small-molecule peptide mimetic, Peptide 021 (P021). P021 is a neurogenic and neurotrophic compound which enhances dentate gyrus neurogenesis and memory processes via inhibiting leukemia inhibitory factor (LIF) signaling pathway and increasing brain-derived neurotrophic factor (BDNF) expression. It robustly inhibits tau abnormal hyperphosphorylation via increased BDNF mediated decrease in glycogen synthase kinase-3β (GSK-3β, major tau kinase) activity. P021 is a small molecular weight, BBB permeable compound with suitable pharmacokinetics for oral administration, and without adverse effects associated with native CNTF or BDNF molecule. P021 has shown beneficial therapeutic effect in several preclinical studies and has emerged as a highly promising compound for AD drug development.

Keywords: Alzheimer's disease, Cognition, Neurotrophic factor small-molecule mimetics, Brain-derived neurotrophic factor (BDNF), Ciliary neurotrophic factor (CNTF), Amyloid beta, Tau, Neurogenesis, Synaptic loss, Neurodegeneration

* Correspondence: khalid.iqbal.ibr@gmail.com
[1]Department of Neurochemistry, and SUNY Downstate/NYSIBR Program in Developmental Neuroscience, New York State Institute for Basic Research (NYSIBR), 1050 Forest Hill Road, Staten Island, NY 10314, USA
Full list of author information is available at the end of the article

Background

Alzheimer's disease (AD) is a chronic, debilitating, neurodegenerative disorder and is the most common form of dementia in the elderly [1, 2]. AD is the sixth leading cause of mortality in the United States, and affects nearly 5.4 million Americans [3, 4]. Approximately 476,000 people age 65 or older are expected to develop AD in the United States in the year 2016, and the total healthcare expenditure for AD and related dementias will be nearly 236 billion dollars, making it one of the costliest chronic diseases in the United States [4]. Worldwide, AD and related dementias affect approximately 47 million people [5]. As yet there is no effective cure for AD [6]. By the year 2050, the prevalence of AD is projected to be 13.8 million in United States [3, 7], and 135 million worldwide [5, 8], lest an effective AD therapy is developed.

AD is clinically characterized by a heterogeneous set of symptoms including progressive memory impairment, visuospatial decline, aphasia, and loss of executive function [1, 9–11]. Short-term memory loss is the most common early symptom of AD [1, 9–11]. Histopathologically, there are two major lesions in AD: senile plaques (diffuse and neuritic) and neurofibrillary tangles (NFTs) [12, 13]. Amyloid β (Aβ) is the main component of the senile plaques whereas abnormally hyperphosphorylated tau protein gives rise to NFTs [12, 13]. Alongside Aβ plaques and NFTs, impairments in adult hippocampal neurogenesis and synaptic plasticity, synaptic deficit, and profound neurodegeneration are also major features of AD [14–25]. Adult hippocampal neurogenesis and synaptic plasticity have been proposed to be essential for learning and memory [26–30]. Alterations in adult hippocampal neurogenesis and synaptic plasticity could thus be the major mechanisms underlying cognitive dysfunction in AD [18, 31]. AD has also been characterized as a consequence of synaptic failure [22, 32]. Several studies have shown that synaptic loss correlates better with cognitive decline than either Aβ plaque load or NFTs [25, 33–35]. Targeting the impairment in adult hippocampal neurogenesis and neuronal and synaptic loss has been proposed as a potential therapeutic approach to rescue cognitive dysfunction in AD [6, 36].

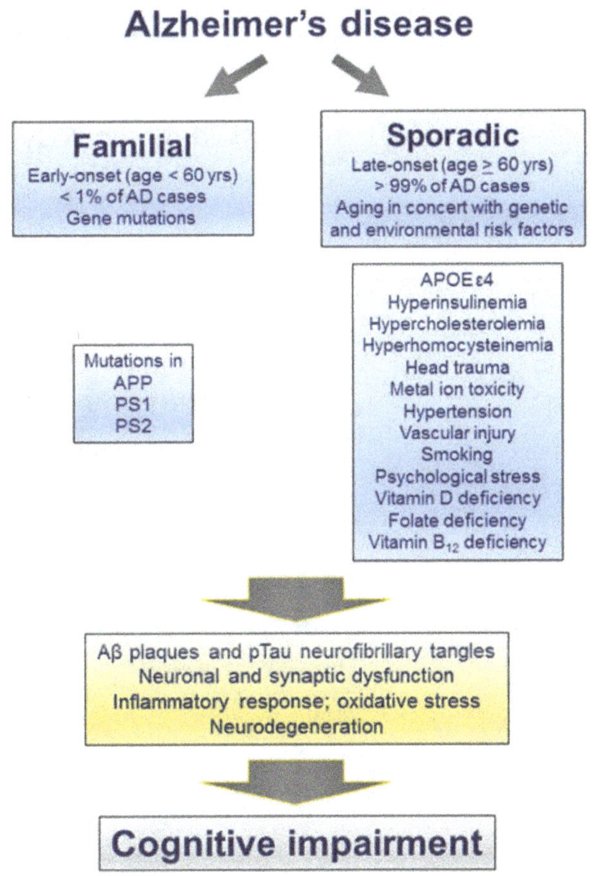

Fig. 1 Multifactorial nature of AD and involvement of several different etiopathogenic mechanisms. Early-onset familial AD caused by mutations in APP, PS1, or PS2 constitutes < 1 % of AD cases. The exact causes of late-onset sporadic AD which accounts for the remaining > 99 % of AD cases are as yet largely unknown. However, aging alongside gene-environment interaction is speculated to contribute to this form of AD. Both forms of AD lead to amyloid plaque and neurofibrillary pathologies, synaptic dysfunction and neurodegeneration, and ultimately cognitive impairment

Main text

Etiopathogenesis of Alzheimer's disease

AD, first described by German psychiatrist Alois Alzheimer in 1907 [37], is a multifactorial and heterogeneous disease, and apparently involves several different etiopathogenic mechanisms (Fig. 1) [6, 38]. The early-onset familial form of AD which is caused by mutations in amyloid β precursor protein (APP), presenilin 1 (PS1), or presenilin 2 (PS2), accounts for <1 % of all cases (Fig. 1) (for review, [39, 40]). The exact causes of the late-onset sporadic form of AD, which accounts for over 99 % of the cases, are not yet understood. The sporadic form of AD probably involves several different etiopathogenic mechanisms in concert with aging such as metabolic derangements, head trauma, metal ion toxicity, hypertension, vascular injury, smoking, psychological stress, and vitamin deficiencies (Fig. 1) [38]. No known mutations are involved in sporadic form of AD, however, the presence of one or two apolipoprotein E epsilon 4 (APOE ε4) alleles increases the disease risk ~3.5-fold or ~10-fold, respectively [39–41].

The histopathological hallmarks in both the sporadic and the familial forms of AD are similar and include amyloid β plaques and NFTs leading to neurodegeneration (Fig. 2) [6]. The immensely popular amyloid cascade hypothesis suggests a major etiological role of Aβ for the NFT pathology, neurodegeneration and cognitive dysfunction in AD [42]. Aβ plaques are produced by amyloidogenic processing of the transmembrane protein, APP, by

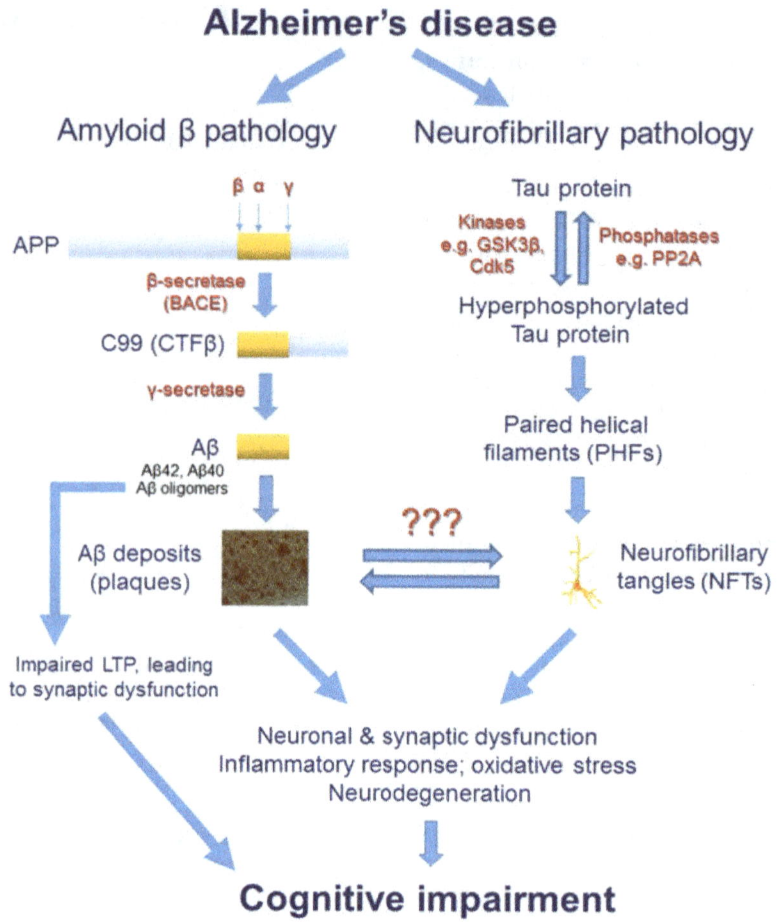

Fig. 2 Aβ plaques and NFTs as hallmarks of AD. AD is characterized by extracellular deposits of Aβ (senile) plaques and intraneuronal NFTs leading to neurodegeneration, and ultimately cognitive impairment and dementia. Aβ plaques are produced by the amyloidogenic processing of APP by β- and γ-secretase enzymes leading to the formation of Aβ peptides (36–43 amino acids) of which the Aβ40 and Aβ42 are the most common. Aβ42 is the most fibrillogenic and thus most amyloidogenic Aβ peptide. Aβ oligomers impair hippocampal LTP, and thus synaptic plasticity, and learning and memory. NFTs are intracellular aggregates of MAP-tau which is abnormally hyperphosphorylated by upregulation of activities of kinases such as GSK3β and Cdk5 or deficit in phosphatases such as PP2A

β- and γ-secretase enzymes resulting in the formation of major toxic products, Aβ40 and Aβ42 peptides (Fig. 2) [12, 43, 44]. The oligomeric form of Aβ has also been suggested as the main neurotoxic state of the peptide [45]. Aβ oligomers are known to inhibit hippocampal long-term potentiation (LTP) [46], a major cellular mechanism underlying synaptic plasticity, and learning and memory [47]. Amyloid cascade hypothesis also derives its major support from the Down syndrome individuals; as part of the trisomy 21, these patients carry 3 copies of APP and almost all of them develop AD neuropathological characteristics by the age of 40 years [48, 49].

Tau which is a neuronal microtubule associated protein (MAP) is a major protein subunit of paired helical filaments that constitute the NFTs (Fig. 2) [50, 51]. Tau in NFTs is abnormally hyperphosphorylated [13]. Tau is a substrate for several protein kinases including cyclin-dependent kinase 5 (Cdk5), glycogen synthase kinase 3 β (GSK-3β), and calcium/calmodulin activated protein kinase II (CaMKII) [52, 53]. The activities of several major tau kinases are regulated by protein phosphatase 2A (PP2A). PP2A can thus regulate the tau phosphorylaiton both directly and by inhibiting the activities of tau protein kinases [54]. PP2A activity is impaired and is possibly a cause of the abnormal hyperphosphorylation of tau in AD brain [55–57].

Stages of Alzheimer's disease

The neuropathologic staging of AD is performed based on three parameters (Aβ, Braak, and Consortium to Establish a Registry for AD, CERAD) to obtain an "ABC" score: histopathologic assessments of Aβ-containing amyloid plaques (A), Braak staging of NFTs (B), and scoring of neuritic amyloid plaques (C). The NFT load in AD brain are known to correlate better with cognitive decline [58]. In the earliest stages of AD (Braak stage I-II, prodromal

AD), NFTs are confined to the entorhinal cortex [59, 60]. Subsequently, NFTs spread to the limbic and medial temporal lobe (Braak stage III-IV; mild cognitive impairment, MCI, or early AD); this stage correlates with early memory related symptoms in AD [61, 62]. During the late stages (Braak stage V–VI, clinical AD), the number of NFTs increase and they occur in neocortical areas leading to impairments in higher cognitive functions such as executive and visuospatial abilities, and speech in concert with AD-related cognitive deficits [60, 63].

AD is a progressive neurodegenerative disorder (Fig. 3). As mentioned before, the earliest neuropathological changes in AD are in the hippocampus and entorhinal cortex, followed by changes in the medial temporal lobe [64–68]. Correspondingly, the earliest detectable cognitive deficit is in the medial temporal lobe dependent episodic memory [62, 69, 70]. Episodic memory deficits are followed by impairment in semantic memory; both memory domains depend on the neural circuitry of medial and lateral temporal lobes and occur prior to deficit in higher cognitive functions such as attention, and executive and visuospatial capabilities [71]. Mild deficits in executive functioning are first detectable near the end of the preclinical phase of AD [72, 73]. As the patient progresses from preclinical stage of AD into MCI, more cognitive functions begin to be impaired including verbal recall and deterioration of general memory domain [71, 74]. As the patient progresses from MCI into mild, moderate, and subsequently the severe stages of AD, general cognition continues to decline with impairment manifesting in all cognitive domains [75].

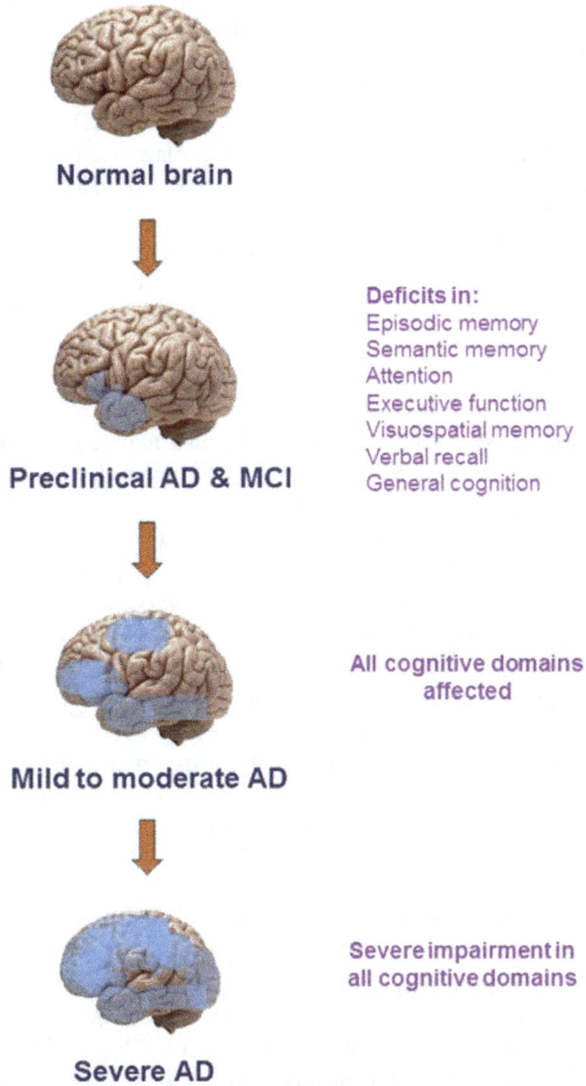

Fig. 3 Progression of neuropathology and cognitive impairment in AD. The earliest AD neuropathology develops in medial temporal lobe and gives rise to episodic memory deficit followed by impairment in semantic memory (preclinical AD). As the patient progresses to MCI stage, higher cognitive domains such as attention, executive function, visuospatial memory, and verbal recall become impaired. Also, general cognition starts to decline. As the patient progresses to mild to moderate AD stages, the neuropathology spreads to frontal and parietal lobes, and all cognitive domains become affected. In severe stage of AD, the neuropathology spreads to involve all brain lobes, and a profound deficit in all cognitive domains is noted

Neurogenic and synaptic failure in Alzheimer's disease

Adult hippocampal neurogenesis plays a pivotal role in learning and memory [26–28, 30, 76]. The essential role of adult-born hippocampal neurons has been suggested in complex forms of spatial and associative memory [27, 77–81]. In rodents, the aberrant hippocampal neurogenesis leads to impairment in different forms of hippocampus dependent learning such as in Morris water maze and contextual fear conditioning tasks [82, 83]. AD and other neurodegenerative diseases are characterized by an imbalance between neurogenesis and neurodegeneration [18, 84]. Consequently, the impairment in neurogenesis has been hypothesized to contribute to learning and memory deficits in AD [17, 18, 84].

In adult hippocampus, the survival, maturation, and integration of new born neurons in the dentate gyrus depends on the appropriate *brain milieu* or microenvironment primarily provided by the neurotrophic factors [85–89]. The dentate gyrus microenvironment in neurodegenerative conditions such as AD is not conducive for the neurogenesis and the survival, maturation, and integration of new born neurons into the hippocampal functional circuitry [90–92]. The AD brain responds to neurodegeneration by stimulating neurogenesis, however, because of the lack of a proper neurotrophic microenvironment of the hippocampus, this effort of the AD brain to replace lost neurons with new neurons is unsuccessful and culminates in failure of neuronal survival, maturation, and integration [16, 17, 36, 93]. As the disease progresses, the neurogenic failure becomes severe, and contributes significantly to cognitive decline [18, 36].

AD has been described as a synaptic failure [22, 32]. AD brains also show dendritic and dendritic spine loss [94]. Quantitative studies on AD brains within 2–4 years after the clinically diagnosed disease showed a 25–35 % decrease in synaptic density and a 15–35 % synaptic loss per neuron in the frontal and temporal lobes of the cerebral cortex [15]. The extent of synaptic loss is even more severe in the hippocampus where it amounts to 44–55 % [19–21, 95, 96]. Remarkably, the synaptic loss in frontal cortex and limbic system is the best correlate of the severity of cognitive dysfunction [25, 33–35]. The profound neuronal, synaptic, and dendritic loss may contribute to impaired synaptic plasticity, including reduced LTP, in AD. Synaptic plasticity is known to be the cellular substrate of learning and memory [29]. Additionally, adult hippocampal neurogenesis has been proposed to play a pivotal role in synaptic plasticity, and subsequently, learning and memory processes in the hippocampus [97]. Both human AD cases and AD transgenic mice exhibit significant alterations in the process of adult hippocampal neurogenesis [16, 93, 98–104]. The synaptic plasticity impairments in AD, thus, may not only be the consequence of synaptic failure but also impaired neurogenesis.

Shifting the balance from neurodegeneration to neural regeneration to treat Alzheimer's disease

The final common outcome of various different etiopathogenic mechanisms involved in AD is neurodegeneration leading to cognitive impairment. Thus, a highly promising therapeutic strategy for AD is to shift the balance from neurodegeneration to neural regeneration [6, 36]. This can be achieved by utilizing means that can enhance adult hippocampal neurogenesis and neuronal and synaptic plasticity. Several different approaches have been employed in rodent models of AD with reasonable success to enhance neurogenesis and neuronal and synaptic plasticity [105]. Neural stem cells-based replacement approach for AD is currently the focus of intense research and has shown promising results in animal models of AD [106, 107]. Neural stem cell implantation in the triple transgenic AD mice (3xTg-AD) that harbor mutated human APP, tau, and PS1, has been reported to rescue cognitive impairment via increased brain derived neurotrophic factor (BDNF) expression [108]. Pharmacological stimulation of neural stem cells with neurotrophic factors and growth factors such as fibroblast growth factor 2 (FGF2) [109], BDNF [110], ciliary neurotrophic factor (CNTF) [111] has also shown promise in mouse models of AD.

Neurotrophic factors — potent neuronal and synaptic repair molecules for the treatment of Alzheimer's disease

Neurotrophic factors can be broadly divided into 3 families: (1) neurotrophins, (2) glial cell-line derived neurotrophic factor (GDNF) family ligands (GFLs), and (3) neuropoeitic cytokines [112]. The neuroprotective effect of various neurotrophic factors via neuroregeneration and synaptic repair is well established [110, 113, 114].

The neurotrophin family comprises nerve growth factor (NGF), BDNF, neurotrophin 3 (NT3), and neurotrophin 4 (NT4) [115]. Neurotrophin signaling is mediated via two receptor types: p75 neurotrophin receptor ($p75^{NTR}$) and tropomysin receptor kinase (Trk) [115]. Each Trk receptor selectively binds to different neurotrophins: NGF binds to TrkA, BDNF and NT4 bind to TrkB, and NT3 binds to TrkC [112, 115]. Neurotrophin signaling occurs via several different pathways including two major tyrosine kinase-mediated pathways: the phosphoinositide 3-kinase (PI3K)-AKT (also known as protein kinase B, PKB) pathway and the mitogen-activated protein kinase (MAPK)-extracellular signal-regulated kinase (ERK) pathway [112, 115]. The neurotrophin signaling mediates neuronal survival, proliferation, and differentiation [115]. Imbalance in the neurotrophin levels in different brain regions has been shown in AD cases [116]. BDNF levels have been shown to be decreased in AD brains suggesting a lack of trophic support that may contribute significantly to neurodegeneration [116–119]. BDNF is essential for basal level of adult hippocampal neurogenesis and also for the survival and integration of new-born neurons into the hippocampal circuitry [120, 121]. BDNF also plays a crucial role in both the early and late phases of LTP, the cellular substrate for learning and memory [122–125]. In mouse and primate models of AD, entorhinal cortex administration of BDNF was found to have a beneficial effect on cognition [110]. In human AD cases, decreased NGF levels have been shown in the nucleus basalis of Meynert [126], a group of neurons in the basal forebrain which has wide ascending projections to the neocortex, is rich in acetylcholine (Ach) and choline acetyltransferase (ChAT), and is well known to undergo degeneration in AD [127]. In animal models, it has been demonstrated that the ascending cholinergic projections in the brain express low- and high-affinity NGF receptors and are NGF-sensitive and probably NGF-dependent [128, 129]. Cholinergic degeneration leads to cognitive dysfunction, and treatment with NGF can improve cognition in animal models [128, 129]. NGF gene therapy has recently been shown to exert a neurotrophic effect in AD patients [130].

The GDNF family of ligands (GFL) comprises of four neurotrophic factors: GDNF, neurturin (NRTN), artemin (ARTN), and persephin (PSPN) [131]. GFL signaling occurs through binding of a particular GFL dimer to a cell surface bound co-receptor, a member of the GFRα protein family, and subsequent activation of a receptor tyrosine kinase molecule, RET ("rearranged during transfection") [131]. The primary ligands for the co-receptors GFRα1, GFRα2, GFRα3, and GFRα4 are GDNF, NRTN, ARTN, and PSPN, respectively [131]. GFLs play a role in several different processes including neuronal survival, differentiation, and migration, and neurite outgrowth [131]. Deficiency of GFRα1, the receptor for GDNF, have been shown in human AD brains [132]. Also, GDNF gene therapy has been reported to protect against AD-like neuropathology in 3xTg-AD mice [133].

Neuropoietic cytokines family of neurotrophic factors exert many similar effects including enhancing neuronal proliferation and differentiation, however, this group signals through cytokine receptors rather than receptor tyrosine kinases [134, 135]. The transforming growth factor β (TGFβ) and interleukin-6 (IL-6) superfamilies are some of the most abundant and influential neuropoeitic cytokines in the brain, particularly during development [134, 135]. The TGFβ superfamily includes brain morphogenic proteins (BMPs) which play a key role in regulating neuron induction [134, 135]. BMPs interact with key neurogenic elements including Wnts and sonic hedgehog, and establish cell-fate determination and subtype differentiation [136–138]. The IL-6 family of cytokines includes CNTF, interleukin-11 (IL-11), leukemia inhibitory factor (LIF), oncostatin-M, cardiotrophin-1, and cardiotrophin-like cytokine [139, 140]. CNTF plays a pivotal role in adult hippocampal and subventricular zone neurogenesis, and the differentiation of neural stem cells [141–143]. CNTF signaling occurs through a tripartite complex of CNTF receptor α (CNTFRα), LIF β receptor (LIFR), and glycoprotein 130 (gp130). CNTF and LIF both signal through tyrosine phosphorylation (Tyr706) of the signal transducers and activators of transcription (STAT) proteins by the membrane associated Janus kinase (JAK) [144]. In the brain, CNTF is expressed in astrocytes in the neurogenic niches [145], while its receptor, CNTFRα, is expressed predominantly in neural progenitor cells and hippocampal neurons, and various other areas of the brain including motor cortex and cerebellum [142, 145]. Overall, CNTF is the most extensively studied neuropoetic cytokine, and its neuroprotective effects are well established [146]. CNTF administration has been shown to alleviate cognitive impairment and to stabilize synaptic protein levels in a transgenic mouse model of AD [111].

Neurotrophic factor small-molecule mimetics for the treatment of Alzheimer's disease

The therapeutic usage of neurotrophic factors such as BDNF and CNTF in AD patients is hindered by limited blood–brain barrier (BBB) permeability, poor plasma stability and unsuitable pharmacokinetics, and unwanted systemic effects [113, 147–149]. The recombinant BDNF or CNTF in clinical trials have shown limited bioavailability and multiple adverse effects [150, 151]. A promising strategy to bypass these limitations to develop neurotrophic factors based drugs for AD which has emerged during the last decade or so is to develop small-molecule mimetics that could exert the therapeutic beneficial effects of neurotrophic factors on neurogenesis, neuronal and synaptic plasticity, and ultimately cognition, with suitable pharmacokinetics and central nervous system (CNS) penetration for drug development, and without unwanted systemic effects produced by the full-length native molecules [148, 149, 152–156]. A major problem associated with the therapeutic usage of whole molecule neurotrophic factors is the pleiotropic actions that derive from their concomitant binding to multiple receptors [154]. The small-molecule mimetics might also allow to modulate various aspects of these signaling pathways in ways that are distinct from the whole molecule neurotrophic factors [154]. By departing from conventional neurotrophic factor signaling, these small-molecule mimetics might provide a novel therapeutic approach to treat AD [154].

Early attempts to develop small-molecule mimetics of neurotrophic factors focused on synthesizing peptidergic compounds consisting of amino acids residues corresponding to various NGF domains [154]. The first small peptide molecule corresponding to an NGF domain demonstrated to exert a neurotrophic effect was the cyclized dimeric form of peptide P7 (amino acid residues, KGKE) which acted through $p75^{NTR}$ receptor [157]. The NGF small peptide mimetics containing KGKE or a homologous sequence have been reported to block Aβ binding to $p75^{NTR}$ and protect against Aβ-induced cell death [158]. Another NGF small peptide mimetic, compound D3, which corresponds to amino acid side chains of NGF β-turn loops and acts through TrkA receptor, has been shown to rescue basal forebrain cholinergic neurodegeneration and spatial reference memory in aged rats [159]. Also, the administration of compound D3 via intracerebroventricular mini pump in J20 mice, which carry APP Swedish and Indiana mutations, has been shown to rescue learning and short-term memory deficits [160].

Small-molecule modulation of BDNF receptor, TrkB, for the treatment of neurodegenerative disorders including AD, has been the focus of intense research in recent years [113, 154, 161]. A naturally occurring flavone, 7,8-dihydroxyflavone (7,8-DHF), which can induce the phosphorylation of TrkB and its downstream mediators, AKT and ERK, has been shown to be neuroprotective and neurotrophic [161–163]. In studies employing transgenic mouse models of AD, 7,8-DHF has shown beneficial effect on learning and memory [164–166]. R7, a prodrug of 7,8-DHF, with considerably improved potency and favorable pharmacokinetics, is currently in preclinical development for the treatment of AD [167]. A BDNF small-molecule mimetic compound, LM22A-4, identified using *in silico* screening with a BDNF loop-domain pharmacophore, was found to promote survival of hippocampal neurons (~85 % of the efficacy of BDNF), induce TrkB phosphorylation, and prevent neuronal death in an in vitro model of AD [168]. Other TrkB small molecule mimetics that have shown promise in preclinical studies include de-oxygedunin [169], N-acetylserotonin [170], adenosine 2A receptor agonist [171, 172], and BDNF loop mimetics [173, 174]. Recently, our lab also identified BDNF tetrapeptides (peptide B1-B5) which can modulate TrkB signaling and exert neurotrophic effect in mouse hippocampal primary neuronal cultures [175].

A $p75^{NTR}$ small-molecule non-peptide mimetic identified through *in silico* screening, LM11A-31, also known as C31, is a highly promising AD drug candidate [154]. LM11A-31 has been shown to block Aβ-induced deleterious signaling, including the activation of calpain-Cdk5, GSK-3β, and c-jun N-terminal kinase (JNK) signaling, and reduce Aβ-induced tau hyperphosphorylation and the inactivation of AKT and cAMP-response element-binding protein (CREB) [176]. LM11A-31 has also been reported to exert beneficial effect both at early and late stages of the AD-like neuropathology in transgenic mice [177, 178]. LM11A-31, has successfully completed a Phase I clinical trial without any significant adverse effects, and is currently undergoing Phase IIa clinical trial in human AD patients.

Neurotrophic factor small-molecule mimetics offer several advantages as compared to native neurotrophic factor molecules including suitable pharmacokinetics and enhanced BBB permeability for drug development. However, there are certain limitations such as insufficient receptor specificity, requirement for continuous dosing, and effects which are not brain region-specific [154]. These limitations need to be taken into consideration for neurotrophic factor small-molecule mimetics based drugs [154].

CNTF small-molecule peptide mimetic, P021, as a drug candidate for Alzheimer's disease

As mentioned before, the neuroprotective effects of CNTF are well established [146], and it has been reported to rescue cognitive dysfunction in AD transgenic mice [111]. However, like other neurotrophic factors, the

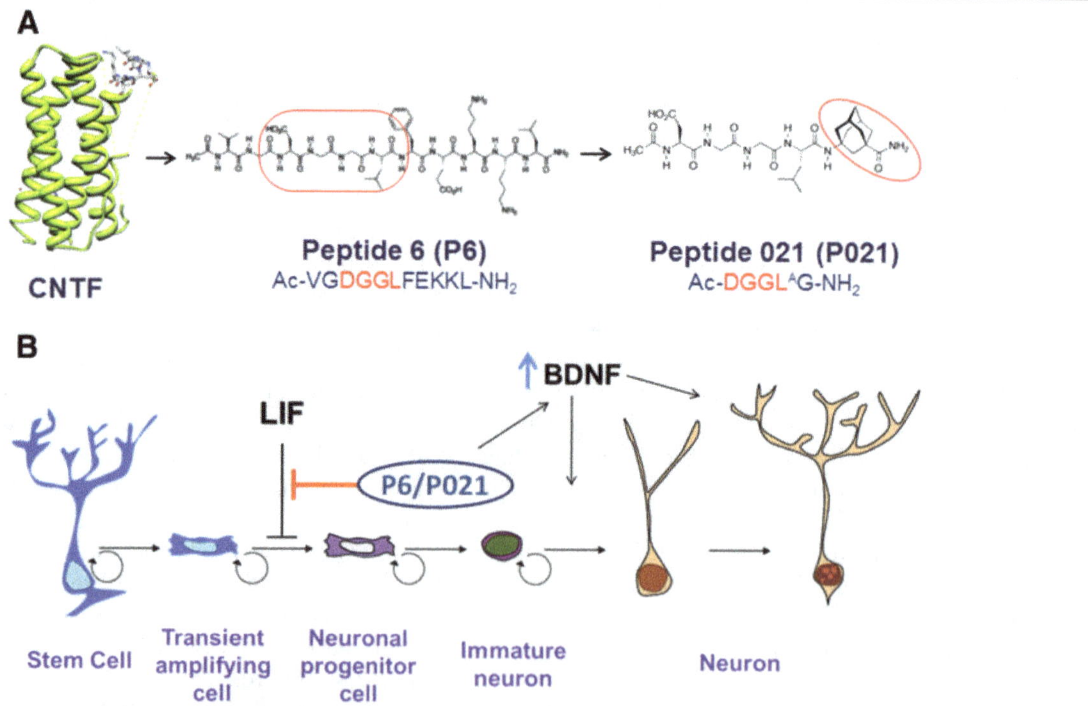

Fig. 4 Design and structures of CNTF small-molecule mimetics and their mechanism of action to enhance formation of NPCs and mature neurons. **a** Protein Data Base rendering of one 4-helix bundle of truncated human CNTF (Residues 2–187), generated from CNTF. Only one protein chain is shown for clarity. Residues 149GGLFEKKL156 are shown as a tube model, while the rest of the sequence are presented as ribbon [98]. The structures of P6 and P021 are also shown. From the neurogenic 11-mer, Ac-VGDGGLFEKKL-NH_2 (P6), a truncated, still neurogenic pentamer, with an adamantylated glycine group (red oval), Ac-DGGLA^G-NH_2 (P021) was designed [191]. **b** P6 and P021 enhance neural progenitor cells (NPCs) formation and maturation and integration of new-born neurons by competitively inhibiting the LIF signaling and increasing BDNF expression respectively [99, 180, 181, 191, 192]

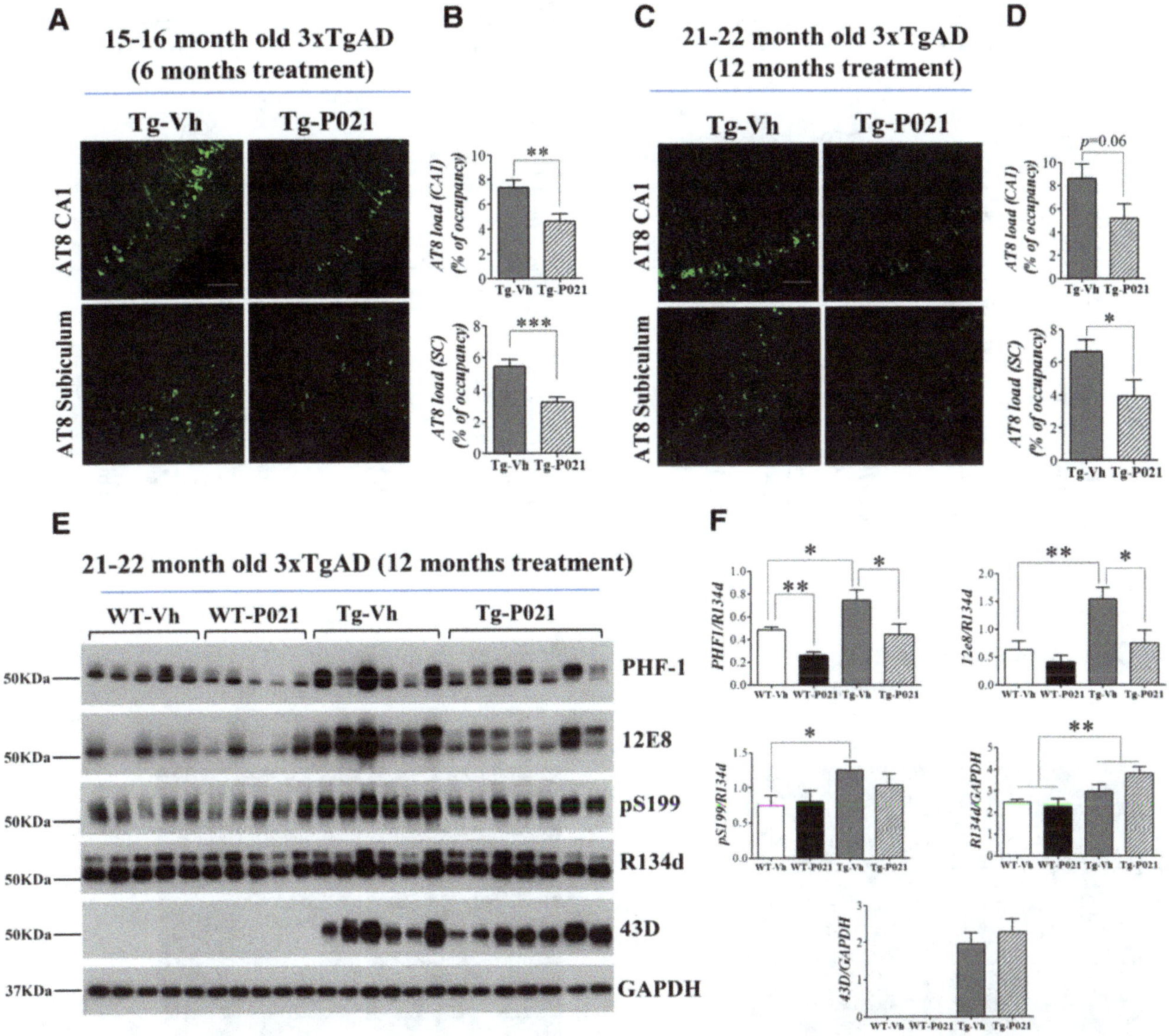

Fig. 5 P021 treatment reduces abnormal hyperphosphorylation of tau in 3xTg-AD mice. Reprinted from Kazim et al. [99] with permission from Elsevier. **a-d** In the subiculum and the CA1 regions of the hippocampus, AT8 (phospho-tau: pSer202, pThr 205) load was significantly reduced by P021 treatment in 3xTg-AD mice (both 15–16 month-old/6 months treatment group and 21–22 month-old/12 months treatment group). **a** Representative photomicrographs illustrating AT8 immunoreactivity in the different regions of hippocampus from the 15–16 month-old/6 months treatment group are shown. **b** The AT8 load was calculated as the percentage of area occupied by immunoreactive label. Quantification of the immunoreactivity is shown as mean ± S.E.M. from Tg-Vh ($n = 7$), and Tg-P021 ($n = 7$). **c** Representative photomicrographs illustrating AT8 immunoreactivity in the different regions of hippocampus from the 21–22 month-old/12 months treatment group are shown. **d** The AT8 load calculated as the percentage of area occupied by immunoreactive label is shown as mean ± S.E.M. from Tg-Vh ($n = 6$), and Tg-P021 ($n = 6$). **e, f** Western blot analyses of tau pathology in 21–22 month old (12 months treatment) group. P021 treatment significantly reduced abnormal hyperphosphorylation of tau at sites pSer396/pSer404 (PHF-1) and pSer262/pSer356 (12E8). Pan-tau antibody, R134d did not show any significant difference between groups. Blots developed with human specific tau antibody 43D showed the protein expression only in 3xTg-AD mice. Quantification of the Western blots is shown as mean ± S.E.M. from WT-Vh ($n = 5$), WT-P021 ($n = 5$), Tg-Vh ($n = 6$), and Tg-P021 ($n = 7$). *$p < 0.05$, **$p < 0.01$, and ***$p < 0.001$. *Scale bar* = 100 μm. WT-Vh = wild-type control mice treated with vehicle diet; WT-P021 = wild-type mice treated with P021 diet; Tg-Vh = 3xTg-AD mice treated with vehicle diet; Tg-P021 = 3xTg-AD mice treated with P021 diet

clinical therapeutic usage of CNTF is restricted due to its short plasma half-life and severe adverse effects including anorexia, skeletal muscle loss, muscle pain and cramps, and hyperalgesia, experienced upon peripheral administration in humans [150].

Our laboratory generated an 11-mer CNTF small-molecule peptide mimetic, Peptide 6 (P6; Ac-VGDGGL FEKKL-NH_2), which corresponds to a biologically active region (amino acid residues 146–156) of human CNTF and was identified using epitope mapping and employing

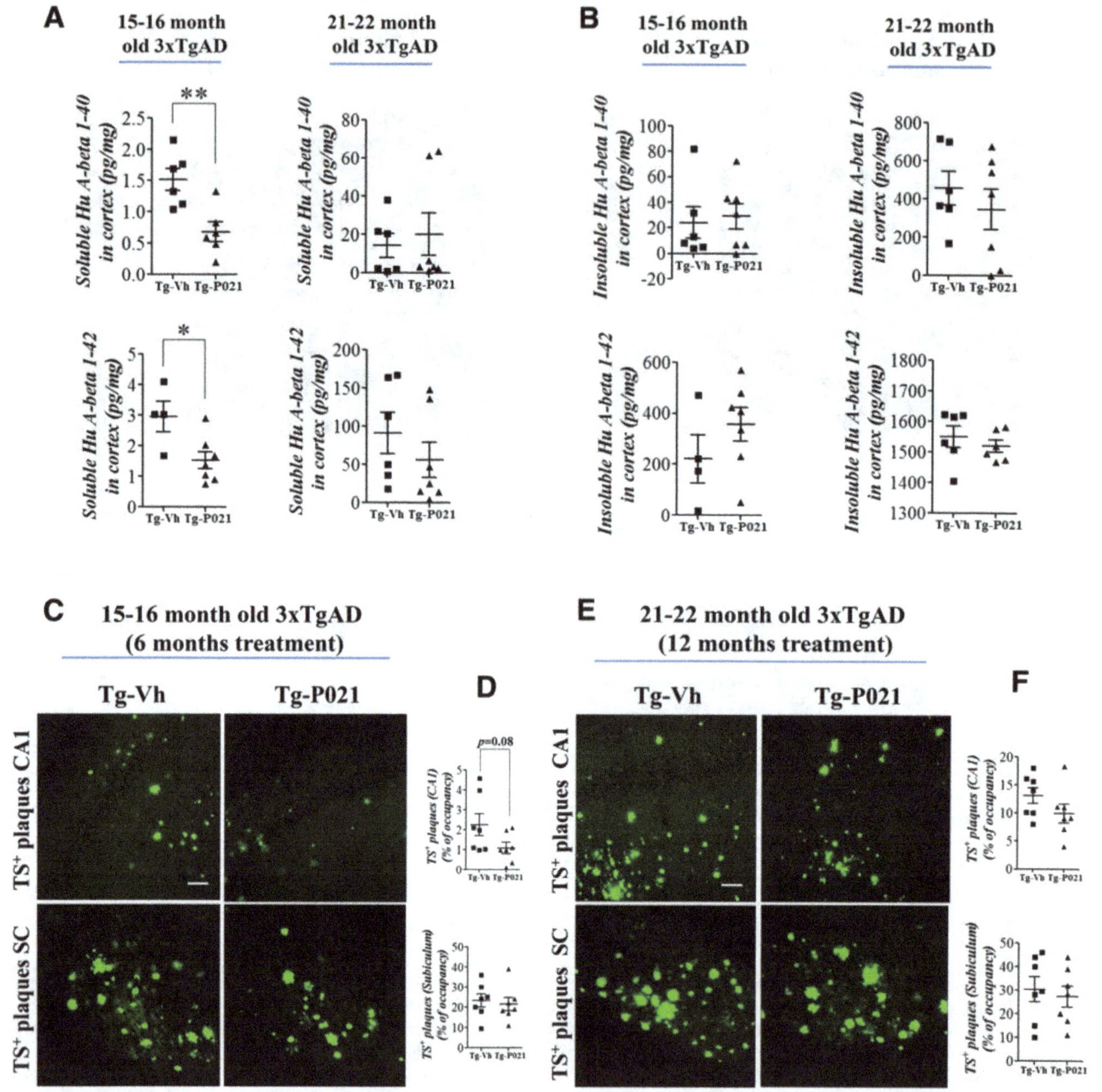

Fig. 6 P021 treatment reduces soluble Aβ in 3xTg-AD mice. Reprinted from Kazim et al. [99] with permission from Elsevier. **a**, **b** ELISA quantification of soluble and insoluble Aβ 1–40 and Aβ 1–42 in the cortex revealed significant reduction of soluble Aβ with P021 treatment in 15–16 month-old/6 months treatment group but not in 21–22 month old/12 months treatment group. No effect on insoluble Aβ was found. Quantification is shown as mean ± S.E.M. from Tg-Vh ($n = 5$–7) and Tg-P021 ($n = 6$–7). **c**, **d** Representative photomicrographs illustrating thioflavin S (TS)$^+$ plaque load in the CA1 and subiculum regions of the hippocampus from 15–16 month old/6 months treatment mice are shown. Quantification of TS$^+$ load is shown as mean ± S.E.M. from Tg-Vh ($n = 7$), and Tg-P021 ($n = 7$). **e**, **f** Representative photomicrographs illustrating TS$^+$ plaque load in the CA1 and subiculum regions of the hippocampus from 21–22 month old/12 months treatment mice are shown. Quantification of TS$^+$ load is shown as mean ± S.E.M. from Tg-Vh ($n = 7$), and Tg-P021 ($n = 6$–7). *$p < 0.05$, **$p < 0.01$. *Scale bar* = 100 μm

neutralizing antibodies (Fig. 4) [179, 180]. P6 has a plasma half-life of over 6 h as compared to ~ 3 min plasma half-life of recombinant CNTF, and is BBB permeable [180]. P6 acts by competitively inhibiting the LIF signaling, thus promoting the formation of neural precursor cells (NPCs), and by increasing BDNF mRNA levels, thus increasing the survival, maturation, and integration of new-born cells (Fig. 4) [180, 181]. Peripheral administration of P6 for 30 days via a subcutaneously implanted slow release bolus, was found to enhance dentate gyrus neurogenesis,

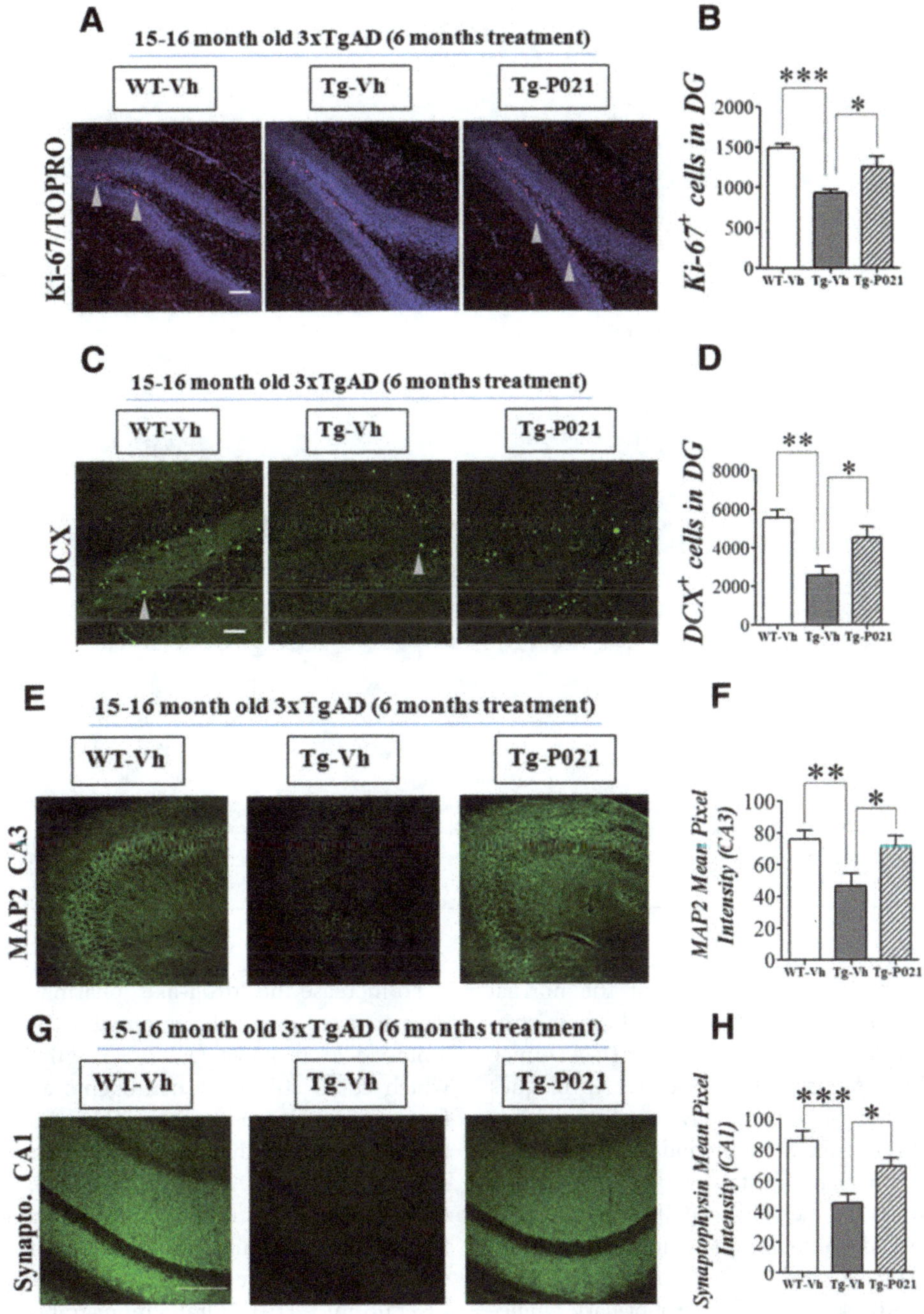

Fig. 7 P021 treatment enhances dentate gyrus neurogenesis and rescues dendritic and synaptic loss in 3xTg-AD mice. Reprinted from Kazim et al. [99] with permission from Elsevier. **a**-**d** DG neurogenesis, as evaluated by counting Ki-67 (cell proliferation maker) and doublecortin (DCX, marker for immature neurons) positive cells, was significantly deficient in 15–16 month-old 3xTg-AD mice, and was corrected by P021 treatment. **a**, **c** Representative photomicrographs illustrating Ki-67+/TOPRO and doublecortin (DCX) + cells in the DG of hippocampus from 15–16 month-old/6 months treatment mice. **b**, **d** Densitometric quantification data of Ki-67+ and DCX+ cells are shown as mean ± S.E.M. from WT-Vh ($n = 6$), Tg-Vh ($n = 7$) and Tg-P021 ($n = 7$), and WT-Vh ($n = 5$), Tg-Vh ($n = 6$), and Tg-P021 ($n = 6$), respectively. Arrow heads indicate positive cells. **e**-**h** The 15–16 month old 3xTg-AD mice showed significantly reduced MAP2 (dendritic marker) and synaptophysin (presynaptic marker) expression level (fluorescence intensity) in the CA3 and CA1 regions of the hippocampus, respectively. P021 treatment significantly ameliorated this deficit. **e** Representative photomicrographs illustrating MAP2 immunoreactivity in the CA3 region. **f** Densitometric quantification of the immunohistochemistry is shown as mean ± S.E.M. fromWT-Vh ($n = 6$), Tg-Vh ($n = 7$), and Tg-P021 ($n = 7$). **g** Representative photomicrographs illustrating synaptophysin immunoreactivity in the CA1 region. **h** Densitometric quantification of the immunohistochemistry is shown as mean ± S.E.M. from WT-Vh ($n = 6$), Tg-Vh ($n = 6$), and Tg-P021 ($n = 6$). $^{*}p < 0.05$, $^{**}p < 0.01$, and $^{***}p < 0.001$. *Scale bar* = 100 μm

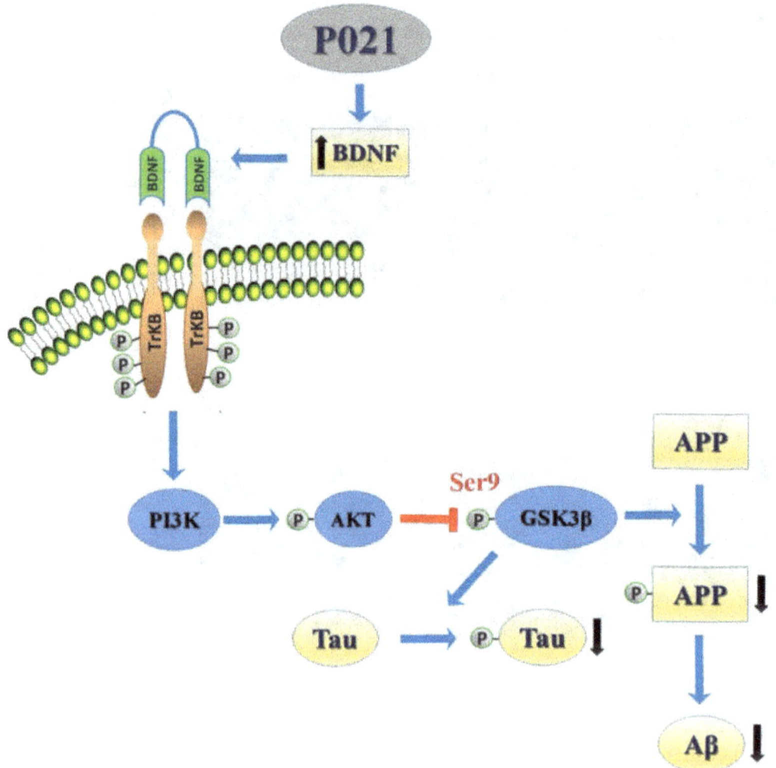

Fig. 8 Mechanism of the disease-modifying effect of P021 in AD. The CNTF small-molecule peptide mimetic compound, P021, increases BDNF expression which via the TrkB-PI3K-AKT pathway leads to inhibitory phosphorylation of GSK3β at Ser9 [99]. GSK3β is major tau kinase and contributes to abnormal hyperphosphorylation of tau at several major sites, and also plays a role in the amyloidogenic processing of APP. P021, via decreasing the GSK3β activity, causes decrease in tau and Aβ pathologies

neuronal plasticity, and spatial memory of the normal adult C57Bl/6 mice [180]. The intraperitoneal administration of P6 for six weeks in 6–7 month-old 3xTg-AD mice (at early stages of the AD pathology prior to Aβ plaques and neurofibrillary tangle-like pathology) ameliorated impairment in spatial reference memory and short-term episodic memory by enhancing dentate gyrus neurogenesis and neuronal plasticity in these mice [98]. The 3xTg-AD mice carry AD-related mutation including human PS1 M146V, human APP Swedish, and human tau P301L [182], and develop Aβ plaques and neurofibrillary tangle-like pathologies in a progressive and age-dependent manner, starting at ~9 and ~12 months respectively but show cognitive impairment as early as 3–5 months of age [182–185]. P6 treatment in 6–7 month-old 3xTg-AD mice could not exert any effect on Aβ and tau pathologies [98], seen in this age mice as intraneuronal Aβ accumulation and tau hyperphosphorylation, and not as plaques and tangles [87, 183]. Other preclinical studies employing P6 showed neurogenic and neurotrophic effects in animal models of sporadic AD [181], familial AD [186], Down syndrome [187], autism [188], and traumatic brain injury [189].

To increase the "drug-like" pharmacokinetic properties, we narrowed down the minimal active region of P6 to 4 amino acid residues (Ac-DGGL-NH_2, Peptide 6c, P6c) which could still exert neurogenic and neurotrophic effects [190]. We subsequently added adamantylated glycine group to P6c to enhance its BBB permeability, and the resultant pentamer (Ac-DGGL^{A}G-NH_2), called Peptide 021 (P021) (Fig. 4), was found to enhance proliferation and differentiation of adult hippocampal progenitors, increase synaptic markers expression, and improve cognition in C57Bl/6 mice [191]. Oral administration of the compound P021 could rescue cognitive aging by enhancing neurogenesis via increased BDNF expression and by decreasing tau levels in aged Fisher rats [192, 193].

In a recent study, we treated 3xTg-AD mice with P021 in diet (60 nmol/g feed) starting at 9–10 months of age (early-moderate stages of the AD-like neuropathology) for 12 months, and evaluated the therapeutic effect of the compound at 15–16 months of age (moderate-severe pathology) and at 21–22 months of age (severe pathology) [99]. P021 treatment significantly reduced tau pathology both at moderate and severe stages of the pathology in 3xTg-AD mice (Fig. 5), however, the effect of P021 on Aβ pathology was limited to a significant decrease in soluble Aβ levels and a trend towards reduction in Aβ plaque load in CA1 region of hippocampus, consistent with reduction in Aβ generation and not clearance (Fig. 6) [99]. P021 treatment also rescued cognitive impairment, enhanced dentate gyrus neurogenesis, and ameliorated synaptic deficit at moderate to severe stage of the pathology in 3xTg-AD mice (Fig. 7). The effect of P021 on tau and probably also on Aβ pathology was via increased BDNF expression mediated activation of TrkB-PI3K-AKT signaling pathway which leads to down-stream inhibition of GSK-3β activity by increase in its inhibitory phosphorylation at Ser9 by AKT (Fig. 8) [99, 194]. GSK3β is a major tau serine/threonine kinase which is known to phosphorylate tau at many different sites including Ser199, Ser202, Thr205, Ser396, and Ser404 [52, 53]. Reduction in GSK3β activity has also been demonstrated to ameliorate Aβ pathology via reduction in amyloidogenic processing of APP [195, 196].

The compound P021 has favorable pharmacokinetics for drug development including plasma half-life of >3 h and stability of >95 % and >90 % in artificial intestinal fluid up till 2 h and in artificial gastric juice up till 30 min, respectively, and is BBB permeable [99]. Up to 1 year of P021 administration did not induce any adverse effect in 3xTg-AD mice or in wild type control [99].

Conclusions

AD is a multifactorial and heterogeneous devastating neurodegenerative disorder which contributes significantly to health care burden worldwide, more so because of the lack of an effective therapy. Independent of the various etiopathogenic mechanisms involved in AD, the neurogenic and synaptic failure are a common feature of AD that play a pivotal role in cognitive dysfunction. The rationale for the use of neurotrophic factors based approach is quite strong by virtue of their well-established pro-neurogenic effects and synaptic repair potential. However, the unfavorable pharmacokinetics, poor brain penetration, and undesired adverse effects associated with the native neurotrophic factor molecules limit their clinical usage. Neurotrophic factor small-molecule mimetics offer a highly promising strategy to overcome these limitations for AD drug development. Preclinical studies have demonstrated therapeutic beneficial effects of several neurotrophic factor small-molecule mimetics particularly the BDNF and CNTF mimetics. These compounds are currently undergoing or will undergo in near-future human clinical trials to assess their therapeutic efficacy in human AD patients. Overall, the neurotrophic factor small-molecule mimetics based neuroregeneration and synaptic repair represents a highly promising therapeutic strategy for AD, and can lead to the development of an effective drug to rescue cognitive impairment.

Abbreviations

3xTg-AD, triple transgenic Alzheimer's disease mice; 7,8-DHF, 7,8-dihydroxyflavone; Ach, acetylcholine; AD, Alzheimer's disease; APOE ε4, apolipoprotein E ε4; APP, amyloid β precursor protein; ARTN, artemin; Aβ, amyloid β; BBB, blood–brain barrier; BDNF, brain-derived neurotrophic factor; BMP, bone morphogenic protein; CaMKII, calcium/calmodulin activated protein kinase II; Cdk5, cyclin-dependent kinase 5; CERAD, consortium to establish a Registry for Alzheimer's disease; ChAT, choline acetyltransferase; CNS, central nervous system; CNTF, ciliary neurotrophic factor; CNTFRα, ciliary neurotrophic factor receptor α; CTFβ, C-terminal fragment β; ERK, extracellular signal-regulated kinase; FGF2, fibroblast growth factor 2; GDNF, glial cell-derived neurotrophic factor; GFL, glial cell-derived neurotrophic factor family ligands; GFRα, glial cell-derived neurotrophic factor family receptor alpha; gp130, glycoprotein 130; GSK-3β, glycogen synthase kinase 3 β; IL-11, interleukin-11; IL-6, interleukin-6; LIF, leukemia inhibitory factor; LIFR, leukemia inhibitory factor β receptor; LTP, long-term potentiation; MAP, microtubule associated protein; MAPK, mitogen-activated protein kinase; MCI, mild cognitive impairment; NFTs, neurofibrillary tangles; NGF, nerve growth factor; NPCs, neural precursor cells; NRTN, neurturin; NT3, neurotrophin 3; NT4, neurotrophin 4; P021, peptide 021; P6, peptide 6; $p75^{NTR}$, p75 neurotrophin receptor; PI3K, phosphoinositide 3-kinase; PKB/AKT, protein kinase B; PP2A, protein phosphatase 2A; PS1, presenilin 1; PS2, presenilin 2; pSer, phosphorylated serine; PSPN, persephin; pTau, abnormally hyperphosphorylated tau protein; pThr, phosphorylated threonine; RET, rearranged during transfection; TGFβ, tansforming growth factor β; Trk, tropomysin receptor kinase.

Acknowledgements

The work on neurotrophic factor small-molecule mimetics in our lab was supported by research grants from Alzheimer's Association, USA; Alzheimer's Drug Discovery Foundation (ADDF), USA; and EVER NeuroPharma GmbH, Unterach, Austria, and in part by the New York State Office of People with Developmental Disabilities. SFK is supported by a doctoral fellowship from SUNY Downstate/NYSIBR Program in Developmental Neuroscience.
We would like to acknowledge late Dr. Inge Grundke-Iqbal who initiated the work with neurotrophic factor small-molecule peptide mimetics in our lab. Dr. Grundke-Iqbal passed away on September 22, 2012. We would also like to acknowledge Dr. M. Omar Chohan, Dr. Julie Blanchard, Dr. Bin Li, and Dr. Silvia Bolognin who contributed significantly to the work on neurotrophic factor small-molecule mimetics in our lab.

Authors' contributions

SFK drafted the first version of this review. KI revised the manuscript for intellectual content. All authors read and approved the final manuscript.

Competing interests

KI has U.S. patents on CNTF small-molecule peptide mimetics for the treatment of AD and related neurodegenerative disorders.

Author details

[1]Department of Neurochemistry, and SUNY Downstate/NYSIBR Program in Developmental Neuroscience, New York State Institute for Basic Research (NYSIBR), 1050 Forest Hill Road, Staten Island, NY 10314, USA. [2]Graduate Program in Neural and Behavioral Science, and Department of Physiology and Pharmacology, State University of New York (SUNY) Downstate Medical Center, 450 Clarkson Avenue, Brooklyn, NY 11203, USA.

References

1. Ballard C, Gauthier S, Corbett A, Brayne C, Aarsland D, Jones E. Alzheimer's disease. Lancet. 2011;377:1019–31.
2. Cornutiu G. The epidemiological scale of Alzheimer's disease. J Clin Med Res. 2015;7:657–66.
3. Hebert LE, Weuve J, Scherr PA, Evans DA. Alzheimer disease in the United States (2010–2050) estimated using the 2010 census. Neurology. 2013;80:1778–83.
4. Alzheimer's A. Alzheimer's disease facts and figures. Alzheimers Dement. 2016;2016:12.
5. Prince MJ, Guerchet MM, Prina M. The Epidemiology and Impact of Dementia: Current State and Future Trends. WHO Thematic Briefing. Geneva; World Health Organization. 2015. APA citation can be accessed at: (https://kclpure.kcl.

ac.uk/portal/en/publications/the-epidemiology-and-impact-of-dementia(538a75cb-1519-49d4-8876-92ae9cfc4151)/export.html)
6. Iqbal K, Grundke-Iqbal I. Opportunities and challenges in developing Alzheimer disease therapeutics. Acta Neuropathol. 2011;122:543–9.
7. Hebert LE, Scherr PA, Bienias JL, Bennett DA, Evans DA. Alzheimer disease in the US population: prevalence estimates using the 2000 census. Arch Neurol. 2003;60:1119–22.
8. Prince M, Guerchet, M, Prina, M. Policy Brief for Heads of Government: The Global Impact of Dementia 2013–2050. London: Alzheimer's Disease Internationall; 2013. APA citation can be accessed at: (https://kclpure.kcl.ac.uk/portal/en/publications/the-global-impact-of-dementia-20132050(893055ed-e533-4d88-9d15-3aa4abdfcc20)/export.html).
9. Burns A, Iliffe S. Alzheimer's disease. BMJ. 2009;338:b158.
10. Cummings JL. Alzheimer's disease. N Engl J Med. 2004;351:56–67.
11. Grady CL, Haxby JV, Horwitz B, Sundaram M, Berg G, Schapiro M, Friedland RP, Rapoport SI. Longitudinal study of the early neuropsychological and cerebral metabolic changes in dementia of the Alzheimer type. J Clin Exp Neuropsychol. 1988;10:576–96.
12. Glenner GG, Wong CW. Alzheimer's disease: initial report of the purification and characterization of a novel cerebrovascular amyloid protein. Biochem Biophys Res Commun. 1984;120:885–90.
13. Grundke-Iqbal I, Iqbal K, Tung YC, Quinlan M, Wisniewski HM, Binder LI. Abnormal phosphorylation of the microtubule-associated protein tau (tau) in Alzheimer cytoskeletal pathology. Proc Natl Acad Sci U S A. 1986;83:4913–7.
14. Crews L, Masliah E. Molecular mechanisms of neurodegeneration in Alzheimer's disease. Hum Mol Genet. 2010;19:R12–20.
15. Davies CA, Mann DM, Sumpter PQ, Yates PO. A quantitative morphometric analysis of the neuronal and synaptic content of the frontal and temporal cortex in patients with Alzheimer's disease. J Neurol Sci. 1987;78:151–64.
16. Demars M, Hu YS, Gadadhar A, Lazarov O. Impaired neurogenesis is an early event in the etiology of familial Alzheimer's disease in transgenic mice. J Neurosci Res. 2010;88:2103–17.
17. Li B, Yamamori H, Tatebayashi Y, Shafit-Zagardo B, Tanimukai H, Chen S, Iqbal K, Grundke-Iqbal I. Failure of neuronal maturation in Alzheimer disease dentate gyrus. J Neuropathol Exp Neurol. 2008;67:78–84.
18. Mu Y, Gage FH. Adult hippocampal neurogenesis and its role in Alzheimer's disease. Mol Neurodegeneration. 2011;6:85.
19. Scheff SW, Price DA. Alzheimer's disease-related alterations in synaptic density: neocortex and hippocampus. J Alzheimers Dis. 2006;9:101–15.
20. Scheff SW, Price DA, Schmitt FA, DeKosky ST, Mufson EJ. Synaptic alterations in CA1 in mild Alzheimer disease and mild cognitive impairment. Neurology. 2007;68:1501–8.
21. Scheff SW, Price DA, Schmitt FA, Mufson EJ. Hippocampal synaptic loss in early Alzheimer's disease and mild cognitive impairment. Neurobiol Aging. 2006;27:1372–84.
22. Selkoe DJ. Alzheimer's disease is a synaptic failure. Science. 2002;298:789–91.
23. Shruster A, Melamed E, Offen D. Neurogenesis in the aged and neurodegenerative brain. Apoptosis. 2010;15:1415–21.
24. Sze CI, Troncoso JC, Kawas C, Mouton P, Price DL, Martin LJ. Loss of the presynaptic vesicle protein synaptophysin in hippocampus correlates with cognitive decline in Alzheimer disease. J Neuropathol Exp Neurol. 1997;56:933–44.
25. Terry RD, Masliah E, Salmon DP, Butters N, DeTeresa R, Hill R, Hansen LA, Katzman R. Physical basis of cognitive alterations in Alzheimer's disease: synapse loss is the major correlate of cognitive impairment. Ann Neurol. 1991;30:572–80.
26. Aimone JB, Deng W, Gage FH. Adult neurogenesis: integrating theories and separating functions. Trends Cogn Sci. 2010;14:325–37.
27. Aimone JB, Wiles J, Gage FH. Potential role for adult neurogenesis in the encoding of time in new memories. Nat Neurosci. 2006;9:723–7.
28. Deng W, Aimone JB, Gage FH. New neurons and new memories: how does adult hippocampal neurogenesis affect learning and memory? Nat Rev Neurosci. 2010;11:339–50.
29. Neves G, Cooke SF, Bliss TV. Synaptic plasticity, memory and the hippocampus: a neural network approach to causality. Nat Rev Neurosci. 2008;9:65–75.
30. Sahay A, Scobie KN, Hill AS, O'Carroll CM, Kheirbek MA, Burghardt NS, Fenton AA, Dranovsky A, Hen R. Increasing adult hippocampal neurogenesis is sufficient to improve pattern separation. Nature. 2011;472:466–70.
31. Battaglia F, Wang HY, Ghilardi MF, Gashi E, Quartarone A, Friedman E, Nixon RA. Cortical plasticity in Alzheimer's disease in humans and rodents. Biol Psychiatry. 2007;62:1405–12.
32. Arendt T. Synaptic degeneration in Alzheimer's disease. Acta Neuropathol. 2009;118:167–79.
33. DeKosky ST, Scheff SW. Synapse loss in frontal cortex biopsies in Alzheimer's disease: correlation with cognitive severity. Ann Neurol. 1990;27:457–64.
34. DeKosky ST, Scheff SW, Styren SD. Structural correlates of cognition in dementia: quantification and assessment of synapse change. Neurodegeneration. 1996;5:417–21.
35. Masliah E, Mallory M, Hansen L, DeTeresa R, Alford M, Terry R. Synaptic and neuritic alterations during the progression of Alzheimer's disease. Neurosci Lett. 1994;174:67–72.
36. Iqbal K, Kazim SF, Bolognin S, Blanchard J. Shifting balance from neurodegeneration to regeneration of the brain: a novel therapeutic approach to Alzheimer's disease and related neurodegenerative conditions. Neural Regen Res. 2014;9:1518–9.
37. About a peculiar disease of the cerebral cortex. By Alois Alzheimer, 1907 (Translated by L. Jarvik and H. Greenson). Alzheimer disease and associated disorders 1987, 1:3–8
38. Iqbal K, Grundke-Iqbal I. Alzheimer's disease, a multifactorial disorder seeking multitherapies. Alzheimers Dement. 2010;6:420–4.
39. Bird TD. Genetic aspects of Alzheimer disease. Genet Med. 2008;10:231–9.
40. Guerreiro R, Hardy J. Genetics of Alzheimer's disease. Neurotherapeutics. 2014;11:732–7.
41. Corder EH, Saunders AM, Strittmatter WJ, Schmechel DE, Gaskell PC, Small GW, Roses AD, Haines JL, Pericak-Vance MA. Gene dose of apolipoprotein E type 4 allele and the risk of Alzheimer's disease in late onset families. Science. 1993; 261:921–3.
42. Hardy JA, Higgins GA. Alzheimer's disease: the amyloid cascade hypothesis. Science. 1992;256:184–5.
43. Kang J, Lemaire HG, Unterbeck A, Salbaum JM, Masters CL, Grzeschik KH, Multhaup G, Beyreuther K, Muller-Hill B. The precursor of Alzheimer's disease amyloid A4 protein resembles a cell-surface receptor. Nature. 1987;325:733–6.
44. Masters CL, Simms G, Weinman NA, Multhaup G, McDonald BL, Beyreuther K. Amyloid plaque core protein in Alzheimer disease and down syndrome. Proc Natl Acad Sci U S A. 1985;82:4245–9.
45. Lambert MP, Barlow AK, Chromy BA, Edwards C, Freed R, Liosatos M, Morgan TE, Rozovsky I, Trommer B, Viola KL, et al. Diffusible, nonfibrillar ligands derived from Abeta1-42 are potent central nervous system neurotoxins. Proc Natl Acad Sci U S A. 1998;95:6448–53.
46. Walsh DM, Klyubin I, Fadeeva JV, Cullen WK, Anwyl R, Wolfe MS, Rowan MJ, Selkoe DJ. Naturally secreted oligomers of amyloid beta protein potently inhibit hippocampal long-term potentiation in vivo. Nature. 2002;416:535–9.
47. Bliss TV, Collingridge GL. A synaptic model of memory: long-term potentiation in the hippocampus. Nature. 1993;361:31–9.
48. Wisniewski KE, Dalton AJ, McLachlan C, Wen GY, Wisniewski HM. Alzheimer's disease in down's syndrome: clinicopathologic studies. Neurology. 1985;35:957–61.
49. Karlinsky H. Alzheimer's disease in down's syndrome. A review J Am Geriatr Soc. 1986;34:728–34.
50. Grundke-Iqbal I, Iqbal K, Quinlan M, Tung YC, Zaidi MS, Wisniewski HM. Microtubule-associated protein tau. A component of Alzheimer paired helical filaments. J Biol Chem. 1986;261:6084–9. (http://www.ncbi.nlm.nih.gov/pubmed/3331112), PMID: 3331112. It's an English translation of original case by Alois Alzheimer.
51. Iqbal K, Wisniewski HM, Shelanski ML, Brostoff S, Liwnicz BH, Terry RD. Protein changes in senile dementia. Brain Res. 1974;77:337–43.
52. Wang JZ, Grundke-Iqbal I, Iqbal K. Kinases and phosphatases and tau sites involved in Alzheimer neurofibrillary degeneration. Eur J Neurosci. 2007;25: 59–68.
53. Wang JZ, Wu Q, Smith A, Grundke-Iqbal I, Iqbal K. Tau is phosphorylated by GSK-3 at several sites found in Alzheimer disease and its biological activity markedly inhibited only after it is prephosphorylated by A-kinase. FEBS Lett. 1998;436:28–34.
54. Iqbal K, Alonso Adel C, Chen S, Chohan MO, El-Akkad E, Gong CX, Khatoon S, Li B, Liu F, Rahman A, et al. Tau pathology in Alzheimer disease and other tauopathies. Biochim Biophys Acta. 2005;1739:198–210.
55. Gong CX, Shaikh S, Wang JZ, Zaidi T, Grundke-Iqbal I, Iqbal K. Phosphatase activity toward abnormally phosphorylated tau: decrease in Alzheimer disease brain. J Neurochem. 1995;65:732–8.
56. Gong CX, Singh TJ, Grundke-Iqbal I, Iqbal K. Phosphoprotein phosphatase activities in Alzheimer disease brain. J Neurochem. 1993;61:921–7.

57. Liu F, Grundke-Iqbal I, Iqbal K, Gong CX. Contributions of protein phosphatases PP1, PP2A, PP2B and PP5 to the regulation of tau phosphorylation. Eur J Neurosci. 2005;22:1942–50.
58. Nelson PT, Alafuzoff I, Bigio EH, Bouras C, Braak H, Cairns NJ, Castellani RJ, Crain BJ, Davies P, Del Tredici K, et al. Correlation of Alzheimer disease neuropathologic changes with cognitive status: a review of the literature. J Neuropathol Exp Neurol. 2012;71:362–81.
59. Braak H, Del Tredici K. The pathological process underlying Alzheimer's disease in individuals under thirty. Acta Neuropathol. 2011;121:171–81.
60. Braak H, Thal DR, Ghebremedhin E, Del Tredici K. Stages of the pathologic process in Alzheimer disease: age categories from 1 to 100 years. J Neuropathol Exp Neurol. 2011;70:960–9.
61. Riley KP, Jicha GA, Davis D, Abner EL, Cooper GE, Stiles N, Smith CD, Kryscio RJ, Nelson PT, Van Eldik LJ, Schmitt FA. Prediction of preclinical Alzheimer's disease: longitudinal rates of change in cognition. J Alzheimers Dis. 2011;25:707–17.
62. Schmitt FA, Davis DG, Wekstein DR, Smith CD, Ashford JW, Markesbery WR. Preclinical" AD revisited: neuropathology of cognitively normal older adults. Neurol. 2000;55:370–6.
63. Webster SJ, Bachstetter AD, Nelson PT, Schmitt FA, Van Eldik LJ. Using mice to model Alzheimer's dementia: an overview of the clinical disease and the preclinical behavioral changes in ten mouse models. Frontiers in Genetics. 2014;5:88.
64. Belleville S, Sylvain-Roy S, de Boysson C, Menard MC. Characterizing the memory changes in persons with mild cognitive impairment. Prog Brain Res. 2008;169:365–75.
65. Khan UA, Liu L, Provenzano FA, Berman DE, Profaci CP, Sloan R, Mayeux R, Duff KE, Small SA. Molecular drivers and cortical spread of lateral entorhinal cortex dysfunction in preclinical Alzheimer's disease. Nat Neurosci. 2014;17:304–11.
66. Liu L, Drouet V, Wu JW, Witter MP, Small SA, Clelland C, Duff K. Trans-synaptic spread of tau pathology in vivo. PLoS One. 2012;7:e31302.
67. Reitz C, Brickman AM, Brown TR, Manly J, DeCarli C, Small SA, Mayeux R. Linking hippocampal structure and function to memory performance in an aging population. Arch Neurol. 2009;66:1385–92.
68. Small SA. Isolating pathogenic mechanisms embedded within the hippocampal circuit through regional vulnerability. Neuron. 2014;84:32–9.
69. Collie A, Maruff P. The neuropsychology of preclinical Alzheimer's disease and mild cognitive impairment. Neurosci Biobehav Rev. 2000;24:365–74.
70. Smith GE, Pankratz VS, Negash S, Machulda MM, Petersen RC, Boeve BF, Knopman DS, Lucas JA, Ferman TJ, Graff-Radford N, Ivnik RJ. A plateau in pre-Alzheimer memory decline: evidence for compensatory mechanisms? Neurology. 2007;69:133–9.
71. Bondi MW, Jak AJ, Delano-Wood L, Jacobson MW, Delis DC, Salmon DP. Neuropsychological contributions to the early identification of Alzheimer's disease. Neuropsychol Rev. 2008;18:73–90.
72. Storandt M, Grant EA, Miller JP, Morris JC. Longitudinal course and neuropathologic outcomes in original vs revised MCI and in pre-MCI. Neurology. 2006;67:467–73.
73. Twamley EW, Ropacki SA, Bondi MW. Neuropsychological and neuroimaging changes in preclinical Alzheimer's disease. J Int Neuropsychol Soc. 2006;12:707–35.
74. Tuokko H, Morris C, Ebert P. Mild cognitive impairment and everyday functioning in older adults. Neurocase. 2005;11:40–7.
75. McKhann GM, Knopman DS, Chertkow H, Hyman BT, Jack Jr CR, Kawas CH, Klunk WE, Koroshetz WJ, Manly JJ, Mayeux R, et al. The diagnosis of dementia due to Alzheimer's disease: recommendations from the National Institute on Aging-Alzheimer's association workgroups on diagnostic guidelines for Alzheimer's disease. Alzheimers Dement. 2011;7:263–9.
76. Bruel-Jungerman E, Rampon C, Laroche S. Adult hippocampal neurogenesis, synaptic plasticity and memory: facts and hypotheses. Rev Neurosci. 2007; 18:93–114.
77. Abrous DN, Wojtowicz JM. Interaction between neurogenesis and hippocampal memory system: New Vistas. Cold Spring Harb Perspect Biol. 2015;7.
78. Drapeau E, Mayo W, Aurousseau C, Le Moal M, Piazza PV, Abrous DN. Spatial memory performances of aged rats in the water maze predict levels of hippocampal neurogenesis. Proc Natl Acad Sci U S A. 2003;100:14385–90.
79. Dupret D, Revest JM, Koehl M, Ichas F, De Giorgi F, Costet P, Abrous DN, Piazza PV. Spatial relational memory requires hippocampal adult neurogenesis. PLoS One. 2008;3:e1959.
80. Leuner B, Gould E, Shors TJ. Is there a link between adult neurogenesis and learning? Hippocampus. 2006;16:216–24.
81. Lledo PM, Alonso M, Grubb MS. Adult neurogenesis and functional plasticity in neuronal circuits. Nat Rev Neurosci. 2006;7:179–93.
82. Deng W, Saxe MD, Gallina IS, Gage FH. Adult-born hippocampal dentate granule cells undergoing maturation modulate learning and memory in the brain. J Neurosci. 2009;29:13532–42.
83. Shors TJ. From stem cells to grandmother cells: how neurogenesis relates to learning and memory. Cell Stem Cell. 2008;3:253–8.
84. Phillips W, Michell AW, Barker RA. Neurogenesis in diseases of the central nervous system. Stem Cells Dev. 2006;15:359–79.
85. Bonfanti L, Peretto P. Adult neurogenesis in mammals–a theme with many variations. Eur J Neurosci. 2011;34:930–50.
86. Gage FH. Neurogenesis in the adult brain. J Neurosci. 2002;22:612–3.
87. Inokuchi K. Adult neurogenesis and modulation of neural circuit function. Curr Opin Neurobiol. 2011;21:360–4.
88. Kempermann G, Gage FH. Neurogenesis in the adult hippocampus. Novartis Found Symp. 2000;231:220–35. discussion 235–241, 302–226.
89. Li Y, Mu Y, Gage FH. Development of neural circuits in the adult hippocampus. Curr Top Dev Biol. 2009;87:149–74.
90. Grote HE, Hannan AJ. Regulators of adult neurogenesis in the healthy and diseased brain. Clin Exp Pharmacol Physiol. 2007;34:533–45.
91. Verret L, Jankowsky JL, Xu GM, Borchelt DR, Rampon C. Alzheimer's-type amyloidosis in transgenic mice impairs survival of newborn neurons derived from adult hippocampal neurogenesis. J Neurosci. 2007;27:6771–80.
92. Verret L, Trouche S, Zerwas M, Rampon C. Hippocampal neurogenesis during normal and pathological aging. Psychoneuroendocrinology. 2007;32 Suppl 1:S26–30.
93. Jin K, Galvan V, Xie L, Mao XO, Gorostiza OF, Bredesen DE, Greenberg DA. Enhanced neurogenesis in Alzheimer's disease transgenic (PDGF-APPSw, Ind) mice. Proc Natl Acad Sci U S A. 2004;101:13363–7.
94. Knobloch M, Mansuy IM. Dendritic spine loss and synaptic alterations in Alzheimer's disease. Mol Neurobiol. 2008;37:73–82.
95. Scheff SW, DeKosky ST, Price DA. Quantitative assessment of cortical synaptic density in Alzheimer's disease. Neurobiol Aging. 1990;11:29–37.
96. Scheff SW, Price DA. Synaptic pathology in Alzheimer's disease: a review of ultrastructural studies. Neurobiol Aging. 2003;24:1029–46.
97. van Praag H, Schinder AF, Christie BR, Toni N, Palmer TD, Gage FH. Functional neurogenesis in the adult hippocampus. Nature. 2002;415:1030–4.
98. Blanchard J, Wanka L, Tung YC, Cardenas-Aguayo Mdel C, LaFerla FM, Iqbal K, Grundke-Iqbal I. Pharmacologic reversal of neurogenic and neuroplastic abnormalities and cognitive impairments without affecting Abeta and tau pathologies in 3xTg-AD mice. Acta Neuropathol. 2010;120:605–21.
99. Kazim SF, Blanchard J, Dai CL, Tung YC, LaFerla FM, Iqbal IG, Iqbal K. Disease modifying effect of chronic oral treatment with a neurotrophic peptidergic compound in a triple transgenic mouse model of Alzheimer's disease. Neurobiol Dis. 2014;71:110–30.
100. Chevallier NL, Soriano S, Kang DE, Masliah E, Hu G, Koo EH. Perturbed neurogenesis in the adult hippocampus associated with presenilin-1 A246E mutation. Am J Pathol. 2005;167:151–9.
101. Dong H, Goico B, Martin M, Csernansky CA, Bertchume A, Csernansky JG. Modulation of hippocampal cell proliferation, memory, and amyloid plaque deposition in APPsw (Tg2576) mutant mice by isolation stress. Neurosci. 2004;127:601–9.
102. Donovan MH, Yazdani U, Norris RD, Games D, German DC, Eisch AJ. Decreased adult hippocampal neurogenesis in the PDAPP mouse model of Alzheimer's disease. J Comp Neurol. 2006;495:70–83.
103. Wang JM, Singh C, Liu L, Irwin RW, Chen S, Chung EJ, Thompson RF, Brinton RD. Allopregnanolone reverses neurogenic and cognitive deficits in mouse model of Alzheimer's disease. Proc Natl Acad Sci U S A. 2010;107:6498–503.
104. Wen PH, Hof PR, Chen X, Gluck K, Austin G, Younkin SG, Younkin LH, DeGasperi R, Gama Sosa MA, Robakis NK, et al. The presenilin-1 familial Alzheimer disease mutant P117L impairs neurogenesis in the hippocampus of adult mice. Exp Neurol. 2004;188:224–37.
105. Enciu AM, Nicolescu MI, Manole CG, Muresanu DF, Popescu LM, Popescu BO. Neuroregeneration in neurodegenerative disorders. BMC Neurol. 2011;11:75.
106. Hunsberger JG, Rao M, Kurtzberg J, Bulte JW, Atala A, LaFerla FM, Greely HT, Sawa A, Gandy S, Schneider LS, Doraiswamy PM. Accelerating stem cell trials for Alzheimer's disease. Lancet Neurol 2015. doi: 10.1016/S1474-4422(15)00332-4.
107. Tang J. How close is the stem cell cure to the Alzheimer's disease: Future and beyond? Neural Regen Res. 2012;7:66–71.
108. Blurton-Jones M, Kitazawa M, Martinez-Coria H, Castello NA, Muller FJ, Loring JF, Yamasaki TR, Poon WW, Green KN, LaFerla FM. Neural stem cells improve cognition via BDNF in a transgenic model of Alzheimer disease. Proc Natl Acad Sci U S A. 2009;106:13594–9.

109. Kiyota T, Ingraham KL, Jacobsen MT, Xiong H, Ikezu T. FGF2 gene transfer restores hippocampal functions in mouse models of Alzheimer's disease and has therapeutic implications for neurocognitive disorders. Proc Natl Acad Sci U S A. 2011;108:E1339–48.
110. Nagahara AH, Merrill DA, Coppola G, Tsukada S, Schroeder BE, Shaked GM, Wang L, Blesch A, Kim A, Conner JM, et al. Neuroprotective effects of brain-derived neurotrophic factor in rodent and primate models of Alzheimer's disease. Nat Med. 2009;15:331–7.
111. Garcia P, Youssef I, Utvik JK, Florent-Bechard S, Barthelemy V, Malaplate-Armand C, Kriem B, Stenger C, Koziel V, Olivier JL, et al. Ciliary neurotrophic factor cell-based delivery prevents synaptic impairment and improves memory in mouse models of Alzheimer's disease. J Neurosci. 2010;30:7516–27.
112. Barbacid M. Neurotrophic factors and their receptors. Curr Opin Cell Biol. 1995;7:148–55.
113. Lu B, Nagappan G, Guan X, Nathan PJ, Wren P. BDNF-based synaptic repair as a disease-modifying strategy for neurodegenerative diseases. Nat Rev Neurosci. 2013;14:401–16.
114. Semkova I, Krieglstein J. Neuroprotection mediated via neurotrophic factors and induction of neurotrophic factors. Brain Res Brain Res Rev. 1999;30:176–88.
115. Chao MV. Neurotrophins and their receptors: a convergence point for many signalling pathways. Nat Rev Neurosci. 2003;4:299–309.
116. Hock C, Heese K, Hulette C, Rosenberg C, Otten U. Region-specific neurotrophin imbalances in Alzheimer disease: decreased levels of brain-derived neurotrophic factor and increased levels of nerve growth factor in hippocampus and cortical areas. Arch Neurol. 2000;57:846–51.
117. Lee J, Fukumoto H, Orne J, Klucken J, Raju S, Vanderburg CR, Irizarry MC, Hyman BT, Ingelsson M. Decreased levels of BDNF protein in Alzheimer temporal cortex are independent of BDNF polymorphisms. Exp Neurol. 2005;194:91–6.
118. Michalski B, Fahnestock M. Pro-brain-derived neurotrophic factor is decreased in parietal cortex in Alzheimer's disease. Brain Res Mol Brain Res. 2003;111:148–54.
119. Phillips HS, Hains JM, Armanini M, Laramee GR, Johnson SA, Winslow JW. BDNF mRNA is decreased in the hippocampus of individuals with Alzheimer's disease. Neuron. 1991;7:695–702.
120. Lee J, Duan W, Mattson MP. Evidence that brain-derived neurotrophic factor is required for basal neurogenesis and mediates, in part, the enhancement of neurogenesis by dietary restriction in the hippocampus of adult mice. J Neurochem. 2002;82:1367–75.
121. Vilar M, Mira H. Regulation of neurogenesis by neurotrophins during adulthood: expected and unexpected roles. Front Neurosci. 2016;10:26.
122. Ji Y, Lu Y, Yang F, Shen W, Tang TT, Feng L, Duan S, Lu B. Acute and gradual increases in BDNF concentration elicit distinct signaling and functions in neurons. Nat Neurosci. 2010;13:302–9.
123. Kang H, Schuman EM. Long-lasting neurotrophin-induced enhancement of synaptic transmission in the adult hippocampus. Science. 1995;267:1658–62.
124. Korte M, Kang H, Bonhoeffer T, Schuman E. A role for BDNF in the late-phase of hippocampal long-term potentiation. Neuropharmacol. 1998;37:553–9.
125. Lu Y, Christian K, Lu B. BDNF: a key regulator for protein synthesis-dependent LTP and long-term memory? Neurobiol Learn Mem. 2008;89:312–23.
126. Scott SA, Mufson EJ, Weingartner JA, Skau KA, Crutcher KA. Nerve growth factor in Alzheimer's disease: increased levels throughout the brain coupled with declines in nucleus basalis. J Neurosci. 1995;15:6213–21.
127. Francis PT, Palmer AM, Snape M, Wilcock GK. The cholinergic hypothesis of Alzheimer's disease: a review of progress. J Neurol Neurosurg Psychiatry. 1999;66:137–47.
128. Iulita MF, Cuello AC. Nerve growth factor metabolic dysfunction in Alzheimer's disease and down syndrome. Trends Pharmacol Sci. 2014;35:338–48.
129. Olson L. NGF and the treatment of Alzheimer's disease. Exp Neurol. 1993;124:5–15.
130. Tuszynski MH, Yang JH, Barba D, HS U, Bakay RA, Pay MM, Masliah E, Conner JM, Kobalka P, Roy S, Nagahara AH. Nerve growth factor gene therapy: activation of neuronal responses in alzheimer disease. JAMA Neurol. 2015; 72:1139–47.
131. Airaksinen MS, Saarma M. The GDNF family: signalling, biological functions and therapeutic value. Nat Rev Neurosci. 2002;3:383–94.
132. Konishi Y, Yang LB, He P, Lindholm K, Lu B, Li R, Shen Y. Deficiency of GDNF receptor GFRalpha1 in Alzheimer's neurons results in neuronal death. J Neurosci. 2014;34:13127–38.
133. Revilla S, Ursulet S, Alvarez-Lopez MJ, Castro-Freire M, Perpina U, Garcia-Mesa Y, Bortolozzi A, Gimenez-Llort L, Kaliman P, Cristofol R, et al. Lenti-GDNF gene therapy protects against Alzheimer's disease-like neuropathology in 3xTg-AD mice and MC65 cells. CNS Neurosci Ther. 2014;20:961–72.
134. Ip NY. The neurotrophins and neuropoietic cytokines: two families of growth factors acting on neural and hematopoietic cells. Ann N Y Acad Sci. 1998;840:97–106.
135. Stolp HB. Neuropoietic cytokines in normal brain development and neurodevelopmental disorders. Mol Cell Neurosci. 2013;53:63–8.
136. Adachi T, Takanaga H, Kunimoto M, Asou H. Influence of LIF and BMP-2 on differentiation and development of glial cells in primary cultures of embryonic rat cerebral hemisphere. J Neurosci Res. 2005;79:608–15.
137. Kasai M, Satoh K, Akiyama T. Wnt signaling regulates the sequential onset of neurogenesis and gliogenesis via induction of BMPs. Genes Cells. 2005;10:777–83.
138. Rowitch DH, Kriegstein AR. Developmental genetics of vertebrate glial-cell specification. Nature. 2010;468:214–22.
139. Senaldi G, Varnum BC, Sarmiento U, Starnes C, Lile J, Scully S, Guo J, Elliott G, McNinch J, Shaklee CL, et al. Novel neurotrophin-1/B cell-stimulating factor-3: a cytokine of the IL-6 family. Proc Natl Acad Sci U S A. 1999;96:11458–63.
140. Shi Y, Wang W, Yourey PA, Gohari S, Zukauskas D, Zhang J, Ruben S, Alderson RF. Computational EST database analysis identifies a novel member of the neuropoietic cytokine family. Biochem Biophys Res Commun. 1999;262:132–8.
141. Ding J, He Z, Ruan J, Ma Z, Liu Y, Gong C, Iqbal K, Sun S, Chen H. Role of ciliary neurotrophic factor in the proliferation and differentiation of neural stem cells. J Alzheimers Dis. 2013;37:587–92.
142. Emsley JG, Hagg T. Endogenous and exogenous ciliary neurotrophic factor enhances forebrain neurogenesis in adult mice. Exp Neurol. 2003;183:298–310.
143. Yang P, Arnold SA, Habas A, Hetman M, Hagg T. Ciliary neurotrophic factor mediates dopamine D2 receptor-induced CNS neurogenesis in adult mice. J Neurosci. 2008;28:2231–41.
144. Davis S, Aldrich TH, Stahl N, Pan L, Taga T, Kishimoto T, Ip NY, Yancopoulos GD. LIFR beta and gp130 as heterodimerizing signal transducers of the tripartite CNTF receptor. Science. 1993;260:1805–8.
145. Sendtner M, Carroll P, Holtmann B, Hughes RA, Thoenen H. Ciliary neurotrophic factor. J Neurobiol. 1994;25:1436–53.
146. Pasquin S, Sharma M, Gauchat JF. Ciliary neurotrophic factor (CNTF): New facets of an old molecule for treating neurodegenerative and metabolic syndrome pathologies. Cytokine Growth Factor Rev. 2015;26(5):507–15.
147. Chen ZY, Cao L, Wang LM, Guo C, Ye JL, Chai YF, Yan ZY. Development of neurotrophic molecules for treatment of neurodegeneration. Curr Protein Pept Sci. 2001;2:261–76.
148. Longo FM, Yang T, Knowles JK, Xie Y, Moore LA, Massa SM. Small molecule neurotrophin receptor ligands: novel strategies for targeting Alzheimer's disease mechanisms. Curr Alzheimer Res. 2007;4:503–6.
149. Massa SM, Xie Y, Longo FM. Alzheimer's therapeutics: neurotrophin domain small molecule mimetics. J Mol Neurosci. 2003;20:323–6.
150. ACTSG. A double-blind placebo-controlled clinical trial of subcutaneous recombinant human ciliary neurotrophic factor (rHCNTF) in amyotrophic lateral sclerosis. ALS CNTF Treatment Study Group. Neurology. 1996;46:1244–9.
151. Ochs G, Penn RD, York M, Giess R, Beck M, Tonn J, Haigh J, Malta E, Traub M, Sendtner M, Toyka KV. A phase I/II trial of recombinant methionyl human brain derived neurotrophic factor administered by intrathecal infusion to patients with amyotrophic lateral sclerosis. Amyotroph Lateral Scler Other Motor Neuron Disord. 2000;1:201–6.
152. Longo FM, Massa SM. Neurotrophin-based strategies for neuroprotection. J Alzheimers Dis. 2004;6:S13–7.
153. Longo FM, Massa SM. Neurotrophin receptor-based strategies for Alzheimer's disease. Curr Alzheimer Res. 2005;2:167–9.
154. Longo FM, Massa SM. Small-molecule modulation of neurotrophin receptors: a strategy for the treatment of neurological disease. Nat Rev Drug Discov. 2013;12:507–25.
155. Massa SM, Xie Y, Longo FM. Alzheimer's therapeutics: neurotrophin small molecule mimetics. J Mol Neurosci. 2002;19:107–11.
156. Xie Y, Longo FM. Neurotrophin small-molecule mimetics. Prog Brain Res. 2000;128:333–47.
157. Longo FM, Manthorpe M, Xie YM, Varon S. Synthetic NGF peptide derivatives prevent neuronal death via a p75 receptor-dependent mechanism. J Neurosci Res. 1997;48:1–17.
158. Yaar M, Zhai S, Panova I, Fine RE, Eisenhauer PB, Blusztajn JK, Lopez-Coviella I, Gilchrest BA. A cyclic peptide that binds p75(NTR) protects neurones from

beta amyloid (1–40)-induced cell death. Neuropathol Appl Neurobiol. 2007; 33:533–43.
159. Bruno MA, Clarke PB, Seltzer A, Quirion R, Burgess K, Cuello AC, Saragovi HU. Long-lasting rescue of age-associated deficits in cognition and the CNS cholinergic phenotype by a partial agonist peptidomimetic ligand of TrkA. J Neurosci. 2004;24:8009–18.
160. Aboulkassim T, Tong XK, Tse YC, Wong TP, Woo SB, Neet KE, Brahimi F, Hamel E, Saragovi HU. Ligand-dependent TrkA activity in brain differentially affects spatial learning and long-term memory. Mol Pharmacol. 2011;80: 498–508.
161. Zeng Y, Wang X, Wang Q, Liu S, Hu X, McClintock SM. Small molecules activating TrkB receptor for treating a variety of CNS disorders. CNS Neurol Disord Drug Targets. 2013;12:1066–77.
162. Jang SW, Liu X, Yepes M, Shepherd KR, Miller GW, Liu Y, Wilson WD, Xiao G, Blanchi B, Sun YE, Ye K. A selective TrkB agonist with potent neurotrophic activities by 7,8-dihydroxyflavone. Proc Natl Acad Sci U S A. 2010;107:2687–92.
163. Liu X, Obianyo O, Chan CB, Huang J, Xue S, Yang JJ, Zeng F, Goodman M, Ye K. Biochemical and biophysical investigation of the brain-derived neurotrophic factor mimetic 7,8-dihydroxyflavone in the binding and activation of the TrkB receptor. J Biol Chem. 2014;289:27571–84.
164. Castello NA, Nguyen MH, Tran JD, Cheng D, Green KN, LaFerla FM. 7,8-Dihydroxyflavone, a small molecule TrkB agonist, improves spatial memory and increases thin spine density in a mouse model of Alzheimer disease-like neuronal loss. PLoS One. 2014;9:e91453.
165. Chen C, Li XH, Zhang S, Tu Y, Wang YM, Sun HT. 7,8-dihydroxyflavone ameliorates scopolamine-induced Alzheimer-like pathologic dysfunction. Rejuvenation Res. 2014;17:249–54.
166. Zhang Z, Liu X, Schroeder JP, Chan CB, Song M, Yu SP, Weinshenker D, Ye K. 7,8-dihydroxyflavone prevents synaptic loss and memory deficits in a mouse model of Alzheimer's disease. Neuropsychopharmacology. 2014;39: 638–50.
167. Liu C, Chan CB, Ye K. 7,8-dihydroxyflavone, a small molecular TrkB agonist, is useful for treating various BDNF-implicated human disorders. Transl Neurodegeneration. 2016;5:2.
168. Massa SM, Yang T, Xie Y, Shi J, Bilgen M, Joyce JN, Nehama D, Rajadas J, Longo FM. Small molecule BDNF mimetics activate TrkB signaling and prevent neuronal degeneration in rodents. J Clin Invest. 2010;120:1774–85.
169. Jang SW, Liu X, Chan CB, France SA, Sayeed I, Tang W, Lin X, Xiao G, Andero R, Chang Q, et al. Deoxygedunin, a natural product with potent neurotrophic activity in mice. PLoS One. 2010;5:e11528.
170. Jang SW, Liu X, Pradoldej S, Tosini G, Chang Q, Iuvone PM, Ye K. N-acetylserotonin activates TrkB receptor in a circadian rhythm. Proc Natl Acad Sci U S A. 2010;107:3876–81.
171. Lee FS, Chao MV. Activation of Trk neurotrophin receptors in the absence of neurotrophins. Proc Natl Acad Sci U S A. 2001;98:3555–60.
172. Lee FS, Rajagopal R, Kim AH, Chang PC, Chao MV. Activation of Trk neurotrophin receptor signaling by pituitary adenylate cyclase-activating polypeptides. J Biol Chem. 2002;277:9096–102.
173. Fletcher JM, Hughes RA. Novel monocyclic and bicyclic loop mimetics of brain-derived neurotrophic factor. J Pept Sci. 2006;12:515–24.
174. O'Leary PD, Hughes RA. Design of potent peptide mimetics of brain-derived neurotrophic factor. J Biol Chem. 2003;278:25738–44.
175. Cardenas-Aguayo Mdel C, Kazim SF, Grundke-Iqbal I, Iqbal K. Neurogenic and neurotrophic effects of BDNF peptides in mouse hippocampal primary neuronal cell cultures. PLoS One. 2013;8:e53596.
176. Yang T, Knowles JK, Lu Q, Zhang H, Arancio O, Moore LA, Chang T, Wang Q, Andreasson K, Rajadas J, et al. Small molecule, non-peptide p75 ligands inhibit Abeta-induced neurodegeneration and synaptic impairment. PLoS One. 2008;3:e3604.
177. Knowles JK, Simmons DA, Nguyen TV, Vander Griend L, Xie Y, Zhang H, Yang T, Pollak J, Chang T, Arancio O, et al. Small molecule p75NTR ligand prevents cognitive deficits and neurite degeneration in an Alzheimer's mouse model. Neurobiol Aging. 2013;34:2052–63.
178. Simmons DA, Knowles JK, Belichenko NP, Banerjee G, Finkle C, Massa SM, Longo FM. A small molecule p75NTR ligand, LM11A-31, reverses cholinergic neurite dystrophy in Alzheimer's disease mouse models with mid- to late-stage disease progression. PLoS One. 2014;9:e102136.
179. Chen H, Tung YC, Li B, Iqbal K, Grundke-Iqbal I. Trophic factors counteract elevated FGF-2-induced inhibition of adult neurogenesis. Neurobiol Aging. 2007;28:1148–62.
180. Chohan MO, Li B, Blanchard J, Tung YC, Heaney AT, Rabe A, Iqbal K, Grundke-Iqbal I. Enhancement of dentate gyrus neurogenesis, dendritic and synaptic plasticity and memory by a neurotrophic peptide. Neurobiol Aging. 2011;32: 1420–34.
181. Bolognin S, Blanchard J, Wang X, Basurto-Islas G, Tung YC, Kohlbrenner E, Grundke-Iqbal I, Iqbal K. An experimental rat model of sporadic Alzheimer's disease and rescue of cognitive impairment with a neurotrophic peptide. Acta Neuropathol. 2012;123:133–51.
182. Oddo S, Caccamo A, Shepherd JD, Murphy MP, Golde TE, Kayed R, Metherate R, Mattson MP, Akbari Y, LaFerla FM. Triple-transgenic model of Alzheimer's disease with plaques and tangles: intracellular Abeta and synaptic dysfunction. Neuron. 2003;39:409–21.
183. Billings LM, Oddo S, Green KN, McGaugh JL, LaFerla FM. Intraneuronal Abeta causes the onset of early Alzheimer's disease-related cognitive deficits in transgenic mice. Neuron. 2005;45:675–88.
184. Davis KE, Eacott MJ, Easton A, Gigg J. Episodic-like memory is sensitive to both Alzheimer's-like pathological accumulation and normal ageing processes in mice. Behav Brain Res. 2013;254:73–82.
185. Stevens LM, Brown RE. Reference and working memory deficits in the 3xTg-AD mouse between 2 and 15-months of age: A cross-sectional study. Behav Brain Res. 2015;278:496–505.
186. Rockenstein E, Ubhi K, Doppler E, Novak P, Moessler H, Li B, Blanchard J, Grundke-Iqbal I, Iqbal K, Mante M, et al. Regional comparison of the neurogenic effects of CNTF-derived peptides and cerebrolysin in AbetaPP transgenic mice. J Alzheimers Dis. 2011;27:743–52.
187. Blanchard J, Bolognin S, Chohan MO, Rabe A, Iqbal K, Grundke-Iqbal I. Rescue of synaptic failure and alleviation of learning and memory impairments in a trisomic mouse model of down syndrome. J Neuropathol Exp Neurol. 2011;70:1070–9.
188. Kazim SF, Cardenas-Aguayo Mdel C, Arif M, Blanchard J, Fayyaz F, Grundke-Iqbal I, Iqbal K. Sera from children with autism induce autistic features which can be rescued with a CNTF small peptide mimetic in rats. PLoS One. 2015;10:e0118627.
189. Chohan MO, Bragina O, Kazim SF, Statom G, Baazaoui N, Bragin D, Iqbal K, Nemoto E, Yonas H. Enhancement of neurogenesis and memory by a neurotrophic peptide in mild to moderate traumatic brain injury. Neurosurg. 2015;76:201–14. discussion 214–205.
190. Blanchard J, Chohan MO, Li B, Liu F, Iqbal K, Grundke-Iqbal I. Beneficial effect of a CNTF tetrapeptide on adult hippocampal neurogenesis, neuronal plasticity, and spatial memory in mice. J Alzheimers Dis. 2010;21:1185–95.
191. Li B, Wanka L, Blanchard J, Liu F, Chohan MO, Iqbal K, Grundke-Iqbal I. Neurotrophic peptides incorporating adamantane improve learning and memory, promote neurogenesis and synaptic plasticity in mice. FEBS Lett. 2010;584:3359–65.
192. Bolognin S, Buffelli M, Puolivali J, Iqbal K. Rescue of cognitive-aging by administration of a neurogenic and/or neurotrophic compound. Neurobiol Aging. 2014;35:2134–46.
193. Khatoon S, Chalbot S, Bolognin S, Puolivali J, Iqbal K. Elevated tau level in aged rat cerebrospinal fluid reduced by treatment with a neurotrophic compound. J Alzheimers Dis. 2015;47:557–64.
194. Elliott E, Atlas R, Lange A, Ginzburg I. Brain-derived neurotrophic factor induces a rapid dephosphorylation of tau protein through a PI-3 Kinase signalling mechanism. Eur J Neurosci. 2005;22:1081–9.
195. DaRocha-Souto B, Coma M, Perez-Nievas BG, Scotton TC, Siao M, Sanchez-Ferrer P, Hashimoto T, Fan Z, Hudry E, Barroeta I, et al. Activation of glycogen synthase kinase-3 beta mediates beta-amyloid induced neuritic damage in Alzheimer's disease. Neurobiol Dis. 2012;45: 425–37.
196. Sereno L, Coma M, Rodriguez M, Sanchez-Ferrer P, Sanchez MB, Gich I, Agullo JM, Perez M, Avila J, Guardia-Laguarta C et al. A novel GSK-3beta inhibitor reduces Alzheimer's pathology and rescues neuronal loss in vivo. Neurobiol Dis. 2009;35:359–67.

9

Pim1 inhibition as a novel therapeutic strategy for Alzheimer's disease

Ramon Velazquez[1], Darren M. Shaw[1,2], Antonella Caccamo[1] and Salvatore Oddo[1,2*]

Abstract

Background: Alzheimer's disease (AD) is the most prevalent neurodegenerative disorder worldwide. Clinically, AD is characterized by impairments of memory and cognitive functions. Accumulation of amyloid-β (Aβ) and neurofibrillary tangles are the prominent neuropathologies in patients with AD. Strong evidence indicates that an imbalance between production and degradation of key proteins contributes to the pathogenesis of AD. The mammalian target of rapamycin (mTOR) plays a key role in maintaining protein homeostasis as it regulates both protein synthesis and degradation. A key regulator of mTOR activity is the proline-rich AKT substrate 40 kDa (PRAS40), which directly binds to mTOR and reduces its activity. Notably, AD patients have elevated levels of phosphorylated PRAS40, which correlate with Aβ and tau pathologies as well as cognitive deficits. Physiologically, PRAS40 phosphorylation is regulated by Pim1, a protein kinase of the protoconcogene family. Here, we tested the effects of a selective Pim1 inhibitor (Pim1i), on spatial reference and working memory and AD-like pathology in 3xTg-AD mice.

Results: We have identified a Pim1i that crosses the blood brain barrier and reduces PRAS40 phosphorylation. Pim1i-treated 3xTg-AD mice performed significantly better than their vehicle treated counterparts as well as non-transgenic mice. Additionally, 3xTg-AD Pim1i-treated mice showed a reduction in soluble and insoluble $A\beta_{40}$ and $A\beta_{42}$ levels, as well as a 45.2 % reduction in $A\beta_{42}$ plaques within the hippocampus. Furthermore, phosphorylated tau immunoreactivity was reduced in the hippocampus of Pim1i–treated 3xTg-AD mice by 38 %. Mechanistically, these changes were linked to a significant increase in proteasome activity.

Conclusion: These results suggest that reductions in phosphorylated PRAS40 levels via Pim1 inhibition reduce Aβ and Tau pathology and rescue cognitive deficits by increasing proteasome function. Given that Pim1 inhibitors are already being tested in ongoing human clinical trials for cancer, the results presented here may open a new venue of drug discovery for AD by developing more Pim1 inhibitors.

Keywords: AD, Pim1 inhibitor, PRAS40, 3xTg-AD, Proteasome, Aβ, tau, mTOR, Aging, Working memory

Background

Alzheimer's disease (AD) is the most prevalent neurodegenerative disorder worldwide. Clinically, AD is characterized by impairments of memory, cognitive and intellectual functions [1]. The buildup of amyloid-β (Aβ) plaques and neurofibrillary tangles (NFTs) are the two prominent pathologies contributing to the progression of cognitive deficits in AD [2]. Aβ is generated from the amyloid precursor protein (APP), which is sequentially cleaved by the β-site APP cleaving enzyme 1 (BACE-1) and the γ-secretase complex to liberate Aβ. NFTs consist of hyperphosphorylated and aggregated tau, a microtubule-binding protein. Over the next few decades, advancing age of the global population will dramatically increase the prevalence of AD to an estimated 20 million by 2050 in the US alone [3]. Currently, there are no effective treatment options to either prevent or reduce the progression of AD. Therefore, there is an urgent need for novel, safe, and efficacious strategies to mitigate this disorder.

Aging is the most important risk factor for AD; thus, it is possible that altered signaling pathways associated with aging may facilitate the development of AD and other age-dependent disorders [4, 5]. Overwhelming evidence has shown that the mammalian target of

* Correspondence: oddo@asu.edu
[1]Neurodegenerative Disease Research Center, Biodesign Institute, School of Life Sciences, Arizona State University, 727 E. Tyler Street, Tempe, AZ 85287-5001, USA
[2]School of Life Sciences, Arizona State University, Tempe, AZ 85287, USA

rapamycin (mTOR), a serine/threonine protein kinase involved in the regulation of protein synthesis and degradation, plays a key role in regulating lifespan and health span [5–7]. mTOR is part of two major complexes, the mTOR complex 1 (mTORC1) and 2 (mTORC2), which have different functions [8, 9]. mTOR signaling is upregulated in AD [10–13]. To this end, we and others have shown that reducing mTOR activity pharmacologically, with rapamycin, or genetically ameliorates Aβ plaque load and NFTs while improving cognitive deficits in multiple animal models of AD [10, 14–17]. However, various studies have found that rapamycin has many side effects, necessitating other treatment options to reduce mTOR hyperactivity in AD [18–20].

The proline-rich Akt substrate 40 kDa (PRAS40) is a constituent of the mTORC1, which physically binds to mTOR and inhibits its activity. Upon phosphorylation at Thr246 by serine/threonine-specific protein kinase (AKT) or proto-oncogene serine/threonine-protein kinase Pim-1 (Pim1), PRAS40 detaches from mTORC1 thereby releasing its inhibitory effects [21, 22]. We have shown that intrahippocampal injection of naturally secreted Aβ is sufficient to increase mTOR signaling in the brains of wild type mice by increasing the phosphorylation of PRAS40 [23].

Pim1 is a kinase member of the proto-oncogene Pim kinase family [24–27]. Pim1 plays a role in cell survival and proliferation; hence, its deregulation can easily transform it to an oncogenic protein. Pim1 has gained much attention due to its upregulation in a variety of cancers [28, 29]. Of note, Pim1 knockout mice have no phenotype [30], suggesting that Pim1 might be a viable therapeutic target. Crystallographic studies revealed a unique architecture within the Pim1 secondary structure, which allowed the synthesis of highly specific inhibitors [31, 32]. Here, we sought to determine the effects of reducing Pim 1 activity on AD-like pathology developed by the 3xTg-AD mice.

Results

Pharmacological characterization of Pim1 inhibitor 1

We have previously shown that the levels of PRAS40 phosphorylated at Thr246 (pPRAS40) are increased in 3xTg-AD mice [23]. To further determine the role of PRAS40 in AD, we assessed the levels of pPRAS40 in the inferior frontal gyrus of human AD brains (Table 1). We found that the levels of pPRAS40 are increased in human AD brains compared to age-matched controls (Fig. 1). We then sought to determine the effects of reducing PRAS40 phosphorylation on the AD-like pathology in 3xTg-AD mice. To achieve our goal, we targeted Pim1, a kinase known to phosphorylate PRAS40 [33]. Several Pim1 kinase inhibitors are commercially available,

Table 1 Descriptive information of patients whose brain tissue was utilized to measure pPRAS40 levels. Gel order indicates the order in which protein samples were loaded in Fig. 1

Age at death	Diagnosis	MMSE score	Braak stage	Gel load order
86	AD	16	IV	1
82	AD	23	IV	2
93	CTL	30	I	3
89	CTL	29	II	4
92	CTL	26	III	5
79	CTL	29	II	6
82	AD	19	V	7
78	AD	0	VI	8
87	CTL	28	III	9
91	CTL	27	II	10
87	CTL	26	III	11
75	CTL	29	III	12
95	CTL	26	III	13
88	AD	9	VI	14
78	AD	-	IV	15
68	AD	0	VI	16
78	CTL	29	III	17
85	AD	23	VI	18
86	AD	20	IV	19

and some are currently in clinical trial for the treatment of cancer (ClinicalTrials.gov Identifier: NCT00848601). The commercially available Pim1 inhibitor, 3-Cyano-4-phenyl-6-(3-bromo-6-hydroxy) phenyl-2 (1*H*)-pyridone (herein referred to as Pim1i; Fig. 2a), exhibits highly specific competitive inhibition to Pim1; IC_{50} 50 nM for Pim1 and 2 μM for Pim2 [33]. We have shown that intracranial delivery of this inhibitor effectively decreases pPRAS40 [23], a downstream substrate of Pim1. We first tested Pim1i bioavailability and measured its brain-to-plasma ratio by LC-MS/MS analysis. To this end, C57BL/6 mice received a single dose of 50 mg/kg Pim1i intraperitoneally (i.p.). We found that maximum plasma concentration of Pim1i was 32166 ± 11220 ng/mL, which was observed at 1 h post dose with half-life of 1.02 h (Fig. 2b). Pim1i was also detectable up to 3 h post dose in brain tissue homogenate samples (Fig. 2c). The maximum brain concentration of 197 ± 48.5 ng/g was observed at 0.5 h post dose.

To determine whether Pim1i engages the target, we injected C57BL/6 mice with 100 mg/kg i.p. and harvested brains at 1, 3, 6, 12 and 24 post injection ($n = 5$ per time-point). Three additional mice were used as our baseline. We decided to increase the dose as no toxicity was detected in mice receiving 50 mg/kg Pim1i. We found that the levels of pPRAS40 were significantly different across the different time points ($F_{(6, 26)} = 11.09$; $p < 0.001$; Fig. 2d). A Bonferroni's multiple comparison

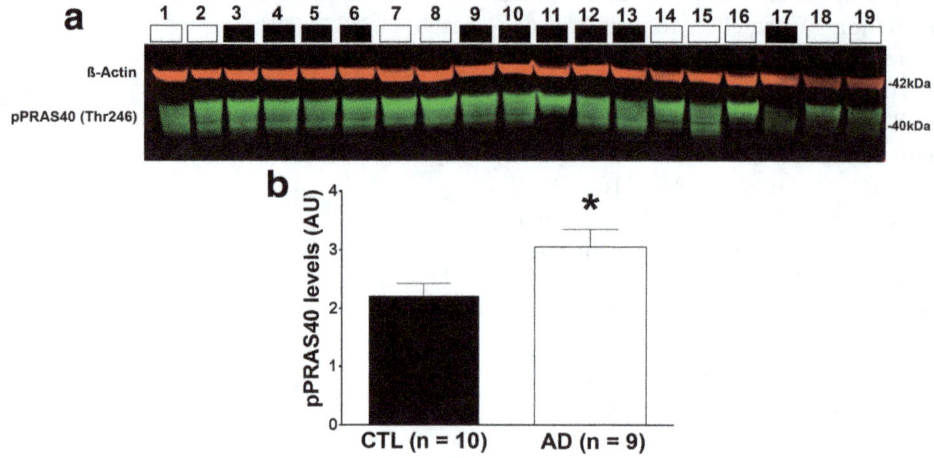

Fig. 1 Phosphorylated PRAS40 levels are increased in AD patients. **a** Western blots of proteins extracted from the inferior temporal gyrus of human control (CTL; $n = 10$) and AD brains ($n = 9$). Blots were probed with the indicated antibodies. The descriptive information for each patient (numbered above the blots) are reported in Table 1. **b** Quantitative analysis of the blot shows that phosphorylated PRAS40 levels were significantly higher in AD compared to CTL cases ($p = 0.0325$). Quantitative analyses of the blots were obtained by normalizing PRAS40 levels to β-Actin, used as a loading control. Error bars represent mean ± SEM

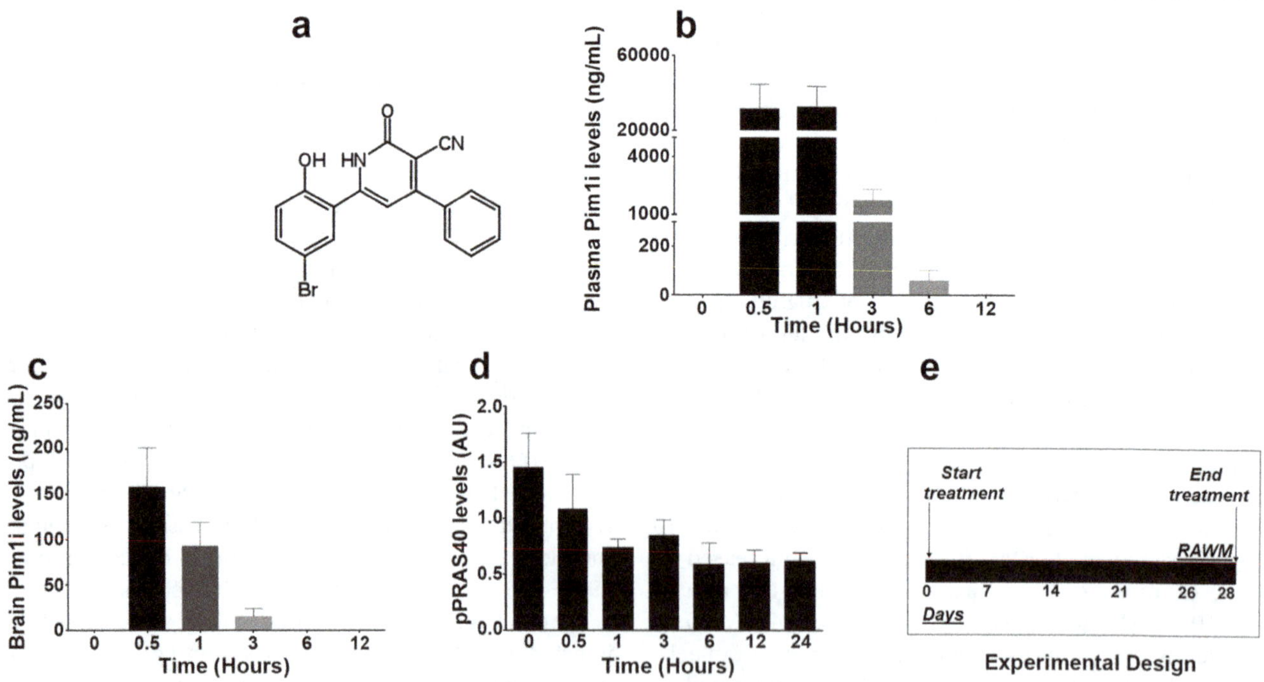

Fig. 2 Pharmacological profile of Pim1i. **a** Chemical structure of the Pim1 inhibitor (Pim1i) used in this study. **b** The Pim1i levels measured in plasma as a function of time after a single intraperitoneal injection of 50 mg/kg. The maximum plasma concentration of Pim1i was 32166 ± 11220 ng/mL observed at 1 h post dose with half-life of 1.02 h. **c** Pim1i measured in the brain as a function of time after a single intraperitoneal injection of 50 mg/kg. Pim1i was also detectable up to 3 h post dose in brain tissue homogenate samples. The maximum brain concentration of 197 ± 48.5 ng/g was observed at 0.5 h post dose. **d** Pim1i reduced phosphorylated PRAS40 levels up to 24 h after a single intraperitoneal injection of 100 mg/kg. **e** Schematic of the experimental design. NonTg and 3xTg-AD mice were injected with either the vehicle or 100 mg/kg Pim1i for 28 days. All animals started behavioral testing in the radial arm water maze task at day 26

test indicated that pPRAS40 levels at the time points 1, 3, 6, 12 and 24 h were significantly different than time 0, our baseline control. These data show that brain levels of pPRAS40 were significantly reduced one hour following the Pim1i injections and stayed low for 24 h.

Pim1 inhibition reduces spatial reference and working memory deficits in 3xTg-AD mice

Given these data, we sought to determine the effects of chronic administration of the Pim1i at a dosage of 100 mg/kg on the AD-like pathology in 3xTg-AD mice. To this end, we used 7-month-old female 3xTg-AD and non-transgenic (NonTg) mice. At this age, 3xTg-AD mice have mild cognitive deficits, which are associated with high soluble Aβ and tau levels [34]. Mice were randomly assigned to one of the following groups: 3xTg-AD Vehicle (Veh), NonTg Veh, 3xTg-AD Pim1i, NonTg Pim1i ($n = 14$/group) and received daily i.p. injections of Pim1i or vehicle for 28 days (Fig. 2e).

We first assessed body weight of the mice at the beginning of treatment and found that the average body weight was 24.21 ± 0.635 g for NonTg mice and 31.46 ± 1.427 g for 3xTg-AD mice. The analysis of mean weight revealed a significant main effect of Genotype ($F_{(1, 42)} = 36.624$, $p < 0.0001$), indicating that 3xTg-AD mice weighed significantly more than NonTg mice. Similarly, 3xTg-AD mice (28.28 ± 1.05 g) weighed more than the NonTg mice (22.48 ± 0.46 g) at completion of treatment. The analysis of mean weight in grams revealed a significant main effect of Genotype ($F_{(1, 42)} = 28.689$, $p < 0.0001$) and Treatment ($F_{(1, 42)} = 5.364$, $p < 0.05$), however no significant Genotype by Treatment interaction ($F_{(1, 42)} = 1.117$, $p > 0.05$). Together, these data indicate that the Pim1i treated mice weighed less at the end of treatment compared to the mice on vehicle, and this difference was independent of genotype. Notably, during the 28 days of treatment, we lost mice in all four groups. The total numbers of mice that did not show any overt toxicity and were tested behaviorally are as follows: 3xTg-AD Veh ($n = 13$), NonTg Veh ($n = 12$), 3xTg-AD Pim1i ($n = 7$), NonTg Pim1i ($n = 13$).

To determine the effect of 28 days of the Pim1i on spatial reference and working memory, we tested all subjects on an 8-arm radial arm water maze (RAWM) task. Mice were tested for two consecutive days: on day one, mice received 15 trials, with trials alternating between visible and hidden platform. On day 2, mice received 15 additional trials but the platform was kept hidden throughout the trials. Entry into an incorrect arm was scored as a spatial reference error. Reentry into a previously visited arm within the trial was considered a working memory error. The number of errors were averaged by block, with each block being equivalent to three trails. Using a mixed model ANOVA, we first examined mean incorrect errors between day 1 and 2 to assess learning. We found a significant effect of Genotype ($F_{(1,42)} = 13.610$; $p < 0.01$), Treatment ($F_{(1,42)} = 18.790$, $p < 0.0001$), day ($F_{(1, 42)} = 107.868$, $p < 0.0001$) and a trend in Genotype by Treatment interaction ($F_{(1, 42)} = 3.755$, $p = 0.0594$; Fig. 3a). Specifically, all groups showed a significant reduction in incorrect errors between day 1 and day 2, indicating that all groups significantly learned the task.

We next analyzed the number of errors during the probe trials (day 2). For reference errors, we found a significant effect of Block ($F_{(4, 42)} = 3.882$, $p < 0.005$, Fig. 3b), Genotype ($F_{(1, 42)} = 8.126$, $p < 0.01$), Treatment ($F_{(1, 42)} = 18.105$, $p < 0.001$) and a significant Genotype by Treatment interaction ($F_{(1, 42)} = 4.496$, $p < 0.05$). Post hoc test with Bonferroni's correction indicated that 3xTg-AD Veh mice committed a higher number of reference errors throughout the 5 blocks of testing when compared to the NonTg Veh group ($p < 0.05$; Fig. 3b for errors across each block; 2C for mean total errors). Notably, 3xTg-AD Pim1i mice made significantly fewer errors compared to 3xTg-AD Veh treated mice, indicating improved spatial reference memory ($p < 0.01$). Furthermore, 3xTg-AD Pim1i mice performed as well as NonTg Veh mice ($p > 0.05$), illustrating a full rescue of spatial reference memory. Interestingly, NonTg mice injected with Pim1i made significantly fewer errors than the vehicle treated NonTg mice ($p < 0.05$). These results show that 28 days of Pim1i administration is sufficient to normalize the spatial reference memory deficits in 3xTg-AD mice to NonTg levels, and to improve performance in NonTg mice.

We then examined reentry errors into a previously entered arm within a trial, which indicate working memory errors. When we compared the mice performance between the two days of training, we found a significant effect of Genotype ($F_{(1, 42)} = 8.045$, $p = 0.01$), Treatment ($F_{(1, 42)} = 10.381$, $p < 0.01$), day ($F_{(1, 42)} = 13.693$, $p < 0.001$), and a Genotype by Treatment interaction ($F_{(1, 42)} = 4.390$, $p < 0.05$; Fig. 3d). Notably, 3xTg-AD Veh mice had the same number of working memory errors between day 1 and day 2 ($p > 0.05$), indicating that although they decreased the number of reference memory errors, they continued to commit working memory errors on day 2. All other groups show a decrease in working memory errors between day 1 and day 2. These data indicate that 3xTg-AD Pim 1i mice performed significantly fewer working memory errors compared to 3xTg-AD Veh. During the probe trials (day 2), we found a significant effect of Genotype ($F_{(1, 42)} = 5.255$, $p < 0.05$), Treatment ($F_{(1, 42)} = 10.131$, $p < 0.01$), and Genotype by Treatment interaction ($F_{(1, 42)} = 4.496$, $p < 0.05$; Fig. 3e). Post hoc test with Bonferroni's correction indicated that 3xTg-AD Veh mice committed a higher number of working memory errors throughout the 5 blocks of testing when compared to the NonTg-AD Veh mice ($p = 0.0147$, Fig. 3e for errors across each block; 3f for

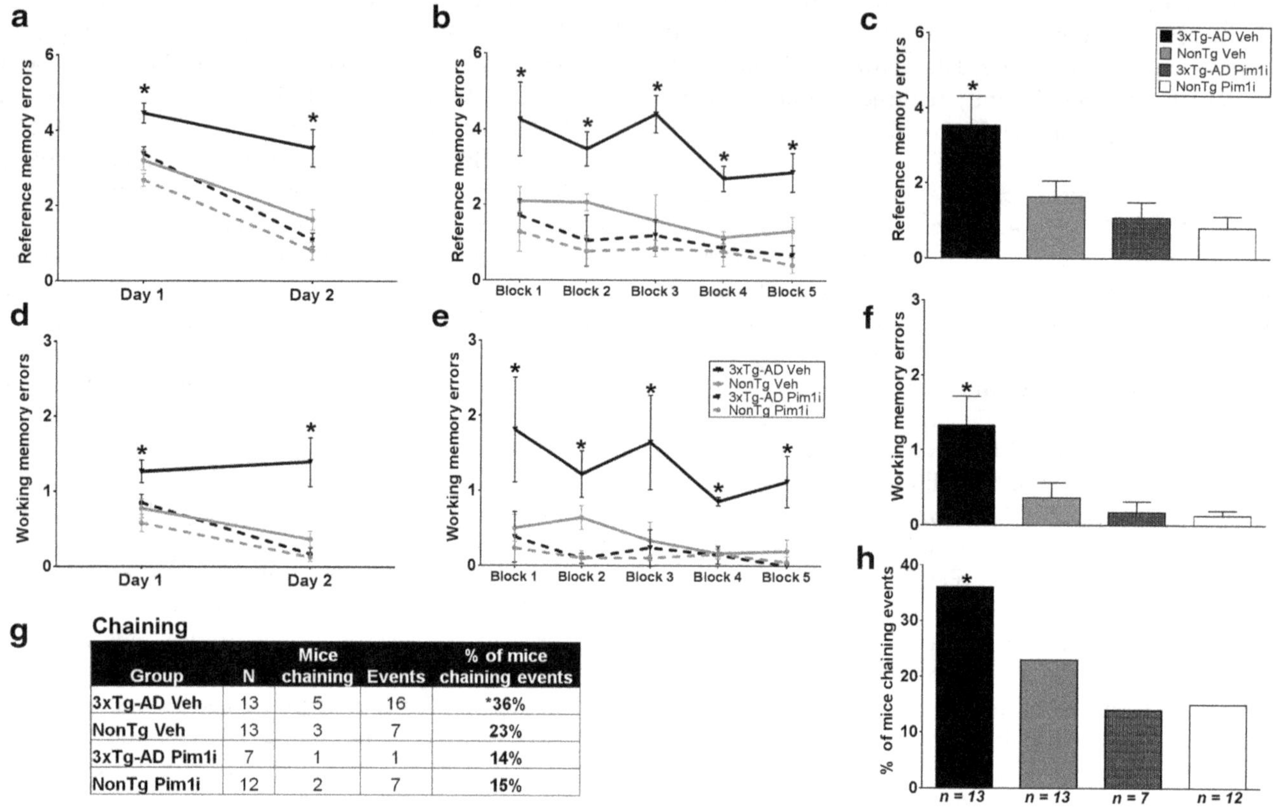

Group	N	Mice chaining	Events	% of mice chaining events
3xTg-AD Veh	13	5	16	*36%
NonTg Veh	13	3	7	23%
3xTg-AD Pim1i	7	1	1	14%
NonTg Pim1i	12	2	7	15%

Fig. 3 Pim1 inhibition reduces spatial reference and working memory deficits in 3xTg-AD mice. NonTg Veh ($n = 13$), 3xTg-AD Veh ($n = 13$), NonTg Pim1i ($n = 12$), 3xTg-AD Pim1i ($n = 7$) were tested in the radial arm water maze (RAWM). **a** Average reference memory errors on day 1 and day 2 RAWM task. All groups show a decrease in total errors in day 2 indicating learning ($F_{(1, 42)} = 107.868$, $p < 0.0001$). **b** Average reference memory errors across the 5 blocks of testing of day 2 (1 block = 3 trials). 3xTg-AD Veh mice committed a higher number of reference errors throughout the 5 blocks of testing compared to all the other groups. **c** Mean total errors of day 2. **d** Working memory errors on day 1 and day 2. Working memory errors are defined as a reentry into a previously visited arm. 3xTg-AD Veh mice had the same number of working memory errors between day 1 and day 2 ($p > 0.05$), whereas all the other groups showed significant learning between the two days. **e** Average working memory errors across the 5 blocks of testing of day 2. 3xTg-AD Veh mice commit a higher number of working memory errors throughout the 5 blocks of testing compared to the other three groups. **f.** Mean working memory errors during day 2. **g** Pim1i significantly reduces the percentage of 3xTg-AD mice using a hippocampal-independent default strategy to find the hidden platform, known as chaining. The panel illustrates the percentage of mice committing chaining events between all groups. **h** The panel illustrates the percentage of animals that committed chaining events between the four groups. Pim 1i significantly reduced the percentage of chaining committed by the 3xTg-AD mice ($X^2 = 7.8045$, $p < 0.01$). Error bars represent mean ± SEM

mean total errors). Pim1i significantly reduced the number of working memory errors in 3xTg-AD mice compared to 3xTg-AD Veh mice ($p < 0.05$). Indeed, the number of working memory errors made by 3xTg-AD Pim1i mice were not statistically significant from errors made by NonTg Veh mice ($p > 0.05$). Collectively, these results show that 28 days of the Pim1 inhibitor is sufficient to reduce spatial reference and working memory deficits in 3xTg-AD mice.

"Chaining" is a commonly used search strategy to find the platform in the RAWM [35]. This method does not require use of spatial cues and instead consists of sequential arm visits until the platform is found. To further determine the nature of the cognitive impairment in 3xTg-AD mice, we examined the use of a chaining strategy for navigation of the maze during the day 2 probe trials. For this analysis, a chaining event was defined as three consecutive arm entries in an anticlockwise or clockwise direction, an operational definition used by [35]. The percentage of chaining events committed per group were analyzed using a chi-square test. We found that 3xTg-AD Veh mice show a significantly higher number of chaining events compared to both NonTg groups and 3xTg-AD Pim1i treated group ($X^2 = 7.8045$, $p < 0.01$, Fig. 3g-h). These data suggest that Pim1 inhibition reduces the usage of the chaining search strategy in 3xTg-AD mice.

Pim1 inhibition lowers Aβ levels and hippocampal CP13 immunoreactivity in 3xTg-AD mice

At the end of the behavioral testing, mice were sacrificed and their brains were used for neuropathological and biochemical assessment. To determine whether peripheral administration of Pim1i reached the brain, we used sandwich enzyme linked immunosorbent assay to measure the levels of pPRAS40 at Thr246, as this epitope is directly phosphorylated by Pim 1 [33]. We found a significant effect for Genotype ($F_{(1,\ 20)} = 4.501$, $p < 0.05$), Treatment ($F_{(1,\ 20)} = 36.593$, $p < 0.0001$), and a non-significant Genotype by Treatment interaction ($F_{(1,\ 20)} = 1.767$, $p > 0.05$; Fig. 4a). The effect of genotype indicated that 3xTg-AD mice show higher levels of pPRAS40 than NonTg mice. Interestingly, the treatment effect reveals that both 3xTg-AD and NonTg Pim1i mice have a reduced pPRAS40 level. Together, these data further confirm that Pim1i crosses the blood brain barrier and decreases the levels of brain pPRAS40.

One of the key neuropathological features of AD is the accumulation of extracellular Aβ plaques [2]. Aβ peptides consist of 36–43 amino acids, where $A\beta_{40}$ and $A\beta_{42}$ are the more abundant Aβ species. $A\beta_{42}$ is more prone to aggregation and toxicity than the $A\beta_{40}$ species [2]. We immunostained sections from 3xTg-AD Veh ($n = 6$) and 3xTg-AD Pim1i ($n = 5$) mice with an $A\beta_{42}$-specific antibody and found that $A\beta_{42}$ immunoreactivity was significantly reduced in the brains of 3xTg-AD mice injected with Pim1i (Fig. 4b-c). Quantitative analysis of the overall $A\beta_{42}$ load indicated a significant decrease of 45.2 % in the brain of 3xTg-AD Pim1i compared with 3xTg-AD mice ($t_{(10)} = 8.419$, $p < 0.05$; Fig. 4d). We next measured Aβ levels by sandwich ELISA and found that both soluble and insoluble $A\beta_{40}$ levels were significantly lower in 3xTg-AD Pim1i mice compared with 3xTg-AD Veh mice (soluble $A\beta_{40}$: $t_{(10)} = 2.442$, $p < 0.05$; insoluble $A\beta_{40}$: $t_{(10)} = 2.681$, $p = 0.0230$; Fig. 5a-b). Furthermore, both soluble and insoluble levels of $A\beta_{42}$ were significantly lower in 3xTg-AD Pim1i compared to 3xTg-AD Veh mice (soluble $A\beta_{42}$: $t_{(10)} = 2.404$, $p = 0.0371$; insoluble $A\beta_{42}$: $t_{(10)} = 3.932$, $p < 0.01$; Fig. 5c-d).

Another hallmark pathology associated with AD is the accumulation of neurofibrillary tangles made of hyperphosphorylated tau [2]. To determine the effects of Pim1 inhibition on tau pathology, we first immunostained sections from 3xTg-AD Veh and 3xTg-Pim1-inh1 mice with CP13, an antibody that recognizes tau phosphorylated at serine 202. We found that CP13 immunoreactivity was reduced in 3xTg-AD Pim1i compared with 3xTg-AD mice (Fig. 6a-b). Quantitative analysis indicated that CP13 immunoreactivity was significantly decreased by 38 % in the brain of 3xTg-AD Pim1i compared with 3xTg-AD Veh mice ($t_{(10)} = 2.785$, $p < 0.05$; Fig. 6c). To further assess the tau pathology, we measured tau levels by western blot

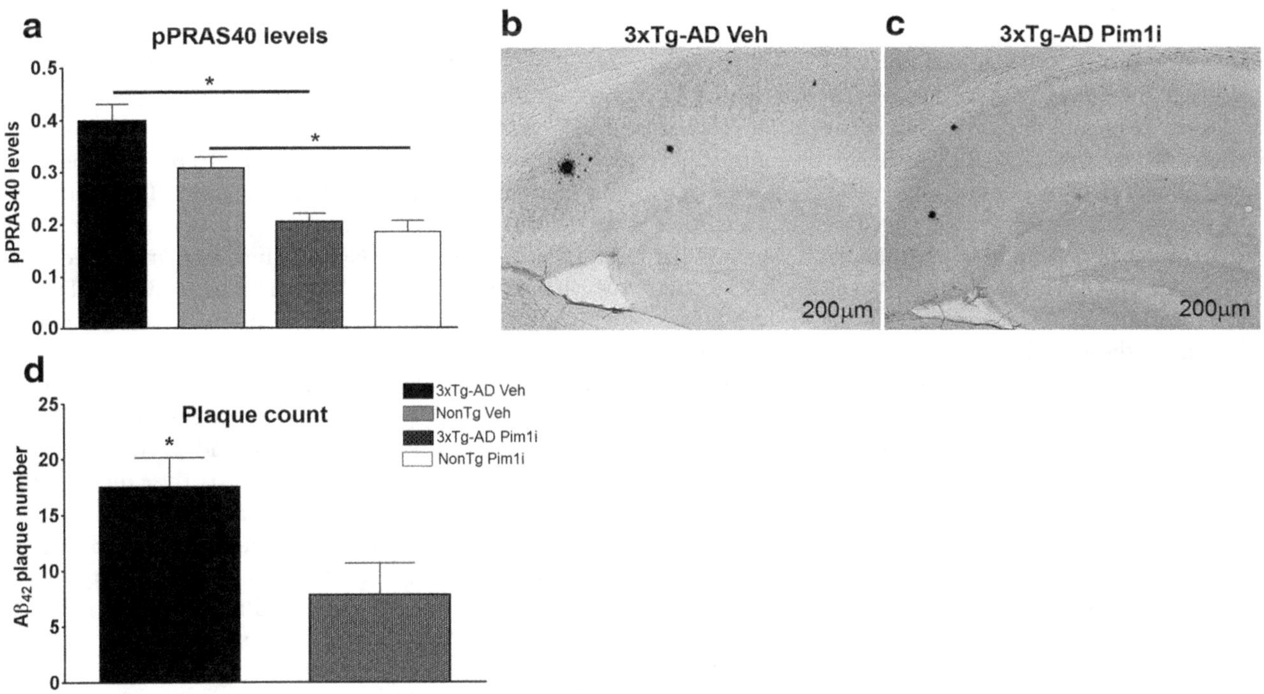

Fig. 4 Pim1i decreases Aβ pathology. **a** The graph shows the phosphorylated levels of PRAS40 levels after 28 days of treatment, measured by sandwich ELISA. The Pim1 inhibitor significantly reduced the pPRAS40 levels of both the 3xTg-AD and NonTg mice as evident by a significant effect of treatment ($F_{(1,\ 42)} = 36.593$, $p < 0.0001$). **b** Representative microphotographs of brain sections from 3xTg-AD mice stained with an $A\beta_{42}$ specific antibody (Millipore, catalog number AB5078P). **d** Quantitative analysis of $A\beta_{42}$ immunoreactivity by unpaired *t*-test reveals that 3xTg-AD mice treated with Pim1i had significantly fewer plaques compared to 3xTg-AD mice treated with vehicle ($t_{(8)} = 8.419$, $p < 0.05$). Error bars represent mean ± SEM

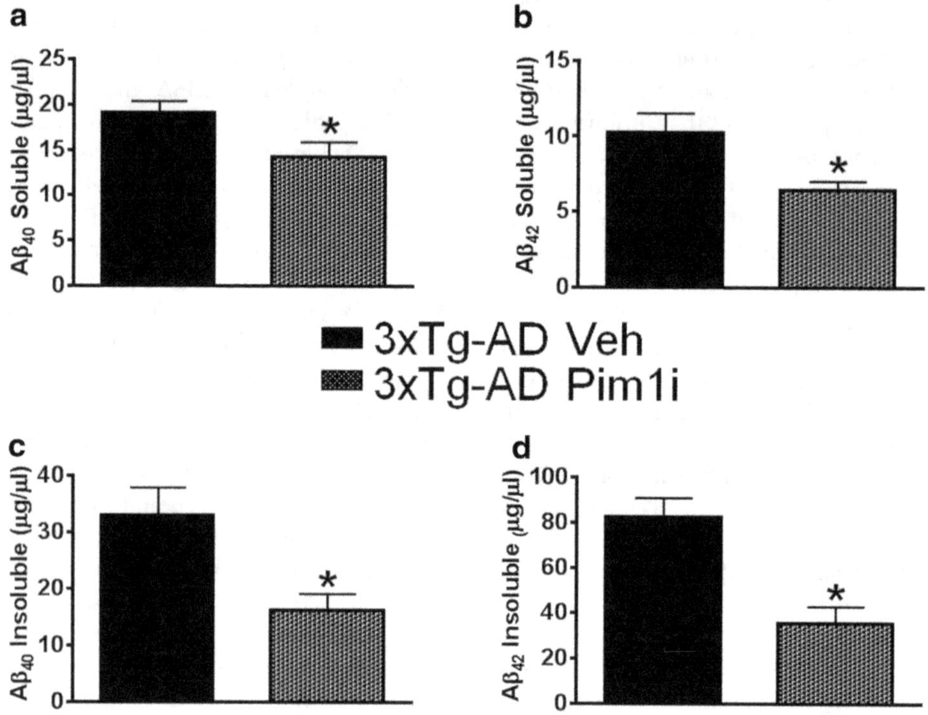

Fig. 5 Pim1i decreases Aβ levels. Sandwich ELISA measurements of insoluble and soluble $A\beta_{40}$ and $A\beta_{42}$ levels in brain extracts from 3xTg-AD veh (n = 7) and 3xTg-AD Pim1i ($n = 5$) mice. **a**, **b** Soluble and insoluble Aβ42 levels were significantly lower in 3xTg-AD mice injected with Pim1i (Soluble $A\beta_{40}$: $t_{(10)} = 2.442$, $p < 0.05$; insoluble $A\beta_{40}$: $t_{(10)} = 2.681$, $p < 0.05$). **c**, **d** Soluble and insoluble $A\beta_{42}$ levels were significantly lower in 3xTg-AD mice treated with Pim1i (soluble $A\beta_{42}$: $t_{(10)} = 2.404$, $p < 0.05$; insoluble $A\beta_{42}$: $t_{(10)} = 3.932$, $p < 0.01$). Error bars represent mean ± SEM

using antibodies against total and phosphorylated tau. We found that the levels of total human tau (measured by HT7) were not significantly different between the Veh and Pim1i-treated groups ($p > 0.05$; Fig. 6d-e). In contrast, we found a main effect of Genotype for CP13 levels ($F_{(1,15)} = 4.563$, $p < 0.05$; Fig. 6d, f). Post hoc analyses indicated that 3xTg-AD mice had significantly higher levels than NonTg mice. The apparent contradiction between the CP13 data obtained by immunohistochemistry and by western blot is likely due to the fact that the immunohistochemistry allows for single cell resolution while the western blot was done by homogenizing different cell types from different brain regions. Overall, these results show that Pim1 inhibition reduces hippocampal tau immunoreactivity in 3xTg-AD mice.

Pim1i increases proteasome activity

Our results indicate that reductions in pPRAS40 via Pim1 inhibition is sufficient to reduce spatial reference and working memory deficits in 3xTg-AD mice. These improvements in cognitive function are associated with a reduction in Aβ levels and phosphorylated tau immunoreactivity. To better elucidate the mechanisms underlying these effects, we first assessed mTOR signaling by measuring the phosphorylation levels of the two major downstream targets of mTOR: p70S6K1 and 4EBP1. For the phosphorylation levels of p70S6K1, there were no significant effects of Genotype ($F_{(1,15)} = 4.067$, $p > 0.05$), treatment ($F_{(1,15)} = 0.428$, $p > 0.05$), and Genotype by Treatment interaction ($F_{(1,15)} = 1.831$, $p > 0.05$; Fig. 7a-b). Interestingly for the downstream target 4EBP1, there was a main effect of Genotype ($F_{(1, 15)} = 5.621$, $p = 0.05$; Fig. 7a, c) where the NonTg mice had increased levels of phosphorylated 4EBP1 compared to 3xTg-AD mice. There was no effect of the Pim1i treatment on these targets.

To further understand what mechanisms may underlie changes in AD pathology and improvements in behavior, we assessed autophagy induction and proteasome function. We focused on these systems as they represent the two major cellular protein degradation systems and are known to be involved in the turnover of Aβ and tau [36]. First, we measured the levels of LC3, Atg3, Atg5, and Atg12, key proteins involved in autophagy induction whose levels are routinely used to monitor it [37]. We found a significant main effect of Genotype ($F_{(1, 15)} = 7.238$, $p < 0.05$) but a non-significant effect of Treatment ($F_{(1, 15)} = 2.230$, $p > 0.05$) or Genotype by Treatment interaction ($F_{(1, 15)} = 0.00042$, $p > 0.05$) for p62 (Fig. 8a-b). In addition, we found a significant main effect of Genotype ($F_{(1, 15)} = 10.851$, $p < 0.01$) but a non-significant effect of Treatment ($F_{(1, 15)} = 0.266$, $p > 0.05$) and the Genotype by

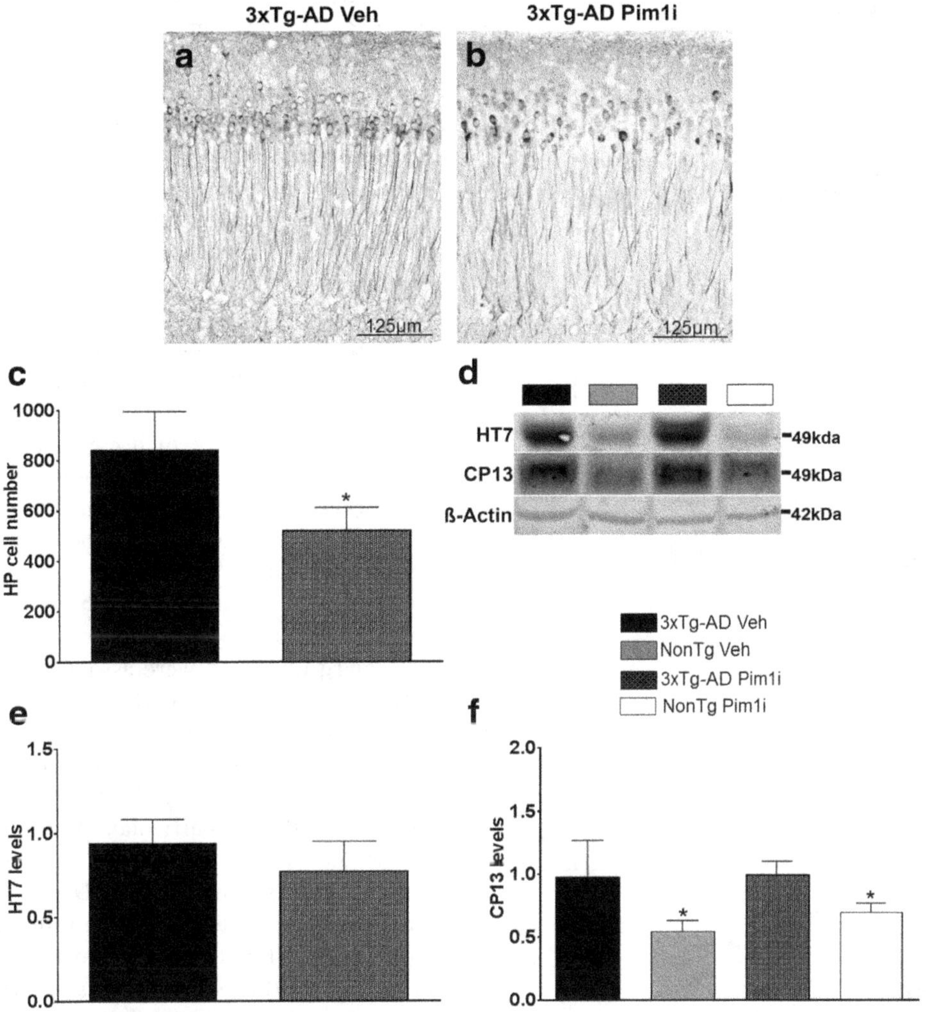

Fig. 6 Reduced Tau pathology in 3xTg-AD Pim1i mice. **a**, **b** Representative microphotographs of CA1 hippocampal neurons from 3xTg-AD Veh and 3xTg-AD Pim1i mice stained with the anti-tau antibody CP13, which recognizes tau phosphorylated at Ser202. **c** Quantitative analysis of the CP13 immunoreactivity by unpaired *t*-test reveals that Pim1i significantly reduced tau immunoreactivity ($t_{(9)} = 2.785$, $p < 0.05$). **d** Representative western blots of protein extracted from 3xTg-AD Veh, NonTg Veh, 3xTg-AD Pim1i, and NonTg Pim1i mice. Blots were probed with the indicated antibodies. The HT7 antibody recognizes total human tau and CP13 antibody recognizes tau phosphorylated at Ser202. **e**, **f** Quantitative analyses of the blots. HT7 levels were not significantly different between the two groups ($t_{(9)} = 0.558$, $p > 0.05$). For CP13, we found a Genotype effect ($t_{(9)} = 4.563$, $p < 0.05$), revealing higher levels of CP13 in 3xTg-AD mice. Quantitative analyses of the blots were obtained by normalizing the levels of the protein of interest to β-Actin, used as a loading control. Error bars represent mean ± SEM

Treatment interaction ($F_{(1, 15)} = 1.607$, $p > 0.05$) for Atg3 (Fig. 8a, c). In contrast, the levels of Atg5 and Atg12 were similar among the four groups (Fig. 8a, d and e). Next, we used the fluorogenic substrates Bz-VGR-AMC, Suc-LLVYAMC, and Z-LLE-AMC to measure trypsin-like, chymotrypsin-like, and caspase-like activities of the proteasome. We found an effect of Treatment for chymotrypsin-like ($F_{(1, 20)} = 10.127$, $p < 0.05$, Fig. 8f), trypsin-like ($F_{(1, 20)} = 16.18$, $p < 0.001$, Fig. 8g) and caspase-like ($F_{(1, 20)} = 19.804$, $p < 0.001$, Fig. 8h) activity. This finding indicates that the Pim1 inhibitor increases the activity of the three substrates for both the 3xTg-AD and NonTg mice over the vehicle treated groups. This suggests that the reductions in Aβ pathology and tau immunoreactivity may be accomplished by an increase in protein degradation.

Discussion

The incidence of AD is quickly increasing and with no effective therapeutics to reduce the associated pathologies, this disorder is bound to have a major socio-economic impact on our society. The data presented here unambiguously show that inhibiting Pim1 activity for 28 days, thereby reducing pPRAS40 levels, has beneficial effects on AD-like pathology in 3xTg-AD mice. Indeed, these data show that

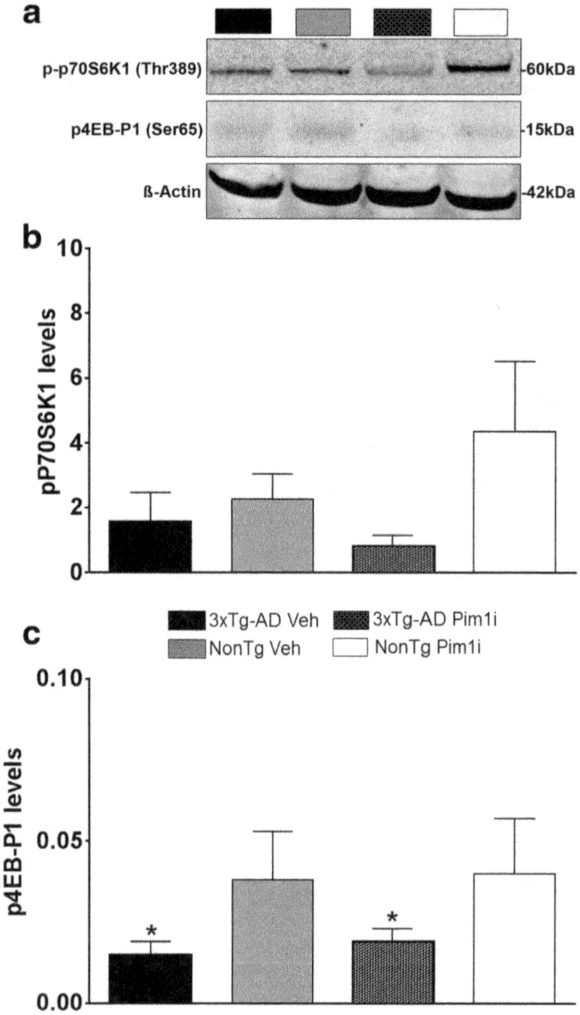

Fig. 7 Pim 1i does not alter mTORC1 signaling. **a** Representative western blots of the phosphorylated levels of downstream mTORC1 targets 4EB-P1, p70S6K1 and β-Actin control. **b, c** Quantitative analyses of the blots show. We found no changes in p-p70S6K1 levels. In contrast, we found that the NonTg groups had higher levels of p4EBP1 compared to the 3xTg-AD groups ($F_{(1, 15)} = 5.621$, $p < 0.05$). Quantitative analyses of the blots were obtained by normalizing the levels of the protein of interest to β-Actin, used as a loading control. Error bars represent mean ± SEM

inhibition of Pim1 reduced spatial reference and working memory errors in 3xTg-AD mice, and improved performance to NonTg levels. This cognitive improvement was associated with a reduction in hippocampal Aβ pathology and hippocampal tau immunoreactivity.

PRAS40 is a component of the mTOR complex 1; it physically binds to mTOR and negatively regulates its activity [33]. Upon phosphorylation, PRAS40 detaches from mTOR releasing its inhibitory effects. Indeed, high levels of pPRAS40 have been associated with high mTOR activity [8, 33]. Notably, the levels of pPRAS40 are elevated in both humans AD patients and 3xTg-AD mice [23]. We have previously shown that the increase in pPRAS40 is due to a buildup in Aβ oligomers [23]. Paradoxically, although we show that Pim1 inhibition reduces the levels of pPRAS40, the activity of mTOR appeared unaffected. Indeed, Pim1 inhibition did not change the phosphorylation levels of p70S6K1 and 4EBP1. These findings suggest that the reduction in Aβ pathology and hippocampal tau immunoreactivity may occur through an mTOR independent pathway. To this end, our data suggest that the mechanism underlying the reduced AD-like pathology is linked to an increase in proteasome activity as evident by the changes in the three proteolytic activities, chymotrypsin-like, trypsin-like and caspase-like, which comprise the catalytic core of the proteasome [38–40]. These results are consistent with previous findings showing that modulation of pPRAS40 levels alter proteasome function independent of mTOR activity [41, 42].

Interestingly, the increase in three proteolytic activities of the proteasome were observed in both the 3xTg-AD and NonTg mice and were associated with inhibition of Pim1 and reduced pPRAS40 levels. The increase in proteasome activity suggests an increase in degradation of Aβ and tau proteins. Proteasome dysfunction has been linked to AD pathology in both AD patients and mouse models [43–45]. In particular, studies have shown that proteasome activity is decreased in the hippocampus, which is more susceptible to AD pathology, and less in areas like the cerebellum, where minimal to no changes in proteasome functions have been detected in AD patients [43]. To this end, work has found accumulation of Aβ and tau after direct inhibition of proteasome activity in the 3xTg-AD mice [45]. Consistent with these observations, we and others have reported that increased proteasome activity is sufficient to degrade Aβ and relieve deficits in cognitive function [44, 46, 47].

Diabetes is a major risk factor of AD [48–50]; however, the molecular pathways linking diabetes to AD remain elusive. Physiologically, PRAS40 is activated by Pim1 and by phosphatidylinositol 3-kinase/Akt (PI3K/Akt), which are further regulated by upstream tyrosine kinase receptor growth factors, including insulin-like growth factor 1 [51]. To this end, insulin signaling facilitates PRAS40 phosphorylation at Thr246 [9, 52, 53]. Glucose-induced hyperphosphorylation of PRAS40 has been implicated in type 2 diabetes [54] and in the progression of diabetic nephropathy [55]. Higher pPRAS40 levels increase activation of mTORC1 and its downstream targets [33]. At the same time, both PRAS40 phosphorylation and mTOR activity are increased in AD patients and in AD animal models, and contribute to the buildup of Aβ and tau [6, 10, 15, 56]. While further studies are needed, these data suggest that PRAS40

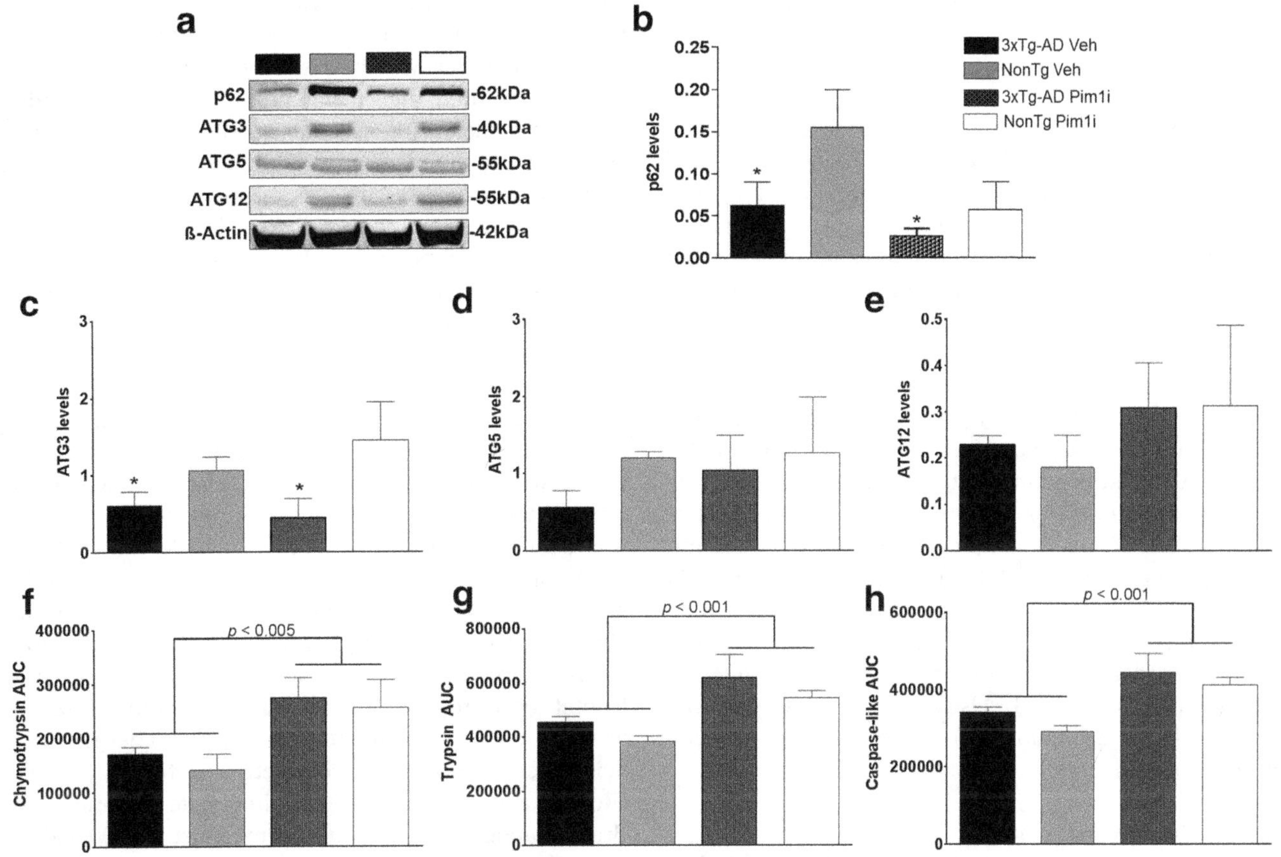

Fig. 8 Pim 1i increases proteasome function. **a** Representative western blots of protein extracted from treated and untreated 3xTg-AD and NonTg mice. Blots were probed with the indicated antibodies. **b** Quantitative analyses of the p62 blots show that p62 levels are reduced in both 3xTg-AD groups compared to the NonTg groups, as indicated by a significant main effect of Genotype ($F_{(1, 15)} = 7.238$, $p < 0.05$). These p62 changes were independent of Pim1 inhibition. **c**. Quantitative analyses of the ATG3 blots show that the ATG3 levels are reduced in both 3xTg-AD groups compared to the NonTg groups, as indicated by a significant main effect of Genotype ($F_{(1, 15)} = 10.851$, $p < 0.01$). **d, e** Quantitative analyses of the ATG5 and ATG12 blots indicate no significant difference among the four groups. **f-h** Proteasome analyses of proteins extracted from the brains of the four groups of mice revealed significant main effects of treatment for chymotrypsin-like ($F_{(1, 20)} = 10.127$, $p < 0.05$), trypsin-like ($F_{(1, 20)} = 16.18$, $p < 0.001$), and caspase-like ($F_{(1, 20)} = 19.804$, $p < 0.001$) activities. Quantitative analyses of the blots were obtained by normalizing the levels of the protein of interest to β-Actin, used as a loading control. Error bars represent mean ± SEM

phosphorylation might represent a molecular link between diabetes and AD.

Conclusions

In conclusion, our data highlight the commercially available Pim1 inhibitor as a potential therapeutic to reduced AD-neuropathology and associated cognitive deficits by decreasing elevated pPRAS40 levels and increasing proteasome activity in the 3xTg-AD mouse model.

Methods

Human and mouse tissue

Human tissue was obtained from the Brain and Body Donation Program at the Banner Sun Health Research Institute, an ongoing longitudinal clinicopathological study of normal aging and neurodegenerative disorders [57]. Human cases were selected randomly by personnel of the Brain and Body Donation program among the tissue available. Groups were matched based on their clinical and neuropathological phenotype. The generation of the 3xTg-AD mice used in the current study has been described previously [34]. All mice were housed 4–5 per cage at 23 °C, kept on a 12 h light/dark cycle, and were given *ad libitum* access to food and water. In our colony of 3xTg-AD mice, males show a large neuropathological variability, even between littermates. In contrast, female 3xTg-AD mice do not show such large variability and their phenotype changes as a function of age in a predictable manner. Therefore, only female mice were used for the experiments described here. All animal procedures were approved by the Arizona State University Institutional Animal Care and Use Committee (IACUC). All behavioral and experiments were performed with the experimenters blind to the genotype and treatment.

Pim1i analysis

Absorption Systems (Philadelphia, PA) performed the detection of the Pim1 inhibitor in the blood and brain of C57BL/6 mice injected with a dosage of 50 mg/kg. Standards were prepared in C57BL/6 mouse plasma containing sodium heparin as an anticoagulant, or in blank homogenized C57BL/6 mouse brain. The calibration curve was prepared to concentrations of 1000, 500, 250, 100, 50, 10, 5, and 2.5 ng/mL by serial dilution. Standard samples were treated identically to the study samples. Plasma and brain homogenate samples were extracted via acetonitrile precipitation on a Tomtec Quadra 96-Model 320 liquid handling system in a 96-well plate format. The procedure for sample extraction were as follows; (1) Add 55 μL of samples or standards into 2 mL polypropylene 96-well plate; (2) Using the Tomtec, add 50 μL of sample to 150 μL of acetonitrile (containing 100 ng/mL warfarin as an internal standard) that has been pre-loaded onto a Sirocco Protein Precipitation plate (Waters Corp.); (3) Using the Tomtec, mix the samples via air aspiration; (4) Apply vacuum and Cap for analysis.

8-arm radial arm water maze

The radial arm water maze (RAWM) task is utilized to assess hippocampal-dependent spatial reference and working memory [58, 59]. The task was performed in a black maze of 66 cm in diameter, made of black ABS Plexiglas. The maze consists of eight radiating arms, which were filled with water kept at 23.5 °C. The water was made opaque with nontoxic white paint. An 8 cm wide platform was kept 1.5 cm under the surface of the water at the end of the arm and was invisible to mice. A white ABS pipe 2.5 cm wide and plastic flag were used for visible trials. The location of the extramazal cues and platform were kept in the same place in space throughout the testing period. Mice were tested between 9:00 A.M. and 3:00 P.M. and started from a different pseudo-randomly chosen arm for each of the 15 daily trials. On the first trial of day one, mice were to locate the platform with the aid of a flag attached to the platform, making this trial visible. On trial 2, the flag was removed, forcing the mice to use extramazal cues (located throughout the room) to find the escape platform. The proceeding trials alternated from visible to hidden until 12 trials were completed, followed by three hidden trials to end day one. On day two, mice received 15 trials, which were all performed with the hidden platform. If mice failed to find the platform within 60 s, they were gently guided to the platform location and allowed to stay on it for 10 s. At the end of each trial, mice were placed in a warm holding cage for 25 s before starting the next trial. A video camera recorded each mouse, and the experimenter, which was blind to the genotype and treatment scored the entries into arms. The dependent variables for learning were incorrect arm entries and re-entries in day one versus two, with a decrease number of errors in day 2 versus day 1 interpreted as learning. The dependent measures for day 2 were incorrect arm entries (reference memory errors), reentries (working memory errors) and chaining events (3 consecutive arm entries into adjacent arms).

Protein extraction

Human and mouse proteins were prepared as previously described [10]. Briefly, mice were sacrificed and their brains were removed and cut in half along the medial longitudinal/sagittal fissure. One hemisphere of the brain was post-fixed in 4 % paraformaldehyde for 48 h and used for immunohistochemical evaluation. The other hemisphere was flash-frozen on dry ice and used for biochemical experiments and stored at −80 °C. The frozen mouse hemispheres as well as 0.1 g of human inferior frontal gyrus tissue were mechanically homogenized in ice-cold T-PER protein extraction buffer (Thermo Fisher Scientific) containing complete protease inhibitor (Roche) and phosphatase inhibitor (Life Technologies). Brain homogenates were ultracentrifuged at 100,000 × g for 1 h at 4 °C. The supernatant was recovered and stored at −80 °C until used for western blots and for both pPRAS40 and soluble Aβ levels by ELISA. The pellet was re-suspended in 70 % formic acid, mechanically homogenized, and centrifuged as described above. The supernatant of this second centrifugation was recovered and stored at −80 °C until used as the insoluble fraction for ELISA experiments.

Western blot

Western blots were performed under reducing conditions using precast Novex gels (Life Technologies). Proteins were transferred to nitrocellulose membranes (iBlot2, Life Technologies) followed by incubation for 60 min in 5 % nonfat powdered milk (Great Value) in Tris-buffered saline with Tween (TBST: 0.1 M Tris, 0.15 M NaCl, and 0.1 % Tween 20). Primary antibodies specific to the experiment were then applied overnight at 4 °C in 5 % milk in TBST. The following day, blots were washed in TBST three times for 15 min and then incubated in the appropriate fluorescent secondary antibody for 1 h at room temperature. The blots were then washed as describe above, and imaged/quantified using a LICOR Odyssey CLx (LI-COR Biosciences) attached to a Dell computer (OptiPlex 7010) running Windows 7 and Image Studio (version 1.0.11, LI-COR Biosciences). Quantitative analyses of the western blots were obtained by normalizing the intensity of the protein of interest with its loading control, β-actin.

Histology

For immunohistochemistry analysis, hemispheres were fixed in 4 % paraformaldehyde for 48 h. Tissue was then sectioned (50 μm thick) using a sliding vibratome, and stored in 0.02 % sodium azide in PBS. The endogenous peroxidase activity was quenched with 3 % H_2O_2 in 10 % methanol for 30 min. For $A\beta_{42}$ staining, tissue was incubated for 7 min in 95 % formic acid to retrieve the epitope. Then, tissue was incubated overnight at 4 °C with an appropriate primary antibody. Sections were washed to remove excess primary antibody and incubated in the appropriate secondary antibody for 1 h at room temperature. Excess secondary antibody was washed and sections were developed with diaminobenzidine substrate using the avidin– biotin horseradish peroxidase system (Vector Labs).

ELISA

The commercially available sandwich ELISA assay by Cell Signaling Technology was used to assess pPRAS40 levels. Fractions of brain homogenates were processed and read in a plate reader (Bio Tek) at 450 nm in pre-coated, flat-bottom 96-well plates according to the kit's instructions. The concentration of pPRAS40 (picograms per milliliter of sample) present in the homogenate was the dependent variable used for statistical analysis. We used the Life Technologies ELISA kit to assess $A\beta_{40}$ and $A\beta_{42}$ levels. Briefly, soluble or insoluble fractions of brain tissue homogenates were processed and read in a plate reader (BioTek) at 450 nm in precoated, flat-bottom 96-well plates according to the kit's instructions. The range of Aβ detection was between 10 and 1000 pg/ml. For each assay kit, cross-reactivity with other species of Aβ, APP, or tau was negligible when concentrations were <10 ng/ml. The concentration of Aβ (picograms per milliliter of sample) present in the homogenate was the dependent variable used for statistical analysis.

Proteasome activity

Proteasome activity was assessed as previously described [10]. Briefly, 10 μl of brain homogenate were incubated with proteasomal substrates Suc-LLVY-AMC, Bz-VGR-AMC, and Z-LLE-AMC (Enzo Life Sciences), which probe for chymotrypsin-like, trypsin-like, and caspase-like activities, respectively. Reactions were performed in 200 μl of assay buffer (25 mM HEPES, pH 7.5, 0.5 mM EDTA, 0.05 % NP-40) using black 96-well plates. Substrates were added immediately before readings. Kinetic readings were taken at 37 °C every 1.5 min for 60 min (excitation, 360 nm; emission, 460 nm) using the Synergy HT multimode microplate reader with Gen5 software (BioTek). Readings were normalized to total protein concentrations assayed via a Coomassie Protein Assay Kit (Bradford, Thermo Scientific) following the manufacturer's instructions.

Antibodies

The following antibodies were purchased from Cell Signaling Technology: pP70S6K1 Thr389 (dilution 1:1000, catalog #9204), p4EB-P1 Ser65 (dilution 1:1000, catalog #9451) β-actin (dilution 1:10000, catalog #3700), Atg3 (dilution 1:1000, catalog #3415), Atg5 (dilution 1:1000, catalog #2630), Atg12 (dilution 1:1000, catalog #2010). The following antibodies were purchased from Millipore: anti-$A\beta_{42}$ (dilution 1:200, catalog #AB5078P). Thermo Fisher Scientific provided HT7 (dilution 1:3000, catalog #MN1000). CP13 (dilution 1:1000) was a gift from Peter Davies.

Statistical analyses

Examination of the data evaluated via mixed (repeated measures) model ANOVAs revealed no violations of any assumptions that would warrant using a statistical test other than the ones described. Assumptions were tested via conventional methods using SPSS 18 (IBM). These included normality (Shapiro–Wilk, p's 0.10), homogeneity of variance (Levene's test, p's 0.05), and sphericity (Mauchly's test, p's 0.26). Learning data which included incorrect (reference) errors and working memory errors were analyzed by a two-way mixed ANOVA, followed by Bonferroni's corrected post hoc tests using Statview for Windows Version 5.0.1. Chaining data were analyzed using a 2x2 contingency Chi-square table. Proteasome activity was analyzed by an omnibus two-way ANOVA. A two-tailed unpaired *t* test was used to analyze select pairwise comparisons (e.g., Western blots in human cases and histology, ELISA for soluble and insoluble Aβ in 3xTg-AD mice), as specified in the results section. These analyses were performed using Stat view for Windows Version 5.0.1. A priori power analysis was not performed but our sample sizes are similar to those reported in previously published papers (Ma et al., 2013; Caccamo et al., 2014; Caccamo et al., 2015). Where representative images are shown, statistical analyses were performed on the entire sample as indicated in each figure legend.

Abbreviations

AD, Alzheimer's disease; Aβ, amyloid beta; APP, amyloid precursor protein; BACE-1, beta-site APP-cleaving enzyme-1; ELISA, enzyme-linked immunosorbent assay; IRS-1, insulin-like growth factor 1; mTOR, mammalian target of rapamycin; mTORC1, mTOR complex 1; NFT, neurofibrillary tangles; PBS, phosphate buffer saline; p, phosphorylation; PRAS40, proline-rick Akt substrate 40 kDa; Pim1, proto-oncogene serine/threonine-protein kinase Pim-1; RAWM, radial arm water maze; AKT, serine/threonine-specific protein kinase; TBST, tris-buffered saline with tween

Acknowledgements

We thank Dr. Joshua Talboom with his help collecting the human data and Mr. Mario Moreno for his help imaging the tau histology slices. This work was supported by grants to S.O. from the National Institute on Aging (R01 AG037637) and the Alzheimer's Drug Discovery Foundation.

Authors contributions

RV carried out the dosing of the mice, the biochemical and histological experiments, analyzed the data and wrote the manuscript. DMS performed the behavioral experiments and contributed to drafting and revising/reviewing the manuscript. AC participated in the design of the study, performed the proteasome and ELISA experiments, and contributed to drafting and revising/reviewing of the manuscript. SO designed the study, analyzed the data and wrote the manuscript.

All authors have read and approved the final version of the manuscript.

Competing interests

The authors have no competing interests in the manuscript.

References

1. LaFerla FM, Oddo S. Alzheimer's disease: Abeta, tau and synaptic dysfunction. Trends Mol Med. 2005;11:170–6.
2. Querfurth HW, LaFerla FM. Alzheimer's disease. N Engl J Med. 2010;362:329–44.
3. Alzheimer's A. Alzheimer's disease facts and figures. Alzheimers Dement. 2015;2015(11):332–84.
4. Moll L, El-Ami T, Cohen E. Selective manipulation of aging: a novel strategy for the treatment of neurodegenerative disorders. Swiss Med Wkly. 2014; 144:w13917.
5. Talboom JS, Velazquez R, Oddo S. The mammalian target of rapamycin at the crossroad between cognitive aging and Alzheimer's disease. NPJ Aging Mech Dis. 2015;1:15008.
6. Johnson SC, Rabinovitch PS, Kaeberlein M. mTOR is a key modulator of ageing and age-related disease. Nature. 2013;493:338–45.
7. Richardson A, Galvan V, Lin AL, Oddo S. How longevity research can lead to therapies for Alzheimer's disease: The rapamycin story. Exp Gerontol. 2015; 68:51–8.
8. Wullschleger S, Loewith R, Hall MN. TOR signaling in growth and metabolism. Cell. 2006;124:471–84.
9. Ma Y, Wu D, Zhang W, Liu J, Chen S, Hua B. Investigation of PI3K/PKB/mTOR/S6K1 signaling pathway in relationship of type 2 diabetes and Alzheimer's disease. Int J Clin Exp Med. 2015;8:18581–90.
10. Caccamo A, Branca C, Talboom JS, Shaw DM, Turner D, Ma L, Messina A, Huang Z, Wu J, Oddo S. Reducing ribosomal protein S6 kinase 1 expression improves spatial memory and synaptic plasticity in a mouse model of Alzheimer's disease. J Neurosci. 2015;35:14042–56.
11. An WL, Cowburn RF, Li L, Braak H, Alafuzoff I, Iqbal K, Iqbal IG, Winblad B, Pei JJ. Up-regulation of phosphorylated/activated p70 S6 kinase and its relationship to neurofibrillary pathology in Alzheimer's disease. Am J Pathol. 2003;163:591–607.
12. Pei JJ, Bjorkdahl C, Zhang H, Zhou X, Winblad B. p70 S6 kinase and tau in Alzheimer's disease. J Alzheimers Dis. 2008;14:385–92.
13. Chang RC, Wong AK, Ng HK, Hugon J. Phosphorylation of eukaryotic initiation factor-2alpha (eIF2alpha) is associated with neuronal degeneration in Alzheimer's disease. Neuroreport. 2002;13:2429–32.
14. Caccamo A, De Pinto V, Messina A, Branca C, Oddo S. Genetic reduction of mammalian target of rapamycin ameliorates Alzheimer's disease-like cognitive and pathological deficits by restoring hippocampal gene expression signature. J Neurosci. 2014;34:7988–98.
15. Caccamo A, Majumder S, Richardson A, Strong R, Oddo S. Molecular interplay between mammalian target of rapamycin (mTOR), amyloid-beta, and Tau: effects on cognitive impairments. J Biol Chem. 2010;285:13107–20.
16. Majumder S, Richardson A, Strong R, Oddo S. Inducing autophagy by rapamycin before, but not after, the formation of plaques and tangles ameliorates cognitive deficits. PLoS One. 2011;6:e25416.
17. Spilman P, Podlutskaya N, Hart MJ, Debnath J, Gorostiza O, Bredesen D, Richardson A, Strong R, Galvan V. Inhibition of mTOR by rapamycin abolishes cognitive deficits and reduces amyloid-beta levels in a mouse model of Alzheimer's disease. PLoS One. 2010;5:e9979.
18. Boers-Doets CB, Epstein JB, Raber-Durlacher JE, Ouwerkerk J, Logan RM, Brakenhoff JA, Lacouture ME, Gelderblom H. Oral adverse events associated with tyrosine kinase and mammalian target of rapamycin inhibitors in renal cell carcinoma: a structured literature review. Oncologist. 2012;17:135–44.
19. Hille U, Soergel P, Makowski L, Dork-Bousset T, Hillemanns P. Lymphedema of the breast as a symptom of internal diseases or side effect of mTor inhibitors. Lymphat Res Biol. 2012;10:63–73.
20. Ersoy A, Koca N. Everolimus-induced lymphedema in a renal transplant recipient: a case report. Exp Clin Transplant. 2012;10:296–8.
21. Sancak Y, Thoreen CC, Peterson TR, Lindquist RA, Kang SA, Spooner E, Carr SA, Sabatini DM. PRAS40 is an insulin-regulated inhibitor of the mTORC1 protein kinase. Mol Cell. 2007;25:903–15.
22. Wang L, Harris TE, Roth RA, Lawrence Jr JC. PRAS40 regulates mTORC1 kinase activity by functioning as a direct inhibitor of substrate binding. J Biol Chem. 2007;282:20036–44.
23. Caccamo A, Maldonado MA, Majumder S, Medina DX, Holbein W, Magri A, Oddo S. Naturally secreted amyloid-beta increases mammalian target of rapamycin (mTOR) activity via a PRAS40-mediated mechanism. J Biol Chem. 2011;286:8924–32.
24. Cuypers HT, Selten G, Quint W, Zijlstra M, Maandag ER, Boelens W, van Wezenbeek P, Melief C, Berns A. Murine leukemia virus-induced T-cell lymphomagenesis: integration of proviruses in a distinct chromosomal region. Cell. 1984;37:141–50.
25. Hoover D, Friedmann M, Reeves R, Magnuson NS. Recombinant human pim-1 protein exhibits serine/threonine kinase activity. J Biol Chem. 1991;266:14018–23.
26. Saris CJ, Domen J, Berns A. The pim-1 oncogene encodes two related protein-serine/threonine kinases by alternative initiation at AUG and CUG. EMBO J. 1991;10:655–64.
27. van der Lugt NM, Domen J, Verhoeven E, Linders K, van der Gulden H, Allen J, Berns A. Proviral tagging in E mu-myc transgenic mice lacking the Pim-1 proto-oncogene leads to compensatory activation of Pim-2. EMBO J. 1995; 14:2536–44.
28. Amson R, Sigaux F, Przedborski S, Flandrin G, Givol D, Telerman A. The human protooncogene product p33pim is expressed during fetal hematopoiesis and in diverse leukemias. Proc Natl Acad Sci U S A. 1989;86:8857–61.
29. van Lohuizen M, Verbeek S, Krimpenfort P, Domen J, Saris C, Radaszkiewicz T, Berns A. Predisposition to lymphomagenesis in pim-1 transgenic mice: cooperation with c-myc and N-myc in murine leukemia virus-induced tumors. Cell. 1989;56:673–82.
30. Laird PW, van der Lugt NM, Clarke A, Domen J, Linders K, McWhir J, Berns A, Hooper M. In vivo analysis of Pim-1 deficiency. Nucleic Acids Res. 1993;21:4750–5.
31. Jacobs MD, Black J, Futer O, Swenson L, Hare B, Fleming M, Saxena K. Pim-1 ligand-bound structures reveal the mechanism of serine/threonine kinase inhibition by LY294002. J Biol Chem. 2005;280:13728–34.
32. Kumar JK, Ping RY, Teong HF, Goh S, Clement MV. Activation of a non-genomic Pim-1/Bad-Pser75 module is required for an efficient pro-survival effect of Bcl-xL induced by androgen in LNCaP cells. Int J Biochem Cell Biol. 2011;43:594–603.
33. Zhang F, Beharry ZM, Harris TE, Lilly MB, Smith CD, Mahajan S, Kraft AS. PIM1 protein kinase regulates PRAS40 phosphorylation and mTOR activity in FDCP1 cells. Cancer Biol Ther. 2009;8:846–53.
34. Oddo S, Caccamo A, Shepherd JD, Murphy MP, Golde TE, Kayed R, Metherate R, Mattson MP, Akbari Y, LaFerla FM. Triple-transgenic model of Alzheimer's disease with plaques and tangles: intracellular Abeta and synaptic dysfunction. Neuron. 2003;39:409–21.
35. Lovasic L, Bauschke H, Janus C. Working memory impairment in a transgenic amyloid precursor protein TgCRND8 mouse model of Alzheimer's disease. Genes Brain Behav. 2005;4:197–208.
36. Vilchez D, Saez I, Dillin A. The role of protein clearance mechanisms in organismal ageing and age-related diseases. Nat Commun. 2014;5:5659.
37. Mizushima N. Methods for monitoring autophagy. Int J Biochem Cell Biol. 2004;36:2491–502.
38. Craiu A, Gaczynska M, Akopian T, Gramm CF, Fenteany G, Goldberg AL, Rock KL. Lactacystin and clasto-lactacystin beta-lactone modify multiple proteasome beta-subunits and inhibit intracellular protein degradation and major histocompatibility complex class I antigen presentation. J Biol Chem. 1997;272:13437–45.
39. Heinemeyer W, Fischer M, Krimmer T, Stachon U, Wolf DH. The active sites of the eukaryotic 20 S proteasome and their involvement in subunit precursor processing. J Biol Chem. 1997;272:25200–9.

40. Layfield R, Cavey JR, Lowe J. Role of ubiquitin-mediated proteolysis in the pathogenesis of neurodegenerative disorders. Ageing Res Rev. 2003;2:343–56.
41. Wiza C, Chadt A, Blumensatt M, Kanzleiter T, Herzfeld De Wiza D, Horrighs A, Mueller H, Nascimento EB, Schurmann A, Al-Hasani H, Ouwens DM. Over-expression of PRAS40 enhances insulin sensitivity in skeletal muscle. Arch Physiol Biochem. 2014;120:64–72.
42. Wiza C, De Wiza Herzfeld D, Nascimento EB, Lehr S, Al-Hasani H, Ouwens DM. Knockdown of PRAS40 inhibits insulin action via proteasome-mediated degradation of IRS1 in primary human skeletal muscle cells. Diabetologia. 2013;56:1118–28.
43. Keller JN, Hanni KB, Markesbery WR. Impaired proteasome function in Alzheimer's disease. J Neurochem. 2000;75:436–9.
44. Oddo S. The ubiquitin-proteasome system in Alzheimer's disease. J Cell Mol Med. 2008;12:363–73.
45. Tseng BP, Green KN, Chan JL, Blurton-Jones M, LaFerla FM. Abeta inhibits the proteasome and enhances amyloid and tau accumulation. Neurobiol Aging. 2008;29:1607–18.
46. Hong L, Huang HC, Jiang ZF. Relationship between amyloid-beta and the ubiquitin-proteasome system in Alzheimer's disease. Neurol Res. 2014;36: 276–82.
47. Medina DX, Caccamo A, Oddo S. Methylene blue reduces abeta levels and rescues early cognitive deficit by increasing proteasome activity. Brain Pathol. 2011;21:140–9.
48. Leibson CL, Rocca WA, Hanson VA, Cha R, Kokmen E, O'Brien PC, Palumbo PJ. The risk of dementia among persons with diabetes mellitus: a population-based cohort study. Ann N Y Acad Sci. 1997;826:422–7.
49. Ott A, Stolk RP, van Harskamp F, Pols HA, Hofman A, Breteler MM. Diabetes mellitus and the risk of dementia: the Rotterdam study. Neurology. 1999;53:1937–42.
50. Qiu CX, Winblad B, Fratiglioni L. Risk factors for dementia and Alzheimer' s disease-findings from a community-based cohort study in Stockholm, Sweden. Zhonghua Liu Xing Bing Xue Za Zhi. 2005;26:882–7.
51. Wang YF, Khan M, van den Berg HA. Interaction of fast and slow dynamics in endocrine control systems with an application to beta-cell dynamics. Math Biosci. 2012;235:8–18.
52. Wang H, Zhang Q, Wen Q, Zheng Y, Lazarovici P, Jiang H, Lin J, Zheng W. Proline-rich Akt substrate of 40 kDa (PRAS40): a novel downstream target of PI3k/Akt signaling pathway. Cell Signal. 2012;24:17–24.
53. Vander Haar E, Lee SI, Bandhakavi S, Griffin TJ, Kim DH. Insulin signalling to mTOR mediated by the Akt/PKB substrate PRAS40. Nat Cell Biol. 2007;9:316–23.
54. Nascimento EB, Fodor M, van der Zon GC, Jazet IM, Meinders AE, Voshol PJ, Vlasblom R, Baan B, Eckel J, Maassen JA, et al. Insulin-mediated phosphorylation of the proline-rich Akt substrate PRAS40 is impaired in insulin target tissues of high-fat diet-fed rats. Diabetes. 2006;55:3221–8.
55. Dey N, Ghosh-Choudhury N, Das F, Li X, Venkatesan B, Barnes JL, Kasinath BS, Ghosh Choudhury G. PRAS40 acts as a nodal regulator of high glucose-induced TORC1 activation in glomerular mesangial cell hypertrophy. J Cell Physiol. 2010;225:27–41.
56. Yates SC, Zafar A, Hubbard P, Nagy S, Durant S, Bicknell R, Wilcock G, Christie S, Esiri MM, Smith AD, Nagy Z. Dysfunction of the mTOR pathway is a risk factor for Alzheimer's disease. Acta Neuropathol Commun. 2013;1:3.
57. Beach TG, Sue LI, Walker DG, Roher AE, Lue L, Vedders L, Connor DJ, Sabbagh MN, Rogers J. The Sun Health Research Institute Brain Donation Program: description and experience, 1987–2007. Cell Tissue Bank. 2008; 9:229–45.
58. Alamed J, Wilcock DM, Diamond DM, Gordon MN, Morgan D. Two-day radial-arm water maze learning and memory task; robust resolution of amyloid-related memory deficits in transgenic mice. Nat Protoc. 2006;1: 1671–9.
59. Penley SC, Gaudet CM, Threlkeld SW. Use of an eight-arm radial water maze to assess working and reference memory following neonatal brain injury. Journal of visualized experiments: JoVE. 2013:50940.

10

Functional alterations of myeloid cells during the course of Alzheimer's disease

Aaron D. Thome, Alireza Faridar, David R. Beers, Jason R. Thonhoff, Weihua Zhao, Shixiang Wen, Belen Pascual, Joseph C. Masdeu and Stanley H. Appel*

Abstract

Background: Neuroinflammation is a hallmark of neurodegenerative disease and a significant component of the pathology of Alzheimer's disease (AD). Patients present with extensive microgliosis along with elevated pro-inflammatory signaling in the central nervous system and periphery. However, the role of peripheral myeloid cells in mediating and influencing AD pathogenesis remains unresolved.

Methods: Peripheral myeloid cells were isolated from peripheral blood of patients with prodromal AD ($n = 44$), mild AD dementia ($n = 25$), moderate/severe AD dementia ($n = 28$), and age-matched controls ($n = 54$). Patients were evaluated in the clinic for AD severity and categorized using Clinical Dementia Rating (CDR) scale resulting in separation of patients into prodromal AD (CDR0.5) and advancing forms of AD dementia (mild-CDR1 and moderate/severe-CDR2/3). Separation of peripheral myeloid cells into mature monocytes or immature MDSCs permitted the delineation of population changes from flow cytometric analysis, RNA phenotype analysis, and functional studies using T cell suppression assays and monocyte suppression assays.

Results: During stages of AD dementia (CDR1 and 2/3) peripheral myeloid cells increase their pro-inflammatory gene expression while at early stages of disease (prodromal AD—CDR0.5) pro-inflammatory gene expression is decreased. MDSCs are increased in prodromal AD compared with controls (16.81% vs 9.53%) and have markedly increased suppressive functions: 42.4% suppression of activated monocyte-produced IL-6 and 78.16% suppression of T cell proliferation. In AD dementia, MDSC populations are reduced with decreased suppression of monocyte IL-6 (5.22%) and T cell proliferation (37.61%); the reduced suppression coincides with increased pro-inflammatory signaling in AD dementia monocytes.

Conclusions: Peripheral monocyte gene expression is pro-inflammatory throughout the course of AD, except at the earliest, prodromal stages when pro-inflammatory gene expression is suppressed. This monocyte biphasic response is associated with increased numbers and suppressive functions of MDSCs during the early stages and decreased numbers and suppressive functions in later stages of disease. Prolonging the early protective suppression and reversing the later loss of suppressive activity may offer a novel therapeutic strategy.

Keywords: Alzheimer's disease, Inflammation, Myeloid cells, Monocyte, Microglia, Myeloid-derived suppressor cells

* Correspondence: sappel@houstonmethodist.org
Department of Neurology, Houston Methodist Neurological Institute, 6560 Fannin St. Suite 802, Houston, TX 77030, USA

Background

Alzheimer's disease (AD) is the most common neurodegenerative disease and is characterized by cognitive impairment, amyloid-β (Aβ) deposition, and neurofibrillary tangle formation [1–5]. Increasing evidence suggests that immune mechanisms contribute to the pathogenesis of AD including reactive microgliosis in postmortem samples, increased microglial activation marker, translocator protein (TSPO), binding on positron emission tomography (PET), [6] and increased pro-inflammatory cytokines such as interleukin (IL)-6, IL-1β, TNF, and IFN-γ in the cerebrospinal fluid and serum [7–11]. Thus, neuroinflammation is potentially a target for immunomodulatory therapies [12, 13].

Genome-wide association studies implicate immune system dysfunction, particularly in myeloid-derived cells, as immune-related genes coding for triggering receptor expressed on myeloid cells 2 (TREM2) and CD33 confer increased risk for AD susceptibility [14–18]. Current studies focus on microglia, resident myeloid cells of the brain, throughout AD pathogenesis, but recent literature in neurodegenerative diseases suggest extensive neuro-immune cross-talk between the brain and peripheral immune system [19–22]. This cross-talk may derive either directly or indirectly from peripheral immune cells in the presence of a compromised blood brain barrier (BBB) such as in neurodegenerative disease [23–25]. Additionally during inflammatory insult and microglial depletion, peripheral macrophage engraftment into the CNS was observed with these cells retaining a distinct and lasting transcriptional and functional identity [26]. Thus peripheral immune myeloid cells could modulate disease progression and outcomes in the CNS. The accessibility of these peripheral myeloid cells, and the lack of accessibility to CNS microglia, prompted a detailed examination of blood monocyte populations during the pathoprogression of AD.

Immature and mature monocytes, here-after denoted as "peripheral myeloid cells," originate from hematopoietic stem cells and mature into peripheral monocytes with the capability of differentiating into macrophages once they enter tissue parenchyma [27–31]. Changes and shifts in peripheral myeloid populations are indicators of disease onset and progression for a multitude of diseases; the pro-inflammatory phenotypes have direct effects on their specific disease [32–40]. A detailed analysis of peripheral monocyte population and phenotype changes have not been documented thoroughly in AD progression.

Myeloid-derived suppressor cells (MDSCs) are immature myeloid cells that exhibit robust suppressive function on T cell proliferation and mature myeloid cell function which has made them a target of multiple immunomodulatory therapies [41–44]. Chronic AD immune signaling provides a practical mechanism where MDSC activation and recruitment potentially promotes an immunosuppressive environment [45]. However, the actual role of MDSCs in AD pathology and progression remains unexplored. A detailed investigation into the role and function of mature and immature peripheral myeloid cells could provide insight into mechanisms of their direct involvement in AD pathogenesis as well as provide clues as to the changes in CNS myeloid cells through disease progression.

In this study, we investigated peripheral myeloid populations and their pro-inflammatory gene expression throughout the course of AD compared with age-matched controls. We also investigated changes in a novel and previously unrecognized cell type in AD, MDSCs, to determine their phenotypes during course of disease. Understanding the role of peripheral myeloid cells in AD-related inflammation and mechanisms of their immune suppression may lead to novel therapeutic interventions for the successful treatment of AD.

Methods

Patient recruitment and AD-defined population

AD patients and aged-matched healthy controls were recruited into the study from the Houston Methodist Nantz National Alzheimer's Center (NNAC) based on National Institute on Aging-Alzheimer's Association (NIA-AA) diagnostic criteria [46, 47]. The study was approved by the Houston Methodist IRB and all participants signed informed consent. Clinical evaluations for prodromal AD (CDR0.5) (n = 44), mild AD dementia (CDR1) (n = 25), moderate/severe AD dementia (CDR2/3) (n = 28), and age-matched, healthy controls (n = 54) were made under the direction of Dr. Joseph Masdeu and colleagues at the NNAC. Staging of dementia severity was based on the Clinical Dementia Rating (CDR) Scale (Table 1).

Immune cell isolation

Immune cells were isolated from peripheral blood of participants using Lymphoprep density gradient (STEMCELL) followed by Human Pan Monocyte Isolation Kit (Miltenyi Biotec) for negative selection of human monocytes. Further isolation using anti-HLA-DR microbeads (Miltenyi Biotec) allowed for the separation of HLA-DR+, mature monocytes, and HLA-DR-, immature MDSCs (Additional file 1: Table S1). T responder cells were isolated from the PBMC pool using CD4 + CD25+

Table 1 Patient demographics

Diagnosis	CDR	Number	M,F	Age, yr. ± SD
Control	CDR 0	54	30, 24	69.81 ± 6.52
Prodromal AD	CDR0.5	44	21, 23	73.57 ± 6.57
Mild AD Dementia	CDR1	25	10, 15	74.48 ± 7.98
Moderate/Severe AD Dementia	CDR2/3	28	9, 19	71.29 ± 8.52

regulatory T Cell Isolation Kit (Miltenyi Biotec) to obtain CD4 + CD25- cells.

Flow cytometry

Fluorescent immune cell probes for the delineation of monocyte subsets included anti-human CD14-V450, anti-human CD16-FITC, anti-human HLA-DR-PerCP-Cy5.5, anti-human CD33-APC, anti-human CD11b-PE, and IgG isotype controls (ebioscience or BD Biosciences). Cells were counted using an LSRII flow cytometer with the data was analyzed with BD FACSDIVA software. The submitted flow cytometry gating paradigm (Additional file 2: Figure S2) depicts cell populations for analysis of mature monocyte populations and the immature MDSC population.

RNA purification, RT-PCR analysis, and Nanostring

RNA was extracted from immune cell populations and in vitro cell experiments using Trizol reagent followed by Direct-zol RNA MiniPrep Kit (Zymo Research). Quantitative RT-PCR (qRT-PCR) experiments were performed using a One-Step RT-PCR kit with SYBR Green and run using Bio-Rad iQ5 Multicolor Real-Time PCR Detection Systems. Primers for the study were purchased from BioRad and the relative expression level of each mRNA was calculated using the ΔΔCt method with normalization to β-actin and relative to control samples. RNA sample QC and Nanostring experiments were performed using Baylor College of Medicine Genomic and RNA Profiling Core. Monocyte RNA was run on the nCounter Human Inflammation Panel (Nanostring, Human v2). The panel consisted of 255 human inflammation-related genes with 15 internal reference genes. Analysis of data QC, normalization, and differential gene expression was performed using nSolver analysis software provided by the company. Normalized data counts generated from Nanostring experiment provided in Additional file 3: Figure S9.

T cell suppression assays

Responder T cells and MDSCs were isolated using Miltenyi Biotec microbeads as previously described. CD4+ T responder cells were placed in a 96 well plate at a density of 50 k cells per well followed by co-culture of MDSCs at a ratio of 1:1, 1:1/2, and 1:1/4 (T cell: MDSC). CD3/CD28 T cell stimulation reagent is then added to the co-culture for five days followed by addition of tritium (Miltenyi). Proliferation measured via tritium incorporation.

Myeloid cell suppression assays

Our lab has recapitulated protocols for the generation of mature monocyte cells from induced pluripotent stem cells (iPS cells). Yanagimachi et al. describes a detailed protocol and discussion of the process [48]. Isolation and polarization of CD14 cells into pro-inflammatory "M1" cells can be found in the culturing paradigm (Additional file 4: Figure S4). Briefly, iPSC-derived macrophages are grown from a control line and polarized to be pro-inflammatory. We then use MDSCs isolated from patients to co-culture with the pro-inflammatory iPSC-derived macrophages overnight (18 h) to look at suppressive function of the MDSCs on myeloid cells. We collected RNA from co-cultured pro-inflammatory macrophages for transcript analysis and cultured media for ELISA protein changes (Invitrogen).

Results

Peripheral myeloid cells have increased pro-inflammatory gene expression in AD dementia but significantly decreased expression in prodromal AD

RNA isolated from the blood-derived peripheral myeloid cells were analyzed using Nanostring chip and qRT-PCR to determine their inflammatory profiles. We detected increased pro-inflammatory RNA in AD dementia patients (CDR1, 2, 3) with increased expression of IL-6, IL-1β, NLRP3, TNF, IL-18, and HLA-DRA, among others. (Fig. 1a). There was little to no increase in inflammation-associated RNA signatures between controls and prodromal AD (CDR0.5) patient cells (Fig. 1b). In fact, there were decreased RNA levels of C-reactive protein (CRP), CXCR4, CCL11, and complement system components (C1s and C8a) in prodromal AD cells compared with controls. Follow-up analysis from additional patients using qRT-PCR corroborated the Nanostring data showing decreased expression of IL-6 and IL-1β in CDR0.5 peripheral myeloid cells but increased expression of these two cytokines in CDR1 and CDR2/3 peripheral myeloid cells (Fig. 1c). Additionally, anti-inflammatory IL-10 expression, as determined by qRT-PCR, was increased in CDR0.5 peripheral myeloid cells compared with controls but not in samples from CDR1 or CDR2/3 patients (Fig. 1c).

Surface level expression of HLA-DR, up-regulated during immune cell activation to promote pro-inflammatory signaling, was increased on mature monocytes from CDR1 and CDR2/3 compared with both controls and CDR0.5 (Fig. 1d). CD33 expression which is known to inhibit activation and cytokine release from myeloid cells was increased on cells from CDR0.5 patient monocytes but not on cells from controls and CDR1 and CDR2/3 patients (Fig. 1e). Gender and age of the controls and patients were not confounding variables in these experiments (Additional file 5: Figure S3 and Additional file 6: Figure S6).

Alterations in mature and immature monocyte populations through AD progression

We observed a progressive decline of the classical monocytes ($CD14^{+}CD16^{-}$) with increasing AD burden

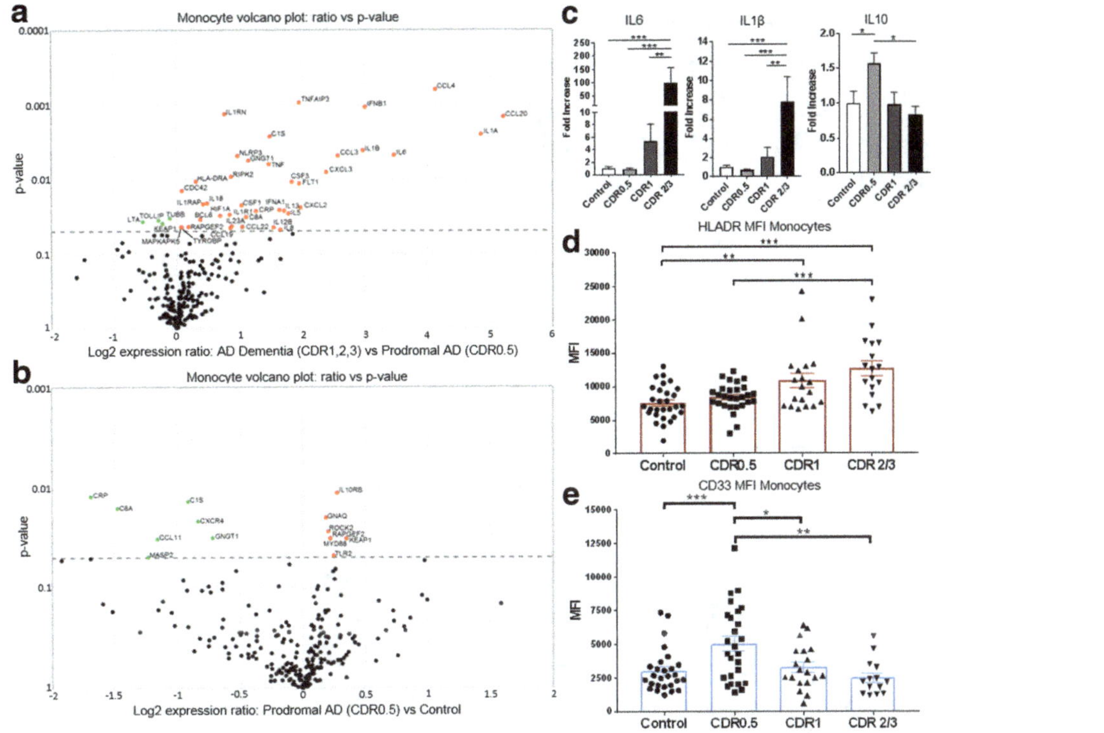

Fig. 1 Peripheral myeloid cells are pro-inflammatory in AD dementia but suppressed/anti-inflammatory in prodromal AD. Volcano plots showing log2 expression ratios vs *p*-values of nCounter human inflammation v2 panel for (**a**) AD dementia (CDR1,2,3) vs prodromal AD (CDR0.5) and (**b**) Prodromal AD (CDR0.5) vs Control (AD Dementia, $n = 10$; Prodromal AD, $n = 6$; C $n = 8$). Analysis and statistics run using nSolver 3.0 analysis software. (**c**) Upregulation of pro-inflammatory gene expression of IL-6 and IL-1β in peripheral myeloid cells in CDR1 and 2/3 while IL-10 is increased in CDR0.5 peripheral myeloid cells (C $n = 20$, CDR0.5 n = 20, CDR1 $n = 8$, CDR2/3 $n = 10$). Numbers shown as averages ± SEM and with one-way ANOVA with Tukey's post hoc test. **d** Flow cytometric median fluorescence intensity of pro-inflammatory HLADR is increased on the surface of CDR1 and CDR2/3 peripheral myeloid cells while (**e**) inhibitory motif, CD33, is increased on the surface of CDR0.5 peripheral myeloid cells and decreases with increasing AD burden. Numbers shown as averages ± SEM and with one-way ANOVA with Tukey's post hoc test (C $n = 30$, CDR0.5 $n = 27$, CDR1 $n = 17$, CDR2/3 $n = 13$). *P*-values are $^{*}p < 0.05$, $^{**}p < 0.01$, and $^{***}p < 0.001$

(Fig. 2a) leading to a redistribution of the populations to intermediate ($CD14^{+}CD16^{+}$) and non-classical populations ($CD14^{low}CD16^{+}$). Intermediate populations in CDR0.5, 1, and 2/3 were increased compared with controls (Fig. 2b). CDR1 and CDR2/3 non-classical populations were increased compared with controls (Fig. 2c). Using $CD14^{+}$, $HLA\text{-}DR^{-}$, $CD11b^{+}$, and $CD33^{+}$ as cell surface marker for MDSCs, there was an increased number of MDSCs in CDR0.5 (16.81%) and CDR1 (17.74%) patients compared with age-matched controls (9.53%). CDR2/3 MDSC levels (9.64%) were similar to control levels (Fig. 2d). Gender and age did not confound monocyte population changes (Additional file 7: Figure S5).

Pro-inflammatory responses of monocytes from AD dementia patients and anti-inflammatory responses of MDSCs from prodromal AD patients

Following separation of MDSCs from monocytes, RNA analysis demonstrated increases in pro-inflammatory signaling in monocytes from AD dementia patients. Specifically, there were increased mRNA expression of IL-6, IL-1β, and TNF in mature monocytes isolated from CDR1 and CDR2/3 patients when compared with controls (Fig. 3a). Additionally, there was a trend for a decrease in IL-6 transcript from CDR0.5 patient monocytes while the IL-1β and TNF were not different than controls. In evaluating anti-inflammatory signaling in MDSC populations, IL-10 and IL-13 transcripts were increased in CDR0.5 but then decreased as the disease progressed to CDR1 and CDR2/3 (Fig. 3b). Interestingly, anti-inflammatory TGF-β was increased in mature monocytes from CDR0.5 patients but not from the monocytes of later stages.

Pro-inflammatory myeloid cells and T cell proliferation are suppressed by prodromal AD MDSCs but not AD dementia MDSCs

We investigated the suppressive capacity of MDSCs on a pro-inflammatory macrophage population. We co-cultured patient-isolated MDSCs with pro-inflammatory iPSC-derived macrophages overnight to examine attenuation of pro-inflammatory IL-6 transcript and protein. MDSCs from CDR0.5 patients attenuated IL-6 transcript expression

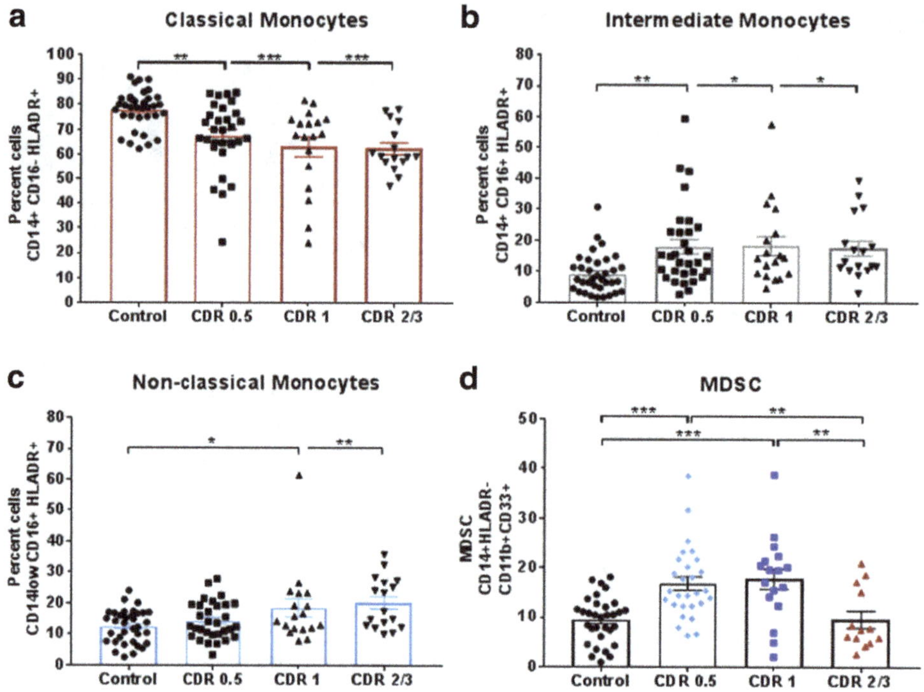

Fig. 2 Monocyte populations shift as AD burden increases. Monocyte population changes via flow cytometric analysis of CD14 and CD16 expression on HLADR+ myeloid immune cells. Decreases in (**a**) classical monocytes (CD14+ CD16-) with increasing disease burden with a redistribution of monocytes into (**b**) intermediate (CD14+ CD16+) and (**c**) non-classical populations (CD14low CD16+). Numbers shown as averages ± SEM and with one-way ANOVA with Tukey's post hoc analysis (Control $n = 35$, CDR0.5 $n = 31$, CDR1 $n = 18$, CDR2/3 $n = 17$). Increased MDSC populations (**d**) in CDR0.5 and CDR1 patients compared with controls as percent of total CD14 cell population. MDSC numbers fall to control levels in CDR2/3 patients (Control $n = 32$, CDR0.5 $n = 28$, CDR1 $n = 17$, CDR2/3 $n = 13$). Numbers shown as averages ± SEM and with one-way ANOVA with Tukey's post hoc test. *P*-values are $^{*}p < 0.05$, $^{**}p < 0.01$, and $^{***}p < 0.001$

(42.4%) compared with control MDSCs (22.09%) (Fig. 4a). This attenuation of IL-6 expression decreased in CDR1 (17.33%) and CDR2/3 (5.22%) patients. In examination of the co-cultured media, we find decreased IL-6 protein when we co-culture pro-inflammatory macrophages (alone-18,208 pg/mL IL-6) with CDR0.5 MDSCs (6154 pg/mL). This suppressive effect decreases as patients advance to CDR1 (10,856 pg/mL) and later into CDR 2/3 (16,348 pg/mL). Control MDSCs in our experiment were able to reduce pro-inflammatory IL-6 output to 12,791 pg/mL while MDSCs alone did not produce IL-6 protein. Gender and age did not affect suppressive capacity of control or patient MDSCs (Additional file 8: Figure S7). Our RNA expression data from isolated mature monocytes and MDSCs displayed increased IL-10 transcript from CDR0.5 MDSCs. Adding an IL-10 neutralizing antibody (IL10ab) to the MDSC: M1 cultures at 5μg/mL significantly reduced suppression of IL-6 transcripts (Fig. 4c), suggesting that secretion of IL-10 contributes to the MDSC-mediated suppression.

The suppression profiles of MDSCs were next examined when co-cultured with $CD4^{+}$ Tresp. CDR0.5 and CDR1 MDSCs showed increased suppression of autologous Tresp proliferation compared with the suppression of control MDSCs. Similar to the decreased numbers of MDSCs, there was decreased MDSC suppressive function in CDR2/3 compared with all groups. At a 1:1 ratio (Tresp: MDSC), CDR0.5 and CDR1 yielded 79.03% and 61.81% suppression, respectively, compared with control 55.7% suppression while CDR2/3 MDSCs dropped to 37.61% (Fig. 4d, e). When examining the expression of arginase-1 (Arg1) as a mechanism to block T cell proliferation, Arg1 expression was increased in CDR0.5 MDSCs compared with controls and subsequently decreased in CDR1 and then in CDR2/3 patients (Fig. 4f). T cell suppression by MDSCs positively correlated with myeloid cell suppression; patients with early disease possess increased suppressive function while suppressive function is progressively impaired as disease advances (Additional file 9: Figure S8).

Discussion

The analyses of peripheral myeloid cells in AD patients provided three important findings. First, pro-inflammatory gene-expressing phenotypes of peripheral monocytes are increased in CDR1,2,3 patients. Second, pro-inflammatory gene-expressing phenotypes of peripheral monocytes are decreased in CDR0.5 patients. Third, MDSCs are increased

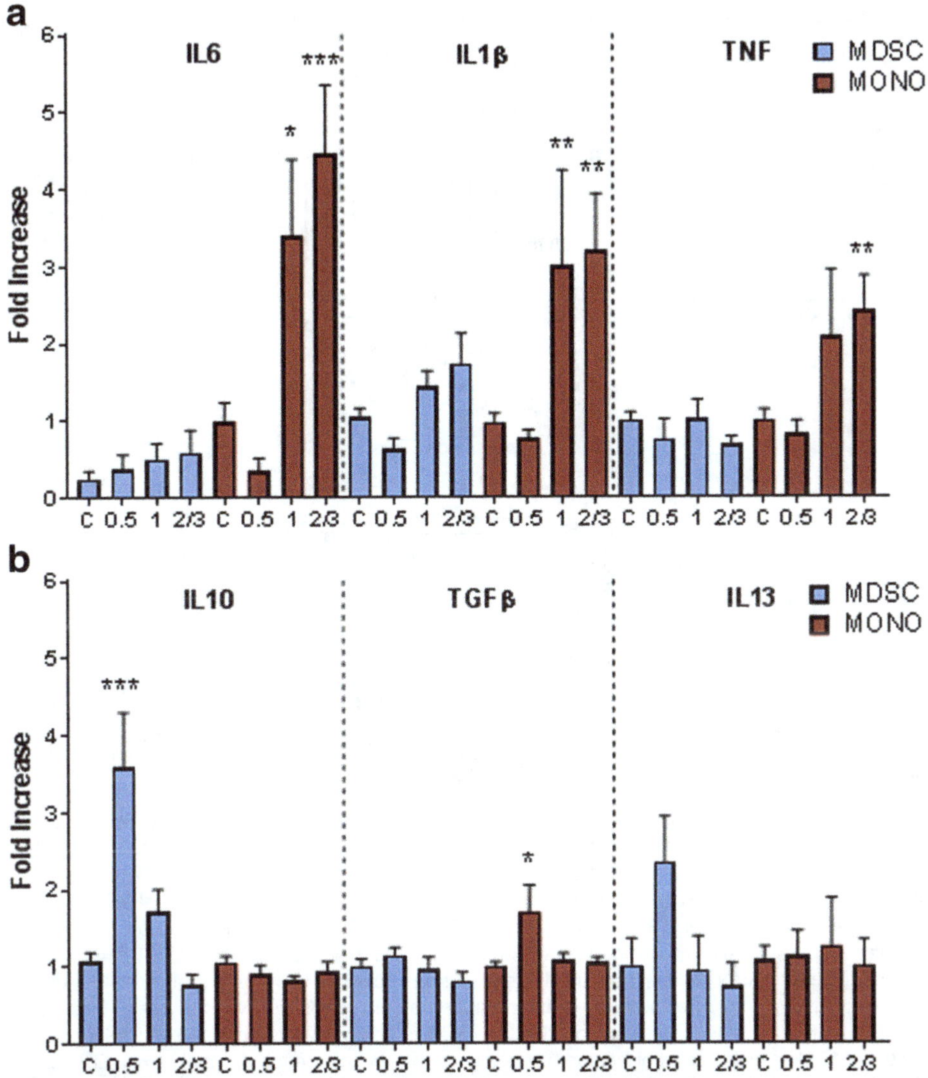

Fig. 3 Mature monocytes are pro-inflammatory in AD dementia while MDSCs are anti-inflammatory in prodromal AD. Isolated mature monocytes and MDSCs displayed differential inflammatory gene expression profiles. **a** Mature monocytes from CDR1 and CDR2/3 display increased pro-inflammatory cytokine expression via IL-6, IL-1β, and TNF. **b** MDSCs from CDR0.5 patients have increased anti-inflammatory IL-10 and IL-13 expression. TGFβ transcripts were increased in CDR0.5 monocytes. One-way ANOVA with Tukey's post hoc analysis (Control $n = 13–14$, CDR0.5 $n = 8$, CDR1 $n = 7$, CDR2/3 $n = 10$). P-values are $^{*}p < 0.05$, $^{**}p < 0.01$, and $^{***}p < 0.001$

in number and suppressive function in CDR0.5 and decreased in CDR2/3. MDSC from CDR0.5 suppressed Tresp proliferation and iPSC-derived pro-inflammatory myeloid cells in vitro more effectively than control MDSCs. MDSCs from CDR2/3 patients had significantly decreased suppressive function for both Tresp proliferation and pro-inflammatory myeloid cells.

Activation of myeloid cells has been extensively studied in humans and animal models of neurodegeneration, including AD, with much of the focus on brain microglia which are difficult to study directly during the course of disease. Peripheral myeloid cells have similar functions to brain microglia including chemotaxis, phagocytosis, and cytokine expression but constitute a cell population that can be collected and studied through simple, minimally-invasive methods [28, 49–51]. Activation of immune cells can be assessed using flow cytometry by analyzing HLA-DR, a MHC class II cell surface receptor that is upregulated upon antigen presenting cell activation. HLA-DR expression was increased on mature monocytes from CDR1 and CDR2/3 patients when compared with controls and CDR0.5 which matches the pro-inflammatory gene expression seen in these patients. CDR0.5 monocytes did not exhibit pro-inflammatory gene expression but displayed increased inhibitory CD33 cell surface expression compared with controls and this expression diminished in CDR1 patients while decreasing below control values in CDR2/3 patients.

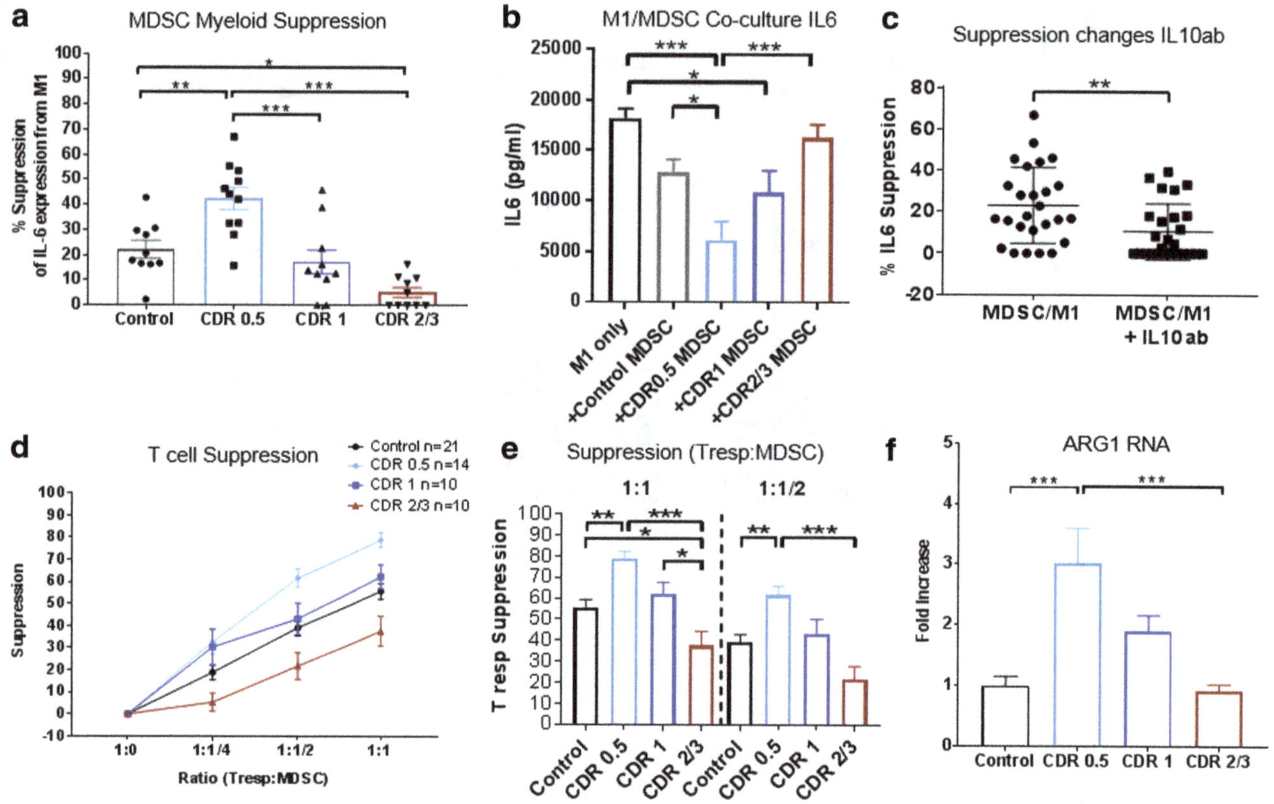

Fig. 4 Stage-specific MDSC suppression of pro-inflammatory myeloid cells and T cell proliferation. Isolated patient MDSCs are co-cultured overnight (18 h) at 1:1 ratio with iPSC-generated M1 pro-inflammatory macrophages. **a** Production of IL-6 transcripts were highly suppressed by MDSCs from CDR0.5 patients while that suppression decreases as the patient advances to CDR1 and CDR2/3. (Control $n = 10$, CDR0.5 $n = 11$, CDR1 $n = 10$, and CDR2/3 $n = 10$). **b** Conditioned media from iPSC-M1 and patient MDSC co-cultures were analyzed via ELISA for changes in IL-6 protein. Changes in protein levels mirrored the IL-6 RNA suppression with CDR0.5 MDSCs causing a decrease in IL-6 protein production by M1 cells. These suppressive effects tapered off with advancing disease condition (Control $n = 6$, CDR0.5 $n = 6$, CDR1 $n = 4$, and CDR2/3 $n = 5$). **c** Addition of 5μg/mL neutralizing antibody for IL-10 reduces the IL-6 suppression in our MDSC: M1 assays. Numbers shown as averages ± SEM and statistics utilized were one-way ANOVA with Tukey post hoc (**a**, **b**) and student's t-test (**c**). Isolated MDSCs were co-cultured with T responder cells at ratios of 1:1/4, 1:1/2, and 1:1 and stimulated for proliferation. **d**, **e** CDR0.5 MDSCs show hypersuppression of T cell proliferation compared with other groups. Late CDR2/3 MDSCs lost their T cell proliferation suppression below that of controls (Control $n = 21$, CDR0.5 $n = 14$, CDR1 $n = 10$, and CDR2/3 $n = 10$). **f** Arg1 expression in isolated MDSCs increase in CDR0.5 but decrease with increasing AD burden (Control $n = 12$, CDR0.5 $n = 8$, CDR1 $n = 8$, CDR2/3 $n = 10$). Numbers shown as averages ± SEM with one-way ANOVA with Tukey's post hoc analysis. *P*-values are $^{*}p < 0.05$, $^{**}p < 0.01$, and $^{***}p < 0.001$

While some studies implicate differential activation and polarization of immune cells due to the age and gender of the patient, we did not observe any significant effects contributed by these factors in our control or AD datasets. Advanced studies into gender and age-specific contributions to neurodegenerative disease are warranted.

The peripheral pattern of immune cell deactivation and reactivation is in accord with the biphasic immune marker profile reported in a study of CSF immune makers in AD [52]; decreases in immune signaling were noted early in the course of disease and a strong increase in immune signaling was noted in later stages of disease. Additionally, a longitudinal imaging study of AD patients found initial microglial activation upon diagnosis followed by a reduction of activation as patients went through mild cognitive impairment stages. As patients progressed into later stages of AD, microglial activation increased again suggesting that there might be two activation stages; the first being a protective activation state while the later peak being a more pro-inflammatory and destructive process [53].

Many studies utilize changes and shifts in monocyte populations to identify and predict inflammatory disease and progression in a multitude of inflammation-based disorders [38–40]. Previous AD studies suggest monocyte involvement in AD although our analysis showed no difference of total monocyte number between controls and through the progression of AD [54–57]. With no studies focused on AD monocyte population shifts, our results present a progressive decline of the classical monocyte population ($CD14^{+}CD16^{-}$) with a subsequent increase in both the intermediate ($CD14^{+}CD16^{+}$) and non-classical ($CD14^{low}CD16^{+}$) subsets as disease progresses. Shifting of populations from the classical population, a patrolling subset, into intermediate and non-classical populations reflects monocyte maturation and pro-inflammatory activation [58]. Identification of mechanisms whereby patient monocytes are shifting to their subsets and how they are inhibited early while being activated with increasing disease burden is needed.

MDSCs are immature myeloid cells that expand under pathological conditions such as cancer and immune disorders but have yet to be fully characterized in patients or animal models of AD. These cells suppress pro-inflammatory immune cells including mature myeloid cells and $CD4^+$/ $CD8^+$ T cells. MDSCs are roughly divided into early-stage, granulocytic, and monocytic MDSCs with the latter being most suppressive and characterized as $CD14^+$/HLA-DR^-/$CD11b^+$/ $CD33^+$ cells [41, 59]. MDSC numbers were increased in CDR0.5 and CDR1 patients, and decreased in CDR2/3 patients. While monocytic MDSCs are undocumented in AD, a previous study documented an increase in granulocytic MDSCs in amnestic mild cognitive impaired patients compared with mild AD patients. However, this previous study did not provide functional data, thus it is not known whether granulocytic MDSCs have differential functions as the course of AD progresses or if AD granulocytic MDSCs have different properties compared to those of healthy controls [60].

MDSCs and mature pro-inflammatory monocytes have opposing roles in inflammation. The former provides strong immunosuppression while the latter contributes to pro-inflammatory signaling. Analyses of these phenotypes and signaling mechanisms in advancing AD would provide important information on the state of the immune system during the progression of AD. Additionally, these cells may directly engraft into the CNS given the evidence of a compromised BBB based upon the leakage of blood-derived constituents in postmortem AD brains [61–63], the increased CSF/ serum or CSF/plasma ratios of albumin [64–66], and imaging showing an age-dependent increase in BBB permeability in the hippocampus, dentate gyrus, and CA1 region [67]. Additionally, dysregulation of the neurovascular unit, responsible for maintaining BBB integrity, is known to accompany AD pathology [68]. Peripheral immune cell involvement and engraftment into the CNS are postulated to play important roles in AD [69, 70]. With that said, roles of infiltrating cells during CNS disease pathogenesis is controversial, contextual, and disease/ stage-dependent [22, 56, 71–73]. Whether and how peripheral myeloid cells dictate progression of AD necessitates further investigation, especially the question of peripheral immune cell migration into the CNS and other mechanisms of neuro-immune cross-talk.

Microglia and monocytes, through genetics and activation status in AD, play a critical role in AD pathogenesis [6, 14–18]. Their responsibilities include phagocytosis, cytokine secretion, and restoration of homeostatic conditions with impairments to these functions being deleterious to sensitive neuronal environments in AD. We have developed CD14 myeloid cells from control iPS cells (unpublished Zhao et al.) and polarized them to be pro-inflammatory to examine differential effects of control/AD MDSCs on activated myeloid cells. Pro-inflammatory polarization of iPS cells provides a consistent, activated cell type to compare suppression between patients without the confounding variable of primed or differentially activated mature monocytes from patients.

MDSCs from CDR0.5 patients were able to suppress pro-inflammatory IL-6 expression and protein from activated cells more than controls while CDR1 and CDR2/3 markedly lost their suppressive function. IL-6 transcript and protein analysis were used due to MDSCs producing no IL-6 while IL-6 is a predominant pro-inflammatory output from activated myeloid cells [74]. The IL-10 data from the RNA studies provided a mechanistic target for MDSC suppression of the myeloid cells. Adding IL-10ab to co-cultures reduced MDSC suppression of myeloid IL-6 transcripts that was most pronounced with CDR0.5 co-cultures but also observed in the other groups. IL-10ab only partially blocked IL-6 suppression leaving other additional mechanisms contributing to suppression, either through soluble signaling or direct cell contact. An extensive study into the intrinsic differences between MDSCs from prodromal and AD dementia is warranted to comprehensively parse out the predominating mechanisms of their suppressive functions and which of these are lost through AD progression.

Co-culture of MDSCs with Tresps showed increased CDR0.5 and CDR1 MDSC suppression compared with controls. The mechanism for MDSC suppression of T cell proliferation is through metabolism of arginine via increased Arg1 transcript in MDSCs [75, 76]. Arg1 gene expression increased in CDR0.5 MDSCs and then diminished as AD advances. Analysis of CDR1 MDSC suppression shows enhanced T cell proliferation but decreased M1 suppression which may suggest a suppressive function transition occurring at this stage.

Limitations of these studies involve lack of direct evidence that peripheral myeloid cells enter the CNS parenchyma and influence disease progression in AD. Nevertheless, the definitive evidence for alterations in the BBB in AD, the comparability of CSF findings and peripheral myeloid cell phenotype alterations, and the PET scan evidence of increasing neuroinflammation during the course of disease are all in accord with extensive neuro-immune cross-talk between the brain and peripheral immune system. Advances in neuroimaging with specialized ligands may provide tools for analyzing central vs peripheral identities as well as the anti vs pro-inflammatory phenotypes contributing to AD pathogenesis. The identification of distinct transcriptional and functional phenotypes could assist in developing these technologies [26]. Additionally, complex networks and signaling cascades involving additional cells outside our examination might assist in dictating inflammatory environments and cell phenotypes. Examination of these cells, both individually and in concert with each other, will help establish a more definitive immune environment during AD and through its course.

Conclusions

This study documents that peripheral monocytes are pro-inflammatory in advancing stages of AD but not in prodromal AD. The pro-inflammatory responses of monocytes from prodromal AD patients are suppressed while advancing AD patients monocytes lose this suppression, and become activated and pro-inflammatory. Numbers and suppressive functions of MDSCs are increased in prodromal AD and decreased in patients with advancing AD and correlate with pro-inflammatory expression of AD monocytes. MDSCs also suppress Tresp which can readily enter the CNS, and loss of T effector suppression can significantly enhance inflammatory disease pathology. These findings provide a novel inflammatory paradigm that may have confounded early therapeutic interventions and provides a new basis for how future studies and treatments should be designed. Additionally, we have documented the significant impact of AD MDSCs on immune cell subsets. Understanding the role of early enhanced immunosuppression in prodromal AD and the subsequent dysfunction of this process in AD dementia may lead to novel therapeutic strategies.

Additional files

Additional file 1: Table S1. Cell Populations.

Additional file 2: Figure S2. Flow cytometry gating schemes for monocyte and MDSC populations. (TIF 539 kb)

Additional file 3: Figure S9. Nanostring dataset for RNA analysis of CDR rated patients and age-matched controls.

Additional file 4: Figure S4. iPSC-derived M1 and MDSC co-culture paradigm.

Additional file 5: Figure S3. (a) Correlation data of inflammatory RNA expression and subject age from peripheral myeloid cells. Data represent analyses of RNA expression with controls only, patients with varying levels of AD, and all groups combined (Control $n = 20$, AD $n = 38$). (b) Analyses of gender contributions to pro-inflammatory RNA expression among controls, CDR0.5, CDR1, and CDR2/3 (Control $n = 10/10$ M/F, CDR0.5 $n = 6/14$ M/F, CDR1 $n = 5/3$ M/F, CDR2/3 $n = 4/6$ M/F). Graphs show average ± SEM with statistics run using two-way ANOVA with Sidak's multiple comparisons test. No statistical difference observed after age and gender data stratification unless signified by $*p < 0.05$, $**p < 0.01$, or $***p < 0.001$.

Additional file 6: Figure S6. (a) Correlation data between age and protein expression of HLADR and CD33 analyzed via flow cytometry (Control $n = 30$, AD $n = 57$). (b) Analyses of gender contributions to HLADR and CD33 expression on mature myeloid cells isolated from controls, CDR0.5, CDR1, and CDR2/3 (Control $n = 14/16$ M/F, CDR0.5 $n = 13/14$ M/F, CDR1 $n = 8/10$ M/F, CDR2/3 $n = 3/10$ M/F). Graphs show average ± SEM with statistics run using two-way ANOVA with Sidak's multiple comparisons test. No statistical difference observed after age and gender data stratification unless signified by $*p < 0.05$, $**p < 0.01$, or $***p < 0.001$.

Additional file 7: Figure S5. (a) Correlation data between age and monocyte population changes. Analyses performed examined the ages of controls, varying levels of AD, and combined groups for correlations in changes in classical monocytes, intermediate monocytes, non-classical monocytes, and MDSCs (Control $n = 35$, AD $n = 66$). (b) Analyses of gender contributions to monocyte population changes among controls, CDR0.5, CDR1, and CDR2/3 (Control n = 20/15 M/F, CDR0.5 $n = 15/16$ M/F, CDR1 $n = 8/10$ M/F, CDR2/3 $n = 5/12$ M/F). Graphs show average ± SEM with statistics run using two-way ANOVA with Sidak's multiple comparisons test. No statistical difference observed after age and gender data stratification unless signified by $*p < 0.05$, $**p < 0.01$, or $***p < 0.001$.

Additional file 8: Figure S7. (a) Analysis of gender contribution to MDSC suppressive function on pro-inflammatory M1 cells (Control $n = 6/4$ M/F, CDR0.5 n = 5/6 M/F, CDR1 $n = 4/6$ M/F, CDR2/3 $n = 3/7$ M/F). Graph shows average ± SEM with statistics run using two-way ANOVA with Sidak's multiple comparisons test. No statistical difference observed after gender data stratification unless signified by $*p < 0.05$, $**p < 0.01$, or $***p < 0.001$.

Additional file 9: Figure S8. (a) Correlation plot graphing T resp. proliferation suppression and myeloid IL-6 transcript suppression at 1:1 ratio of responding cells to MDSCs ($R = .7288$ $p = 0.004$). (b) IL-6 control experiment whereby MDSCs from controls ($n = 6$) and AD patients from various stages ($n = 12$) do not express IL-6 transcript when cultured alone in LPS/IFNγ treatments. Corroboration with no IL-6 protein in the MDSC only treated media when analyzed via ELISA (data not shown).

Acknowledgements

We would like to thank the Stanley H. Appel Department of Neurology, the Nantz National Alzheimer Center, and Houston Methodist Hospital for their contributions and patient organization/recruitment. Individually, we acknowledge Douglas Casey, Jinghong Wang, and Neha Pal for their time and efforts in the completion of this project. We also thank patients and their families for their participation and involvement in the study.

Funding

This study was funded by the Ting Tsung and Wei Fong Chao Foundation in Houston, TX.

Author's contributions

ADT and SHA conceived and designed research; ADT, AF, JRT, WZ, and SW performed experiments; ADT, DRB, JRT, WZ, and SHA analyzed and interpreted the data. AF, BP, and JCM recruited, organized clinical operations for sample collection, and rated/categorized patients; ADT wrote manuscript with input from all authors. All authors read and approved the final version of the manuscript.

Competing interests

The authors of this manuscript declare that they have no competing interests.

References

1. Brion JP. Neurofibrillary tangles and Alzheimer's disease. Eur Neurol. 1998;40: 130–40.

2. Hardy JA, Higgins GA. Alzheimer's disease: the amyloid cascade hypothesis. Science. 1992;256:184–5.
3. Larson EB, Kukull WA, Katzman RL. Cognitive impairment: dementia and Alzheimer's disease. Annu Rev Public Health. 1992;13:431–49.
4. Hardy J, Selkoe DJ. The amyloid hypothesis of Alzheimer's disease: progress and problems on the road to therapeutics. Science. 2002;297:353–6.
5. Holtzman DM, Morris JC, Goate AM. Alzheimer's disease: the challenge of the second century. Sci Transl Med. 2011;3:77sr71.
6. Kreisl WC, Lyoo CH, Liow JS, Wei M, Snow J, Page E, Jenko KJ, Morse CL, Zoghbi SS, Pike VW, et al. (11)C-PBR28 binding to translocator protein increases with progression of Alzheimer's disease. Neurobiol Aging. 2016;44:53–61.
7. Akiyama H, Barger S, Barnum S, Bradt B, Bauer J, Cole GM, Cooper NR, Eikelenboom P, Emmerling M, Fiebich BL, et al. Inflammation and Alzheimer's disease. Neurobiol Aging. 2000;21:383–421.
8. Cuello AC. Early and late CNS inflammation in Alzheimer's disease: two extremes of a continuum? Trends Pharmacol Sci. 2017;38:956–66.
9. Hopperton KE, Mohammad D, Trepanier MO, Giuliano V, Bazinet RP. Markers of microglia in post-mortem brain samples from patients with Alzheimer's disease: a systematic review. Mol Psychiatry. 2018;23:177–98.
10. Wyss-Coray T, Rogers J. Inflammation in Alzheimer disease-a brief review of the basic science and clinical literature. Cold Spring Harb Perspect Med. 2012;2:a006346.
11. Zimmer ER, Leuzy A, Benedet AL, Breitner J, Gauthier S, Rosa-Neto P. Tracking neuroinflammation in Alzheimer's disease: the role of positron emission tomography imaging. J Neuroinflammation. 2014;11:120.
12. Schwab C, Klegeris A, McGeer PL. Inflammation in transgenic mouse models of neurodegenerative disorders. Biochim Biophys Acta. 2010;1802:889–902.
13. Wilcock DM, Zhao Q, Morgan D, Gordon MN, Everhart A, Wilson JG, Lee JE, Colton CA. Diverse inflammatory responses in transgenic mouse models of Alzheimer's disease and the effect of immunotherapy on these responses. ASN Neuro. 2011;3:249–58.
14. Bradshaw EM, Chibnik LB, Keenan BT, Ottoboni L, Raj T, Tang A, Rosenkrantz LL, Imboywa S, Lee M, Von Korff A, et al. CD33 Alzheimer's disease locus: altered monocyte function and amyloid biology. Nat Neurosci. 2013;16:848–50.
15. Griciuc A, Serrano-Pozo A, Parrado AR, Lesinski AN, Asselin CN, Mullin K, Hooli B, Choi SH, Hyman BT, Tanzi RE. Alzheimer's disease risk gene CD33 inhibits microglial uptake of amyloid beta. Neuron. 2013;78:631–43.
16. Guerreiro R, Wojtas A, Bras J, Carrasquillo M, Rogaeva E, Majounie E, Cruchaga C, Sassi C, Kauwe JS, Younkin S, et al. TREM2 variants in Alzheimer's disease. N Engl J Med. 2013;368:117–27.
17. Jonsson T, Stefansson H, Steinberg S, Jonsdottir I, Jonsson PV, Snaedal J, Bjornsson S, Huttenlocher J, Levey AI, Lah JJ, et al. Variant of TREM2 associated with the risk of Alzheimer's disease. N Engl J Med. 2013;368: 107–16.
18. Malik M, Simpson JF, Parikh I, Wilfred BR, Fardo DW, Nelson PT, Estus S. CD33 Alzheimer's risk-altering polymorphism, CD33 expression, and exon 2 splicing. J Neurosci. 2013;33:13320–5.
19. Goldeck D, Witkowski JM, Fulop T, Pawelec G. Peripheral immune signatures in Alzheimer disease. Curr Alzheimer Res. 2016;13:739–49.
20. Kipnis J. Multifaceted interactions between adaptive immunity and the central nervous system. Science. 2016;353:766–71.
21. Le Page A, Dupuis G, Frost EH, Larbi A, Pawelec G, Witkowski JM, Fulop T. Role of the peripheral innate immune system in the development of Alzheimer's disease. Exp Gerontol. 2018;107:59–66.
22. Varvel NH, Neher JJ, Bosch A, Wang W, Ransohoff RM, Miller RJ, Dingledine R. Infiltrating monocytes promote brain inflammation and exacerbate neuronal damage after status epilepticus. Proc Natl Acad Sci U S A. 2016; 113:E5665–74.
23. Carvey PM, Hendey B, Monahan AJ. The blood-brain barrier in neurodegenerative disease: a rhetorical perspective. J Neurochem. 2009;111:291–314.
24. de Vries HE, Kooij G, Frenkel D, Georgopoulos S, Monsonego A, Janigro D. Inflammatory events at blood-brain barrier in neuroinflammatory and neurodegenerative disorders: implications for clinical disease. Epilepsia. 2012;53(Suppl 6):45–52.
25. Erickson MA, Dohi K, Banks WA. Neuroinflammation: a common pathway in CNS diseases as mediated at the blood-brain barrier. Neuroimmunomodulation. 2012;19:121–30.
26. Cronk JC, Filiano AJ, Louveau A, Marin I, Marsh R, Ji E, Goldman DH, Smirnov I, Geraci N, Acton S, et al. Peripherally derived macrophages can engraft the brain independent of irradiation and maintain an identity distinct from microglia. J Exp Med. 2018;215:1627–47.
27. Ginhoux F, Lim S, Hoeffel G, Low D, Huber T. Origin and differentiation of microglia. Front Cell Neurosci. 2013;7:45.
28. London A, Cohen M, Schwartz M. Microglia and monocyte-derived macrophages: functionally distinct populations that act in concert in CNS plasticity and repair. Front Cell Neurosci. 2013;7:34.
29. Perry VH, Teeling J. Microglia and macrophages of the central nervous system: the contribution of microglia priming and systemic inflammation to chronic neurodegeneration. Semin Immunopathol. 2013;35:601–12.
30. Yang J, Zhang L, Yu C, Yang XF, Wang H. Monocyte and macrophage differentiation: circulation inflammatory monocyte as biomarker for inflammatory diseases. Biomark Res. 2014;2(1):1. https://doi.org/10.1186/2050-7771-2-1.
31. Ziegler-Heitbrock L, Ancuta P, Crowe S, Dalod M, Grau V, Hart DN, Leenen PJ, Liu YJ, MacPherson G, Randolph GJ, et al. Nomenclature of monocytes and dendritic cells in blood. Blood. 2010;116:e74–80.
32. Boyette LB, Macedo C, Hadi K, Elinoff BD, Walters JT, Ramaswami B, Chalasani G, Taboas JM, Lakkis FG, Metes DM. Phenotype, function, and differentiation potential of human monocyte subsets. PLoS One. 2017;12:e0176460.
33. Gawdat K, Legere S, Wong C, Myers T, Marshall JS, Hassan A, Brunt KR, Kienesberger PC, Pulinilkunnil T, Legare JF. Changes in circulating monocyte subsets (CD16 expression) and neutrophil-to-lymphocyte ratio observed in patients undergoing cardiac surgery. Front Cardiovasc Med. 2017;4:12.
34. Kim WK, Sun Y, Do H, Autissier P, Halpern EF, Piatak M Jr, Lifson JD, Burdo TH, McGrath MS, Williams K. Monocyte heterogeneity underlying phenotypic changes in monocytes according to SIV disease stage. J Leukoc Biol. 2010;87:557–67.
35. Mukherjee R, Kanti Barman P, Kumar Thatoi P, Tripathy R, Kumar Das B, Ravindran B. Non-classical monocytes display inflammatory features: validation in Sepsis and systemic lupus erythematous. Sci Rep. 2015;5:13886.
36. Ong SM, Hadadi E, Dang TM, Yeap WH, Tan CT, Ng TP, Larbi A, Wong SC. The pro-inflammatory phenotype of the human non-classical monocyte subset is attributed to senescence. Cell Death Dis. 2018;9:266.
37. Stansfield BK, Ingram DA. Clinical significance of monocyte heterogeneity. Clin Transl Med. 2015;4:5.
38. Wildgruber M, Aschenbrenner T, Wendorff H, Czubba M, Glinzer A, Haller B, Schiemann M, Zimmermann A, Berger H, Eckstein HH, et al. The "intermediate" CD14(++)CD16(+) monocyte subset increases in severe peripheral artery disease in humans. Sci Rep. 2016;6:39483.
39. Grozdanov V, Bliederhaeuser C, Ruf WP, Roth V, Fundel-Clemens K, Zondler L, Brenner D, Martin-Villalba A, Hengerer B, Kassubek J, et al. Inflammatory dysregulation of blood monocytes in Parkinson's disease patients. Acta Neuropathol. 2014;128:651–63.
40. Zhao W, Beers DR, Hooten KG, Sieglaff DH, Zhang A, Kalyana-Sundaram S, Traini CM, Halsey WS, Hughes AM, Sathe GM, et al. Characterization of gene expression phenotype in amyotrophic lateral sclerosis monocytes. JAMA Neurol. 2017;74:677–85.
41. Bronte V, Brandau S, Chen SH, Colombo MP, Frey AB, Greten TF, Mandruzzato S, Murray PJ, Ochoa A, Ostrand-Rosenberg S, et al. Recommendations for myeloid-derived suppressor cell nomenclature and characterization standards. Nat Commun. 2016;7:12150.
42. Greten TF, Manns MP, Korangy F. Myeloid derived suppressor cells in human diseases. Int Immunopharmacol. 2011;11:802–7.
43. Kong YY, Fuchsberger M, Xiang SD, Apostolopoulos V, Plebanski M. Myeloid derived suppressor cells and their role in diseases. Curr Med Chem. 2013;20: 1437–44.
44. Tamadaho RSE, Hoerauf A, Layland LE. Immunomodulatory effects of myeloid-derived suppressor cells in diseases: role in cancer and infections. Immunobiology. 2018;223:432–42.
45. Salminen A, Kaarniranta K, Kauppinen A. The potential importance of myeloid-derived suppressor cells (MDSCs) in the pathogenesis of Alzheimer's disease. Cell Mol Life Sci. 2018;75:3099. https://doi.org/10.1007/s00018-018-2844-6.
46. Albert MS, DeKosky ST, Dickson D, Dubois B, Feldman HH, Fox NC, Gamst A, Holtzman DM, Jagust WJ, Petersen RC, et al. The diagnosis of mild cognitive impairment due to Alzheimer's disease: recommendations from the National Institute on Aging-Alzheimer's Association workgroups on diagnostic guidelines for Alzheimer's disease. Alzheimers Dement. 2011;7:270–9.

47. McKhann GM, Knopman DS, Chertkow H, Hyman BT, Jack CR Jr, Kawas CH, Klunk WE, Koroshetz WJ, Manly JJ, Mayeux R, et al. The diagnosis of dementia due to Alzheimer's disease: recommendations from the National Institute on Aging-Alzheimer's Association workgroups on diagnostic guidelines for Alzheimer's disease. Alzheimers Dement. 2011;7:263–9.
48. Yanagimachi MD, Niwa A, Tanaka T, Honda-Ozaki F, Nishimoto S, Murata Y, Yasumi T, Ito J, Tomida S, Oshima K, et al. Robust and highly-efficient differentiation of functional monocytic cells from human pluripotent stem cells under serum- and feeder cell-free conditions. PLoS One. 2013;8:e59243.
49. Guillemin GJ, Brew BJ. Microglia, macrophages, perivascular macrophages, and pericytes: a review of function and identification. J Leukoc Biol. 2004;75: 388–97.
50. Prinz M, Priller J. Microglia and brain macrophages in the molecular age: from origin to neuropsychiatric disease. Nat Rev Neurosci. 2014;15:300–12.
51. Yamasaki R, Lu H, Butovsky O, Ohno N, Rietsch AM, Cialic R, Wu PM, Doykan CE, Lin J, Cotleur AC, et al. Differential roles of microglia and monocytes in the inflamed central nervous system. J Exp Med. 2014;211:1533–49.
52. Meyer PF, Savard M, Poirier J, Labonte A, Rosa-Neto P, Weitz TM, Town T, Breitner J. Alzheimer's disease neuroimaging I, group P-AR: bi-directional Association of Cerebrospinal Fluid Immune Markers with stage of Alzheimer's disease pathogenesis. J Alzheimers Dis. 2018;63:577–90.
53. Fan Z, Brooks DJ, Okello A, Edison P. An early and late peak in microglial activation in Alzheimer's disease trajectory. Brain. 2017;140:792–803.
54. Feng Y, Li L, Sun XH. Monocytes and Alzheimer's disease. Neurosci Bull. 2011;27:115–22.
55. Martin E, Boucher C, Fontaine B, Delarasse C. Distinct inflammatory phenotypes of microglia and monocyte-derived macrophages in Alzheimer's disease models: effects of aging and amyloid pathology. Aging Cell. 2017;16:27–38.
56. Saresella M, Marventano I, Calabrese E, Piancone F, Rainone V, Gatti A, Alberoni M, Nemni R, Clerici M. A complex proinflammatory role for peripheral monocytes in Alzheimer's disease. J Alzheimers Dis. 2014;38:403–13.
57. Theriault P, ElAli A, Rivest S. The dynamics of monocytes and microglia in Alzheimer's disease. Alzheimers Res Ther. 2015;7:41.
58. Wong KL, Tai JJ, Wong WC, Han H, Sem X, Yeap WH, Kourilsky P, Wong SC. Gene expression profiling reveals the defining features of the classical, intermediate, and nonclassical human monocyte subsets. Blood. 2011;118: e16–31.
59. Youn JI, Gabrilovich DI. The biology of myeloid-derived suppressor cells: the blessing and the curse of morphological and functional heterogeneity. Eur J Immunol. 2010;40:2969–75.
60. Le Page A, Garneau H, Dupuis G, Frost EH, Larbi A, Witkowski JM, Pawelec G, Fulop T. Differential phenotypes of myeloid-derived suppressor and T regulatory cells and cytokine levels in amnestic mild cognitive impairment subjects compared to mild Alzheimer diseased patients. Front Immunol. 2017;8:783.
61. Wisniewski HM, Kozlowski PB. Evidence for blood-brain barrier changes in senile dementia of the Alzheimer type (SDAT). Ann N Y Acad Sci. 1982;396: 119–29.
62. Wisniewski HM, Vorbrodt AW, Wegiel J. Amyloid angiopathy and blood-brain barrier changes in Alzheimer's disease. Ann N Y Acad Sci. 1997;826: 161–72.
63. Zipser BD, Johanson CE, Gonzalez L, Berzin TM, Tavares R, Hulette CM, Vitek MP, Hovanesian V, Stopa EG. Microvascular injury and blood-brain barrier leakage in Alzheimer's disease. Neurobiol Aging. 2007;28:977–86.
64. Alafuzoff I, Adolfsson R, Bucht G, Winblad B. Albumin and immunoglobulin in plasma and cerebrospinal fluid, and blood-cerebrospinal fluid barrier function in patients with dementia of Alzheimer type and multi-infarct dementia. J Neurol Sci. 1983;60:465–72.
65. Blennow K, Wallin A, Fredman P, Karlsson I, Gottfries CG, Svennerholm L. Blood-brain barrier disturbance in patients with Alzheimer's disease is related to vascular factors. Acta Neurol Scand. 1990;81:323–6.
66. Skoog I, Wallin A, Fredman P, Hesse C, Aevarsson O, Karlsson I, Gottfries CG, Blennow K. A population study on blood-brain barrier function in 85-year-olds: relation to Alzheimer's disease and vascular dementia. Neurology. 1998;50:966–71.
67. Montagne A, Barnes SR, Sweeney MD, Halliday MR, Sagare AP, Zhao Z, Toga AW, Jacobs RE, Liu CY, Amezcua L, et al. Blood-brain barrier breakdown in the aging human hippocampus. Neuron. 2015;85:296–302.
68. Yamazaki Y, Kanekiyo T. Blood-brain barrier dysfunction and the pathogenesis of Alzheimer's disease. Int J Mol Sci. 2017;18.
69. Prinz M, Priller J. The role of peripheral immune cells in the CNS in steady state and disease. Nat Neurosci. 2017;20:136–44.
70. Rezai-Zadeh K, Gate D, Town T. CNS infiltration of peripheral immune cells: D-day for neurodegenerative disease? J NeuroImmune Pharmacol. 2009;4: 462–75.
71. El Khoury J, Toft M, Hickman SE, Means TK, Terada K, Geula C, Luster AD. Ccr2 deficiency impairs microglial accumulation and accelerates progression of Alzheimer-like disease. Nat Med. 2007;13:432–8.
72. Harms AS, Delic V, Thome AD, Bryant N, Liu Z, Chandra S, Jurkuvenaite A, West AB. Alpha-Synuclein fibrils recruit peripheral immune cells in the rat brain prior to neurodegeneration. Acta Neuropathol Commun. 2017;5:85.
73. Harms AS, Thome AD, Yan Z, Schonhoff AM, Williams GP, Li X, Liu Y, Qin H, Benveniste EN, Standaert DG. Peripheral monocyte entry is required for alpha-Synuclein induced inflammation and neurodegeneration in a model of Parkinson disease. Exp Neurol. 2018;300:179–87.
74. Beury DW, Parker KH, Nyandjo M, Sinha P, Carter KA, Ostrand-Rosenberg S. Cross-talk among myeloid-derived suppressor cells, macrophages, and tumor cells impacts the inflammatory milieu of solid tumors. J Leukoc Biol. 2014;96:1109–18.
75. Bronte V, Zanovello P. Regulation of immune responses by L-arginine metabolism. Nat Rev Immunol. 2005;5:641–54.
76. Rodriguez PC, Ochoa AC. Arginine regulation by myeloid derived suppressor cells and tolerance in cancer: mechanisms and therapeutic perspectives. Immunol Rev. 2008;222:180–91.

11

Modifying Rap1-signalling by targeting Pde6δ is neuroprotective in models of Alzheimer's disease

Michael Dumbacher[1,10], Tom Van Dooren[1], Katrien Princen[1], Koen De Witte[1], Mélissa Farinelli[2], Sam Lievens[3,4], Jan Tavernier[4], Wim Dehaen[5], Stefaan Wera[6], Joris Winderickx[7], Sara Allasia[8], Amuri Kilonda[8], Stéphane Spieser[8], Arnaud Marchand[8], Patrick Chaltin[8,9], Casper C. Hoogenraad[10] and Gerard Griffioen[1*]

Abstract

Background: Neuronal Ca^{2+} dyshomeostasis and hyperactivity play a central role in Alzheimer's disease pathology and progression. Amyloid-beta together with non-genetic risk-factors of Alzheimer's disease contributes to increased Ca^{2+} influx and aberrant neuronal activity, which accelerates neurodegeneration in a feed-forward fashion. As such, identifying new targets and drugs to modulate excessive Ca^{2+} signalling and neuronal hyperactivity, without overly suppressing them, has promising therapeutic potential.

Methods: Here we show, using biochemical, electrophysiological, imaging, and behavioural tools, that pharmacological modulation of Rap1 signalling by inhibiting its interaction with Pde6δ normalises disease associated Ca^{2+} aberrations and neuronal activity, conferring neuroprotection in models of Alzheimer's disease.

Results: The newly identified inhibitors of the Rap1-Pde6δ interaction counteract AD phenotypes, by reconfiguring Rap1 signalling underlying synaptic efficacy, Ca^{2+} influx, and neuronal repolarisation, without adverse effects *in-cellulo* or in-vivo. Thus, modulation of Rap1 by Pde6δ accommodates key mechanisms underlying neuronal activity, and therefore represents a promising new drug target for early or late intervention in neurodegenerative disorders.

Conclusion: Targeting the Pde6δ-Rap1 interaction has promising therapeutic potential for disorders characterised by neuronal hyperactivity, such as Alzheimer's disease.

Keywords: Alzheimer's disease, Hyperexcitability, Neuroprotection, Pde6δ, Rap1

Background

Neuronal hyperactivity and chronically elevated cytosolic calcium $[Ca^{2+}]_i$ are among the earliest pathological events in both familial and sporadic Alzheimer's disease (AD) [1–4]. Amyloid-beta (Aβ), a peptide which progressively aggregates around neurons during the disease, appears to play an important role in driving these aberrations, as in the vicinity of Aβ accumulations (or plaques), where concentrations of soluble oligomeric Aβ (Aβo) are highest, neurons have a tendency to be hyperactive [5]. These AD associated changes in neuronal activity appear to involve, at least in part, a direct or indirect modulation of Ca^{2+} permeable receptors and ion channels as well as the disruption of lipid barriers by Aβo [6].

Apart from Aβ, also Tau, the second major aggregating protein crucial for AD progression, has signalling functions, involving Ca^{2+}, and plays a role in excitability and network synchronisation [7, 8]. Of particular interest in this regard is dendritic Tau, which facilitates Ca^{2+} influx during Aβ induced neurotoxicity [7, 9]. An additional indication for the prominent role of Tau in AD is that, in animal models of the disease, the depletion of the former protein prevented Aβ associated neuronal hyperactivity and cognitive deficits [10, 11]. Thus, the interplay between Aβ and Tau in AD is essential for driving Ca^{2+} aberrations and excessive neuronal activity.

Moreover, neuronal hyperactivity and Ca^{2+} dyshomeostasis are not only the consequences of pathological Aβ and

* Correspondence: gerard.griffioen@remynd.com
1reMYND NV, Gaston Geenslaan 1, Leuven-Heverlee 3001, Belgium
Full list of author information is available at the end of the article

Tau but in turn also accelerate their formation. Aberrant Ca^{2+} signalling was shown to facilitate Tau phosphorylation [12] and Aβo production [13, 14], the precursors of the well-known AD hallmarks – neurofibrillary tangles and amyloid plaques respectively. Hence, it can be envisaged that risk factors for sporadic AD, which impair Ca^{2+} homeostasis (most notably ageing) [1, 6], set-off a neurotoxic cascade leading to neuronal hyperexcitability and aberrant network activity resulting in enhanced formation of Aβo and Tau phosphorylation. These aberrations in turn reinforce the disease cascade in a feed-forward fashion, bringing about progressive neuronal degeneration [15]. In case of familial AD, the same pathological sequence of events can be directly and potently initiated by genetic mutations which increase Aβo formation [16, 17].

The importance of excessive neuronal activity in light of the pathology is emphasised by recent findings linking enhanced cognitive deficits, accelerated symptoms and greater neuronal loss in AD to patients suffering from spontaneous non-motoric seizures (10–22% of AD population), compared to other AD patients [18]. In addition, treatments targeting abnormal neuronal activity, including the antiepileptic drug levetiracetam, have shown to improve cognitive performance in mouse models of the disease [10, 19] and are currently under investigation in patients with AD during clinical trials (e.g.: NCT02002819) [20].

Collectively, these mechanistic underpinnings indicate that normalising Ca^{2+} homeostasis and hyperactivity represent a promising therapeutic paradigm. However, given the fundamental nature of Ca^{2+} signalling in cell physiology, targeting such deregulations in a safe fashion represents a major challenge. Here we addressed this problem by screening directly for therapeutic compounds using a neuronal cell based phenotypic screen that mimics crucial mechanisms underlying AD and by subsequently identifying their corresponding cellular target conferring neuroprotection.

Methods

Mice, drug treatment, behavioural testing and termination

Human mutant transgenic APP-V717I [21] (hAPP) and APP-V717I*PS1-A246E [22] (hAPP*PS1) mice in FVB/NxC57Bl/6 J background and age-, sex- and background-matched wild-type (WT) mice with ad libitum access to food and water were used. Breeding and housing for electrophysiological studies was in conventional 12 h light/dark cycle. Housing of mice for behaviour and biochemistry was in inverted 12 h light/dark cycle. All animals used in this study were female and four mice were housed per cage. Overexpression of human transgenes is steered by the mouse neuron-specific Thyl gene promotor. All experimental procedures were performed in accordance with the Guide for the Care and Use of Laboratory Animals (NRC, 2011) and the European Communities Council Directive of September 22nd, 2010. REM0043039 was dissolved in liposomes (Phares, Switzerland).

For chronic treatment of REM, hAPP and hAPP*PS1 mice were injected daily subcutaneously (sc) with vehicle or compound at 20 mg/kg. For acute REM effects, mice were dosed orally at 30 mg/kg achieving (similarly to sc dosing) a sufficiently high free compound concentration in brain. Pharmacokinetic assessments, prior to the commencement of studies, had indicated that both dosing regimens resulted in sufficient compound levels for target engagement (data not shown).

hAPP*PS1 used for biochemistry were dosed during 14 consecutive days before termination at the age of 6 months. For behaviour studies, daily treatment of hAPP and control mice started at the age of 4.5 months. After 8 weeks treatment (around 8 months of age) hAPP and control mice were tested in the Morris water maze (MWM) paradigm. Therefore, mice were trained to find the hidden escape platform (10 cm diameter, 1.5 cm submerged below the surface) in a pool (160 cm diameter) filled with white opaque water (23–24 °C) during 4 consecutive days and 4 trials per day (with a maximum of 90 s trial and an inter-trial interval of 120 min). Both intra- and extra-maze cues were present. During the first day mice were allowed to sit on the platform for 10 s before being taken out of the pool. Mice that did not mount the platform were gently guided to it. The platform location remained constant throughout the 4 training days. However, the drop location of the mice varied semi-randomly among trials. For the probe trial on day 5 the platform was removed, and mice were allowed to swim for 60 s. The swimming pattern of the mice was video-monitored using a CCD camera and analysed using dedicated software (EthoVision, Noldus, The Netherlands). Search path (cm) and the annulus crossing index (ACI, defined as the frequency of crossing the target platform region minus the averaged imaginary platform regions in the other quadrants) were used as primary read-out during learning and probe trial, respectively. At the end of the study, all mice were terminated.

Cell culture

For construction of hTAU-P301L cells a TAU expression plasmid was constructed by sub-cloning the cDNA of human TAU-P301L (encoding for TAU with proline 301 substituted by a leucine residue) into mammalian expression vector pcDNA3.1 resulting in plasmid pcDNA3.1-TAU P301L. Plasmid pcDNA3.1-TAU-P301L were transfected into human BE(2)-M17neuroblastoma cells (ATCC No. CRL-2267) with the plasmids stably integrated into the genome were selected. These resulted in the cell line referred to as hTau-P301L. Expression of the hTAU-P301L gene in the cell lines was confirmed by Western blot analysis (Additional file 1: Figure S1a).

hTAU-P301L cells were cultured in culture medium containing Opti-MEM Reduced Serum Medium with phenol red supplemented with 1 mM sodium pyruvate, 1 x non-essential amino acids, 500 µg/ml G418 0,5 x antibiotic/antimycotic, antibiotics and 10% foetal calf serum (FCS).

For the cellular toxicity assay hTAU-P301L cells were seeded at 2500 cells/cm^2 in 96-well microplates, in experiment medium containing Opti-MEM Reduced Serum Medium without phenol red supplemented with 1 mM sodium pyruvate, 1 x non-essential amino acids, 500 µg/ml G418 0,5 x antibiotic/antimycotic, antibiotics and 1% FCS. After 3 h of incubation at 37 °C/5% CO_2, 100 µl of experiment medium without FCS supplemented with all-trans retinoic acid (ATRA) (final concentration 3.75 µM) and compound dissolved in dimethyl sulfoxide (DMSO) or vehicle alone (final concentration DMSO 2%) was added. The cells were further incubated for 7 days at 37 °C/5% CO_2. Subsequently, Lactate dehydrogenase (LDH) activity was determined using Promega Cytotox 96 Non-Radioactive cytotoxicity assay (Cat. G1780), according the supplier's instructions and the percentage LDH in the growth medium was calculated as a measure for toxicity using the following formula (slopes are calculated from the measured kinetic A492 values in function of time):

$$Toxicity = \frac{slope\ of\ released\ LDH\ (dead\ cells)}{slope\ of\ total\ LDH\ (dead + viable\ cells)}.$$

Primary hippocampal cultures were prepared from CD-1 (Swiss) embryonic day 16 (E16) mouse brains and plated on culture plates or glass coverslips coated with (0.1 mg/ml) poly-D-lysine (PDL) and (0.002 mg/ml) laminin or PDL pre-coated plates (Greiner) were used. Cultures were grown in serum free Neurobasal medium (NB, Gibco) supplemented with B27 (Gibco), glutamax (Gibco) and penicillin/streptomycin (50 u/ml) in multi-well plates at a density of 0.15 × 10^6 cells per ml. Culture medium was refreshed twice a week.

siRNA transfection

For gene silencing experiments hTAU-P301L neuroblastoma cells were plated out 24 h before transfection in 6-well plates. Cells were with Lipofect-amine® RNAiMAX (Thermo Fisher) according to the Thermo Fisher's "forward transfection protocol" with a final siRNA concentration of 25 pmol. RNA sequences used were siRNA Rap1A (Thermo Fisher, #4390771, s11779), siRNA retinal rod rhodopsin-sensitive cGMP 3′,5′-cyclic phosphodiesterase subunit delta (Pde6δ, protein ID: O43924) (Thermo Fisher, #4390771, s10207) and scrambled negative siRNA control (Thermo Fisher, #4390843). Twenty-four hours post-transfection the cells were re-plated into 96-well microplates for the toxicity assay.

Biochemical pull-down: Pde6δ and REM-MTX interaction assay

The cDNA encoding PDE6δ was sub-cloned into the vector pPR-IBA102 in frame with the upstream Strep tag. The resulting construct was used to express protein using a Mini Expressway cell-free *E. coli* expression system (Life Technologies) according to the manufacturer's instructions. Correct expression was confirmed using Western blot analysis with the StrepMAB-Classic antibody (data not shown).

For the interaction assay, *E. coli* cell-free lysate containing Strep-PDE6δ and methotrexate fused REM compound (REM-MTX) or the corresponding amount of DMF were mixed and incubated on ice for 3 h to achieve binding of the compound to the target. Subsequently, equilibrated Strep-Tactin Sepharose beads were added and incubated for 90 min at 4 °C with over-end rotation. Excess compound was removed by washing the beads 3 times with wash buffer (20 mM Tris-Cl pH 7.4, 150 mM NaCl). After removal of the last wash *E. coli* cell-free lysate containing His-DHFR in wash buffer was added to each sample, followed by incubation for 60 min at 4 °C with over-end rotation. After flow through removal and 3 subsequent washes, the beads were eluted with elution buffer containing 10 mM Desthiobiotin for 30 min on ice. Samples were mixed with SDS sample buffer for SDS-PAGE analysis and Western blot and analysed with an Anti-HisG antibody.

Affinity purification coupled with mass spectrometry to identify interactors with Pde6δ

The cDNA encoding human Pde6δ was fused with a Strep-HA tag encoding DNA sequence and sub-cloned into a standard expression vector. The bait sequence was verified by sequencing. For constitutive overexpression, the expression vector containing the gene encoding the bait Pde6δ-Strep-HA was transfected into HEK293 cells and selected for stable integration. Bait expression and solubility was monitored by immunoblotting using anti-HA antibodies. For affinity purification, protein extracts were prepared from control (HEK293 cells not expressing Pde6δ-Strep-HA), vehicle (DMSO) and compound treated Pde6δ-Strep-HA bearing cells under specific lysis conditions and the fusion protein was pulled-down using Strep-Tactin Sepharose beads. Affinity purification and mass spectrometry analysis of Pde6δ-Strep-HA expressed in HEK293 cells was performed with three biological replicates. For label free quantitative mass spectrometry analysis samples were analysed on a Thermo LTQ Orbitrap XL spectrometer using a C18 column, ESI and a 60 min gradient. The signals' intensity is provided as 2 Log values and correlates to the concentration of the detected mass (number/amount of peptide). The variation within the biological replicates for control, vehicle-treated Pde6δ pulldown, and REM treated Pde6δ pulldown was below 10%. A Co-precipitation threshold of 2 (Pde6δ vehicle /control value) is set to decide on the interacting properties of a protein to Pde6δ. For interacting proteins, signals were background corrected and REM treated samples were normalised to the DMSO control samples to identify for Pde6δ-protein interactions inhibited by REM.

Ca^{2+} recordings

For basal Ca^{2+} measurement in the neuroblastoma toxicity model, cells were loaded with Fura-2 AM (Sigma-Aldrich), a cell permeable fluorescent probe for Ca^{2+} at day 6 of the experiment. Briefly, Fura-2-AM was dissolved in DMSO plus 20% pluronic acid (0.025% final assay concentration (Invitrogen)) in a 1:1 ratio and diluted in medium to a final concentration of 0.5 μM. Probenecid (Sigma-Aldrich) is added to this loading medium at a final concentration of 2.5 μM. Then, culture medium is replaced by loading medium and after incubation for 1 h at 37 °C cells in the dark were washed and incubated in HBSS (Gibco) supplemented with 0.2% FCS (Gibco) and 0.02 M HEPES (Gibco) before Ca^{2+} being recorded in the FlexStation 3 (Molecular Devices). Cells were excited at 340 nm (Ca^{2+} bound Fura-2) and 380 nm (Ca^{2+} unbound Fura-2) of the FlexStation 3 with emission at 510 nm (cut-off filter 475 nm) in well scan modus (9 points/well).

Days in-vitro (DIV) > 14 hippocampal neurons were treated 24 h prior to experiment with 1.5 μM REM or equivalent amount of vehicle and were present throughout the experiment. One hour prior to Ca^{2+} recordings, primary neurons were incubated with loading medium containing 2 μM of the cell permeable Ca^{2+}-indicator Fura-2 AM, 0.02% pluronic acid (F-127) (Invitrogen) and 2.5 μM Probenecid (Sigma-Aldrich) for 30 min at 37 °C in the dark. After loading, cells were washed and incubated in HBSS (Gibco) supplemented with 10 mM HEPES (Gibco) (with or without 12.5 μM nifedipine/vehicle) and/or 1.5 μM REM/vehicle for 30 min, in the dark, at room temperature. Cells were then excited at 340 nm and 380 nm in time with the flex mode of the FlexStation 3, recording 4 reads per well every 3.6 s. Emissions were collected at 510 nm (cut-off filter 475 nm). After 60 s of "background reading", HBSS-HEPES containing high KCl (with adjusted monovalent ion concentration – variable amounts of NaCl/KCl, as previously described [23]) or HBSS-HEPES "control solution" was added to the cells and emissions were read further for four minutes.

Overall, changes in $[Ca^{2+}]_i$ were quantified, by making the ratio of changes in the amount of cytosolic Ca^{2+} bound Fura-2 (fluorescence intensity at 340 nm) relative to the amount of Ca^{2+} unbound Fura-2 (fluorescence intensity at 380 nm). Area under the curves (AUC) was calculated after normalising the data to the average baseline (first 60 s of recording) values. Data was processed with SoftMax Pro 5.4.6 software (Molecular Devices).

Electrophysiology (acute brain slices, sAP, firing rate, LTD)

Acute sagittal brain slices from WT or hAPP mice were prepared by decapitation of the mice after isoflurane anaesthesia. Brains were removed quickly and immersed during 3–4 min in ice-cold freshly prepared cutting artificial cerebrospinal fluid (cutting aCSF) containing (in mM) 214 sucrose, 2.5 KCl, 2 $CaCl_2$, 2 $MgSO_4$, 1.25 NaH_2PO_2, 26 $NaHCO_3$ and 10 glucose and oxygenated with 95% O_2/ 5% CO_2. Sagittal 350 μm slices were generated using a vibratome (VT 1000S; Leica Microsystems) and were incubated in standard carboxygenated aCSF (in mM: 125 NaCl, 2.5 KCl, 2 $CaCl_2$, 2 $MgSO_4$, 1.25 NaH_2PO_2, 26 $NaHCO_3$ and 10 glucose, osmolarity 305 mOsm) at 34 °C for 20 min. The incubation continued at room temperature (RT) for another hour before each slice was transferred to a submerged recording chamber and perfused continuously with carboxygenated aCSF.

Somatic or dendritic (approximately 250 μm from the soma) current-clamp recordings were performed on slices from mice aged 3–4 months at RT (24 to 28 °C). The slices were continuously perfused with carboxygenated standard aCSF. Depending on the experiment, aCSF was supplemented with control or test article REM0043039 at 2 μM. For whole-cell recordings, patch pipettes were filled with a solution containing (in mM) 140 K-gluconate, 5 NaCl, 2 $MgCl_2$, 10 HEPES, 0.5 EGTA, 2 MgATP, 0.4 NaGTP, osmolarity 305, pH adjusted to 7.25 with KOH. The soma or dendrite of large CA1 pyramidal neurons were identified and patch-clamped after visual approach of the recording pipette using a combination of infrared light and differential interference contrast (DIC) optics. Patch electrodes had a resistance of around 5 and 14 MΩ when filled for somatic and dendritic recording, respectively. Recordings were terminated when the series resistances exceeded 40 MΩ. Signals were digitised, and low-pass filtered at 10 kHz. The signal was amplified with an Axopatch 200B amplifier, digitised by a Digidata 1550 interface and sampled with Clampex 10 (Molecular Devices).

For the single AP experiment, a single spike was elicited by injecting a 2 milliseconds depolarising current pulse. The following action potential (AP) parameters were analysed: AP area, AP amplitude, AP delay, AP half-width, AP rising slope, AP decay slope, afterhyperpolarisation (AHP) amplitude (calculated by subtracting the minimum value following the AP from the resting membrane potential), AHP half-width and AHP time-to-peak. Somatic single AP recordings were performed at baseline and after 25 min vehicle or compound perfusion. Dendritic single AP recording occurred after at least one hour vehicle or compound incubation and throughout the experiment in perfusion.

Dendritic firing rate of CA1 cells was recorded in response to hyperpolarising and depolarising steps (– 0.2 to + 0.45 nA, steps of 0.05 nA) after at least one hour incubation with vehicle or compound at 2 μM and throughout the experiment in perfusion. The mean number of action potentials (firing rate) was plotted in function of current step intensity. In addition, AP amplitude, AP onset, AP threshold, AHP amplitude, input resistance and current-voltage relation were analysed. Results were corrected for vehicle effect.

Somatic voltage-clamp recording of CA1 cells was performed to determine total (P1) and I_A-type potassium (K^+) currents (P2). Electrodes were filled with an intracellular solution containing (in mM) 145 KCl, 1 $MgCl_2$, 10 EGTA, 0.2 $CaCl_2$, and 10 HEPES buffer (Sigma). Tetrodotoxin (TTX; 1 mM) and $CdCl_2$ (0.3 mM) were added into the aCSF to block Na^+ voltage dependent channels and Ca^{2+} channels, respectively. Membrane potential was held at – 60 mV. Depolarising potential steps were preceded by 300 milliseconds hyperpolarising pulse at – 120 mV (voltage protocol P1) to evoke outward currents including I_A. I_A was inactivated by a 50 milliseconds prepulse at + 10 mV (voltage protocol P2). I_A was obtained by subtracting the current evoked from P2 from that evoked from P1 (Klee et al. 1997; Numann et al. 1987). The amplitude of I_A was measured at the peak of the current (at 20 milliseconds after the onset of testing pulses).

MGluR-mediated long-term depression (LTD) was induced by perfusion of 50 μM (S)-3,4-dihydroxyphenylglycine (DHPG; Tocris) to WT (C57Bl/6 J background, 6–8 weeks old) brain slices for 5 min. DHPG was dissolved in H_2O at a stock concentration of 50 mM and aliquots were stored at – 80 °C until dilution into aCSF. Field excitatory postsynaptic potentials (fEPSPs) recordings were performed in the stratum radiatum using a borosilicate micropipette filled with aCSF in a submerged chamber continuously perfused with a CSF at 1.1 ml/minute. The signal was amplified with an Axopatch 200B amplifier, digitised by a Digidata 155 interface and sampled with Clampex 10 (Molecular Devices). Before baseline fEPSP recording and perfusion of DHPG, brain slices were preincubated in aCSF supplemented with vehicle or compound at 2 μM for 80 min. Perfusion of vehicle or compound continued during fEPSP recording up to 60 min after DHPG addition.

For the biochemical analysis of DHPG-induced LTD in primary cells, DIV 19–22 hippocampal neurons were pre-treated > 30 min prior to 50 μM DHPG with 1 μM TTX (Tocris) as well as 1.5 μM REM0043039 or vehicle (DMSO). DHPG was weighed freshly to make up a stock of 25 mM in sterile H_2O. After 30 min, DHPG added to the cells at a final concentration of 50 μM for 10 min. Cells were lysed on ice for ten minutes in RIPA Buffer (Thermo Fisher) containing 1× Halt^{TM} Protease and Phosphatase Inhibitor Cocktail (Thermo Fisher) and debris was removed by centrifuging the homogenate at 14.000 x g for 10 min at 4 °C. Samples were stored at – 80 °C until further use.

Tissue/cell processing and Western blot analysis

Cortex samples of hAPP*PS1 mice were homogenised using a potter-type mechanical homogeniser (VOS 14 S40, rate ~ 750 rpm VWR) in 6.5 weight-volumes of cold tris-protease-phosphatase-inhibition buffer (TPPI--buffer) containing (in mM) 50 Tris-HCl (pH 8.1), 250 saccharose, 3 $MgCl_2$, 1 EDTA, 1 EGTA and a cocktail of Halt^{TM} protease and phosphatase inhibitors (Thermo Fisher). Whole extract was aliquoted and stored at – 80 ° C until further use.

Tissue whole protein extracts were diluted with an equal volume of SDS-PAGE sample buffer (containing final concentrations of 1% (*w*/*v*) SDS and 2.5% (*v*/*v*) 2-mercaptoethanol) and were denatured and reduced by incubation at 95 °C for 10 min. The same was done for Cell extracts after adjusting amounts of protein and volume for each sample (determined using Biorad's DC protein assay (Biorad)). Proteins were separated on 4–12% Bis-Tris or 7.5% Tris-HCl gels (Criterion XT Precast Gel, 26 well, 15 μl, 1.0 mm; Biorad). After semi-dry electrotransfer (iBlot™, Invitrogen) to PVDF-membranes (iBlot™ Gel Transfer Stacks, PVDF, Regular, Invitrogen), the membranes were incubated 2 h or overnight in tris-buffered saline (TBS, pH 7.6) with 0.1% (v/v) Tween-20 containing either 5% (*w*/*v*) non-fat dry milk or 5% bovine serum albumin (BSA) (depending on primary antibody). The next day, the blots were incubated with primary antibody for 2 h or overnight. After washing and incubation for at least 2 h with an HRP-conjugated secondary antibody (goat-anti-mouse or goat-anti-rabbit IgG, DAKO; goat-anti-rabbit IgG, Cell Signaling) blots were developed by the ECL detection system (LiteAblotR Plus ECL substrate, EuroClone; or SuperSignal West Femto Maximum Sensitivity Substrate, product 34096, Thermo Fisher) and images were recorded digitally (VisionWorks Acquisition, UVP) at different exposure times. Dedicated software (VisionWorks Analysis, UVP) was used for densitometric analysis.

Primary antibodies used: rabbit p44/42MAPK (ERK1/2) (Cell Signaling, #4695), rabbit phospho-p44/42MAPK (ERK1/2) (Thr202/Thr204) (Cell Signaling, #4370), rabbit alpha-Tubulin (Abcam, ab24246), rabbit GAPDH (Abcam), rabbit Rap1A (Novus Biologicals, NBP1–97-489), rabbit Pde6δ (Genetex, GTX109240), mouse

AD2 (Biorad, #56484), pS262 Tau (ProSci, XBP-4276), pan-Tau (Tau5, Calbiochem, #577801), HT7 Tau (human Tau, Thermo Fisher, MN1000). HRP-conjugated secondary goat anti-rabbit (Dako), goat anti-mouse (Dako) and goat-anti-rabbit (Cell Signaling) antibodies were used.

Docking procedures

All calculations were carried out using Schrodinger Suite software [24] with default parameters except when otherwise specified. High resolution X-ray crystal structure of farnesylated Rheb in complex with Pde6δ [25], PDB code 3T5G, was selected to perform molecular modelling calculations. Rheb protein atoms were deleted to give the starting structure of isolated Pde6δ in complex with farnesyl moiety fused to terminal Rheb cysteine residue. Protein preparation was then performed in order to add hydrogen atoms, to remove water molecules or to identify possible interacting water, to fix missing sidechain atoms or missing residues, to assess protonation state of ionisable amino acids. Docking simulations were performed using GlideXP (extra precision).

Statistical analysis and data collection

To assess whether the means of two groups are statistically different from each other, we used an unpaired two-tailed t-test unless specified otherwise. Ordinary two-way ANOVA was applied to compare differences in the mean between groups with two independent variables followed by Sidak's test for multiple comparisons as post-hoc analysis unless stated otherwise. Where appropriate, the Grubb's method (alpha = 0.05) was used to identify outliers.

For all ex-vivo electrophysiology and in-vivo studies both animals and treatment were randomly allocated to a treatment group (digital randomisation occurred in Excel using the rand-function). In-vivo and ex-vivo practicalities and analysis of data was always performed in a blind manner after which the treatment groups were decoded by the study director.

All statistical analysis was done with the Prism 7 software (GraphPad). Values are given as mean ± standard error of the mean unless indicated otherwise. Error probabilities of $P < 0.05$ were considered statistically significant. Indication of p-value summaries: $^{*}p < 0.05$, $^{**}p < 0.01$, $^{***}p < 0.001$, $^{****}p < 0.0001$ or $\#\#\#\#p < 0.0001$.

Target identification screen

A three-hybrid approach used to identify the target as described [26, 27]. To this end REM0043037 (B1) was fused with methotrexate, finally resulting in REM0044931 (B3), as a tool compound for identifying interacting proteins was prepared (see "Preparation of fusion compound used for the target identification screen").

Preparation of fusion compound used for the target identification screen

Abbreviations: CC – Column chromatography; DCM – Dichloromethane; TEA – Triethylamine; DMF – N,N-dimethylformamide; BOP: (benzotriazol-1-yloxy) tris (dimethylamino) -phosphonium hexafluorophosphate; TLC – Thin layer chromatography; DMSO. Analysis by LC-MS-UV was carried out on an Agilent system with a 3 × 150 mm Phenomenex Luna 5 µm column, flow 0.8 ml/minute; UV detection at 240 nm and 300 nm, neg. And pos. MS detection (150–1500 amu, fast mode); ambient temperature; gradient made from ACN and aq. 10 mM ammonium formate pH 9. MS (pos.), MS (neg.) and DAD information was recorded online. For MS spectra only the most abundant isotope signal is indicated; for UV spectra, only signals > 220 nm are indicated

Preparation of compound 38

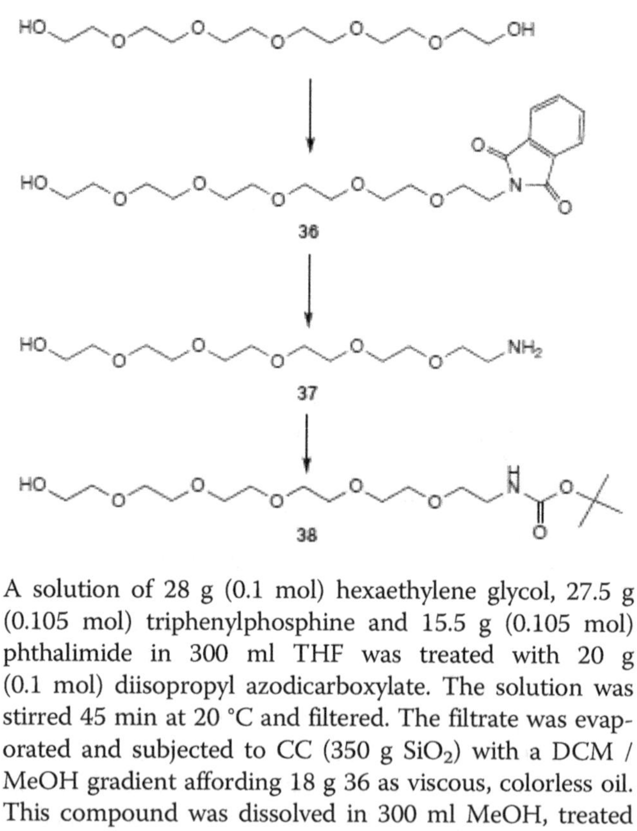

A solution of 28 g (0.1 mol) hexaethylene glycol, 27.5 g (0.105 mol) triphenylphosphine and 15.5 g (0.105 mol) phthalimide in 300 ml THF was treated with 20 g (0.1 mol) diisopropyl azodicarboxylate. The solution was stirred 45 min at 20 °C and filtered. The filtrate was evaporated and subjected to CC (350 g SiO_2) with a DCM / MeOH gradient affording 18 g 36 as viscous, colorless oil. This compound was dissolved in 300 ml MeOH, treated with 15 ml hydrazine monohydrate and kept overnight at 50 °C. The suspension was filtered and evaporated: 11.5 g 37 as colorless oil. This oil was suspended in 75 ml CHCl3, filtered and evaporated. The residue was dissolved in 300 ml DCM and treated with 10 g (0.1 mol) TEA and 11 g (0.05 mol) di-tert-butyl dicarbonate. After 30 min at 20 °C, the solution was evaporated, and the residue was subjected to CC (200 g SiO_2) with a DCM / MeOH gradient, yielding 15 g (40% overall) of 38 as a viscous, colorless oil.

Preparation of compound 39 (= B2)

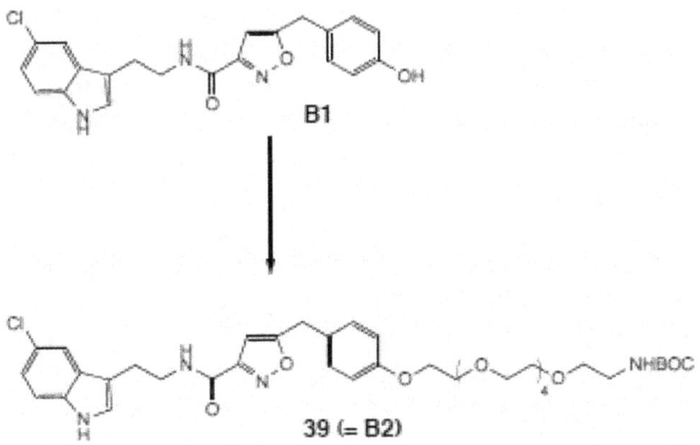

B1

39 (= B2)

A suspension of 150 mg (0.375 mmol) compound B1 (synthesised by CISTIM), 150 mg (0.4 mmol) 38 and 190 mg (0.75 mmol) 1,1′-(azodicarbonyl)dipiperidine in 5 ml THF was heated at 50 °C and then treated with a solution of 150 mg (0.75 mmol) tributylphosphine in 1 ml THF. After 45 min at 50 °C, the suspension was filtered, and the filtrate was evaporated. The residue was subjected to CC (6 g SiO_2) with a hexane / EtOAc gradient. The product-containing fractions were evaporated affording 250 mg of a white solid (containing about 30 wt % reduced 1,1′-(azodicarbonyl)dipiperidine). Fifty mg of this mixture were subjected to prep. TLC with EtOAc as eluent. The product-containing band was scratched off and eluted with EtOAc / MeOH 9:1 yielding 18 mg 39 as a colorless oil.

Preparation of compound 40

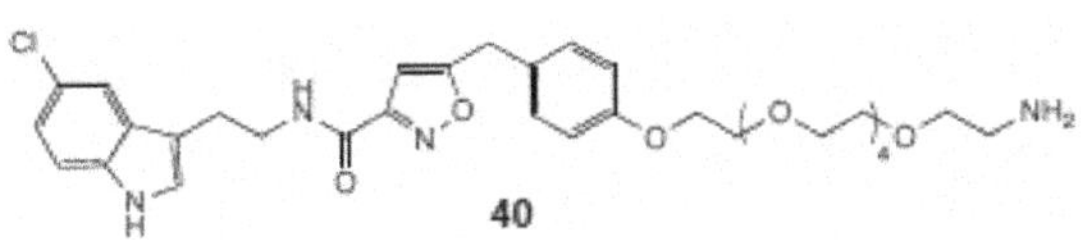

40

At 20 °C, 200 mg of the material obtained above (containing about 70% 39) were dissolved in 2.5 ml TFA / H_2O 9:1. After 45 min, 10 ml toluene were added, and the mixture was evaporated. The residue was subjected to CC (6 g SiO_2) with a DCM / MeOH gradient; after elution of by-products with 4% MeOH, 2% TEA was added to the eluent to elute the product. The product-containing fractions were evaporated, giving 125 mg 40 as colourless, viscous oil (63% yield based on B1).

Preparation of compound 41

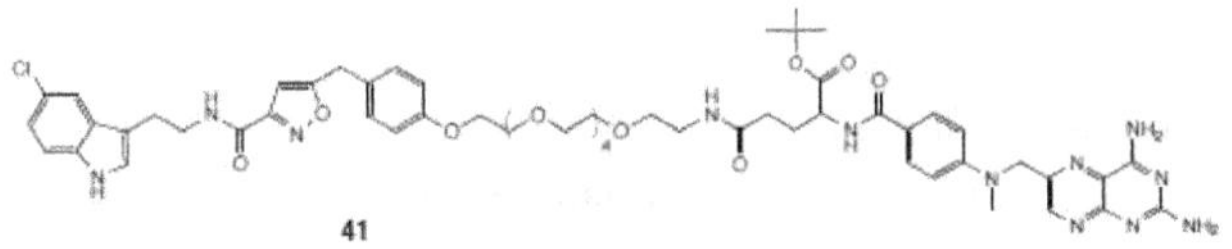

41

A solution of 125 mg (0.19 mmol) 40 and 105 mg (0.2 mmol) MTX (COOtBu) COOLi in 1.0 ml DMF was treated with 100 mg (0.22 mmol) BOP. After 30 min at RT, LC-MS indicated completion of the reaction. The reaction mixture was diluted with 8 ml MeOH/H_2O 1:1 and purified by MPLC (250 ml MeOH / aq. 10 mM NH_3 1:3, 250 ml ACN / aq. 10 mM NH_3 4:6, 500 ml ACN / aq. 10 mM NH_3 1:1). The product containing fractions (analysed by LC-MS) were evaporated, co-evaporated with MeOH and then with DCM and dried: 170 mg (78%) product 41 as yellow, solid foam. LC (10–100% in 15 min): 8.2 min (96%) UV: 230 nm (max), 260 nm, 305 nm, 375 nm MS (pos): 1150 (M + 1) MS (neg): no signal detected.

Preparation of fusion compound used for the target identification screen (alias 42)

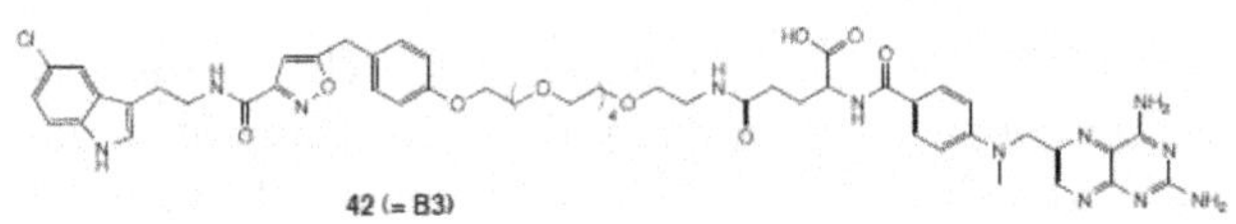

42 (= B3)

Solid 41 (170 mg, 0.145 mmol) was dissolved in 2.0 ml TFA/H_2O 9:1 and stirred 50 min at 20 °C. The reaction mixture was cooled to 4 °C and neutralised by drop-wise addition of conc. aq. NH_3 solution, diluted with 5 ml MeOH/H_2O 1:1 and purified by MPLC (500 ml MeOH / aq. 10 mM NH_3 1:9, 500 ml ACN / aq. 10 mM NH_3 7:3). The product containing fractions were evaporated, co-evaporated with MeOH and dried: 120 mg (75%) of product 42 (REM0044931) as a yellow solid. ^{1}H-NMR (300 MHz, CD_3OD / $CDCl_3$ 2:1): LC (10–100% in 15 min): 5.6 min (98%), UV: 230 nm (max), 260 nm, 305 nm, 375 nm, MS (neg.): 1092 (M-1), MS (pos): 1094 (M + 1).

Results

Identification of small molecule modifiers counteracting mechanisms underlying neurotoxicity in AD

In order to identify new drug targets and therapeutics underlying AD we implemented a neuronal cell-based model of Ca^{2+}-driven neurodegeneration. For this reason, we used neuroblastoma cells containing mutant human tau (TAU-P301L) as these cells were found to be more susceptible to toxic stimuli compared to control cells (Additional file 1: Figure S1a). Neurotoxicity in the model was induced by incubating the cells with ATRA [28]. Upon chronic exposure to ATRA a significant increase in toxicity within seven days in culture was consistently detected (Fig. 1a; Additional file 1: Figure S1b).

Quantification of Ca^{2+} indicator fura-2 fluorescence in the cells following ATRA challenge (Fig. 1b) revealed a significant increase in $[Ca^{2+}]_i$ concurring with toxicity. We thus assessed whether the rise in $[Ca^{2+}]_i$ levels is causal to toxicity and restrained Ca^{2+} influx from the extracellular environment through silencing STIM1 expression, an activator of the Orai channels facilitating influx of extracellular Ca^{2+} into the cytosol. Decreasing STIM1 expression in these cells led to a robust reduction of ATRA induced toxicity (Fig. 1c). In addition, isradipine, a voltage-gated Ca^{2+} channel (VGCC) inhibitor with neuroprotective potential [29], also rescued cell death in the model (Additional file 3: Figure S2a). Thus, ATRA induced toxicity is reduced by lowering $[Ca^{2+}]_i$ in this model.

Deregulated kinase activity has been associated with neuronal dysfunction in AD. Thus, $[Ca^{2+}]_i$ which is a known regulator of mitogen-activated protein kinase (MAPK) signalling [30], may thus mechanistically may underlie the elevated extracellular signal-regulated kinase (ERK1/2) activity observed in preclinical AD models as well as patients [31, 32]. We therefore quantified ERK1/2 activity throughout the ATRA incubation period. The first four days ERK1/2 activity remained relatively low (data not shown), however, the following days, when toxicity started to rise, its activation was found to be significantly increased compared to control conditions (Fig. 1d). To further validate that MAPK ERK deregulation contributes ATRA induced cell death, we applied the MEK inhibitor U0126. Indeed, addition of U0126 counteracted ATRA induced toxicity in a concentration dependent manner (Additional file 3: Figure S2b). This indicates that ERK1/2 signalling, likely as a result of deregulated $[Ca^{2+}]_i$ observed in the model, plays an important role in mediating cell death as a consequence of ATRA exposure.

Taken together, the model features a rise in $[Ca^{2+}]_i$ and aberrant downstream signalling (at least ERK1/2) leading to cell death. The assay therefore recapitulates some key characteristics of AD-like neurotoxicity and represents an attractive in-vitro system for identifying mediators and modulators of neurodegeneration.

Subsequently, the model was used to screen library (compiled and provided by reMYND NV) of small molecules for their potential to inhibit toxicity. This led to the identification of structurally highly similar tryptamine-derivatives REM0042826 and REM0043039 (collectively referred to as REM) (Fig. 1e), which potently and concentration dependently lowered cell loss (Fig. 1f and Additional file 1: Figure S1) as well as reducing elevated levels of $[Ca^{2+}]_i$ (Fig. 1g). In order to emphasise the relevance of the phenotypic screening system described above for identifying novel neuroprotective compounds, we also tested REM in a more conventional AD model involving rat hippocampal neurons challenged with Aβo's. Incubating the neurons with Aβo's resulted in pronounced cell death. However, in the presence of REM, the soluble Aβo-elicited cytotoxicity was countered, independently illustrating the compound's neuroprotective activity (Additional file 4: Figure S3). Altogether, we identified novel compounds that restore Ca^{2+} homeostasis through which they appear to convey their protective effects in cellular models of AD.

Binding of REM in the prenyl-binding pocket of Pde6δ is required for mitigating toxicity

Following the identification of the REM, we set out to identify the corresponding target mediating their neuroprotective effects. To this end we coupled REM to methotrexate (resulting in REM0044931, see Methods) and used it as bait in a yeast-based 3-hybrid system [27] to determine interacting proteins using a human cDNA expression library (constructed by Dualsystems Biotech). This led to the identification of several cDNA fragments encoding (parts of) Pde6δ. We independently confirmed the interaction of the compound with full length human Pde6δ in MASPIT [26], a mammalian cell based 3-hybrid assay, and revealed a concentration-dependent interaction with a half-maximal concentration for binding of 45 nM (Fig. 2a). A direct interaction between REM and Pde6δ was validated further in a cell free context by co-immunoprecipitation (Fig. 2b).

In order to confirm that Pde6δ mediates the neuroprotective properties of REM, we silenced PDE6δ in the toxicity cell model (Fig. 2c). Silencing reduced cell death, indicating that Pde6δ mediates (at least in part) toxicity in the model. Although the remaining toxicity in silenced cells was slightly reduced by the compound, an effect which is presumably due to a residual Pde6δ presence, it was not decreased below the level obtained with REM in non-silenced control cells. Thus, the toxicity-mitigating effect of REM requires the presence of Pde6δ.

To better understand the interaction between REM and its target we aligned the cDNA's identified in the three-hybrid screens. This revealed that the minimal region of Pde6δ required for interaction with REM corresponds to a part of its prenyl-binding pocket (data not shown). The latter hydrophobic cavity accommodates fatty acid chains of small GTPases and is necessary to extract and transport these between cellular membranes [33–35]. In-silico modelling then further elucidated that the identified compounds align closely with prenyl-chains (Fig. 2d). This common topology raised the possibility that it was possible for REM to fit inside Pde6δ's hydrophobic pocket. Using the cavity's position to define the docking search space, we assessed

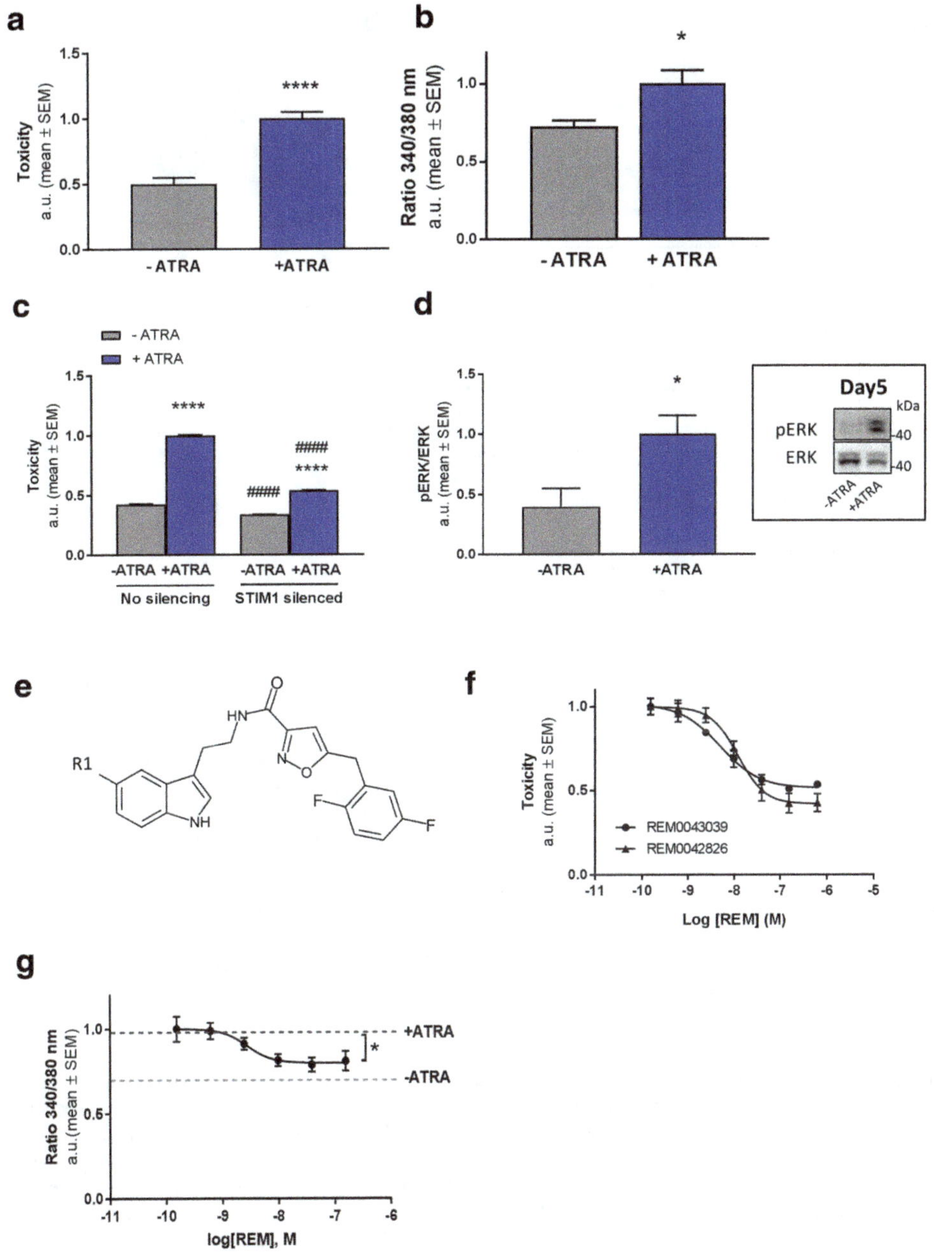

Fig. 1 Development of an AD model for identifying neuroprotective compounds. **a** Toxicity was determined by quantifying LDH release in the medium in BE (2)-M17 neuroblastoma cells incubated for 7 days with or without ATRA. The ATRA induced toxicity in the cells represents the "toxicity assay" used in all following experiments ($n = 5$; +/− ATRA: $P < 0.0001$; $t = 7{,}346$ DF = 8). **b** Cytosolic Ca^{2+} levels quantified by Ca^{2+}-indicator Fura-2 fluorescence ratio (340 nm/380 nm) in hTAU-P301L cells after 6 days with and without ATRA treatment in the toxicity assay ($n = 3$; $P = 0.0435$; $t = 2.915$; DF = 4). **c** Genetic silencing of STIM1 reduces toxicity in the toxicity assay. # denotes the effect of STIM1 silencing compared to unsilenced cells, * indicates the effect of ATRA treatment (silencing: $P < 0.0001$; DF = 1; F (1, 36)=4048; ATRA treatment: $P < 0.0001$; DF = 1; F (1, 36)=8006; Corrected for multiple comparison using Tukey's test: +/−ATRA - silencing: $P < 0.0001$; q = 132.4; DF = 36; −ATRA +/− silencing: $P < 0.0001$; q = 20.68; DF = 36; +/−ATRA + silencing: P < 0.0001; q = 46.53; DF = 36; +ATRA +/− silencing: P < 0.0001; q = 106.6; DF = 36). **d** Increased MAPK signalling prior to toxicity measured by western blot in the cells treated with or without ATRA (day 5). Data are normalised to the "control" (−ATRA) condition ($n = 4$; $P = 0.0322$, $t = 2.775$, $DF = 6$). A representative immunoblot is shown in the inset next to the graph. **e** The chemical structure of the REM compounds. R1 could be either Cl (REM0042826) or F (REM0043039) (Additional file 2: Supplementary Methods). **f** Concentration-response curves of ATRA-toxicity reducing effect REM0042826 (EC_{50} = 12 nM) and REM0043039 (EC_{50} = 5 nM) in the toxicity assay (n = 7 or 5 for REM0043039 or REM0042826 respectively). **g** Concentration-response curve (n = 3) of the cytosolic Ca^{2+} reducing effect of REM, (EC_{50} of 3 nM) in the toxicity assay. The dotted grey line represents the average basal Ca^{2+} levels of vehicle treated cells in the model (One-way ANOVA, REM treatment: $P = 0.0387$; $F = 3.386$; $DF = 5$)

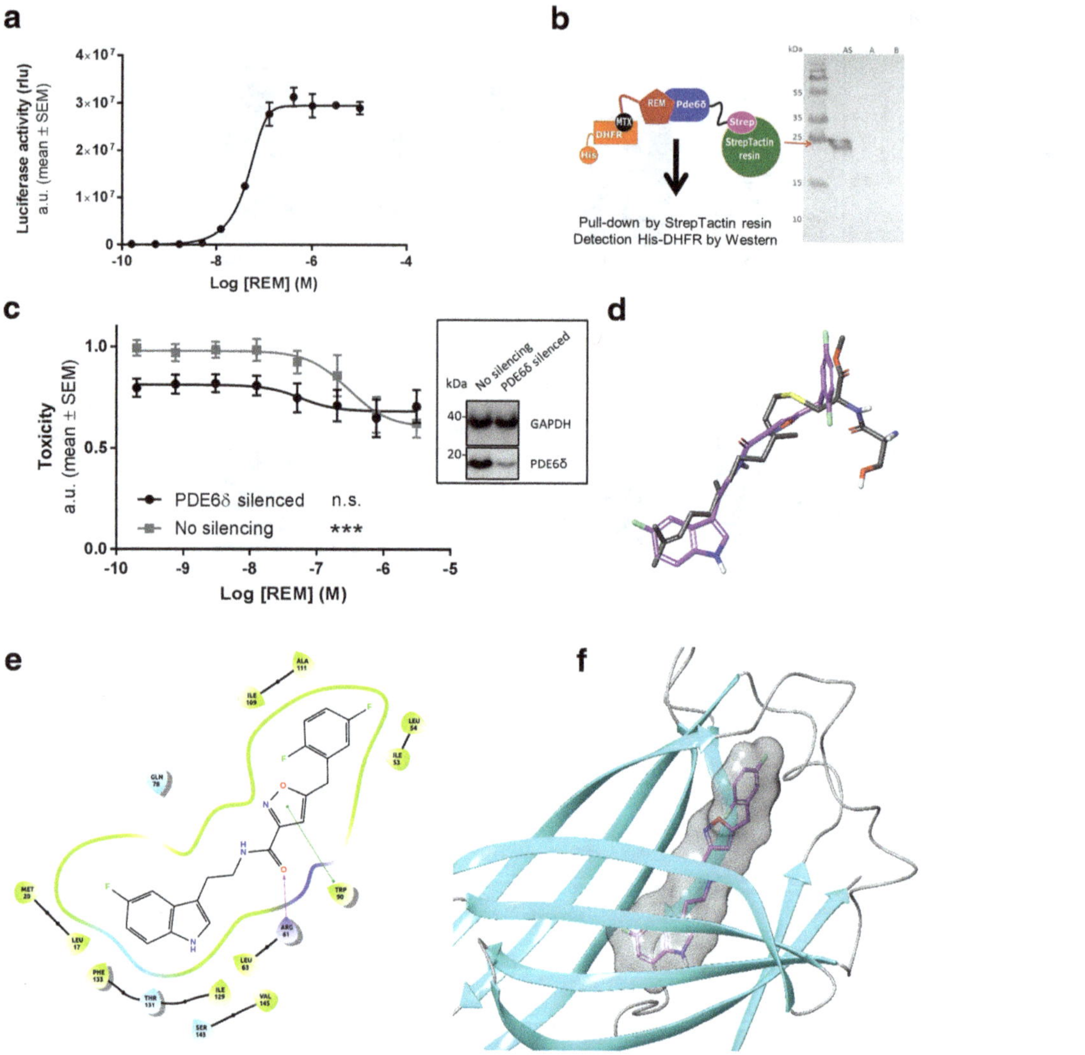

Fig. 2 REM bind to the prenyl-binding pocket of Pde6δ. **a** Concentration-dependent interaction of methotrexate fused REM compound (REM0044931) to full-length Pde6δ in the mammalian 3-hybrid assay MASPIT (EC_{50} = 45 nM; *n* = 3). **b** Pde6δ-Strep and REM compound interaction assay. *Left,* schematic representation: *E. coli* lysates producing Pde6δ-Strep, *E. coli* lysates with His-tagged DHFR and 10 μM REM were mixed and subjected to a Strep-Tactin pull-down. *Right,* co-precipitation of DHFR-His was assessed by Western analysis. Pull-down with all compounds as described above (lane AS), without REM-MTX (lane A) or without Pde6δ-Strep (lane B). **c** *Left,* genetic silencing of PDE6δ in the toxicity assay in function of increasing concentrations REM (*n* = 6). Box on the *right,* efficiency of silencing validated by Western blot ((representative immunoblots; immunostaining of GAPDH was determined as a loading control; Pde6δ expression was reduced on average by 88% ± 3%; Average ± SEM) (One-way ANOVA (REM treatment); siNC: *P* = 0.0002; F = 5.29; DF = 7; siPDE6δ: n.s.)). **d** Superimposition of REM compound (purple) and farnesyl (grey). **e** REM docking into the Pde6δ prenyl-binding pocket showing all interacting amino acids. In green indicates hydrophobic amino acids, in dark blue positively charged amino acids and in cyan neutral polar amino acids. **f** REM docked in Pde6δ's prenyl-binding pocket (ribbon)

whether REM interacts with the pocket. Validation of the docking procedure came from re-docking the farnesyl moiety into the Pde6δ structure. The best docked pose showed a root-mean-square deviation of less than 0.5 Å (all heavy atoms) compared to the published X-ray farnesyl position (Additional file 5: Figure S4a). Taken together, docking of REM revealed that the compound fits well and with high affinity in this cavity (Fig. 2ef and f).

Closer analysis found that the indole group extends deep into the pocket overlapping with the dimethylallyl end of farnesyl and that the indole nitrogen atom is oriented toward Ile129 and Thr131, creating weak interactions, while the amide oxygen atom is engaged in a hydrogen bond with the Arg61 side chain. Furthermore, REM's oxazole ring forms a pi-pi stacking with Trp90 and the di-fluoro phenyl group occupies the highly hydrophobic entrance of the pocket. The modelling data thus indicate that REM can bind into the prenyl-binding cavity and as a result may prevent Pde6δ's prenylated substrates from interacting with it.

REM binding to Pde6δ disrupts the interaction with Rap1 GTPase required for lowering $[Ca^{2+}]_i$ and toxicity

Since the modelling data indicated that REM might compete for Pde6δ substrate binding, we set out to identify such anticipated interactor(s) in an affinity purification coupled with mass spectrometry assay [36] (Fig. 3a) and assessed whether these interactions are impacted by REM. In absence of the compound, a host of previously described Pde6δ binding partners were identified, including Arl3 and RPGR [33, 37, 38] as well as apparently novel interactors like Lamin B2 and Fbxo10. Also, Rab28 and Rap1A representing prenylated GTPases were found to interact with Pde6δ. Importantly, of all detected interactions, only the Pde6δ-Rap1A interaction was significantly and robustly reduced by REM.

Moreover, disruption of the Pde6δ-Rap1A interaction was found to be specific as the interaction with non-prenylated binding partners of Pde6δ such as Arl3 and RPGR, remained unchanged. In fact, there appears to be further specificity regarding the nature of the poly-isoprene lipid group, illustrated by the distinct effects on Pde6δ substrates Rap1A and Rab28. In the presence of REM, Pde6δ's interaction with geranylgeranylated (C20) Rap1A is inhibited, contrary to that with farnesylated (C15) Rab28. This selectivity of the compound may be a reflection of the intrinsically higher affinity of Pde6δ towards farnesyl over

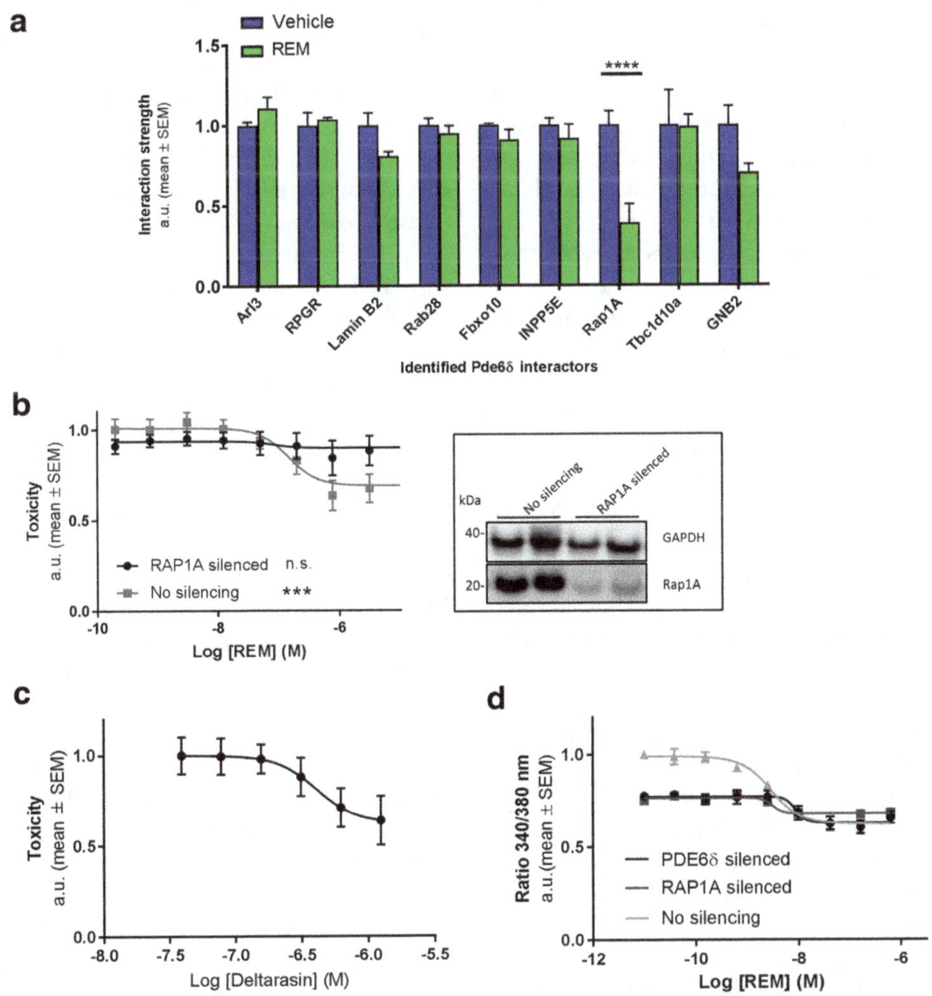

Fig. 3 REM reduces toxicity and $[Ca^{2+}]_i$ by selectively abrogating the interaction of Rap1 with Pde6δ. **a** Affinity purification coupled with mass spectrometry assay to identify interactors associating with Pde6δ in a REM dependent fashion. Signals for each interactor were normalised to the vehicle condition (n = 3; Treatment: $P = 0.01$; DF = 1; F (1, 32)=7.508; Rap1A: $P < 0.0001$; $t = 5.284$; DF = 32). **b** *Left,* the impact of genetic silencing of RAP1A in the toxicity assay in function of increasing concentrations REM ($n = 6$). Box at the *right,* efficiency of silencing validated by Western analysis (representative immunoblots; immunostaining of GAPDH was determined as a loading control; Rap1A expression was reduced on average by 66% ± 8%; Average ± SEM). (One-way ANOVA (REM treatment); siNC: $P = 0.0004$; F = 4.615; DF = 8; siRAP1A: n.s.). **c** Concentration-response curve of deltarasin in the toxicity assay ($EC_{50} = 480$ nM; $n = 3$). **d** The impact of genetic silencing of PDE6δ or RAP1A in the neuroblastoma cells on cytosolic Ca^{2+} levels in the toxicity assay in function of increasing REM concentrations ($n = 2$ per concentration; one representative experiment of three is shown)

geranylgeranyl [39]. Thus, the experimental data confirmed the *in-silico* docking results and revealed that REM binds to and occludes Pde6δ's hydrophobic pocket, preventing the interaction specifically with a geranylgeranylated substrate which we identified as Rap1A.

From these data we envisaged that the toxicity-lowering effects of REM are brought about by abrogating the interaction of Rap1A with Pde6δ. To test this hypothesis, we assessed whether toxicity in our model required Rap1A. Silencing RAP1A completely prevented any REM compound induced decrease in toxicity (Fig. 3b), indicating that REM requires Rap1A for its effect. We independently confirmed this result by using deltarasin, a compound structurally unrelated to REM, which also binds in Pde6δ's prenyl-binding pocket [40] and, similarly to REM, showed a trend towards counteracting cell-death in our model of neurotoxicity (Fig. 3c).

Having established that REM targets the Rap1-Pde6δ interaction for lowering neuronal toxicity in our model, we tested whether decreasing elevated $[Ca^{2+}]_i$ requires both proteins. To this end, we measured $[Ca^{2+}]_i$ levels in Pde6δ and Rap1A silenced cells in function of REM treatment in the neurotoxicity model. This revealed that silencing of both PDE6δ and RAP1A reduced $[Ca^{2+}]_i$ levels to a similar extent (Fig. 3d), indicating that both Pde6δ and Rap1A are required for elevated $[Ca^{2+}]_i$ in the model. Furthermore, in both Pde6δ and Rap1A silenced cells, the already low levels of $[Ca^{2+}]_i$ were not reduced below the levels recorded in non-silenced cells by REM. Thus, the REM mediated decrease of $[Ca^{2+}]_i$ in the model is, like toxicity, dependent on Pde6δ and Rap1A.

Taken together, we revealed geranylgeranylated Rap1A as a novel substrate of Pde6δ's prenyl-binding pocket and that this interaction is involved in Ca^{2+} dyshomeostasis and associated cytotoxicity.

Disruption of the Pde6δ-Rap1 interaction has distinct effects on spatially discrete Rap1-functions

Pde6δ is known to act as a cytosolic chaperone controlling the subcellular membrane localisation (and thereby their function) of prenylated substrates [25, 34, 37, 41], such as Rap1. In particular, Rap1 was shown to regulate signalling of MAPK-ERK1/2 at spatially discrete subcellular locations [42–46]. In resting neurons for instance, basal levels of Ca^{2+} and cAMP [47] control a membrane pool of Rap1-ERK1/2, which phosphorylates (inactivates) protein Kv4.2, the main A-type K^+ channel driving the fast transient outward K^+ current (I_A) involved in action potential AHP and repolarisation in pyramidal neurons [48]. On the other hand, upon depolarisation a different subcellular pool of Rap1-ERK1/2 has been implicated in signalling towards nuclear targets mediating gene transcription [49], whereas an exclusively intracellular pool of mGluR-Rap1-ERK1/2 mediates the internalisation of surface AMPA receptors during LTD [50–52].

Given that Pde6δ regulates the subcellular membrane localisation of prenylated substrates, we hypothesised that Pde6δ mediated control over Rap1 functions at spatially discrete pools specifies its signalling outcome. Accordingly, disruption of the Rap1-Pde6δ interaction by REM should alter activity of distinct ERK1/2 signalling pathways. To test this hypothesis, we assessed basal and mGluR driven Rap1-ERK1/2 activity.

As shown previously in the toxicity model, basal ERK1/2 activity was found to be strongly increased under conditions of cell death (Fig. 4a). However, in the presence of REM, this ERK1/2 over-activation was strongly reduced (Fig. 4a). Also, in hippocampal neurons, where synaptic activity was eliminated using the Na^+ channel blocker TTX, REM treatment led to a reduction in basal ERK1/2 activity (Fig. 4b). Conversely, upon stimulation with the selective group 1 mGluR agonist DHPG the fold Rap1-ERK1/2 activation in cells incubated with REM was increased compared to vehicle treated cells (Fig. 4b). Collectively, these results indicate that the basal activity of Rap1-ERK1/2 signalling in resting cells, which is considered to represent the membrane-associated pool [49], is decreased by REM, while activation of an intracellular DHPG responsive pool [53] of Rap1-ERK1/2 signalling is increased.

We then tested whether such REM-induced changes on different pools of Rap1-ERK1/2 resulted in functional changes in an AD model. Previous studies have shown that lowering basal Rap1-ERK1/2 signalling reduces the phosphorylation of plasma membrane Kv4.2 channels and thereby increases neuronal repolarisation [49, 54]. This regulation appears highly relevant for AD because in $A\beta_{1-42}$ exposed hippocampal primary neurons and in numerous human transgenic APP mouse models the activity of Kv4.2 is reduced [10, 55]. As a result of this, transgenic APP models were shown to feature an A-type K^+ channel-deficiency driving neuronal hyperactivity [10, 56] and therefore we anticipated REM to mitigate this phenotype. To test this, we quantified the I_A in function of REM treatment. Hippocampal CA1 somatic voltage-clamp recordings were performed in acute slices excised from human transgenic APP[V717I] (hAPP) [21] mice orally administered with vehicle or a single dose of REM at 30 mg/kg. The recorded I_A current (as isolated by subtraction of the 4-AP insensitive from the total K+ current (Additional file 6: Figure S5a)) was significantly increased at higher depolarising pulses by REM compared to the vehicle group (Fig. 4c).

Furthermore, to test the impact of REM on neuronal repolarisation, single action potentials (AP) were assessed by somatic patch-clamp of hippocampal CA1 pyramidal

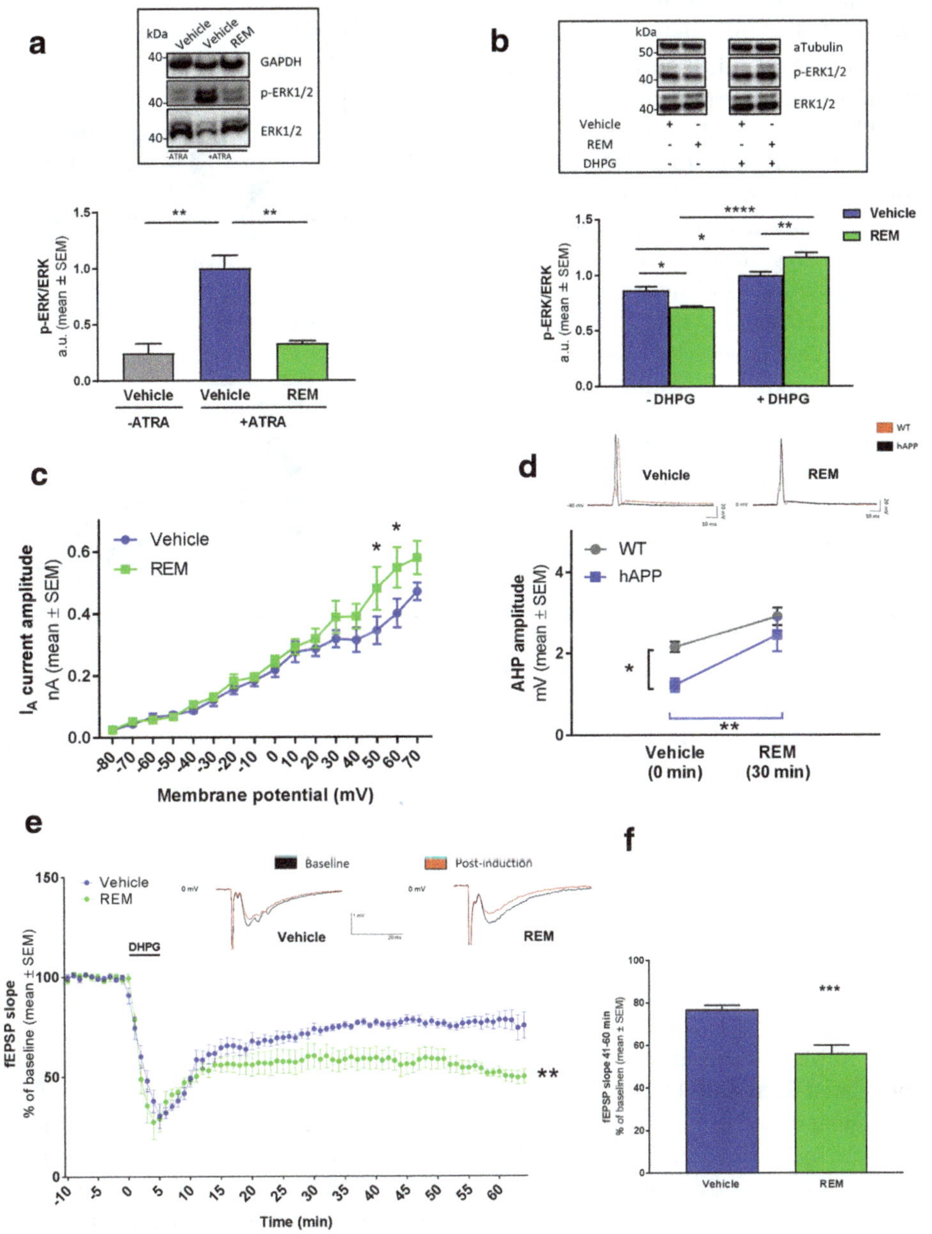

Fig. 4 REM modulates spatially discrete Rap1-ERK1/2 signalling processes. **a** Western blot analysis of ERK1/2 phosphorylation in neuroblastoma cells after 7 days with or without ATRA toxicity challenge and with or without (0.25 μM) REM ($n = 3$; Vehicle +/− ATRA: $P = 0.0066$; $t = 5.191$; DF = 4; Vehicle/REM + ATRA: $P = 0.0052$; $t = 5.55$; DF = 4). Representative Western blots are shown in inset above the graph. **b** Western blot analysis of ERK1/2 phosphorylation ratio to total ERK1/2 in DIV ≥19 mouse primary hippocampal neurons treated with or without 50 μM DHPG and REM/Vehicle as indicated ($n = 6$; ordinary two-way ANOVA followed by Tukey's multiple comparison test; $P < 0{,}0001$; DF = 1; F (1, 20) = 27,41; vehicle +/− DHPG: $P = 0{,}0248$; q = 4,431; DF = 20; REM +/− DHPG: $P < 0.0001$; q = 14,9; DF = 20; vehicle/REM - DHPG: $P = 0{,}0107$; q = 4,975; DF = 20; vehicle/REM + DHPG: $p = 0{,}0047$; q = 5,497; *DF* = 20). Representative Western blot images are shown in insets above graph. **c** K^+ current analysis in hAPP mice treated with a single dose of REM or vehicle show that application of REM increases the I_A contribution at higher membrane potentials (50–60 mV) (n = 7 per condition; RM-two way ANOVA Interaction: $P = 0.056$; DF = 15; F(15,180) = 1.691; Sidak's multiple comparison: membrane potential 50 mV Vehicle/REM: $P = 0.0326$; $t = 3.122$; DF = 192; membrane potential 60 mV Vehicle/REM: $P = 0.0130$; $t = 3.401$; DF = 192). **d** Analysis of AHP amplitudes in function of REM treatment obtained by longitudinal somatic recordings of single APs in WT and hAPP slices that were incubated with vehicle or 2 μM REM. (Two-way ANOVA repeated measures, followed by Sidak's multiple comparison test; n = 7 WT mice or $n = 8$ hAPP mice; Treatment: $P = 0.0015$; DF = 1; F (1, 13)=15.91; Genotype: $P = 0.0279$; DF = 1; F (1, 13)=6.127; WT/APP + Vehicle: $P = 0.0376$; $t = 2.502$; DF = 26; hAPP + Vehicle/REM: $P = 0.006$; $t = 3.635$; *DF* = 13.) Examples of recorded traces are shown above the graph. **e** CA3-CA1 LTD: quantification of fEPSP slopes from hippocampal slices. Slices were continuously perfused with artificial CSF containing vehicle or REM for (at least) one hour prior to (pre-incubation), as well as during and after the addition of DHPG (two-way ANOVA repeated measures; $n = 6$ mice per condition; Treatment: $P = 0.0032$; DF = 1; F (1, 10)=14.91). Example traces are shown above the graph. **f** Graph shows the summary of mean fEPSP slopes during the 41–60 min interval from **d** ($n = 6$ mice per condition; $P = 0.0008$; $t = 4.725$; DF = 10)

neurons from acute brain slices of hAPP and WT mice. These recordings revealed that the AHP amplitude was significantly decreased in hAPP mice compared to WT mice, (Fig. 4d). After these baseline measurements, treatment of the same hAPP slices with REM significantly increased (normalised) the AHP amplitude (Fig. 4d). No significant impact of REM was observed on other AP parameters in hAPP slices (data not shown). Since Kv4.2 plays a key role in regulating dendritic AP shape and propagation, we also assessed CA1 dendritic single AP's (recorded > 200 μm from soma) in hAPP acute brain slices. These recordings likewise revealed that REM robustly increased the AHP amplitude (Additional file 6: Figure S5b).

Collectively, these data indicate that REM predominantly facilitates the K^+ channel driven component of AP's. This is consistent with the hypothesis that lowering basal Rap1-ERK1/2 signalling by REM treatment increases K^+ channel activity and neuronal repolarisation.

In addition, we assessed the functional impact of a REM-driven increase in intracellular mGluR5-Rap1-ERK1/2 signalling (Fig. 4b) and ensuing LTD. As expected, DHPG induced a significant and robust decrease in fEPSP slopes compared to baseline, indicating a depression of synaptic efficacy through AMPA receptor removal (Fig. 4d) [57]. Pre-incubation with REM led to a significantly greater reduction in fEPSP slopes 40 min after the induction compared to vehicle (Fig. 4d and e), revealing that mGluR driven LTD is enhanced by the compound. Thus, these data indicate that Pde6δ controls intracellular Rap1-ERK1/2 signalling regulating synaptic plasticity.

Altogether, we demonstrated that Pde6δ modifies the outcome of different subcellular Rap1-ERK1/2 signalling pathways. Accordingly, REM, by neutralising Pde6δ's control over Rap1, reduces basal Rap1-ERK1/2 activity in resting neurons, which enhances the K^+ channel driven component of AP's; while increasing mGluR-Rap1-ERK1/2 signalling, leading to greater synaptic depression.

Abrogation of the Rap1-Pde6δ interaction by REM reduces VGCC activity

Previous studies demonstrated that Rap1-ERK1/2 signalling regulates the surface expression and consequently the activity of L-type VGCC [58]. We therefore tested whether inhibiting Pde6δ's control over Rap1 alters the activity of VGCC's, measuring Ca^{2+} influx after depolarisation induced by high extracellular K^+ in function of REM treatment. Here, the addition of potassium chloride (KCl) to the extracellular medium produced a concentration-dependent increase in $[Ca^{2+}]_i$ (Fig. 5a). This Ca^{2+} influx was shown to be in part mediated by L-type VGCC's, since the influx was reduced by approximately 50% in the presence of L-type channel specific inhibitor nifedipine (Fig. 5b). Incubation with REM significantly lowered Ca^{2+} influx only at KCl concentrations above 25 mM (Fig. 5a), indicating that REM specifically inhibits VGCC's that are active during relatively strong depolarisations such as L-type channels [59].

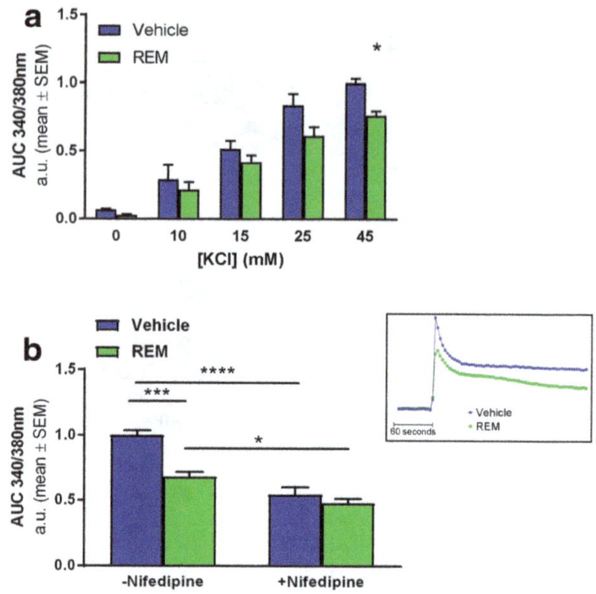

Fig. 5 REM represses VGCC activity in primary hippocampal neuron cultures. **a** Quantification of $[Ca^{2+}]_i$ influx using Ca^{2+} indicator Fura-2 after KCl instigated depolarisation at increasing concentrations in function of 1.5 μM REM treatment. Graphs represent the normalised mean Area's Under the Curve's (AUC) over a 4 min period after the addition of KCl ($n = 3$; Treatment: $P = 0.0015$; DF = 1; F (1, 20)=13.47; KCl concentration: $P < 0.0001$; DF = 4; F (4, 20)= 68.45; Multiple comparisons test: 45 mM KCl Vehicle/REM: $P = 0.0454$; $t = 2.881$; DF = 20). **b** AUC's are determined as in (a) after exposure to 45 mM KCl in presence or absence of 12.5 μM nifedipine as indicated. A representative Ca^{2+} trace (+/–REM) is depicted in the small inset next to the graph. ($n = 5$; REM Treatment: $P = 0.0003$; DF = 1; F (1, 16)=20.87; +/– Nifedipine: $P < 0.0001$; DF = 1; F (1, 16)=60.32; Interaction: $P = 0.008$; DF = 1; F(1.16) = 9.156; Multiple comparisons test: Vehicle/REM – nifedipine: P = 0.0004; $t = 5.37$; DF = 16; Vehicle +/– nifedipine: $P < 0.0001$; $t = 7.631$; DF = 16; REM +/– nifedipine: $P = 0.0241$; $t = 3.352$; DF = 16)

Co-application of nifedipine together with REM produced no additional inhibition compared to nifedipine alone, indicating that the compound acts on nifedipine sensitive channels (Fig. 5b and Additional file 7: Figure S6). Thus these data show that Rap1-ERK1/2 signalling controls VGCC surface activity and consequently neurotransmitter release upon depolarisation [58]. Further we show that Pde6δ modifies Rap1 mediated VGCC activity.

Inhibition of the Pde6δ-Rap1 interaction with REM restores spike frequency adaptation in hAPP mice

Our data thus far demonstrated that REM facilitates neuronal repolarisation, decreases synaptic efficacy and lowers VGCC activity, each process on its own geared towards restraining neuronal excitability under conditions of strong stimulation. We therefore assessed the neuronal firing rate in mouse hippocampal CA1pyramidal cells by apical dendritic current-clamp. Thus, in an initial experiment we set out to compare WT mice with their hAPP transgenic counterparts. The results show that in WT mice, the firing rate increased with each current step intensity until 250 pA, after which the firing frequency started to decline. This decline at high depolarising currents indicates a functional spike frequency adaptation process, a natural safety mechanism protecting neurons from overstimulation. Contrary to what was observed in WT cells, neurons from hAPP mice did not demonstrate a decrease in firing frequency at depolarising currents above 250 pA, meaning that mechanisms underlying spike frequency adaptation in these neurons are dysfunctional (Fig. 6a).

Having shown that overexpression of mutant hAPP led to enhanced neuronal activity, we conducted a second experiment to assess the impact of REM on the neuronal firing rates in these mice. Application of REM restored spike frequency adaptation in hAPP mice as opposed to vehicle treatment (Fig. 6b).It has to be noted however that the addition of the vehicle DMSO led to an overall increase in firing rate, an effect that has been previously documented [60, 61]. This action of DMSO is further supported by the lack of action potentials generated at the lowest injected current (50 pA) in absence of vehicle (Fig. 6a) contrary to their presence following DMSO treatment (Fig. 6b). Nevertheless, regardless of this DMSO effect, the spike frequency adaptation process in hAPP mice was restored by REM treatment.

In-depth analysis of action potentials evoked at the first depolarisation current (50 pA) revealed a significant increase in the AHP amplitude in hAPP neurons treated with REM (Fig. 6c) confirming the single AP findings. Altogether, our data demonstrate that REM normalises

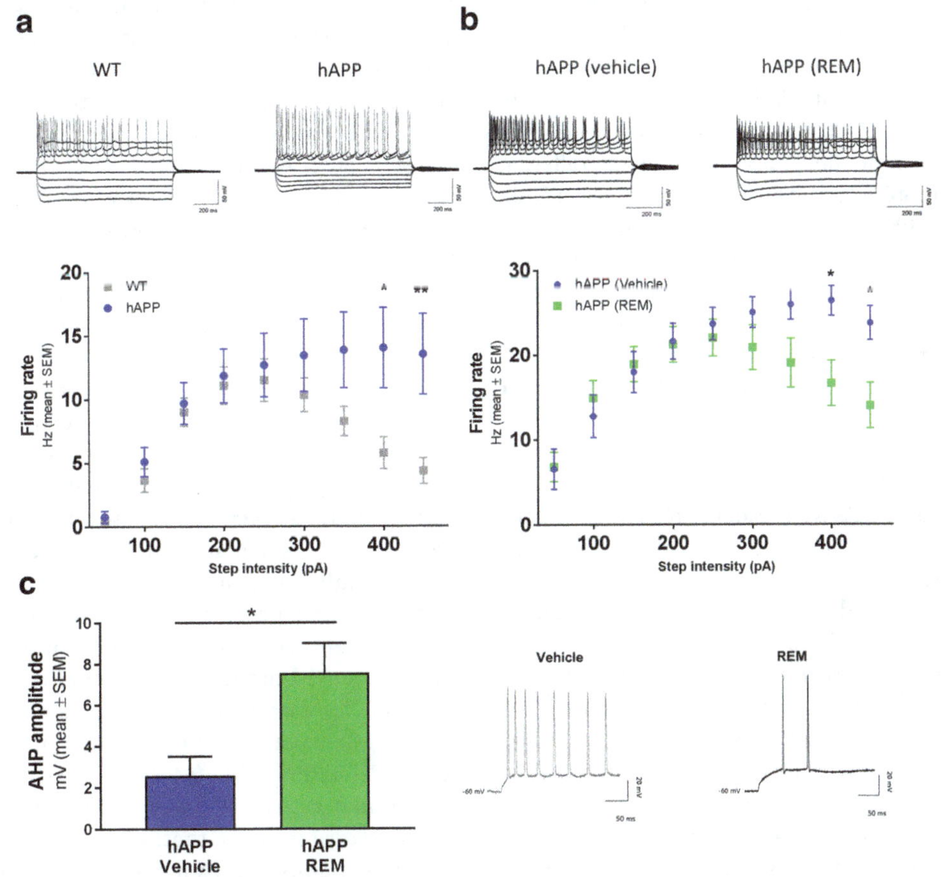

Fig. 6 hAPP deficit in spike frequency adaptation is rescued by REM. **a** Dendritic firing rate of hippocampal CA1 pyramidal neurons in WT and hAPP slices in response to increasing depolarising step current injections (50–450 pA; $n = 12$ mice per genotype; repeated measures two-way ANOVA: Interaction: $P = 0.0006$; DF = 8; F(8,176) = 3.649; Sidak's multiple comparison: 400 pA: $P = 0.0218$; $t = 3.069$; DF = 198; 450 pA: $P = 0.0071$; $t = 3.41$; DF = 189). **b** Dendritic firing rate of hippocampal CA1 pyramidal neurons in WT and hAPP slices perfused with either vehicle or 2 μM REM in response to depolarising step current step injections (50–450 pA). (Vehicle: $n = 12$ mice; REM: $n = 15$ mice; repeated measures two-way ANOVA: Interaction: $P < 0.0001$; DF = 8; F(8,200) = 5.082; Sidak's multiple comparison: 400 pA: $P = 0.0168$; $t = 3.146$; DF = 225; 450 pA: $P = 0.0079$; $t = 3.372$; DF = 225). Note that the overall firing rates were increased in the second experiment (b) compared to the first one (a). This is likely due to the addition of the vehicle DMSO which was shown previously to enhance neuronal activity [60, 61]. **c** Dendritic AHP amplitude in CA1 neurons in response to the first depolarising current that induced an AP in hAPP slices with or without REM (Vehicle: n = 12 mice; REM: $n = 16$ mice; $P = 0.0128$; $t = 2.673$; DF = 26)

spike frequency adaptation in hAPP CA1 neurons and increases their repolarisation as evidenced by enhanced AHP.

Modulation of the Pde6δ-Rap1 interaction and ERK1/2 signalling by REM decreases phosphorylation of tau and rescues behavioural deficits in different mouse models for AD

We showed earlier that abrogation of the Pde6δ-Rap1 interaction by REM reduced $[Ca^{2+}]_i$ and ERK1/2 signalling in resting neurons. Since MAPK are important Tau kinases involved in hyperphosphorylation of the protein in an AD context, REM treatment is expected to lower pathological Tau phosphorylation. Hence, in-vivo efficacy of REM was assessed in hAPP*PS1 transgenic mice [22] and two different hTAU transgenic mouse strains [62, 63]. Following two weeks sc administration of REM to hAPP*PS1 mice, Western blot analysis of brain extracts revealed a significant decrease in ERK1/2 activity (Fig. 7a), similar to the *in-cellulo* observations presented earlier (Fig. 4a). Moreover, pathological phosphorylation of endogenous Tau on different epitopes was reduced (pS262 epitope; Fig. 7b; AT8, pT231 and AD2 data not shown). Similarly, REM treatment of hTAU-P301L or hTAU-R406W transgenic mice resulted in a significant decrease in the phosphorylation of different epitopes of Tau (pS626-Tau, hTau-P301L: Fig. 7c; pS202 and pT205, hTau-R406W: Additional file 8: Figure S7a). No impact was observed on total levels of Tau protein. As such, it is reasonable to assume that, since MAPK's are known to be involved in Tau phosphorylation [31], the reduction of the latter is a downstream effect of REM's action on ERK. Nevertheless, we cannot exclude the contribution of other Ca^{2+}-dependent Tau kinases at this point.

Finally, we set-out to assess cognitive deficits in AD mice in function of REM treatment. To this end, hAPP and WT mice were tested in a MWM paradigm to assess (hippocampal based) spatial learning and memory after chronic REM or vehicle treatment. Following four days of training, in which the REM treated hAPP mice showed a reduced escape latency (Fig. 7d) and search path (Additional file 9: Figure S8a). During the probe task on day five, REM treated hAPP mice demonstrated a fully normalised cognitive performance, similar to that of WT mice (Fig. 7e), as opposed to the vehicle treated ones. After completion of the probe test, pharmacologically relevant exposure of REM in the brain of treated animals was confirmed by liquid chromatography-tandem mass spectrometry (Additional file 9: Figure S8b). Furthermore, although no MWM-based learning deficit was observed in R406W-Tau mice compared to WT mice (data not shown), the transgenic mice showed a significantly reduced mobility (swim speed), which may represent a motoric deficit observed in most transgenic Tau models as a consequence of Tau pathology in the hind brain. This motoric deficit was fully normalised after a four weeks treatment with REM (Additional file 8: Figure S7b). In addition, neither short-, nor long-term treatment with REM at the predetermined effective dose led to any side effects in the mice.

Altogether, these data demonstrate that, by modulation of the Pde6δ-Rap1 interaction, REM treatment reduces phosphorylation of protein Tau and rescues behavioural deficits in different AD-like mouse models.

Discussion

We report the development of a cell-based assay of neuronal degeneration featuring elevated levels of $[Ca^{2+}]_i$, deregulation of intracellular signalling and cytotoxicity. As such the model recapitulates key aspects of neurodegeneration in AD and represents a promising system for assessing underlying disease mechanisms and for identifying new therapies. To this end we have discovered novel compounds (REM), which selectively abrogate the binding of Pde6δ to small GTPase Rap1, thus representing a valuable pharmacological tool to study this interaction in more detail. Analysis of REM activity revealed that its target Pde6δ -by controlling Rap1- impacts Ca^{2+} homeostasis, plasticity and excitability, processes fundamentally underlying neuronal function and survival. Accordingly, normalising these processes by REM treatment mitigates neuronal toxicity, reduces in-vivo Tau phosphorylation and improves cognitive performance in animal models of AD.

Pde6δ as a GDI-like solubilisation factor facilitates non-vesicular inter-membrane transport of prenylated proteins [64]. As such, Pde6δ ensures the correct spatial organisation of cargo proteins for interaction with their respective effectors and/or modulators and thus determines the functional outcome of their signalling [25, 41]. In contrast to what the somewhat misleading name suggest, Pde6δ has no phosphodiesterase activity but participates in intracellular trafficking of cognate substrates and is more appropriately coined prenyl-binding protein δ (PrBP/δ) [64]. We here provide further evidence that Pde6δ interacts with Rap1 via its prenyl-binding pocket, confirming earlier findings [35]. In case of Ras, Pde6δ was shown to facilitate shuttling between different membrane locations in the cell by shielding the GTPase's prenyl-chain from the hydrophilic cytosol in its hydrophobic pocket [25, 41]. We therefore propose that, like for Ras, Pde6δ mediates the inter-membrane transport of Rap1 determining its subcellular distribution and consequently its function (Fig. 8).

According to this model, Pde6δ driven transport would enhance Rap1 enrichment at membranes destined for the PM (Fig. 8). The mechanism of Rap1 removal from the PM remains to be determined. Nevertheless, it seems reasonable to assume that it, like for Ras, follows endocytosis [25]. Thus, we

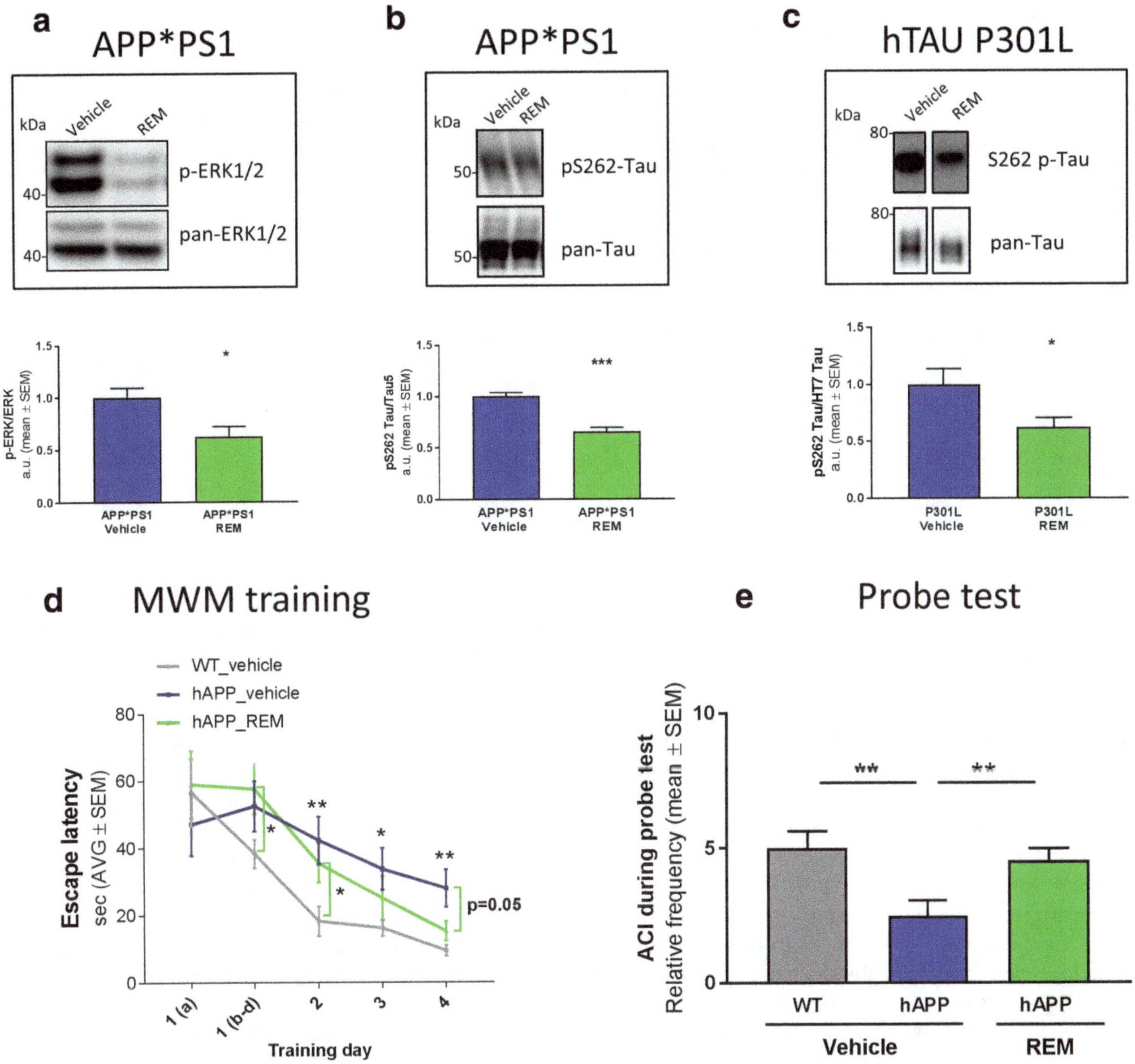

Fig. 7 REM treatment reduces ERK1/2 signalling, Tau phosphorylation and cognitive impairments in mouse models of AD. **a** Western blot analysis quantifying p-ERK1/2 ratio to total ERK1/2 (n = 6 vehicle or 5 REM treated mice; P = 0.0220; t = 2.763; DF = 9) or **b** phosphorylated Tau at epitope: pS262 ratio to total tau (Vehicle: n = 4 mice; REM: n = 5 mice; P = 0.0007; t = 5.735; DF = 7) in cortex of transgenic hAPP*PS1 mice treated for 2 weeks with vehicle or REM0043039. Representative immunoblots are shown in inset above the graph. **c** REM significantly decreases pathological tau phosphorylation on epitope S262 compared to total tau also in the brainstem of tau P301L transgenic mice (n = 9 vehicle and 13 REM treated mice; P = 0.0217; t = 2.491; DF = 20). **d** Escape latency during MWM training comparing WT to hAPP mice with or without REM (n = 12 mice per condition; t-test: WT Vehicle/hAPP Vehicle: day 2 P = 0.0083; t = 2.901; DF = 22; day 3 P = 0.0153; t = 2.629; DF = 22; day 4 P = 0.00431; t = 3.183; DF = 22; hAPP Vehicle/REM: day 4 P = 0.056; t = 2.015; DF = 22; WT Vehicle/hAPP REM: day 1(b-d) P = 0.034; t = 2.256; DF = 22; day 2 P = 0.0264; t = 2.381; DF = 22 **e** Graphs showing the annulus crossing index (ACI) representing the number of crossings over the platform site in the target area adjusted for crossings over corresponding areas in other quadrants during the probe test (n = 12 mice per condition; ACI: Vehicle WT/ Vehicle hAPP: P = 0.0069; t = 2.98; DF = 22; hAPP Vehicle/REM: P = 0.0098; t = 2.829; DF = 22)). (One data-point from hAPP vehicle group is below 0 and is included in the analysis but not shown in the graph)

envisage that under conditions of elevated neuronal activity and concomitant high rate of endocytosis, transport of Rap1 towards intracellular membranes is enhanced. In other words, in active neurons Rap1 is removed from the PM and concentrated on intracellular membranes. This relocalisation of Rap1 then reconfigures its functions towards more efficient reduction of neuronal excitability. The endomembrane

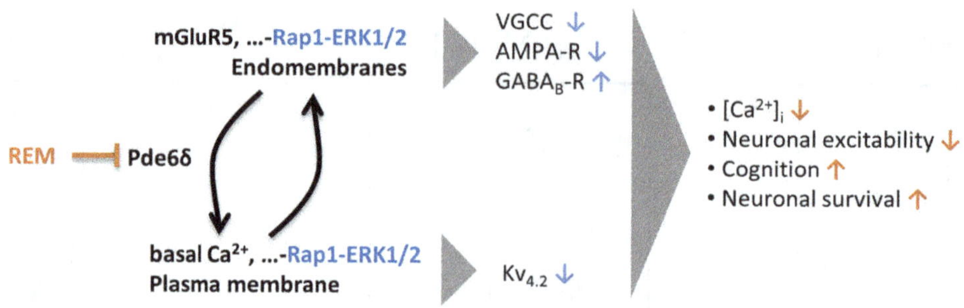

Fig. 8 Model illustrating how Pde6δ links different pools of Rap1 to Ca^{2+} homeostasis, neuronal excitability, cognition and neuronal survival. The Rap1-ERK1/2 cascade emanating from endomembranes represses VGCC and AMPA-R but increases $GABA_B$ receptor activity, thus favouring a reduction in neuronal activity. On the other hand, a plasma membrane associated pool of basal Rap1-ERK1/2 activity inhibits Kv4.2 channels, which promotes neuronal activity. Assuming that like for Ras [41], removal of Rap1 from the plasma membrane is endocytosis dependent, neuronal activity coinciding with endocytosis will redistribute Rap1 towards endomembranes. This Rap1 redistribution is geared towards lowering neuronal excitability, it could represent a natural feedback control to keep neuronal activity and VGCC mediated Ca^{2+} influx within certain limits and protecting neurons. Rap1 recycling from endomembranes to the plasma membrane is facilitated by Pde6δ. Thus, inhibition of Rap1 plasma membrane recycling by REM augments the small GTPase's presence and activity at endomembranes, while depleting it from the plasma membrane. As a result, under conditions of persistent excessive neuronal activity (such as in AD and epilepsy), REM rearranges the different pools of Rap1 towards restraining Ca^{2+} influx and neuronal excitability, resulting in neuroprotection. (In blue: Rap1-ERK1/2 actions at different membranes; orange arrows indicate Rap1-ERK1/2 functions altered by REM)

directed transport of Rap1 on the other hand is countered by Pde6δ, which actively enhances the small GTPase's recycling to the PM. REM antagonises this function of Pde6δ and thereby increases Rap1 on endomembranes at the expense of a PM localised pool, gearing the small GTPase's functions towards restraining neuronal excitability. Indeed, following high stimulation (electrically or chemically), REM, through blockage of Pde6δ mediated Rap1 recycling, decreases Ca^{2+} influx and excessive neuronal activity (Fig. 8).

Taken together, the subcellular membrane distribution of Rap1 may represent a dynamic auto-regulatory system containing neuronal excitability within physiological limits. During excessive stimulation such control would prevent neuronal hyperactivity and associated excitotoxicity, whereas at the same time keeping neurons sensitive for activation following less strong stimulations. Such a mechanism does not necessarily imply that Pde6δ-Rap1 functionality is altered in or causal to AD. However, under conditions of neuronal hyperexcitability, such as occurring during AD, REM would simply gear Rap1-ERK signalling towards a reduction of excessive activity.

Considering that neuronal activity is closely associated with Aβ production as well as its release and thereby aggregation and spread [65]; we anticipate that REM treatment, by mitigating neuronal hyperactivity, has beneficial effects on the amyloid burden. Although we have not yet addressed this aspect of REM action, it remains an interesting possibility to be explored in future studies.

Moreover, hyperexcitability underlies the susceptibility of hAPP mice to suffer from epileptic seizures [66], a phenomenon which is also observed in AD patients [20]. Here we show that REM by abrogating the Rap1-Pde6δ interaction can normalise neuronal excitability in hAPP mice. This outcome is not unexpected, since many Rap1 functions affected by REM treatment also represent major target classes for known anti-epileptic drugs [67], e.g. voltage-dependent Ca^{2+} and K^+ channels and ionotropic glutamate AMPA receptor. Moreover, Kv4.2, the main A-type K^+ channel, appears to be highly involved in the most prevalent form of epilepsy in adults, namely temporal lobe epilepsy [68] and experimental models thereof [69]. We therefore envisage that reducing neuronal hyperexcitability by inhibiting the interaction between Pde6δ and Rap1 has therapeutic potential not only in AD, but also seizure disorders such as epilepsy.

Along the same lines and, an intracellular pool of Rap1 was previously shown to control the surface expression and therefore activity of the inhibitory neurotransmitter receptor gamma-aminobutyric acid receptor B ($GABA_B$) [70]. Accordingly, we anticipate that increasing Rap1 on endomembranes by REM promotes $GABA_B$ surface expression, providing an additional mechanism of controlling neuronal activity (Fig. 8). As such, it would be interesting to evaluate such a REM effect in follow-up studies.

As discussed above, Rap1-ERK1/2 signalling controls a host of spatially discrete processes underlying neuronal function and survival. Hence under pathological conditions, where cytosolic Ca^{2+} levels are chronically elevated, the ensuing inappropriate activation of basal Rap1-ERK1/2 may lead to a reduction in Kv4.2 activity [49] and thus contribute to the neuronal hyperexcitability observed in the AD models [10, 19]. In agreement with this notion, we showed that REM diminishes basal Ca^{2+} driven Rap1-ERK1/2 signalling originating at the

PM and thereby restores AP repolarisation and the AP firing pattern in AD models possibly by increasing the I_A–type K^+ current. In addition, REM prevented Ca^{2+} induced chronic ERK1/2 activation, a process which can induce apoptosis [71]. Accordingly, we show that down-regulating basal Rap1-ERK1/2 activity, by inhibiting the Pde6δ-Rap1 interaction, is neuroprotective in models of AD. This is in agreement with previous findings where more general ERK1/2 inhibition approaches conferred neuroprotection [72–75].

Conclusion

The data presented here indicate that Pde6δ is an important regulator of Rap1-ERK1/2 signalling by controlling the latter's spatial organisation in the cell. Consequently, the newly identified neuroprotective REM compounds, by targeting Pde6δ mediated Rap1 inter-membrane shuttling, restrains critical aspects of neuronal functionality, including Ca^{2+} influx and excitability, which ultimately improve neuronal health and survival under conditions of excessive stimulation. Thus, targeting Pde6δ has promising therapeutic potential for disorders characterised by neuronal hyperactivity, such as AD and epilepsy.

Additional files

Additional file 1: Figure S1. ATRA induced cell death in the model is enhanced by expression of a cDNA encoding mutant human Tau and is prevented by REM. **a** Left: Western blot analysis confirmed successful tau overexpression (approximately 2-fold) in neuroblastoma cells containing the hTAU-P301L plasmid. Right: Toxicity was determined by quantifying LDH release in the medium in BE (2)-M17 neuroblastoma cells with (hTAU-P301L) and without (Control) expression of a cDNA encoding hTAUP301L incubated for 7 days with or without ATRA. The ATRA induced toxicity in hTAU-P301L cells represents the "toxicity assay" used in all following experiments (two-way ANOVA: +/− ATRA: $P < 0.0001$, F(1, 36)=4276, DF = 1; +/− hTAU-P301L: $P < 0.0001$, F (1, 36)=255.3, DF = 1; Sidak's multiple comparison test: control +/− ATRA: P < 0.0001, $t = 27.54$, DF = 36; hTAU-P301L +/− ATRA: $P < 0.0001$, $t = 64.93$, DF = 36; $n = 10$). # denotes the effect of hTAU-P301L expression silencing compared to control cells, * indicates the effect of ATRA treatment. **b** Representative images of neuroblastoma cells exposed to ATRA for six days treated with either REM or vehicle. **c** Treating hTAU-P301L cells in the toxicity assay with tau aggregation inhibitor methylthioninium rescues cell death ((EC50 = 23 nM; $n = 3$) One-way ANOVA, Methylthioninium treatment: $P < 0.0001$, F = 109.7, DF = 4).

Additional file 2: Supplementary Methods [76, 77]. (DOCX 17 kb)

Additional file 3: Figure S2. Reduction in Ca^{2+} influx through VGCCs reduces ATRA induced toxicity. **a** The effect of isradipine (VGCC inhibitor) in the toxicity assay (EC_{50} = 971 nM; $n = 2$). **b** The effect of U0126 (ERK1/2 kinase kinase (MEK) inhibitor) in the toxicity assay ((EC_{50} = 55.88 nM; n = 4) One-way ANOVA, U0126 treatment: $P < 0.0001$, F = 95.21, DF = 5).

Additional file 4: Figure S3. REM rescues ADDL induced cytotoxicity in primary hippocampal neurons. Viability assessment using live (yellow)/dead (purple) assay (representative pictures below the graphs – i, Control; ii, vehicle; iii, REM) of rat primary hippocampal neurons (Additional file 2: Supplementary Methods) exposed for 24 h to 1 μM ADDL's treated with vehicle or 0.25 μM REM0043039 (($n = 3$) Control/Vehicle: p = 0.0175, $t = 3.9$, DF = 4; Vehicle/REM: $P = 0.0208$, $t = 3.704$, DF = 4).

Additional file 5: Figure S4. The farnesyl group of Rheb fits into Pde6δ's hydrophobic pocket. **a** Rheb's farnesyl moiety sequestered in Pde6δ internal hydrophobic cavity as solved in X-ray crystal structure. Pde6δ shown in ribbon (left) or solid surface (right), and farnesyl moiety fused to terminal cysteine shown in stick bonds. **b** Superimposition of the farnesyl moiety (purple) and farnesyl group as solved in the crystal structure (grey).

Additional file 6: Figure S5. REM increases somatic and dendritic action potential AHP in hAPP brain slices. **a** K^+ current analysis: left graph shows the total K^+ current; right graph shows the 4-AP (I_A channel blocker) insensitive current ($n = 7$ mice per condition; RM-two way ANOVA 4-AP insensitive current amplitude: Interaction: $P = 0.0294$; F(15,180) = 1.865; DF = 15; Sidak's multiple comparison test: 60 mV: P = 0.0496; $t = 2.988$; DF = 192; 70 mV: $P = 0.0088$; $t = 3.512$; DF = 192). **b** Dendritic single AP parameters in hAPP brain slices after at least one hour vehicle or REM incubation; example traces are shown in the insets next to the graphs. ($n = 8$ mice per condition; AHP amplitude: P = 0.0003; $t = 4.816$; DF = 14; AP decay slope: $P = 0.0317$; $t = 2.387$; DF = 14).

Additional file 7: Figure S6. REM decreases KCl depolarisation induced Ca^{2+} influx by modulation of L-type channels**.** Summary of Fura-2 fluorescence traces (ratio 340/380 nm over time) after normalising to the mean of the first minute "baseline" recording. (+ nifedipine: n = 8; − nifedipine $n = 16$).

Additional file 8: Figure S7. REM reduces behaviour deficits and phosphorylated Tau in R406W mice. **a** Western blot analysis showing the ratio of phosphorylated Tau on epitope AT8 (pS202, pT205) to total Tau in cortex of R406W transgenic mice treated with either vehicle or REM subcutanously for 4 weeks. Examples of the immunoblots are shown above the graph. (n = 8 or 9 vehicle or REM treated respectively; P = 0,0328; t = 2,324; DF = 17). **b** Average velocity of R406W Tau transgenic mice during a MWM test after 4 weeks treatment with REM. (n = 16 or 18 or 17 WT + Vehicle or R406W + Vehicle or R406W + REM respectively; WT + Vehicle/R406W + Vehicle: P = 0,0033; t = 3,181; DF = 32; R406W + REM/ +Vehicle: $P = 0{,}0307$; t = 2,258; DF = 33).

Additional file 9: Figure S8. REM reaches effective concentrations in brains of hAPP mice and improves their ability to learn during a MWM test. **a** Search path length during the 4 training days in a MWM setting. ($n = 12$ mice per condition; multiple t-test: WT/hAPP Vehicle day 4: P = 0.033; $t = 2.277$; DF = 22; hAPP Vehicle/REM day 4: $P = 0.05$; $t = 2.072$; DF = 22). **b** Brain exposure levels of REM in hAPP mice 3 h post last dose.

Abbreviations

ACI: Annulus crossing index; aCSF: Artificial cerebrospinal fluid; AD: Alzheimer's disease; AHP: Afterhyperpolarisation; AP: Action potential; ATRA: All-trans retinoic acid; AUC: Area under the curve; Aβ: Amyloid-beta; Aβo: Soluble oligomeric Aβ; BSA: Bovine serum albumin; Ca^{2+}: Calcium; DHPG: (S)-3,4-dihydroxyphenylglycine; DIC: Differential interference contrast; DIV: Days in-vitro; DMSO: Dimethyl sulfoxide; E: Embryonic day; ERK1/2: Extracellular signal-regulated kinase; FCS: Foetal calf serum; fEPSPs: Field excitatory postsynaptic potentials; $GABA_B$: Gamma-aminobutyric acid receptor B; hAPP: Human mutant transgenic APP-V717I; hAPP*PS1: Human mutant transgenic APP-V717I*PS1-A246E; I_A: Fast transient outward K^+ current; K^+: Potassium; KCl: Potassium chloride; LDH: Lactate dehydrogenase; LTD: Long-term depression; MAPK: Mitogen-activated protein kinase; ms: Millisecond; MWM: Morris water maze; NB: Neurobasal medium; PDL: Poly-D-lysine; REM-MTX: Methotrexate fused REM compound; RT: Room temperature; sc: Subcutaneous; TBS: Tris-buffered saline; TTX: Tetrodotoxin; WT: Wild-type

Acknowledgements

The authors are indebted to Dr. Michael Kreutz for critically reading the manuscript.

Funding

This work was supported by the People Program (Marie Curie Actions) of the European Union's Seventh Framework Program FP7/2007–2013 under REA grant agreement n [289581] NPlast and by a fund of the "Agentschap Innoveren en Ondernemen" of Flanders. JT holds an ERC Advanced Grant, CYRE N°340941.

Authors' contributions

MD, TVD, KP, GG designed experiments and wrote the manuscript. MD, TVD, KP performed most of the experiments. MF generated electrophysiology data. AM, PC, SA and AK designed the chemistry. SS did the molecular modelling. CCH supervised and contributed to the design of experiments. GG directed the study. All authors read and approved the final manuscript.

Competing interests

MD, TVD, KP, KDW and GG are employed by reMYND. TVD, KP, KDW, GG, SW and JW own reMYND warrants and/or stocks. MF employed by E-Phy-Science and owns stocks. SL is employed by Orionis Biosciences. SW employed by ViroVet and owns stocks.

Author details

[1]reMYND NV, Gaston Geenslaan 1, Leuven-Heverlee 3001, Belgium. [2]E-Phy-Science, IPMC, 660 route des Lucioles, 06560 Sophia Antipolis, France. [3]Orionis Biosciences, Technologiepark 12B, Zwijnaarde-Ghent 9052, Belgium. [4]Cytokine Receptor Lab, Flanders Institute of Biotechnology, Medical Biotechnology Center, Faculty of Medicine and Health Sciences, Ghent University, Albert Baertsoenkaai 3, 9000 Ghent, Belgium. [5]Department of Chemistry, KU Leuven, Celestijnenlaan 200f - box 2404, Leuven-Heverlee 3001, Belgium. [6]ViroVet NV, Ambachtenlaan 1, Leuven-Heverlee 3001, Belgium. [7]Department of Biology, Functional Biology, KU Leuven, Kasteelpark Arenberg 31 box 2433, Leuven-Heverlee 3001, Belgium. [8]Cistim Leuven vzw, Gaston Geenslaan 2, Leuven-Heverlee 3001, Belgium. [9]Center for Drug Design and Development (CD3), KU Leuven, Waaistraat 6, 3000 Leuven, Belgium. [10]Cell Biology, Department of Biology, Faculty of Science, Utrecht University, 3584CH Utrecht, The Netherlands.

References

1. LaFerla FM. Calcium dyshomeostasis and intracellular signalling in Alzheimer's disease. Nat Rev Neurosci. 2002;3:862–72.
2. Bookheimer SY, et al. Patterns of brain activation in people at risk for Alzheimer's disease. N Engl J Med. 2000;343:450–6.
3. Elman J a, et al. Neural compensation in older people with brain amyloid-β deposition. Nat Neurosci. 2014;17:1316–8.
4. Sperling RA, et al. Amyloid deposition is associated with impaired default network function in older persons without dementia. Neuron. 2009;63:178–88.
5. Busche MA, et al. Clusters of hyperactive neurons near amyloid plaques in a mouse model of Alzheimer's disease. Science. 2008;321:1686–9.
6. Bezprozvanny I, Mattson MP. Neuronal calcium mishandling and the pathogenesis of Alzheimer's disease. Trends Neurosci. 2008;31:454–63.
7. Morris M, Maeda S, Vossel K, Mucke L. The many faces of tau. Neuron. 2011;70:410–26.
8. Holth JK, et al. Tau loss attenuates neuronal network Hyperexcitability in mouse and Drosophila genetic models of epilepsy. J Neurosci. 2013;33:1651–9.
9. Ittner LM, Götz J. Amyloid-β and tau--a toxic pas de deux in Alzheimer's disease. Nat Rev Neurosci. 2011;12:65–72.
10. Hall AM, et al. Tau-dependent Kv4.2 depletion and dendritic hyperexcitability in a mouse model of Alzheimer's disease. J Neurosci. 2015;35:6221–30.
11. Roberson ED, et al. Reducing endogenous tau ameliorates amyloid beta-induced deficits in an Alzheimer's disease mouse model. Science. 2007;316:750–4.
12. Zempel H, Thies E, Mandelkow E, Mandelkow E-M. Abeta oligomers cause localized ca(2+) elevation, missorting of endogenous tau into dendrites, tau phosphorylation, and destruction of microtubules and spines. J Neurosci. 2010;30:11938–50.
13. Haass C, Selkoe DJ. Soluble protein oligomers in neurodegeneration: lessons from the Alzheimer's amyloid beta-peptide. Nat. Rev. Mol. Cell Biol. 2007;8:101–12.
14. Spires-Jones TL, Hyman BT. The intersection of amyloid beta and tau at synapses in Alzheimer's disease. Neuron. 2014;82:756–71.
15. Van Dooren, T., Princen, K., De Witte, K. & Griffioen, G. Derailed intraneuronal signalling drives pathogenesis in sporadic and familial Alzheimer's disease. Biomed Res Int (2014) 2014, 167024.
16. Hardy JA, Higgins GA. Alzheimer's disease: the amyloid cascade hypothesis. Science. 1992;256:184–5.
17. Hardy J, Selkoe DJ. The amyloid hypothesis of Alzheimer's disease: Progress and problems on the road to therapeutics. Science. 2002;297:353–6.
18. Vossel KA, et al. Seizures and epileptiform activity in the early stages of Alzheimer disease. JAMA Neurol. 2013;70:1158–66.
19. Sanchez PE, et al. Levetiracetam suppresses neuronal network dysfunction and reverses synaptic and cognitive deficits in an Alzheimer's disease model. Proc Natl Acad Sci. 2012;109:E2895–903.
20. Vossel KA, Tartaglia MC, Nygaard HB, Zeman AZ, Miller BL. Epileptic activity in Alzheimer's disease: causes and clinical relevance. Lancet Neurol. 2017;16:311–22.
21. Moechars D, et al. Early phenotypic changes in transgenic mice that overexpress different mutants of amyloid precursor protein in brain. J Biol Chem. 1999;274:6483–92.
22. Dewachter I, et al. Aging increased amyloid peptide and caused amyloid plaques in brain of old APP/V717I transgenic mice by a different mechanism than mutant presenilin1. J Neurosci. 2000;20:6452–8.
23. Everett KL, Cooper DMF. An improved targeted cAMP sensor to study the regulation of adenylyl cyclase 8 by Ca2+ entry through voltage-gated channels. PLoS One. 2013;8:1–11.
24. Schrödinger LLC. In: LLC S, editor. Small-molecule drug discovery suite 2016–2. New York; 2016.
25. Chandra A, et al. The GDI-like solubilizing factor PDEδ sustains the spatial organization and signalling of Ras family proteins. Nat Cell Biol. 2012;14:148–58.
26. Risseeuw MDP, et al. A "clickable" MTX reagent as a practical tool for profiling small-molecule-intracellular target interactions via MASPIT. ChemMedChem. 2013;8:521–6.
27. Rezwan M, Auerbach D. Yeast "N"-hybrid systems for protein–protein and drug–protein interaction discovery. Methods. 2012;57:423–9.
28. Jämsä A, Hasslund K, Cowburn RF, Bäckström A, Vasänge M. The retinoic acid and brain-derived neurotrophic factor differentiated SH-SY5Y cell line as a model for Alzheimer's disease-like tau phosphorylation. Biochem Biophys Res Commun. 2004;319:993–1000.
29. Anekonda TS, et al. L-type voltage-gated calcium channel blockade with isradipine as a therapeutic strategy for Alzheimer's disease. Neurobiol Dis. 2011;41:62–70.
30. Grewal SS, et al. Neuronal calcium activates a Rap1 and B-Raf signaling pathway via the cyclic adenosine monophosphate-dependent protein kinase. J Biol Chem. 2000;275:3722–8.
31. Pei J-J, et al. Up-regulation of mitogen-activated protein kinases ERK1/2 and MEK1/2 is associated with the progression of neurofibrillary degeneration in Alzheimer's disease. Mol Brain Res. 2002;109:45–55.
32. Marambaud P, Dreses-Werringloer U, Vingtdeux V. Calcium signaling in neurodegeneration. Mol Neurodegener. 2009;4:20.
33. Hanzal-Bayer M, Renault L, Roversi P, Wittinghofer A, Hillig RC. The complex of Arl2-GTP and PDE delta: from structure to function. EMBO J. 2002;21:2095–106.
34. Hancock JF. Ras proteins: different signals from different locations. Nat Rev Mol Cell Biol. 2003;4:373–85.
35. Nancy V, et al. The delta subunit of retinal rod cGMP phosphodiesterase regulates the membrane association of Ras and rap GTPases. J Biol Chem. 2002;277:15076–84.
36. Glatter T, Wepf A, Aebersold R, Gstaiger M. An integrated workflow for charting the human interaction proteome: insights into the PP2A system. Mol Syst Biol. 2009;5(237).
37. Ismail S a, et al. Arl2-GTP and Arl3-GTP regulate a GDI-like transport system for farnesylated cargo. Nat Chem Biol. 2011;7:942–9.
38. Wätzlich D, et al. The interplay between RPGR, PDEδ and Arl2/3 regulate the ciliary targeting of farnesylated cargo. EMBO Rep. 2013;14:465–72.
39. Baehr W. Membrane protein transport in photoreceptors: the function of PDEδ: the Proctor lecture. Invest Ophthalmol Vis Sci. 2014;55:8653–66.
40. Zimmermann G, et al. Small molecule inhibition of the KRAS–PDEδ interaction impairs oncogenic KRAS signalling. Nature. 2013;497:638–42.
41. Schmick M, et al. KRas localizes to the plasma membrane by spatial cycles of Solubilization, trapping and vesicular transport. Cell. 2014;157:459–71.
42. York RD, et al. Rap1 mediates sustained MAP kinase activation induced by nerve growth factor. Nature. 1998;392:622–6.
43. Mochizuki N, et al. Spatio-temporal images of growth-factor-induced activation of Ras and Rap1. Nature. 2001;411:1065–8.

44. Wu GY, Deisseroth K, Tsien RW. Spaced stimuli stabilize MAPK pathway activation and its effects on dendritic morphology. Nat Neurosci. 2001;4:151–8.
45. Ohba Y. Mechanism of the spatio-temporal regulation of Ras and Rap1. EMBO J. 2003;22:859–69.
46. Wang Z, et al. Rap1-Mediated Activation of Extracellular Signal-Regulated Kinases by Cyclic AMP Is Dependent on the Mode of Rap1 Activation Rap1-Mediated Activation of Extracellular Signal-Regulated Kinases by Cyclic AMP Is Dependent on the Mode of Rap1 Activation. Mol Cell Biol. 2006;26:2130–45.
47. de Rooij J, et al. Epac is a Rap1 guanine-nucleotide-exchange factor directly activated by cyclic AMP. Nature. 1998;396:474–7.
48. Kim J, Wei D, Hoffman DA. Kv4 potassium channel subunits control action potential repolarization and frequency-dependent broadening in rat hippocampal CA1 pyramidal neurones. J Physiol. 2005;569:41–57.
49. Morozov A, et al. Rap1 couples cAMP signaling to a distinct pool of p42/44MAPK regulating excitability, synaptic plasticity, learning, and memory. Neuron. 2003;39:309–25.
50. Purgert C a, et al. Intracellular mGluR5 can mediate synaptic plasticity in the Hippocampus. J Neurosci. 2014;34:4589–98.
51. Gladding CM, Fitzjohn SM, Molnár E, Molnar E. Metabotropic glutamate receptor-mediated long-term depression: molecular mechanisms. Pharmacol Rev. 2009;61:395–412.
52. Gallagher SM. Extracellular signal-regulated protein kinase activation is required for metabotropic glutamate receptor-dependent long-term depression in hippocampal area CA1. J Neurosci. 2004;24:4859–64.
53. Jong Y-JI, Sergin I, Purgert C, O'Malley KL. Location-dependent signaling of the group 1 metabotropic glutamate receptor mGlu5. Mol Pharmacol. 2014; 86:774–85.
54. Yuan L, Adams JP, Swank M, Sweatt JD, Johnston D. Protein kinase modulation of dendritic K+ channels in hippocampus involves a mitogen-activated protein kinase pathway. J Neurosci. 2002;22:4860–8.
55. Scala F, et al. Intraneuronal Aβ accumulation induces hippocampal neuron hyperexcitability through A-type K+ current inhibition mediated by activation of caspases and GSK-3. Neurobiol Aging. 2015;36:886–900.
56. Ping Y, et al. Linking Abeta42-induced Hyperexcitability to neurodegeneration, learning and motor deficits, and a shorter lifespan in an Alzheimer's model. PLoS Genet. 2015;11:1 25.
57. Snyder EM, et al. Internalization of ionotropic glutamate receptors in response to mGluR activation. Nat Neurosci. 2001;4:1079–85.
58. Subramanian J, Dye L, Morozov A. Rap1 signaling prevents L-type calcium channel-dependent neurotransmitter release. J Neurosci. 2013;33:7245–52.
59. Catterall WA. Voltage-Gated Calcium Channels. Cold Spring Harb. Perspect. Biol. 3; 2011. p. a003947.
60. Sawada M, Sato M. The effect of dimethyl sulfoxide on the neuronal excitability and cholinergic transmission in Aplysia ganglion cells. Ann N Y Acad Sci. 1975;243:337–57.
61. Morley P, Whitfield JF. The differentiation inducer, dimethyl sulfoxide, transiently increases the intracellular calcium ion concentration in various cell types. J Cell Physiol. 1993;156:219–25.
62. Terwel D, et al. Changed conformation of mutant tau-P301L underlies the moribund Tauopathy, absent in progressive, nonlethal Axonopathy of tau-4R/2N transgenic mice. J Biol Chem. 2005;280:3963–73.
63. Zhang B, et al. Retarded axonal transport of R406W mutant tau in transgenic mice with a neurodegenerative tauopathy. J Neurosci. 2004;24:4657–67.
64. Zhang H, Constantine R, Frederick JM, Baehr W. The prenyl-binding protein PrBP/δ: a chaperone participating in intracellular trafficking. Vis Res. 2012;75:19–25.
65. Bero AW, et al. Neuronal activity regulates the regional vulnerability to amyloid-β deposition. Nat Neurosci. 2011;14:750–6.
66. Palop JJ, et al. Aberrant excitatory neuronal activity and compensatory remodeling of inhibitory hippocampal circuits in mouse models of Alzheimer's disease. Neuron. 2007;55:697–711.
67. Meldrum BS, Rogawski MA. Molecular targets for antiepileptic drug development. Neurotherapeutics. 2007;4:18–61.
68. Bernard C, et al. Acquired dendritic channelopathy in temporal lobe epilepsy. Science. 2004;305:532–5.
69. Lugo JN, et al. Altered phosphorylation and localization of the A-type channel, Kv4.2 in status epilepticus. J Neurochem. 2008;106:1929–40.
70. Zhang Z, et al. GABAB receptor promotes its own surface expression by recruiting a Rap1-dependent signaling cascade. J Cell Sci. 2015;128:2302–13.
71. Cagnol S, Chambard J-C. ERK and cell death: mechanisms of ERK-induced cell death--apoptosis, autophagy and senescence. FEBS J. 2010;277:2–21.
72. Chong YH, et al. ERK1/2 activation mediates Abeta oligomer-induced neurotoxicity via caspase-3 activation and tau cleavage in rat organotypic hippocampal slice cultures. J Biol Chem. 2006;281:20315–25.
73. Satoh T, et al. Neuroprotection by MAPK / ERK kinase inhibition with U0126 against oxidative stress in a mouse neuronal cell line and rat primary cultured cortical neurons. Neurosci Lett. 2000;288:163–6.
74. Amadoro G, et al. NMDA receptor mediates tau-induced neurotoxicity by calpain and ERK/MAPK activation. Proc Natl Acad Sci U S A. 2006;103:2892–7.
75. Feld M, et al. Decrease of ERK/MAPK overactivation in prefrontal cortex reverses early memory deficit in a mouse model of Alzheimer's disease. J Alzheimers Dis. 2014;40:69–82.
76. Yau KW, et al. Microtubule minus-end binding protein CAMSAP2 controls axon specification and dendrite development. Neuron. 2014;82:1058–73.
77. Klein WL. Abeta toxicity in Alzheimer's disease: globular oligomers (ADDLs) as new vaccine and drug targets. Neurochem Int. 2002;41:345–52.

12

Molecular and functional signatures in a novel Alzheimer's disease mouse model assessed by quantitative proteomics

Dong Kyu Kim[1†], Joonho Park[2†], Dohyun Han[3†], Jinhee Yang[1], Ahbin Kim[1], Jongmin Woo[1], Youngsoo Kim[2*] and Inhee Mook-Jung[1,4*]

Abstract

Background: Alzheimer's disease (AD), the most common neurodegenerative disorder, is characterized by the deposition of extracellular amyloid plaques and intracellular neurofibrillary tangles. To understand the pathological mechanisms underlying AD, developing animal models that completely encompass the main features of AD pathologies is indispensable. Although mouse models that display pathological hallmarks of AD (amyloid plaques, neurofibrillary tangles, or both) have been developed and investigated, a systematic approach for understanding the molecular characteristics of AD mouse models is lacking.

Methods: To elucidate the mechanisms underlying the contribution of amyloid beta (Aβ) and tau in AD pathogenesis, we herein generated a novel animal model of AD, namely the AD-like pathology with amyloid and neurofibrillary tangles ($ADLP^{APT}$) mice. The $ADLP^{APT}$ mice carry three human transgenes, including amyloid precursor protein, presenilin-1, and tau, with six mutations. To characterize the molecular and functional signatures of AD in $ADLP^{APT}$ mice, we analyzed the hippocampal proteome and performed comparisons with individual-pathology transgenic mice (i.e., amyloid or neurofibrillary tangles) and wild-type mice using quantitative proteomics with 10-plex tandem mass tag.

Results: The $ADLP^{APT}$ mice exhibited accelerated neurofibrillary tangle formation in addition to amyloid plaques, neuronal loss in the CA1 area, and memory deficit at an early age. In addition, our proteomic analysis identified nearly 10,000 protein groups, which enabled the identification of hundreds of differentially expressed proteins (DEPs) in $ADLP^{APT}$ mice. Bioinformatics analysis of DEPs revealed that $ADLP^{APT}$ mice experienced age-dependent active immune responses and synaptic dysfunctions.

Conclusions: Our study is the first to compare and describe the proteomic characteristics in amyloid and neurofibrillary tangle pathologies using isobaric label-based quantitative proteomics. Furthermore, we analyzed the hippocampal proteome of the newly developed $ADLP^{APT}$ model mice to investigate how both Aβ and tau pathologies regulate the hippocampal proteome. Because the $ADLP^{APT}$ mouse model recapitulates the main features of AD pathogenesis, the proteomic data derived from its hippocampus has significant utility as a novel resource for the research on the Aβ-tau axis and pathophysiological changes in vivo.

Keywords: Alzheimer's disease, Animal disease model, Aβ, Tau, Quantitative proteomics, 10-plex tandem mass tag

* Correspondence: biolab@snu.ac.kr; inhee@snu.ac.kr
[†]Equal contributors
[2]Interdisciplinary Program in Bioengineering, College of Engineering, Seoul National University, 1 Gwanak-ro, Seoul 151-742, South Korea
[1]Department of Biomedical Sciences, Seoul National University, College of Medicine, 103 Daehak-ro, Seoul 110-799, South Korea
Full list of author information is available at the end of the article

Background

Alzheimer's disease (AD) is the most common neurodegenerative disorder and is characterized by extracellular amyloid plaque deposition, intracellular neurofibrillary tangle (NFT) development, and memory impairments [1, 2]. Although the disease has been extensively studied over the past several decades, the exact mechanisms and pathological causes of AD remain unclear. Genetically modified mouse models that recapitulate the major features of AD pathologies are invaluable in determining the underlying disease mechanisms and evaluating new therapeutic approaches. Few transgenic mouse models, such as the triple transgenic mice, 3xTg-AD model, have been introduced to develop the concomitant manifestation of both amyloid plaques and NFT formation [3]. Because this model showed no neuronal cell death in the hippocampus, the development of a new mouse model that fully mimics AD pathologies is still needed.

One of the most widely used models in AD research is the 5xFAD (Tg6799) model, which contains five familial AD mutations within the *APP* and *PSEN1* genes. The 5xFAD model is considered to be an effective AD model because of the rapid progression of the amyloid pathology [4]. The JNPL3 mouse model, which expresses P301L-mutant human tau, has been widely used to examine intraneuronal NFTs [5]. To recapitulate the main features of AD pathogenesis, we herein developed a new mouse model that carries six mutations within transgenes encoding human amyloid precursor protein (APP), presenilin-1 (PSEN1), and tau. The resulting transgenic mouse model, Alzheimer's disease-like pathology with *APP, PSEN1,* and *MAPT* transgenes ($ADLP^{APT}$), exhibited Aβ accumulation, NFTs, early neuronal loss in the brain, and subsequent memory impairments. The pathological phenotypes of $ADLP^{APT}$ mice, which feature both Aβ deposition and NFTs, were compared with those of $ADLP^{APP/PS1}$ (Aβ deposition, no NFTs) and $ADLP^{Tau}$ (no Aβ deposition, NFTs) mice of the same genetic background. Understanding the interplay between Aβ accumulation and NFTs is imperative for elucidating the pathogenesis of AD. Thus, the $ADLP^{APT}$ mouse model, which shows both robust amyloid and NFT pathologies, should be an excellent model for examining the Aβ-tau axis in vivo.

The hippocampus is known to play an important role in memory formation [6]. Thus, understanding the pathological status of the hippocampus under AD is crucial for studying the mechanisms of AD-related memory impairments. Although some mechanisms that contribute to AD pathogenesis have been uncovered by studies on individual genes or proteins, systematic analysis of the pathological changes of the hippocampus is lacking. Mass spectrometry (MS)-based proteomics is expected to be an appropriate tool for systematic analysis [7, 8]. Although MS-based proteomics have been limited because of the incomplete coverage of the proteome, recent technological advances allowed researchers to study comprehensively up to 10,000 proteins from a single cell line [9]. However, this level of coverage requires extensive pre-fractionation, large samples, and several months of instrument time [10]. In addition, the reliable MS-based quantitation under several perturbation states requires the use of biological and technical replicates, thus increasing the complexity of MS experiments. Importantly, these shortcomings can be overcome by an isobaric labeling strategy, such as the application of tandem mass tags (TMTs) [11]. The recent expansion of multiplexing capacity up to 10 samples per MS injection has markedly increased the scope of quantitative proteomics [12]. In TMT experiments, protein quantification is accomplished by comparing the intensities of reporter ions produced during MS/MS [11]. Since this approach enables sensitive and precise protein quantification, many research groups have successfully used TMT-based strategies [13–16].

With the aid of 10-plex TMT quantification strategy combined with high-resolution MS, we constructed a comprehensive proteome map of the newly developed mouse models. We have successfully discovered nearly 10,000 proteins and quantified 7000 proteins from the hippocampus of wild type, $ADLP^{APP/PS1}$, $ADLP^{Tau}$, and $ADLP^{APT}$ mice. The protein abundances of $ADLP^{APT}$ mice were compared with those of other single transgenic mice to discover differentially expressed proteins and characterize functional signatures of $ADLP^{APT}$ mice via bioinformatics analysis. Furthermore, our network analysis could suggest the presence of interacting proteins that connect between amyloid and NFT pathologies. In conclusion, new $ADLP^{APT}$ mice and their hippocampal proteome dataset may help to offer a novel insight of pathogenesis of AD in further studies targeting the concurrent molecular network of amyloid and NFT pathologies.

Methods

Experimental design

The aim of this study was to construct a mouse model of Alzheimer's disease that carries mutant human genes and to introduce its molecular and functional characteristics. The protein expressions of newly constructed mouse models were assessed by quantitative proteomics combined with LC-MS/MS and TMT isobaric labeling. A total of 36 hippocampi samples were used in the proteomic experiments. (4 mouse types * 3 age-points * biological triplicates), which were randomly divided into four 10-plex TMT experimental sets. All samples were analyzed twice via MS. Three to twelve mice were sacrificed accordingly to the type of biochemical experiment, which includes western blotting and immunostaining. Behavioral tests of the AD model mice were performed by investigators in blind with respect to genotypes. No data were excluded.

Reagents and materials

Tandem mass tag (TMT) 10-plex isobaric reagents, bicinchoninic acid (BCA) assay kit - reducing agent compatible, tris (2-carboxyethyl) phosphine (TCEP), and LC/MS-grade solvents such as acetone, acetonitrile (ACN), and water were purchased from Thermo Fisher Scientific (Waltham, MA). Other reagents and materials were purchased from the following companies: Dithiothreitol (DTT) and urea from AMRESCO (Solon, OH), Sodium dodecyl sulfate (SDS), Trizma base from USB (Cleveland, OH) and sequencing-grade modified trypsin from Promega Corporation (Madison, WI), POROS20 R2 bead from Applied Biosystems (Foster City, CA). High-purity (>97%) mass spectrometry (MS) grade ovalbumin from Protea (Morgantown, WV), HLB OASIS column from Waters (Milford, MA). All other reagents, unless noted, were purchased from Sigma-Aldrich (St. Louis, MO).

Transgenic mice

5XFAD mice (Tg6799; Jackson Laboratory, Stock#006554) express both mutant human *APP* with the Swedish, Florida, and London mutations and mutant human *PSEN1* with the M146 L and L286 V mutations under the murine Thyl promoter. JNPL3 mice (TauP301L-JNPL3; Taconic, Stock#2508 homozygote) carry mutant human tau with the P301L mutation under the murine prion protein promoter. Due to the mixed genetic background of JNPL3 mice, JNPL3 mice were backcrossed with B6SJL (C57BL/6 X SJL) mice. The resulting JNPL3 mice on the B6SJL genetic background were crossed with 5XFAD mice to create a novel animal model, ADLP animal model. This carries the three human mutant genes and its corresponding mutations mentioned before. Only female mice were used for pathological characterization due to earlier signs of aggravated pathologies and memory deficit than male mice.

Immunohistochemistry (IHC)

Mice were anesthetized and perfused with 4% paraformaldehyde (PFA) solution in phosphate-buffered saline (PBS). The brain tissues were fixed with 4% PFA for 20 h at 4 °C, incubated in 30% sucrose (wt/vol) for 72 h and then frozen. The frozen brains were cut into 30 μm coronal sections using a Leica CM 1850 Cryostat. Brain slices were washed with PBS and then incubated in 70% formic acid in PBS for 20 min to perform antigen retrieval when amyloid plaques and NFTs were stained. Brain slices were permeabilized and blocked with blocking solution (0.3% Triton X-100, 5% horse serum, and 0.05% BSA solution) for 1 h at 20 °C prior to incubating it with primary antibodies overnight. Amyloid plaques were stained with the biotin-4G8 antibody (1:700, COVANCE), followed by the streptavidin-488-conjugated secondary antibody (Invitrogen). Hyperphosphorylated tau was examined by using the AT8 (1:300, Thermo Scientific) and AT180 (1:300, Thermo Scientific) antibody, which recognize the Ser202/Thr205 epitopes and Thr231 of human tau, followed by biotinylated anti-mouse IgG (Vector Laboratories) and streptavidin-594-conjugated secondary antibody (Invitrogen). To visualize astrocytes and microglia, anti-GFAP (1:1000, Invitrogen) for astrocytes and anti-Iba-1 (1:500, Wako) antibodies were used respectively. Hippocampal neurons of the CA1 layer were visualized by staining with anti-NeuN (1:1000, Millipore) antibody. Stained brain slices were incubated with goat anti-rat Alexa 488, donkey anti-rabbit Alexa 488, and donkey anti-mouse Alexa 647 antibody (1:500, Life Technologies) for 1 h at 20 °C. Images were obtained using LSM 700 (Carl Zeiss). At least six serial sections of each sample were imaged to consider the volume of cells in brain slices. When the number of neuronal cells in CA1 layer stained by anti-NeuN antibody were counted, one middle region of the hippocampus tissue was imaged to avoid an overlap of CA1 pyramidal neurons. All images were quantified using ImageJ software (NIH).

Sarkosyl-insoluble tau fractionation

One side of the hippocampus was homogenized in 8 volumes of Tris buffer solution (TBS) including phosphatase inhibitors and protease by tissue grinder [TBS solution; 25 mM Tris/HCl, pH 7.4, 150 mM NaCl, 1 mM EDTA, 1 mM EGTA, phenylmethylsulfonyl fluoride (PMSF), protease 1, and 2]. The homogenates were centrifuged at 14,000 x g at 4 °C for 15 min. The supernatant was collected for further fractionation. The supernatant was incubated with N-Lauroylsarcosine sodium salt solution 20% solution (1% final concentration) at 37 °C rotator for 1 h and then ultracentrifuged at 150,000 x g at 25 °C for 1 h. The resulting sarkosyl-insoluble pellets were resuspended in TBS solution for washing pellets. The mixture was concentrated by ultracentrifuge again at 150,000 x g at 25 °C for 1 h. The resulting pellets containing tau aggregates were suspended with 5xSample buffer (Serva Blue G) and heated at 70 °C for 10 min to prevent further aggregation.

Behavioral test

For Y-maze test, after introduction to the middle of the maze, the mouse was allowed to freely explore new environments for 8 min. Spatial memory function was measured as the percent of spontaneous alteration [17]. The number of total arm entries and the sequence of the Y-maze arm into which mice entered were recorded in order to calculate the percentage of spontaneous alteration. The number of alternations was counted when the mouse entered into the three different maze arms consecutively. The percent of spontaneous alteration was calculated as the number of alterations divided by the total entry number multiplied by 100.

RT-PCR analysis

To verify the amount of mouse or human tau mRNA levels in ADLP^{Tau} and ADLP^{APT} mice, RT-PCR analysis was carried out with 10-month-old ADLP model mice. Total RNA was extracted from the hippocampus with the RNeasy Mini kit (QIAGEN). All RNA samples were converted into cDNA using Maxime RT PreMix Kit (iNtRON BIOTECH). Quantitative RT-PCR was carried out in triplicates using KAPA SYBR FAST ABI Prism qPCR kit (KAPA Biosystems). For mouse Tau, the primers 5'-AGCCCTAAGACTCCTCCA-3′ and 5'-TGCTGTAGCC GCTTCGTTCT-3′ were used. Human tau was amplified with the primers 5'-CTCCAAAATCAGGGGATCGC-3′ and 5'-CCTTGCTCAGGTC AACTGGT-3′. The mRNA levels of mouse Tau and human Tau were normalized with GAPDH which was amplified with the primers 5'-GGCCTTGACTGTGCCGTTGAATTT-3′ and 5'-ACA GCCGCATC TTCTTGTGCAGTG-3′. Once the reaction was completed, the RT-PCR products were evaluated/analyzed via gel-electrophoresis to measure/calculate the specificity of human tau primers.

Western blot analysis

Western blot analysis was used to confirm tau aggregates from sarkosyl-insoluble tau fractionation and the validation of proteomic analysis results. After isolated tau aggregates were heated at 70 °C for 10 min to prevent further tau protein aggregation, the same volume of sarkosyl-insoluble tau aggregate samples was loaded per lane of 4–12% Bis-Tris polyacrylamide precast gels (NuPAGE system, Invitrogen). Following electrophoresis, proteins were transferred to a PVDF membrane. Membranes were blocked with 5% skim milk solution and then incubated with primary antibodies against human tau (Tau13, Abcam, 1:1000) and total tau (endogenous tau and human tau) (Tau5, Abcam, 1:1000). Primary antibodies against ABCA1 (Abcam, 1:500), Ptprc (CD45, Abcam, 1:1000) and Hcls1 (HS1, CST, 1:1000) were used for the validation of proteomic analysis. For confirmation of kinase expression levels, CK1δ (Abcam, 1:5000), RSK1 (CST, 1:2000) and GSK-3β (CST, 1:2000) were used as primary antibodies. Anti-mouse or rabbit IgG conjugated HRP was used to detect primary antibodies and West Save Gold (Ab frontier) was used for their visualization. Since sarkosyl-insoluble fractionation only extracts protein aggregates, certain proteins generally used for normalization such as GAPDH and β-actin were not detected in the sarkosyl-insoluble pellets. Thus, total antibody signals of tau aggregates or each signal for distinct sizes of tau aggregates were quantified for quantification.

Mass spectrometry-based proteomics

Mouse hippocampus tissues were resected and subjected to the previously described sample preparation methods with some modifications [18–20]. Detailed procedures including protein digestion, peptide labeling, fractionation, and MS analysis are described in Additional file 1: Supplementary Methods.

Quantification of protein abundance and statistics

The quantification and statistical processing methods described below are related to proteomic data. First of all, among the 9814 identified proteins, only 6964 proteins satisfying the following criteria were used for subsequent quantitative analysis; identification in all channels (7022 proteins), high protein confidence (6970 proteins, assessed by Proteome Discoverer), and possessing 1 or more unique peptides (6964 proteins). The protein abundance ratio of individual samples to pooled sample (named "normalized protein abundance") was generated by dividing the reporter ion intensity of each channel by the intensity of the pooled sample channel in its corresponding experimental TMT set (Additional file 2: Figure S3B). There was no significant difference between the values of the pooled sample channels (Additional file 2: Figure S5E). Thus, the denominators were considered to be common and eliminated. The fold-change values used in the bioinformatics analysis were generated by dividing the normalized protein abundance of each transgenic mouse by the value of the age-matched wild type mouse. The distribution of ratiometric data was almost normal (Additional file 2: Figure S5G) but this was not thoroughly tested.

Statistical processes for the proteomic data were performed based on the normalized protein abundance using Perseus [21]. Initially, total identified proteins were filtered based on the 6964 proteins that quantified in all mouse samples. The statistical cut-off value for significance was set to p-value <0.05 for the Student's t-test, while Benjamini-Hochberg FDR adjusted p-value cut-off [22] of 0.05 was applied for the ANOVA test. The normalized protein abundances were subjected to z-normalization followed by hierarchical clustering. The statistical tests for the other biochemical experiments were described in each figure legend.

Bioinformatics analysis

The Gene Ontology (GO) of the proteins was classified using DAVID bioinformatics tool (version 6.8) [23]. The GO classification was evaluated by Fisher's exact test to obtain a set of P-values, which were then filtered at a cut-off value of 0.01. Canonical pathways, downstream biological functions, and upstream regulators were enriched using Ingenuity Pathway Analysis (IPA, QIAGEN) [24]. The analytical algorithms embedded in IPA uses input protein list (here differentially expressed proteins) to predict putative upstream regulators such as transcription factors and growth factors, as well as downstream effects on known biological pathways. IPA derives these protein set-pathway (or regulator) relationships from their own large-scale causal network database, named Ingenuity Knowledge Base. Because the algorithm cannot determine with certainty which causalities in its database can explain our experimental results, the tool performs statistical tests (i.e. Fisher's exact test) to assess the reliability of predicted upstream genes and pathways. Finally, IPA also assigns activation states (activated or inhibited) to putative regulators or pathways based on the quantitative values of protein members. The user will be given a confidence in the *P*-value obtained from the Fisher's exact test and the magnitude of activation as a Z-score, respectively. In this study, the *P*-value cut-off criteria for the enrichment was 0.01 for Fig. 6a and b and the predictive activation Z-score cut-off was 1. For the Fig. 4b, the cut-off value was 0.05 and the predictive activation Z-score cut-off was 1. The initial pathway diagrams were obtained by IPA but were manually modified. Protein-protein interactions (PPIs) for the network analysis was interrogated from STRING database (http://www.string-db.org) [25]. The PPIs in network model were visualized using Cytoscape [26].

Results

Pathological symptoms of ADLP^{APT} mice

Four mouse models with the same genetic background were generated: wild-type, ADLP$^{APP/PS1}$ (Aβ accumulation only), ADLP^{Tau} (NFTs only), and ADLP^{APT} (both Aβ and NFTs) mice. To confirm the amyloid plaque burden in the hippocampus of the ADLP mice, we stained coronal brain sections of 4-, 7-, and 10-month-old ADLP mice with the biotin-4G8 antibody that recognizes amino acids 17–24 of Aβ peptides. Both ADLP$^{APP/PS1}$ and ADLP^{APT} mice started showing slight extracellular accumulation of Aβ at 4 months and exhibited large amyloid plaques at 7 months; no significance was observed between-model difference in their amyloid plaque burdens (Fig. 1a and c).

To investigate the NFT pathology in the hippocampus, we first stained phosphorylated tau using the AT8 antibody, which detects residue Ser202/Thr205 of phosphorylated tau in paired helical filaments (PHFs). Intense immunoreactivity of PHFs against phosphorylated tau was observed in the hippocampal CA1 area of 7- and 10-month-old ADLP^{APT} mice compared with ADLP^{Tau} mice (Fig. 1b and d). Subsequently, we used the AT180 antibody to detect the residue Thr231 of phosphorylated tau. The residue Thr231 was strongly stained at the soma and dendrites of CA1 neurons starting from 4 months of age. In 10-month-old mice, we observed phosphorylated tau localized only at the soma region as a form of NFTs, indicating that ADLP^{APT} mice developed severe NFT pathology compared with ADLP^{Tau} mice (Additional file 2: Figure S1A).

To validate the expression of tau in the hippocampus, mRNA levels of endogenous mouse tau were confirmed by RT-PCR analysis. The results indicated no significant differences among the ADLP mouse models. Furthermore, the human tau mRNA expression was not different between ADLP^{Tau} and ADLP^{APT} mice, indicating accelerated NFT pathology in ADLP^{APT} mice without quantitative difference in tau protein (Additional file 2: Figure S1B–1D). Subsequently, we isolated NFTs from the hippocampus of 7- and 10-month-old ADLP^{Tau} and ADLP^{APT} mice using sarkosyl-insoluble tau fractionation. Tau aggregates in ADLP^{APT} mice were composed of higher molecular weight of tau at both 7 and 10 months of age, and they appeared at regular intervals above the 55 kDa of human tau. The proportion of the higher molecular weight tau increased in 10-month-old ADLP^{APT} mice as compared to age-matched ADLP^{Tau} mice (Fig. 1e). However, ADLP^{Tau} mice had only low-molecular-weight tau as a main constituent until 10 months of age (Fig. 1e and f). This suggests that the phosphorylation of human tau was increased by the amyloid pathology in ADLP^{APT} mice. Using the Tau5 antibody, which reacts to both mouse and human tau, we confirmed that sarkosyl-insoluble tau fractionation was the appropriate method for specifically extracting tau aggregates from the hippocampus of ADLP^{Tau} and ADLP^{APT} mice (Additional file 2: Figure S1E).

We also examined whether the accelerated NFT pathology observed in the hippocampal CA1 area of ADLP^{APT} mice was associated with neuronal loss in the CA1 layer. Neuronal quantification using NeuN immunostaining revealed a significant decrease in the number of CA1 neurons in 10-month-old ADLP^{APT} mice, but not in the other models, indicating that the amyloid pathology of this model aggravated neuronal death via the NFT pathology (Fig. 1g and h). Because spatial memory impairment is an essential feature in AD animal models [27], we used the alternation Y-maze task to evaluate spatial memory in ADLP mice at different ages. Although there was no memory deficit in 4-month-old ADLP^{APT} mice, they showed significant deficits in spatial memory beginning at 7 months (Fig. 1i). Altogether, these data indicated that ADLP^{APT} mice exhibit an accelerated NFT pathology, amyloid pathology, neuronal loss, and age-related memory impairment. Thus, this model appears to comprehensively reflect the pathophysiological changes in AD.

Constructing a Hippocampal proteome database of the ADLP mouse models

To obtain insights into the molecular basis of AD pathogenesis, we performed quantitative proteomic analysis using three replicates of hippocampus resected from each mouse model at three time points (4, 7, and 10 months of age; Fig. 2a). Briefly, each hippocampus was homogenized and digested via filter-associated sample preparation [28],

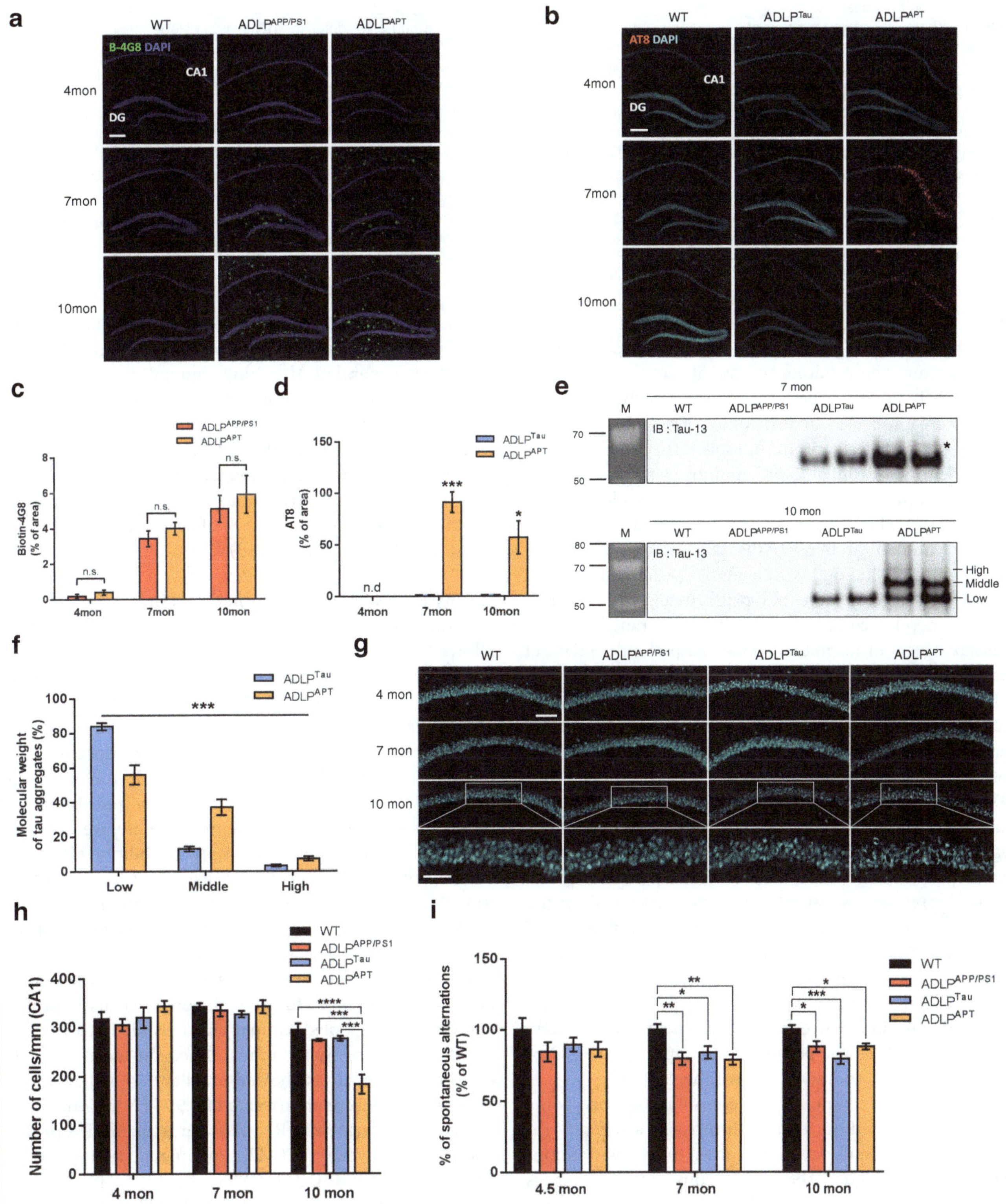

Fig. 1 (See legend on next page.)

(See figure on previous page.)

Fig. 1 Pathological characterization of a novel animal model of Alzheimer's disease. **a** and **c** For detection of amyloid plaques, hippocampal regions of ADLP mice were immunostained with the biotin-4G8 antibody at 4-, 7-, and 10-month-old. The percentage of amyloid plaques area was not significantly different between ADLP$^{APP/PS1}$ and ADLP^{APT} mice (Student's t-test, $n = 3–4$ per group). Scale bar represents 200 μm. **b** and **d**) The hippocampal CA1 layer of ADLP mice was stained with the AT8 antibody against phosphorylated tau (Ser202/Thr205). A significant increase in AT8 immunoreactivity was observed in ADLP^{APT} mice compared with age-matched ADLP^{Tau} mice (Student's t-test, $n = 3–4$ per group). Scale bar represents 200 μm. **e** Sarkosyl-insoluble tau fractions from 7 and 10 months ADLP mice hippocampus were analyzed by western blot analysis using human tau specific antibody (Tau13). **f** Each distinct size of sarkosyl-insoluble tau was quantified in 10 months old ADLP^{Tau} and ADLP^{APT} mice (Chi-square test; $n = 6$ mice per genotypes). **g** The CA1 pyramidal neurons of ADLP mice were stained with anti-NeuN antibody to determine degrees of neuronal loss. Scale bars represents 100 μm or 50 μm (enlarged figures). **h** Quantification of the number of CA1 neurons in 7- and 10-month-old ADLP mouse model (one-way ANOVA in each age of ADLP mouse model). **i** ADLP model mice showed memory impairment compared with wild-type mice, which examined by the Y-maze test (one-way ANOVA in each age of ADLP mouse model, $n = 9–11$ per group). Results are expressed as mean ± SEM. * $P < 0.05$, ** $P < 0.01$, *** $P < 0.001$, **** $P < 0.0001$

and the peptide samples were labeled with TMT reagents. The labeled samples were analyzed using Q Exactive mass spectrometer. The resulting 96 raw files (12 peptide fractions × 4 TMT-mix experimental sets × technical duplicates) were processed in Proteome Discoverer based on the SEQUEST-HT algorithm. In total, 9814 protein groups were identified from 125,683 unique peptides; among them, 7022 protein groups were successfully identified in all 36 samples (Fig. 2b and c). The expression levels of the mutated human proteins (APP, PSEN1, and tau) were clearly verified by our MS analysis (Additional file 2: Figure S1F–H). Our proteomic platform allowed us to discover in-depth proteome which dynamic range covered over six orders of magnitude. This comprehensive dataset included a number of well-known risk factors of AD (http://www.alzgene.org), such as *Apoe* [29], *Clu* [30], and TDP-43 (*Tardbp*) [31, 32], which were quantified in all samples. Notably, we also detected low-abundance risk factors, such as *Gab2* [33–35], *Trem2* [36], and *Abca7* [37], indicating that our proteome exhibited a profound quantification depth (Fig. 2d). The other genes shown in Fig. 2d were reported as AD risk factors in other studies [38–47]. Thus, our extensive proteome profiling of the mouse hippocampus yielded a database that could form a solid foundation for further biological interpretations. All protein identification data are presented in Additional file 3: Table S1. The proteins quantified in all 36 channels are listed in Additional file 4: Table S2. In addition, we have provided the interactive plot that shows the protein changes over three age points for the input gene in "Profile plot" sheet of Additional file 4: Table S2 [48].

To assess the comprehensiveness of the proteome data, we compared our data with those in a recently reported mouse brain proteome atlas (http://www.mousebrainproteome.com) [9]. The comparative analysis showed that approximately 87% of the protein groups in this dataset, which is the largest to date, were also identified in our study. Notably, despite using less instrument time than the label-free method used in constructing the mouse brain atlas, our TMT-based proteomics technique has constructed a proteome dataset of comparable depth. Furthermore, 2344 genes were uniquely identified in our dataset, indicating that our data expanded the hippocampal proteome to a great extent using a single type of sample on a more time-efficient platform (Additional file 2: Figure S4A). In addition, we compared the efficiency of protein identification with those reported in other proteomic studies of transgenic AD mouse models; our dataset contained the highest number of protein identifications (Additional file 2: Figure S4B).

Quality assessment of the proteomic data

The multiplexing capacities of the TMT-based workflow allowed us to characterize the quantitative variations within and between hippocampal samples. Our analysis of a non-homologous (i.e., ovalbumin) spiked-in standard for inter- and intrabatch normalization revealed a coefficient of variation of 6.3% during repetitive MS analysis (Additional file 2: Figure S5A). Although the intensity variations among non-normalized biological replicates showed a suitable reproducibility, we observed a slight improvement of reproducibility when the normalization was performed using ovalbumin (Additional file 2: Figure S5B and C). Thus, the reporter ion intensities of proteins were initially normalized with respect to the intensity of ovalbumin.

To investigate the quantitative reproducibility (technical and experimental set-to-set variations), we used protein abundances in pooled sample channels (131) to perform cross-correlation examinations. Based on the results, the duplicate MS analysis showed excellent consistency, with an average R^2 correlation value of 0.994 (Additional file 2: Figure S5D). The mean R^2 value of the quantified protein abundance between the TMT experimental sets was excellent at 0.992 (range, 0.988–0.995) (Additional file 2: Figure S5E). Furthermore, the results indicated good correlation among the biological replicates, with a mean Pearson's correlation value of 0.991 (Additional file 2: Figure S5F). Thus, the observed differences in protein expression reflected the molecular diversity among the mouse histotypes, not the effect of our TMT-based strategy [49].

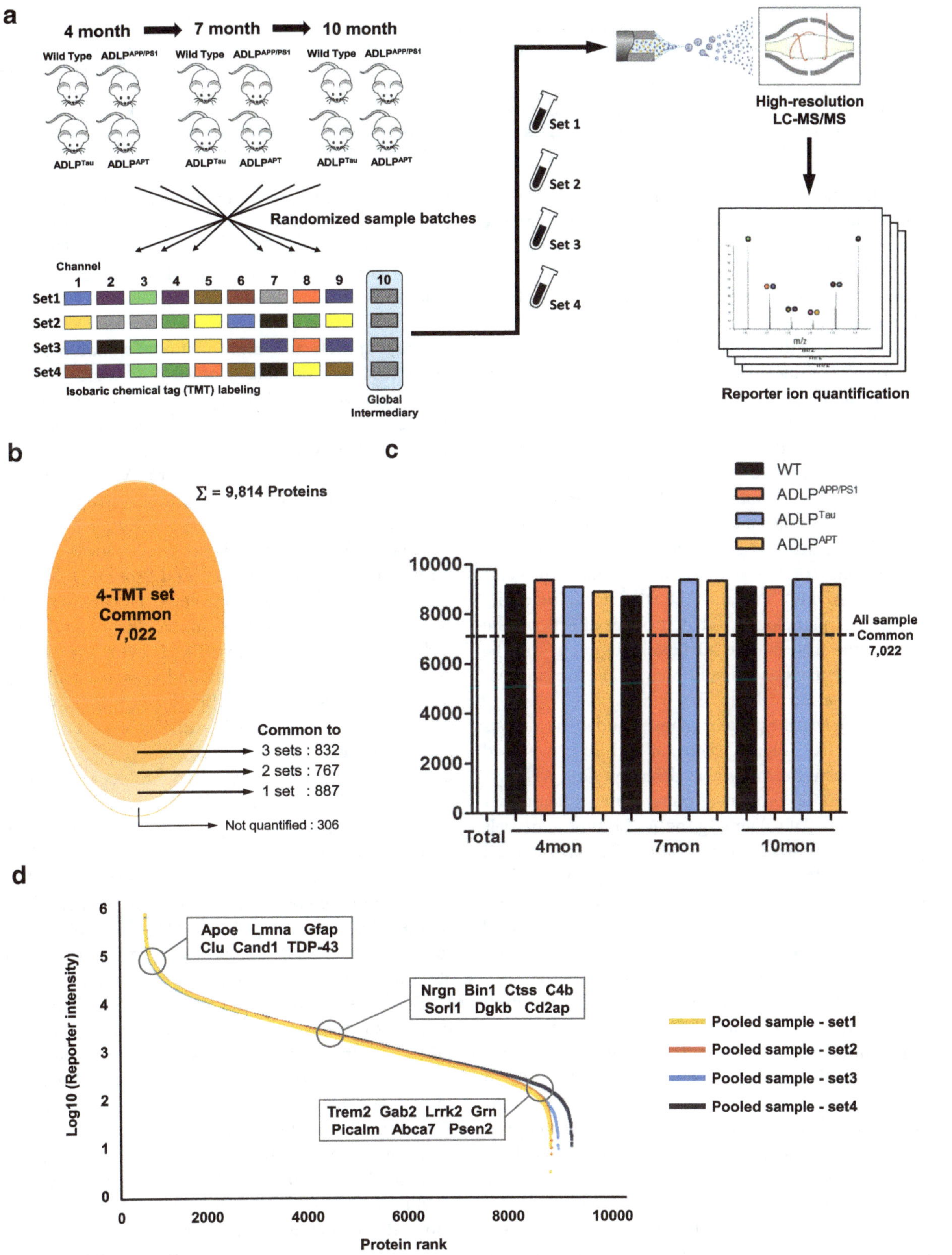

Fig. 2 (See legend on next page.)

(See figure on previous page.)
Fig. 2 Hippocampal proteome analysis of ADLP model mice. **a** Graphical illustration of the workflow used for our TMT-based proteomic analysis. The detailed sample assignments for TMT labeling are shown in Fig. S2A. **b** A total of 9814 protein groups were identified in our study; of them, 7022 protein groups were identified and quantified in all experimental sets. The "Not quantified" proteins were identified via search algorithm, but their reporter ions were not detected and were excluded from subsequent quantitative analysis. **c** A bar chart showing the number of proteins identified in the hippocampus of each ADLP model. **d** Dynamic range of protein abundance, spanning six orders of magnitude. Normalized reporter ion intensities of pooled samples in each experimental set were used. Proteins known as AD risk factors are annotated in the plot

Proteome alterations in ADLP hippocampus

To resolve the regulated proteins in each ADLP mouse model, we quantitatively analyzed the protein expression in a ratiometric manner (see Methods). Based on the fold-change in the normalized protein abundance, we identified 63, 178, and 245 proteins that were significantly regulated in 4-, 7-, and 10-month-old ADLP$^{APP/PS1}$ mice, respectively (Student's *t*-test, *p*-value <0.05, fold-change >1.25). In comparison, 3, 42, and 4 proteins were significantly regulated in 4-, 7-, and 10-month-old ADLP^{Tau} mice, respectively, whereas 62, 131, and 311 proteins were significantly regulated in 4-, 7-, and 10-month-old ADLP^{APT} mice, respectively. The scatter plots showed that more proteins were up-regulated during the progression of amyloid pathology than during that of NFT pathology. Interestingly, the overall tendencies of the significantly regulated proteins were similar in ADLP$^{APP/PS1}$ and ADLP^{APT} mice, indicating that the amyloid pathology exerted stronger effects on the overall proteome than did the NFT pathology (Fig. 3). The proteins with significant change in each model are summarized in Additional file 5: Table S3.

To identify the specific protein changes under the various AD pathologies (Aβ, Tau, or both Aβ and Tau), we used ANOVA to investigate the global diversity. Our ANOVA indicated that 1094 protein groups were differentially expressed proteins (DEPs) among the ADLP mouse models (FDR cut-off <0.05; Additional file 6: Table S4). Hierarchical clustering divided these proteins into three groups, including up-regulated proteins (cluster 2; 681 proteins) and down-regulated proteins (cluster 3; 121 proteins). ADLP^{Tau} mice had relatively few DEPs, whereas ADLP$^{APP/PS1}$ and ADLP^{APT} mice shared DEPs that showed drastic age-related perturbations (Fig. 4a). This suggests that tau itself is insufficient to drive the hippocampal proteome regulation during the stage up to 10 months of AD pathogenesis.

We subsequently investigated how these DEPs affected downstream pathways in an unbiased manner. The ingenuity pathway analysis (IPA) platform identified five canonical pathway categories (nervous system signaling, immune response, cell cycle/apoptosis, cancer/disease signaling, and intracellular signaling pathways) that were significantly enriched by the DEPs (*p*-value <0.05; activation Z-score > 1; Fig. 4b). The primary enriched pathway categories were nervous system signaling and the immune response, which are known to be associated with AD pathogenesis. While the signaling pathways of the nervous system tend to become inactive with age, most identified immune response pathways were predicted to be activated as the disease progressed. The exact Z-scores and *p*-values for the IPA results are listed in Additional file 7: Table S5.

Identifying molecular and functional signatures associated with pathology of ADLP^{APT} mice

We next investigated the age-dependent dysregulation of biological functions in ADLP^{APT} mice. We identified 732 proteins that were differentially expressed with respect to ADLP^{WT} mice (DEPs^{APT}, ANOVA FDR cut-off <0.05; Additional file 8: Table S6). Our hierarchical clustering analysis divided the DEPs^{APT} into five clusters, including gradually down-regulated proteins (cluster 2; 79 proteins) and gradually up-regulated proteins (cluster 5; 499 proteins; Fig. 5a). Gene ontology (GO) enrichment analysis revealed that the proteins in cluster 2 were particularly involved in synapses and cytoskeleton binding, suggesting that the AD pathologies gradually damage the synaptic plasticity in the hippocampus of ADLP^{APT} mice (Fig. 5a, right panel, and Fig 5b). The proteins of cluster 5 were primarily assigned to the inflammatory and degradation systems, such as leukocyte-mediated immunity, phagocytosis, endosomes, and lysosomes, indicating that AD pathologies could activate both inflammation and degradation systems to remove Aβ plaques and NFTs (Fig. 5c and Additional file 9: Table S7).

To define biological activities that contribute to the pathological phenotypes of ADLP^{APT} mice, we performed bioinformatics analysis using IPA to identify upstream regulators as well as downstream functions of DEPs^{APT} (Additional file 10: Table S8). The IPA predicted 25 relevant upstream regulators to modulate DEPs^{APT}. In addition, DEPs^{APT} were assigned to 27 downstream biological functions associated with the immune response and the nervous system (p-value <0.01; Fig. 6a). To further explore the predictive biological pathways significantly altered in ADLP^{APT} mice, we investigated relevant canonical pathways (p-value <0.01; Additional file 10: Table S8). Among these, one of the most dysregulated immune response-related pathways was the leukocyte extravasation signaling pathway. Adhesion-related proteins, which are mainly expressed in peripheral immune cells and endothelial cells, were differentially expressed in 10-month-old ADLP^{APT} mice

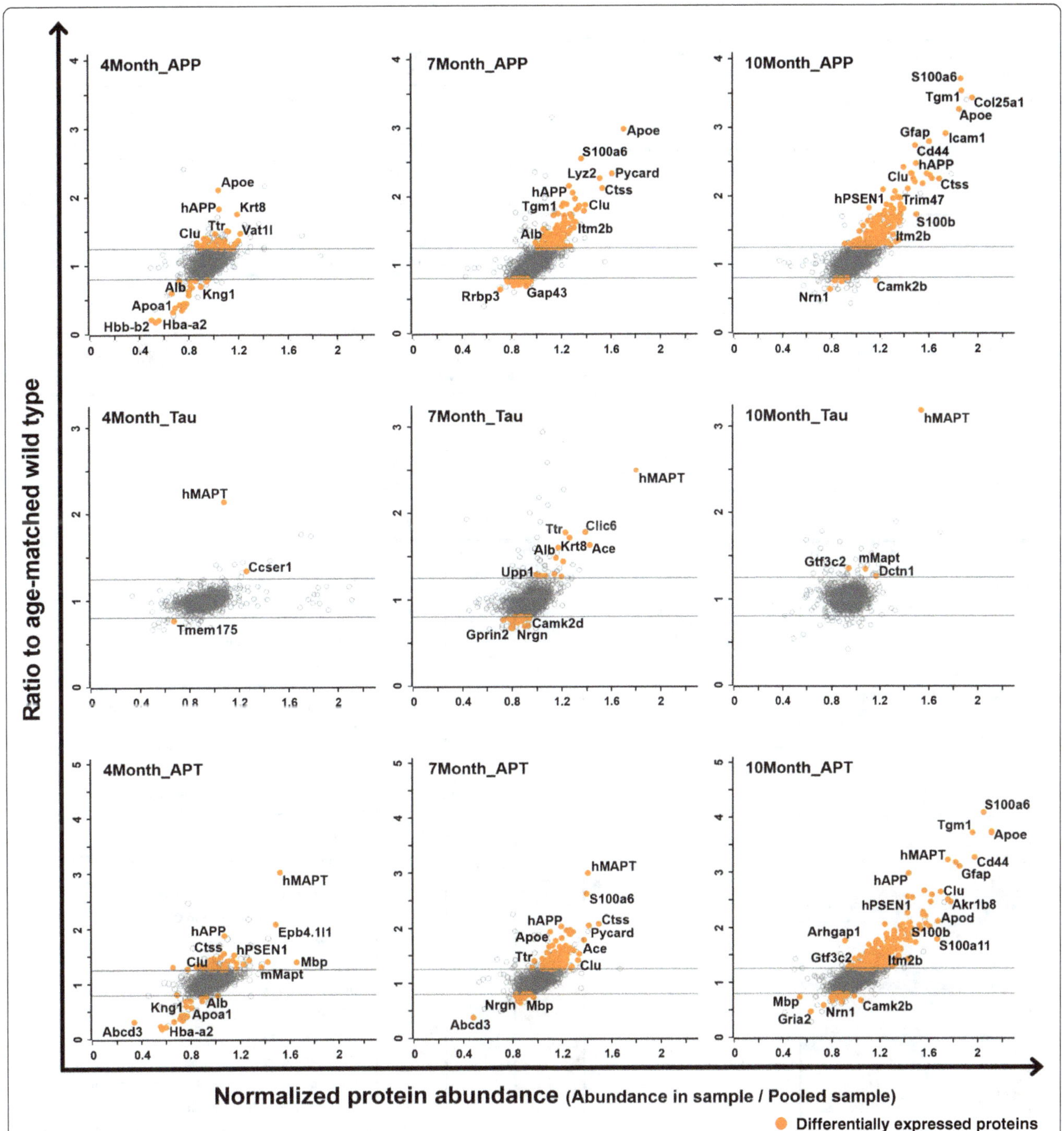

Fig. 3 Abundant and enriched proteins in the hippocampus of transgenic ADLP model mice. Scatter plot of relative protein expression levels in ADLP versus wild-type mice (y-axis). The x-axis represents the normalized protein abundance (ratio to pooled sample). Each graph was vertically placed along with ADLP model type and horizontally placed in order of age/disease progression. Significantly regulated proteins (Student's T-test *p*-value <0.05 and fold-change cut-off: 1.25) are shown as orange circles. *APP = $ADLP^{APP/PS1}$, Tau = $ADLP^{Tau}$, APT = $ADLP^{APT}$ mice

(Fig. 6b). We speculate that changes in endothelial cells are likely to reflect the AD pathology in the brain parenchyma and that such changes recruit peripheral immune cells into the brain parenchyma. Among the canonical pathways related to the nervous system, synaptic long-term potentiation (LTP) was a representative pathway altered in $ADLP^{APT}$ mice (Fig. 6c). Post-synaptic proteins of this pathway were mainly dysregulated by the extracellular amyloid pathology and the intracellular NFT pathology. Thus, the biological pathway alterations seen

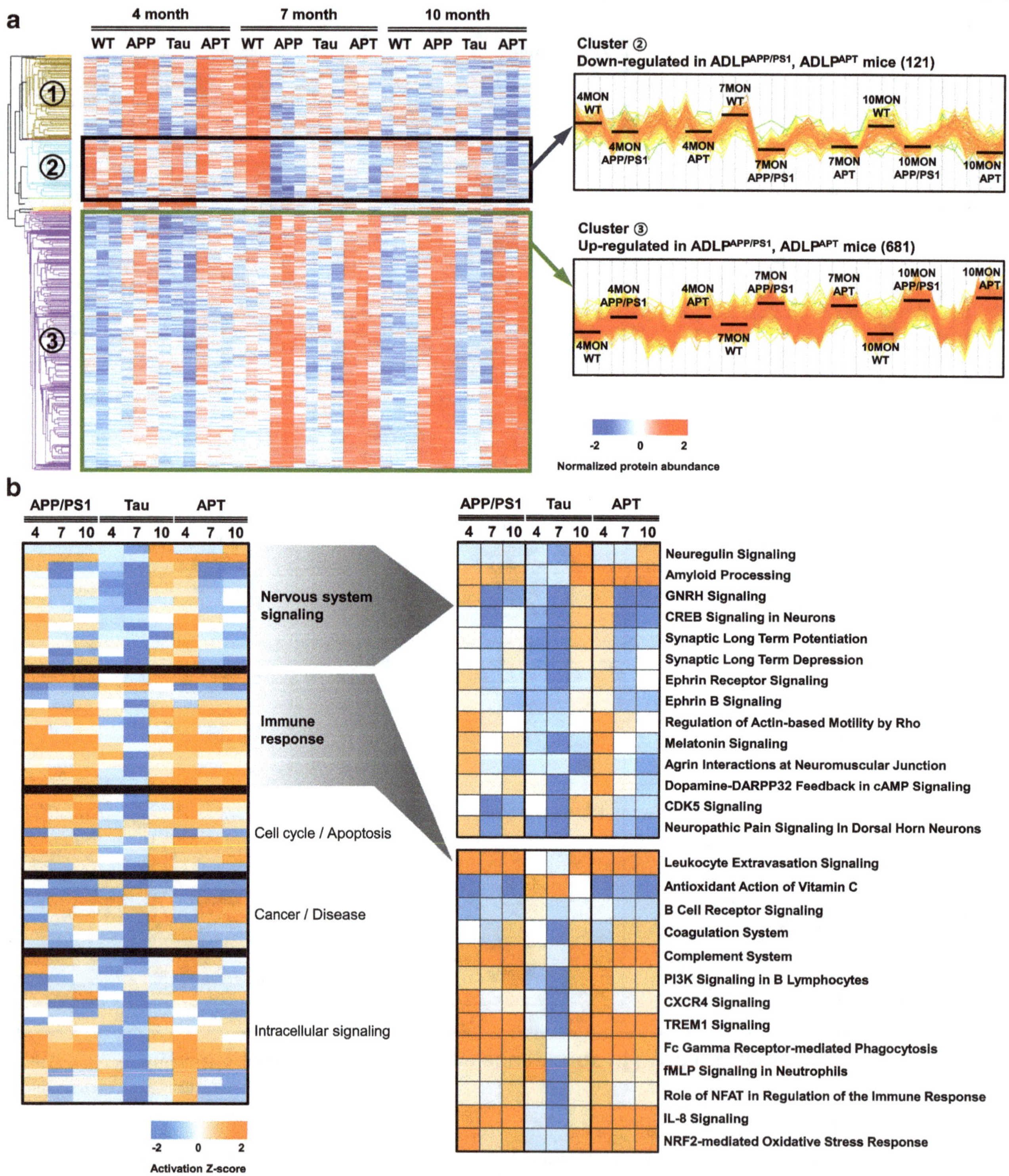

Fig. 4 Protein quantitation overview and comparative pathway enrichment analysis of ADLP model mice. **a** Hierarchical clustering of differentially expressed proteins (DEPs) across different transgenic types and ages (ANOVA FDR < 0.05). Protein expression profiles were largely clustered into three patterns; The decreasing pattern (Cluster 2) and the increasing pattern (Cluster 3) of the mouse models with human *APP* (ADLP $^{APP/PS1}$, ADLP ^{APT}) are prominent. The right panel shows the Z-normalized protein abundance according to the mouse samples as profile plots. **b** Canonical pathway enrichment for DEPs. The categories of nervous system signaling and immune response were overrepresented (~50%) and are highlighted. The significant pathways (Fisher's exact test *p*-value <0.05) were deduced using Ingenuity Pathway Analysis (IPA) and their predictive activation/inhibition status is represented as the Z-score. *APP/PS1 = ADLP$^{APP/PS1}$, Tau = ADLP^{Tau}, APT = ADLP^{APT} mice

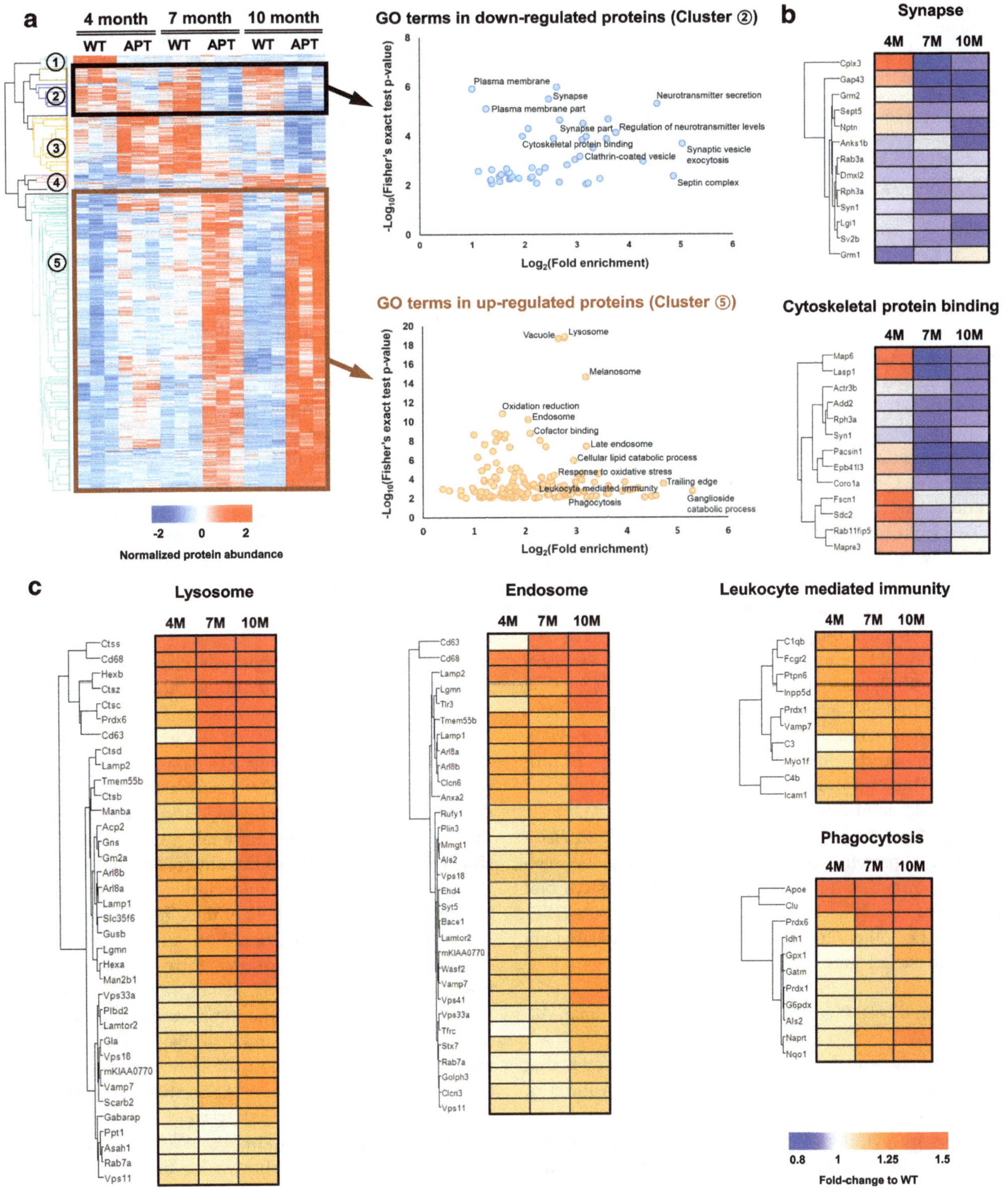

Fig. 5 (See legend on next page.)

(See figure on previous page.)
Fig. 5 Protein clustering reveals major biological and molecular signatures of ADLP^{APT} mice. **a** Hierarchical clustering of differentially expressed proteins (DEP^{APT}s) between ADLP^{APT} and wild-type mice (732 proteins; ANOVA FDR < 0.05). The DEPs^{APT} were clustered into five types of expression pattern. The protein expression level is the normalized protein abundance represented after Z-normalization. Scatter plot of enriched Gene Ontology (GO) terms in protein cluster 2 (down-regulated proteins) and cluster 5 (up-regulated proteins) are shown in the right panel. The -log10 (*P*-value) is plotted against the fold-enrichment of each GO term. **b** Heatmaps showing the expression levels of the proteins involved in the GO terms, such as synapse proteins and cytoskeleton binding proteins, in cluster 2 (down-regulated proteins). **c** Heatmaps for the expression levels of co-regulated proteins corresponding to the GO terms, such as lysosome, endosome, leukocyte-mediated immunity, and phagocytosis, in cluster 5 (up-regulated proteins)

in ADLP^{APT} mice are consistent with the pathological changes seen in the nervous system of patients with AD.

Network analysis of unique proteome changes in ADLP^{APT} mice

To identify ADLP^{APT} mouse-specific protein changes, we investigated the exclusive DEPs^{APT} in 4- (early) and 10-month-old (late) ADLP^{APT} mice (Fig. 7a and Additional file 11: Table S9). Using the STRING database, we organized a protein–protein interaction map of the exclusive DEPs^{APT} representing expression changes by age and the GO categories into which these proteins could be classified. Our GO analysis revealed that the exclusive DEPs^{APT} were classified in the categories related to the immune response (e.g., cell–cell adhesion and inflammatory responses) and neuronal functions (e.g., syntaxin binding, lysosomes, and neuron projection development) (Fig. 7b). Subsequently, we examined the correlation of exclusive DEPs^{APT} with 2 AD-causative molecules, *App* and *Mapt*, in an effort to depict how the amyloid and NFT pathologies interconnect with one another. The constructed *App–Mapt* network showed the direct or indirect connections of proteins with *App* and *Mapt*, suggesting that these molecular targets could influence specific pathologies of ADLP^{APT} mice (Fig. 7c). The expression of *Abca1*, *Ptprc*, and *Hcls1* that form a protein–protein interaction bridge between *App* and *Mapt* were further validated by the western blot analysis (Fig. 7d). The expression levels of exclusive DEPs^{APT} in the other transgenic mice are presented in Additional file 2: Figure S6.

Comparison of ADLP^{APT} mouse proteome with human AD proteome

We ultimately aimed to construct a mouse model that fully recapitulates the molecular and functional features of AD. To investigate how the ADLP^{APT} mouse model reflects AD, we performed a comparative analysis with the proteome data of a recently published human AD study [50]. This group performed proteomic analysis using brain tissues from patients with AD, elucidating molecular features and protein networks. Our dataset encompassed approximately 92% of the proteins identified in the human AD proteomics study. The expression patterns of DEPs common to both studies (Student's *t*-test *p*-value <0.05) overlapped by 41 and 25% in up-regulated and down-regulated proteins, respectively (Additional file 2: Figure S4C). Although the numerical correlation between the two data was low ($R^2 < 0.3$), the commonly significant proteins have been classified into functional categories related to AD. Particularly, 10 up-regulated proteins, such as *Clu*, *Mao-b*, *Cyp46a1*, and *Vps26a*, were deduced to have significant associations with AD (Additional file 12: Table S10). These results implicated that our mouse model adequately reflects the known molecular characteristics of AD and can thus be further utilized in the researches to discover new drug targets. Furthermore, the other proteins in the categories related to neurodegeneration may play a significant role in future studies. The results of the comparative analysis with human proteomic data are listed in Additional file 4: Table S2.

Discussion

The amyloid cascade hypothesis claims that Aβ is the initial trigger for further pathological changes, including tau hyper-phosphorylation and NFT formation, which accelerate AD progression [51]. To investigate the prominent role of Aβ in causing AD pathogenesis, we developed ADLP^{APT} mice, a novel animal model of AD that develops more robust amyloid and NFT pathologies than do other available animal models. This model showed no aggravation of the amyloid pathology beyond that seen in ADLP$^{APP/PS1}$ mice, indicating that the development of the NFT pathology does not affect the amyloid pathology. However, based on sarkosyl-insoluble tau fractionation for the aggregated form of tau and immunostaining for phosphorylated tau, the accelerated NFT pathology appeared in the hippocampus of ADLP^{APT} mice starting from 7 months of age in the absence of any observable difference in the transcription/expression of the human *MAPT* gene. Abnormal tau phosphorylation is a crucial event that triggers tau aggregation in AD brains [52]. Various kinases have been suggested to be involved in tau phosphorylation process. Among external stimuli to activate kinases, the role of Aβ for activating tau kinases has been reported in a downstream of Aβ toxicity [53]. In order to investigate whether increased kinase expression levels are causative factors for accelerating NFT pathology, we have confirmed the expression levels of three kinases (*Csnk1d*, *Gsk3-beta* and *Rps6ka1*) involved in tau phosphorylation by western

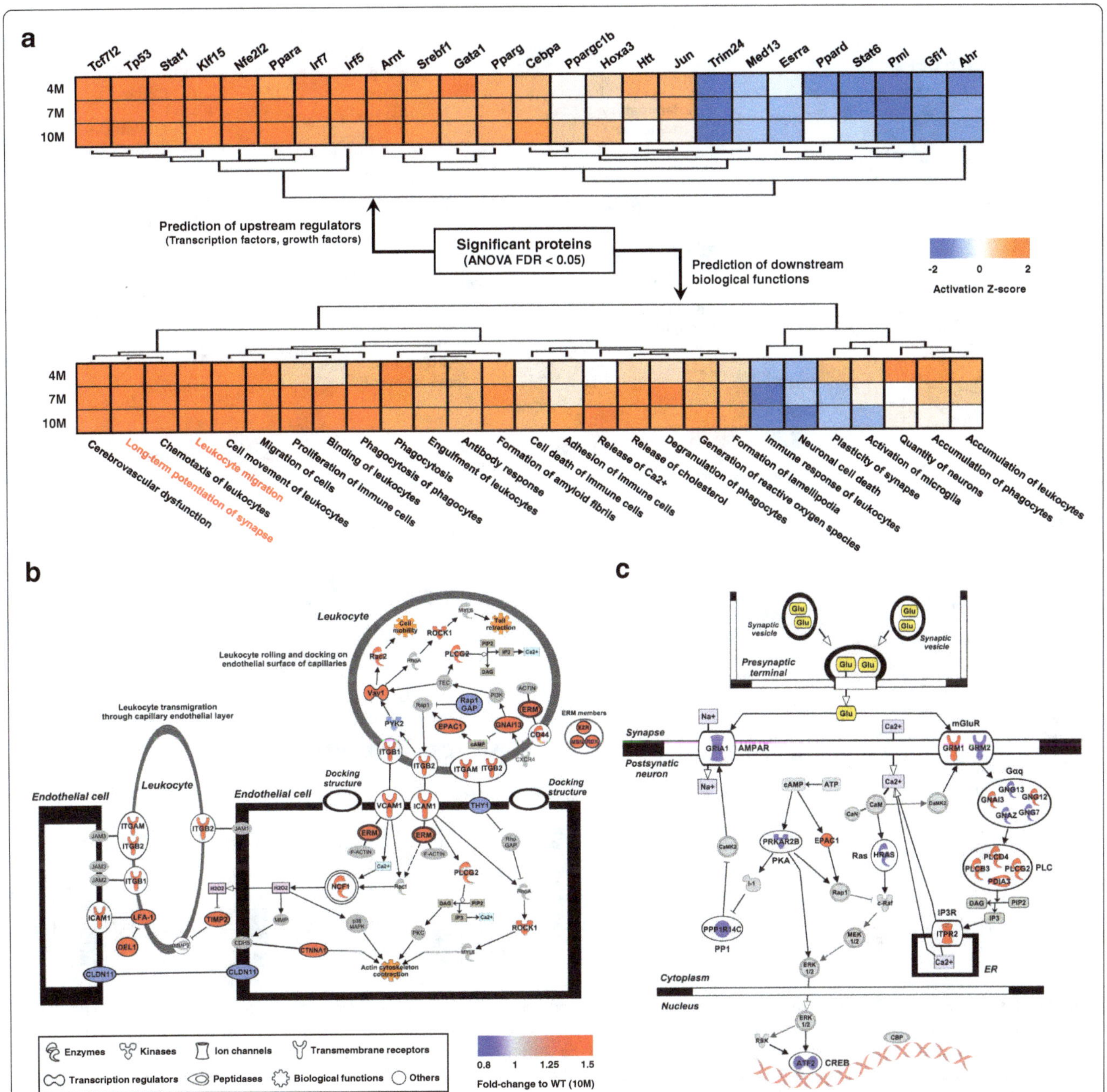

Fig. 6 Prediction of molecular responses to AD pathology in ADLP^{APT} mice. **a** Hierarchical clustering of downstream biological functions (lower panel) and the upstream regulators (upper panel) assessed by IPA using 732 DEPs^{APT} (ANOVA FDR < 0.05). The predictive activation/inhibition status is shown as a Z-score. **b** Graphical representation of the protein expression levels of members of the leukocyte extravasation pathway and (**c**) the synaptic long-term potentiation pathway in 10-month-old ADLP^{APT} mice. Individual proteins' fold-change values to the wild type were visualized in color (blue: down-regulation, red: up-regulation). Glu = Glutamate, PIP2 = Phosphatidylinositol 4,5-bisphosphate, DAG = Diacylglycerol, IP3 = Inositol 1,4,5-trisphosphate, ATP = Adenosine triphosphate, cAMP = Cyclic adenosine monophosphate

blot analysis [54–56]. Notably, no differences were observed in the kinase levels between wild-type and ADLP^{APT} mice with the disease progression. In addition to western blot analysis, the MS results also indicated no changes in kinase expression levels. As for the kinases not checked by western blot analysis (e.g. *Cdk5*, *Src*, *Fyn* and *Abl1*), they were not changed among all groups, as confirmed by our hippocampal proteome data. These results support that accelerated NFT pathology in ADLP^{APT} mice hippocampus is not accompanied by changes of tau kinases (Additional file 2: Figure S7). Previous studies have hypothesized that Aβ is the initiator of the NFT pathology [53, 57, 58]. Indeed, Aβ affects tau kinase activity or localization resulting in tau toxicity in

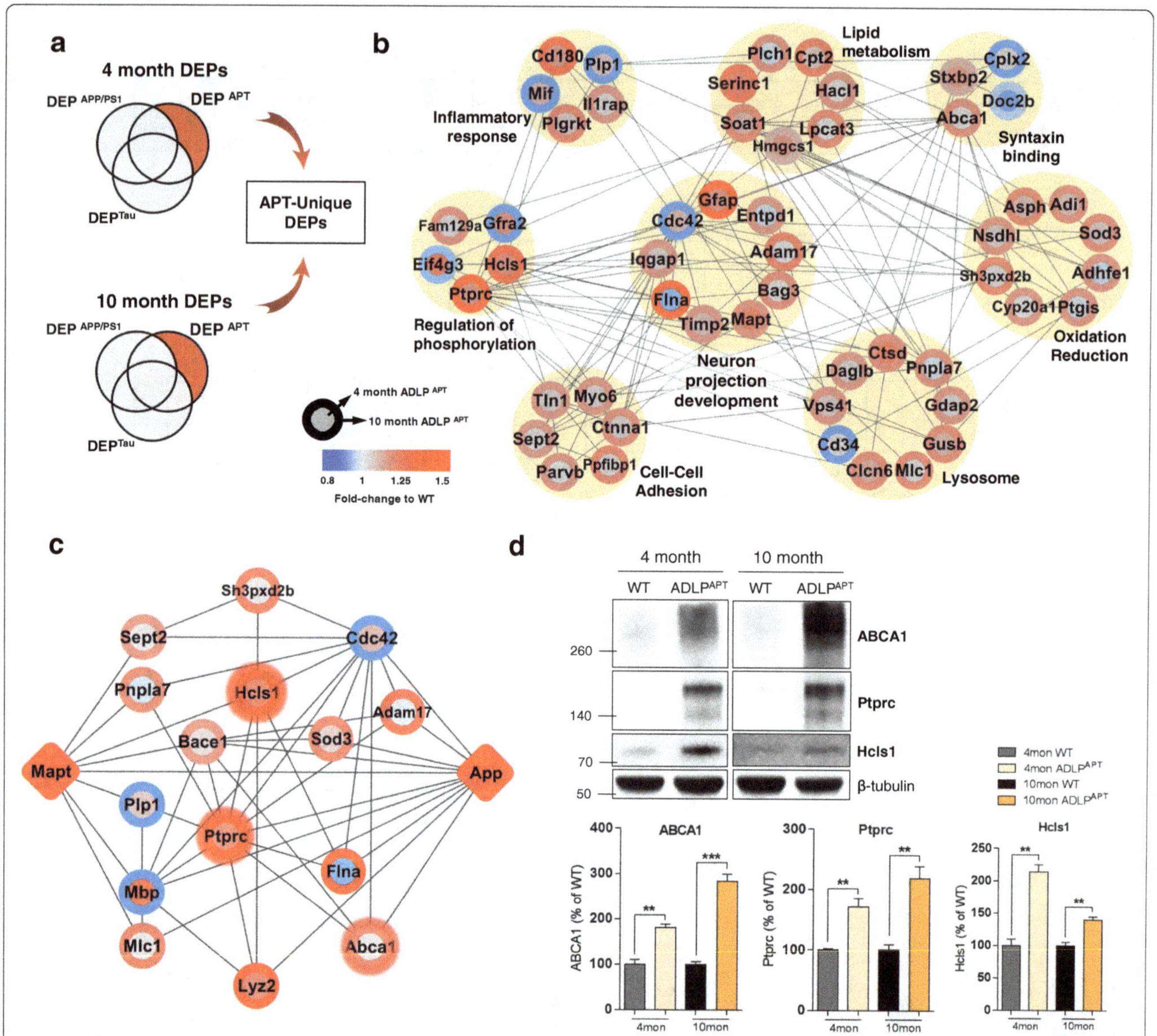

Fig. 7 Exclusive DEPs in ADLP^{APT} mice and their related functional networks. **a** Proteins that were significantly altered in early or late ADLP^{APT} mice (Student's t-test *p*-value <0.05 and fold-change >1.25) but not in the other models (fold change <1.25) were selected as exclusive DEPs^{APT}. **b** The biological functions derived from the GO analysis are shown along with their networking with associated proteins. **c** The knowledge database-derived protein network of *App*, *Mapt*, and exclusive DEPs^{APT}. The fold-change values of individual protein nodes were visualized in color circles (blue: down-regulation, red: up-regulation). The color of the inner circle is the fold-change of the 4-month ADLP^{APT} mouse, and the color of the outer circle represents that of the 10-month ADLP^{APT} mouse. **d** Three proteins that form bridge between *App* and *Mapt* (*Hcls1*, *Ptprc* and *Abca1*) were validated by western blot analysis. Representative western blot images are shown herein. The expression levels of the proteins are quantified compared with wild type mice ($n = 3$ per genotype for 4 and 10 months; Student's t test). Results are expressed as the mean ± SEM. $^{**}P < 0.01$; $^{***}P < 0.001$

neurons. Moreover, the amyloid pathology in the cortex accelerates tau propagation process throughout the entorhinal cortex and aggravates the NFT pathology [57]. Because the underlying molecular mechanisms of the pathophysiological interaction between Aβ and tau are unclear, ADLP^{APT} mice may enable further exploration of the Aβ-tau axis hypothesis on the progression of AD pathogenesis.

To further investigate the biological functions altered in the hippocampus of ADLP^{APT} mice, we first constructed a hippocampal proteomic database of ADLP animal models using LC-MS. Notably, as the disease progressed, the protein expression profiles of ADLP^{Tau} mice resembled those of wild type mice, indicating that the relatively slow NFT pathology had a small impact on the proteomic changes during the early stage of the disease. In contrast, $ADLP^{APT}$ mice showed dramatic proteome-wide changes with a pattern similar to that of $ADLP^{APP/PS1}$ mice. One of the main explanations for the high similarity between $ADLP^{APP/PS1}$ and $ADLP^{APT}$ mice is the presence of inflammatory responses in the hippocampus. Almost all immune-related pathways exhibited similar changes over time in $ADLP^{APP/PS1}$ and $ADLP^{APT}$ mice, indicating that Aβ is one of the main factors for active inflammatory responses in the hippocampus (Fig. 4b). In both mice, the immune response categories exhibited changes at 4 months of age, even before the first deposition of amyloid plaques in the hippocampus. Immunohistochemical analysis confirmed similarities in the inflammation status between $ADLP^{APP/PS1}$ and $ADLP^{APT}$ mice, as evidenced by the staining with astrocytes and microglia markers in the hippocampus (Additional file 2: Figure S2). These findings indicate that the immune responses in the hippocampus were mainly influenced by the amyloid pathology regardless of the NFT pathology.

Moreover, GO analysis of the gradually up-regulated DEPs in $ADLP^{APT}$ mice identified many glial cell type-related categories, such as phagocytosis, cell chemotaxis, and macrophage infiltration (cluster 5, Fig. 5a). One of the main dysregulated pathways in $ADLP^{APT}$ mice was the leukocyte extravasation signaling pathway. Various adhesion-related molecules (*Icam-1, Vcam-1, Itgb-1/2*, and *Cd44*) were up-regulated in the hippocampus of $ADLP^{APT}$ mice (Fig. 6a and b), indicating that AD pathologies can modulate endothelial cells in the brain parenchyma and recruit peripheral immune [59]. Both amyloid plaques and neurofibrillary tangles can activate inflammatory responses, thereby inducing the secretion of cytokines from microglia and astrocytes. Moreover, these serial pathologies also affect endothelial cells and disrupt the blood–brain barrier (BBB) integrity in AD [60]. A disrupted BBB with increased inflammatory cytokines finally results in the recruitment of peripheral immune cells toward brain parenchyma in AD. Several previous reports have suggested communication between peripheral immune cells and brain parenchyma as a pathological phenotype of AD, even if their functional roles remain unclear. Laurent C et al. have reported that CD8-positive T cells infiltrate the hippocampus. They have also demonstrated that the infiltration of CD8-positive lymphocytes in the cortical region of patients with frontotemporal dementia who develop tauopathy resulted from P301L mutation within the *tau* gene [61]. Previously, using two-photon microscopy, we have observed that neutrophils can extravasate from blood vessels into the brain parenchyma where amyloid plaques are present. In the brain parenchyma, the neutrophils adhere to amyloid plaques and phagocyte them [62]. Moreover, Zenaro E et al. have reported that the number of neutrophils adhere both inside blood vessels and in the brain parenchyma of patients with AD [63]. Depleting temporarily neutrophils at the early stage of disease progression in a transgenic mouse model of AD prevented memory impairments, suggesting that the infiltration of neutrophils contributes to the pathogenesis of AD. The up-regulation of the proteins involved in the leukocyte extravasation signaling in $ADLP^{APT}$ mice suggested that peripheral immune cells may interact with capillary endothelial cells for infiltration into the brain parenchyma.

When glial or peripheral immune cells detect extracellular amyloid plaques, they clear the amyloid deposits through phagocytosis [64]. In addition to extracellular amyloid plaques, when neurons host NFTs in the cytosol, they activate the degradation system including the autophagy-lysosome system to eliminate them [65, 66]. Consistent with these, the GO analysis revealed that the gradually upregulated $DEPs^{APT}$ included many components of the degradation system (cluster 5, Fig. 5c). In addition, constituents of the endosome GO category were upregulated, demonstrating that the endocytic pathway via endocytosis was also activated in $ADLP^{APT}$ mice. Thus, although we could not clarify which cell types exhibited these protein changes, the results of the GO analysis of up-regulated proteins collectively suggested that AD pathologies trigger a sequential response that moves from phagocytosis to degradation via the endocytic pathway.

Several nervous system signaling pathways appear to differ between $ADLP^{APP/PS1}$ and $ADLP^{APT}$ mice. The two canonical pathways, cAMP response element-binding protein (CREB) signaling in neurons and synaptic LTP, were inactivated only in the 10-month-old $ADLP^{APT}$ mice (Fig. 6c). It is established that CREB signaling contributes to cognitive functions by modulating synaptic plasticity [67]. Proteins associated with LTP processes are increased by CREB signaling in the hippocampus; in AD, alterations in Ca^{2+} signaling lead to decreased CREB signaling and altered LTP [68]. Similarly, our $ADLP^{APT}$ mice showed downregulated CREB signaling and LTP compared with $ADLP^{Tau}$ and $ADLP^{APP/PS1}$ mice. Thus, these two pathways are predicted to be disturbed simultaneously by both Aβ accumulation and NFTs. This suggests that $ADLP^{APT}$ mice have pathological symptoms similar to those of patients with AD [69].

To investigate the putative mechanisms underlying the molecular pathogenesis of $ADLP^{APT}$ mice, we sorted exclusive DEPs in $ADLP^{APT}$ to identify unique molecular alterations. The protein–protein interaction map of exclusive $DEPs^{APT}$ showed their direct or indirect interactions with each other and categories that each protein belongs to. We further investigated the molecular interactions of exclusive $DEPs^{APT}$ with *App* and *Mapt* (Fig. 7c). The generated *App–Mapt* network contained 15 components that have been reported to interact among each other, although little is known about their relevance to the Aβ-tau axis. For example, *Ptprc* is a well-known microglia marker that has a strong association with Aβ oligomerization [70]. However, to our knowledge, the regulation of this protein in the hippocampus of AD mouse models is not well studied. In contrast, *Abca1*, a risk factor for AD, has been reported to play a significant role in Aβ clearance [71]. In addition, *Hcls1* is a leukocyte-specific actin-binding protein involved in immune response mechanisms [72]. We found that these proteins are involved in immune responses in the hippocampus, forming an interaction bridge on our *App-Mapt* network. Furthermore, western blot analysis clearly confirmed the regulation of these proteins in $ADLP^{APT}$ mice. Since our *App-Mapt* protein network provides information on DEPs affected by both Aβ and tau, it may help researchers to identify novel molecular mechanisms in the Aβ-tau axis.

To verify whether $ADLP^{APT}$ mice and its proteome data could be applied to further AD researches, we performed a comparative analysis with existing AD proteome datasets. First, the proteome data of $ADLP^{APT}$ mice were compared with that of human AD brain generated by Seyfried and Levey [50]. As a result, approximately 92% of the identified proteins were overlapped with the human AD proteome and approximately 30% of significantly regulated proteins in human AD data showed identical expression patterns with those of $ADLP^{APT}$ mice (p-value <0.05 in both studies, respectively). We also assessed the commonality between our mouse model and the previously established 3xTg AD mouse model [73–75]. Notably, the comparative analysis indicated that our DEPs were largely different from those of other studies of 3xTg AD mice (data not shown). Most of our DEPs were neither detected nor showed consistent expression patterns in other studies. This may be attributed to the fact that the results of other studies were generated from 2-DIGE analysis [73] or the vesicular proteome isolated from the forebrain [74]. To the best of our knowledge, this study is the first to perform proteomic analysis in hippocampi developing both amyloid and NFT pathologies. These results indicate that the pathological relevance of our mouse model for AD research is valid at the protein level and in severe hippocampal pathologies.

Conclusion

We herein described a novel mouse model for AD, namely $ADLP^{APT}$ mouse. This model exhibited a rapid progression of AD pathology, including neuronal death and an accelerated NFT pathology that are particularly accelerated by the amyloid pathology. Thus, this model recapitulated the progression of human AD. Using LC-MS with 10-plex TMT isobaric labeling, we further constructed a hippocampal proteome database of ADLP mouse models. We used this database to understand the biological functions that were altered in each transgenic mouse model. This proteomic database also offers extensive resource of various molecular phenotypes in response to amyloid and NFT pathologies. Based on the bioinformatics analysis, we propose potential molecular targets for mechanistic studies and therapeutic development based on the proteomic database generated from our novel animal model.

Additional files

Additional file 1: Supplementary Methods.

Additional file 2: Figure S1. Pathological characterization of a novel animal model of Alzheimer's disease. **Figure S2.** Activated neuroinflammation in a novel animal model of Alzheimer's disease. **Figure S3.** TMT-based protein quantification strategy. **Figure S4.** The comparative analysis between $ADLP^{APT}$ and other AD proteome datasets. **Figure S5.** The quality assessment of MS analysis. **Figure S6.** The expression levels of exclusive $DEPs^{APT}$ in other ADLP mice. **Figure S7.** Longitudinal expression changes of kinases involved in phosphorylation of tau protein.

Additional file 3: Table S1. All identified protein groups.

Additional file 4: Table S2. All quantified protein groups.

Additional file 5: Table S3. Significantly regulated proteins from t-test.

Additional file 6: Table S4. DEPs from ANOVA test.

Additional file 7: Table S5. Canonical pathways enriched by IPA analysis.

Additional file 8: Table S6. DEPs in $ADLP^{APT}$ mice, $DEPs^{APT}$.

Additional file 9: Table S7. GO analysis results in $ADLP^{APT}$ mice.

Additional file 10: Table S8. IPA analysis results in $ADLP^{APT}$ mice.

Additional file 11: Table S9. Exclusive $DEPs^{APT}$.

Additional file 12: Table S10. GO analysis of commonly significant proteins in human and $ADLP^{APT}$.

Abbreviations

ADLP: Alzheimer's disease-like pathology; APP: Amyloid precursor protein; Aβ: Amyloid beta; BPRP: Basic pH reverse phase; DEPs: Differentially expressed proteins; GO: Gene ontology; IPA: Ingenuity pathway analysis; LC-MS: Liquid chromatography - Mass spectrometry; LTP: Long term potentiation; NFT: Neurofibrillary tangle; PPI: Protein-protein interaction; TMT: Tandem mass tag

Acknowledgements

Not applicable.

Funding

This work was supported by the National Research Foundation grant (No. 2011–0030740 and 2017M3C9A5031597) to YK and NRF (2015R1A2A1A05001794, 2014M3C7A1046047, 2015M3C7A1028790, and MRC [2011–0030738]) to IM-J. DKK received a scholarship from the BK21-plus education program provided by the National Research Foundation of Korea.

Authors' contributions

DKK, JP, DH participated equally in the overall work. DKK, JP, DH, YK, and IM-J designed the research and experiments. DKK performed the immunohistochemistry, sarkosyl-insoluble tau fractionation, RT-PCR, and behavioral tests and wrote the manuscript. JP performed proteomics experiment and wrote the manuscript. DH contributed to the proteomics experiments and revised the manuscript. JY contributed to design sarkosyl-insoluble tau fractionation experiment and carry out the immunohistochemistry. AK contributed to do behavioral tests and prepare for biological experiments. JW contributed to analyze the MS-based proteomics data. YK and IM-J revised manuscript. All authors have read and approved the final manuscript.

Competing interests

The authors declare that they have no competing interests.

Author details

[1]Department of Biomedical Sciences, Seoul National University, College of Medicine, 103 Daehak-ro, Seoul 110-799, South Korea. [2]Interdisciplinary Program in Bioengineering, College of Engineering, Seoul National University, 1 Gwanak-ro, Seoul 151-742, South Korea. [3]Biomedical Research Institute, Seoul National University Hospital, 101 Daehak-ro, Seoul 110-744, South Korea. [4]Neuroscience Research Institute, Seoul National University, College of Medicine, Seoul 110-799, South Korea.

References

1. Braak H, Braak E. Staging of Alzheimer's disease-related neurofibrillary changes. Neurobiol Aging. 1995;16:271–8. discussion 278-284
2. Hardy J, Selkoe DJ. The amyloid hypothesis of Alzheimer's disease: progress and problems on the road to therapeutics. Science. 2002;297:353–6.
3. Oddo S, Caccamo A, Shepherd JD, Murphy MP, Golde TE, Kayed R, Metherate R, Mattson MP, Akbari Y, LaFerla FM. Triple-transgenic model of Alzheimer's disease with plaques and tangles: intracellular Abeta and synaptic dysfunction. Neuron. 2003;39:409–21.
4. Oakley H, Cole SL, Logan S, Maus E, Shao P, Craft J, Guillozet-Bongaarts A, Ohno M, Disterhoft J, Van Eldik L, et al. Intraneuronal beta-amyloid aggregates, neurodegeneration, and neuron loss in transgenic mice with five familial Alzheimer's disease mutations: potential factors in amyloid plaque formation. J Neurosci. 2006;26:10129–40.
5. Lewis J, McGowan E, Rockwood J, Melrose H, Nacharaju P, Van Slegtenhorst M, Gwinn-Hardy K, Paul Murphy M, Baker M, Yu X, et al. Neurofibrillary tangles, amyotrophy and progressive motor disturbance in mice expressing mutant (P301L) tau protein. Nat Genet. 2000;25:402–5.
6. Bird CM, Burgess N. The hippocampus and memory: insights from spatial processing. Nat Rev Neurosci. 2008;9:182–94.
7. Aebersold R, Mann M. Mass-spectrometric exploration of proteome structure and function. Nature. 2016;537:347–55.
8. Choudhary C, Mann M. Decoding signalling networks by mass spectrometry-based proteomics. Nat Rev Mol Cell Biol. 2010;11:427–39.
9. Sharma K, Schmitt S, Bergner CG, Tyanova S, Kannaiyan N, Manrique-Hoyos N, Kongi K, Cantuti L, Hanisch UK, Philips MA, et al. Cell type- and brain region-resolved mouse brain proteome. Nat Neurosci. 2015;18:1819–31.
10. Zhang Y, Fonslow BR, Shan B, Baek MC, Yates JR 3rd. Protein analysis by shotgun/bottom-up proteomics. Chem Rev. 2013;113:2343–94.
11. Thompson A, Schafer J, Kuhn K, Kienle S, Schwarz J, Schmidt G, Neumann T, Johnstone R, Mohammed AK, Hamon C. Tandem mass tags: a novel quantification strategy for comparative analysis of complex protein mixtures by MS/MS. Anal Chem. 2003;75:1895–904.
12. McAlister GC, Huttlin EL, Haas W, Ting L, Jedrychowski MP, Rogers JC, Kuhn K, Pike I, Grothe RA, Blethrow JD, Gygi SP. Increasing the multiplexing capacity of TMTs using reporter ion isotopologues with isobaric masses. Anal Chem. 2012;84:7469–78.
13. Christoforou A, Mulvey CM, Breckels LM, Geladaki A, Hurrell T, Hayward PC, Naake T, Gatto L, Viner R, Martinez Arias A, Lilley KSA. Draft map of the mouse pluripotent stem cell spatial proteome. Nat Commun. 2016;7:8992.
14. Murphy JP, Stepanova E, Everley RA, Paulo JA, Gygi SP. Comprehensive temporal protein dynamics during the Diauxic shift in Saccharomyces Cerevisiae. Mol Cell Proteomics. 2015;14:2454–65.
15. Weekes MP, Tomasec P, Huttlin EL, Fielding CA, Nusinow D, Stanton RJ, Wang EC, Aicheler R, Murrell I, Wilkinson GW, et al. Quantitative temporal viromics: an approach to investigate host-pathogen interaction. Cell. 2014;157:1460–72.
16. Chick JM, Munger SC, Simecek P, Huttlin EL, Choi K, Gatti DM, Raghupathy N, Svenson KL, Churchill GA, Gygi SP. Defining the consequences of genetic variation on a proteome-wide scale. Nature. 2016;534:500–5.
17. Gotz J, Ittner LM. Animal models of Alzheimer's disease and frontotemporal dementia. Nat Rev Neurosci. 2008;9:532–44.
18. Han D, Moon S, Kim Y, Kim J, Jin J, Kim Y. In-depth proteomic analysis of mouse microglia using a combination of FASP and StageTip-based, high pH, reversed-phase fractionation. Proteomics. 2013;13:2984–8.
19. Han D, Jin J, Woo J, Min H, Kim Y. Proteomic analysis of mouse astrocytes and their secretome by a combination of FASP and StageTip-based, high pH, reversed-phase fractionation. Proteomics. 2014;14:1604–9.
20. Kulak NA, Pichler G, Paron I, Nagaraj N, Mann M. Minimal, encapsulated proteomic-sample processing applied to copy-number estimation in eukaryotic cells. Nat Methods. 2014;11:319–24.
21. Tyanova S, Temu T, Sinitcyn P, Carlson A, Hein MY, Geiger T, Mann M, Cox J. The Perseus computational platform for comprehensive analysis of (prote)omics data. Nat Methods. 2016;13:731–40.
22. Benjamini Y, Hochberg Y. Controlling the false discovery rate - a practical and powerful approach to multiple testing. J Roy Stat Soc B Met. 1995;57:289–300.
23. Huang d W, Sherman BT, Lempicki RA. Systematic and integrative analysis of large gene lists using DAVID bioinformatics resources. Nat Protoc. 2009;4:44–57.
24. Kramer A, Green J, Pollard J Jr, Tugendreich S. Causal analysis approaches in ingenuity pathway analysis. Bioinformatics. 2014;30:523–30.
25. Szklarczyk D, Franceschini A, Wyder S, Forslund K, Heller D, Huerta-Cepas J, Simonovic M, Roth A, Santos A, Tsafou KP, et al. STRING v10: protein-protein interaction networks, integrated over the tree of life. Nucleic Acids Res. 2015;43:D447–52.
26. Shannon P, Markiel A, Ozier O, Baliga NS, Wang JT, Ramage D, Amin N, Schwikowski B, Ideker T. Cytoscape: a software environment for integrated models of biomolecular interaction networks. Genome Res. 2003;13:2498–504.
27. Wong PC, Cai H, Borchelt DR, Price DL. Genetically engineered mouse models of neurodegenerative diseases. Nat Neurosci. 2002;5:633–9.
28. Wisniewski JR, Zougman A, Nagaraj N, Mann M. Universal sample preparation method for proteome analysis. Nat Methods. 2009;6:359–62.
29. Verghese PB, Castellano JM, Holtzman DM, Apolipoprotein E. In Alzheimer's disease and other neurological disorders. Lancet Neurol. 2011;10:241–52.
30. JT Y, Tan L. The role of clusterin in Alzheimer's disease: pathways, pathogenesis, and therapy. Mol Neurobiol. 2012;45:314–26.
31. Brouwers N, Bettens K, Gijselinck I, Engelborghs S, Pickut BA, Van Miegroet H, Montoya AG, Mattheijssens M, Peeters K, De Deyn PP, et al. Contribution of TARDBP to Alzheimer's disease genetic etiology. J Alzheimers Dis. 2010;21:423–30.
32. Shibata N, Ohnuma T, Baba H, Arai H. Genetic association analysis between TDP-43 polymorphisms and Alzheimer's disease in a Japanese population. Dement Geriatr Cogn Disord. 2009;28:325–9.
33. Schjeide BM, Hooli B, Parkinson M, Hogan MF, DiVito J, Mullin K, Blacker D, Tanzi RE, Bertram L. GAB2 as an Alzheimer disease susceptibility gene: follow-up of genomewide association results. Arch Neurol. 2009;66:250–4.
34. Feulner TM, Laws SM, Friedrich P, Wagenpfeil S, Wurst SH, Riehle C, Kuhn KA, Krawczak M, Schreiber S, Nikolaus S, et al. Examination of the current top candidate genes for AD in a genome-wide association study. Mol Psychiatry. 2010;15:756–66.
35. Sleegers K, Bettens K, Brouwers N, Engelborghs S, van Miegroet H, De Deyn PP, Van Broeckhoven C. Common variation in GRB-associated binding protein 2 (GAB2) and increased risk for Alzheimer dementia. Hum Mutat. 2009;30:E338–44.
36. Rayaprolu S, Mullen B, Baker M, Lynch T, Finger E, Seeley WW, Hatanpaa KJ, Lomen-Hoerth C, Kertesz A, Bigio EH, et al. TREM2 in neurodegeneration: evidence for association of the p.R47H variant with frontotemporal dementia and Parkinson's disease. Mol Neurodegener. 2013;8:19.
37. Kim WS, Weickert CS, Garner B. Role of ATP-binding cassette transporters in brain lipid transport and neurological disease. J Neurochem. 2008;104:1145–66.
38. Naj AC, Jun G, Beecham GW, Wang LS, Vardarajan BN, Buros J, Gallins PJ, Buxbaum JD, Jarvik GP, Crane PK, et al. Common variants at MS4A4/MS4A6E, CD2AP, CD33 and EPHA1 are associated with late-onset Alzheimer's disease. Nat Genet. 2011;43:436–41.
39. Hol EM, Roelofs RF, Moraal E, Sonnemans MA, Sluijs JA, Proper EA, de Graan PN, Fischer DF, van Leeuwen FW. Neuronal expression of GFAP in patients with Alzheimer pathology and identification of novel GFAP splice forms. Mol Psychiatry. 2003;8:786–96.
40. Potkin SG, Guffanti G, Lakatos A, Turner JA, Kruggel F, Fallon JH, Saykin AJ, Orro A, Lupoli S, Salvi E, et al. Hippocampal atrophy as a quantitative trait in

39. Hol EM, Roelofs RF, Moraal E, Sonnemans MA, Sluijs JA, Proper EA, de Graan PN, Fischer DF, van Leeuwen FW. Neuronal expression of GFAP in patients with Alzheimer pathology and identification of novel GFAP splice forms. Mol Psychiatry. 2003;8:786–96.
40. Potkin SG, Guffanti G, Lakatos A, Turner JA, Kruggel F, Fallon JH, Saykin AJ, Orro A, Lupoli S, Salvi E, et al. Hippocampal atrophy as a quantitative trait in a genome-wide association study identifying novel susceptibility genes for Alzheimer's disease. PLoS One. 2009;4:e6501.
41. Grupe A, Abraham R, Li Y, Rowland C, Hollingworth P, Morgan A, Jehu L, Segurado R, Stone D, Schadt E, et al. Evidence for novel susceptibility genes for late-onset Alzheimer's disease from a genome-wide association study of putative functional variants. Hum Mol Genet. 2007;16:865–73.
42. Zorzetto M, Datturi F, Divizia L, Pistono C, Campo I, De Silvestri A, Cuccia M, Ricevuti G. Complement C4A and C4B gene copy number study in Alzheimer's disease patients. Curr Alzheimer Res. 2017;14:303–8.
43. Tarawneh R, D'Angelo G, Crimmins D, Herries E, Griest T, Fagan AM, Zipfel GJ, Ladenson JH, Morris JC, Holtzman DM. Diagnostic and prognostic utility of the synaptic marker Neurogranin in Alzheimer disease. JAMA Neurol. 2016;73:561–71.
44. Lee JH, Cheng R, Barral S, Reitz C, Medrano M, Lantigua R, Jimenez-Velazquez IZ, Rogaeva E. St George-Hyslop PH, Mayeux R. Identification of novel loci for Alzheimer disease and replication of CLU, PICALM, and BIN1 in Caribbean Hispanic individuals. Arch Neurol. 2011;68:320–8.
45. Jayadev S, Leverenz JB, Steinbart E, Stahl J, Klunk W, CE Y, Bird TD. Alzheimer's disease phenotypes and genotypes associated with mutations in presenilin 2. Brain. 2010;133:1143–54.
46. Brouwers N, Sleegers K, Engelborghs S, Maurer-Stroh S, Gijselinck I, van der Zee J, Pickut BA, Van den Broeck M, Mattheijssens M, Peeters K, et al. Genetic variability in progranulin contributes to risk for clinically diagnosed Alzheimer disease. Neurology. 2008;71:656–64.
47. Zhao Y, Ho P, Yih Y, Chen C, Lee WL, Tan EK. LRRK2 variant associated with Alzheimer's disease. Neurobiol Aging. 2011;32:1990–3.
48. Ersing I, Nobre L, Wang LW, Soday L, Ma Y, Paulo JA, Narita Y, Ashbaugh CW, Jiang C, Grayson NE, et al. A temporal proteomic map of Epstein-Barr virus Lytic replication in B cells. Cell Rep. 19:1479–93.
49. Hughes CS, McConechy MK, Cochrane DR, Nazeran T, Karnezis AN, Huntsman DG, Morin GB. Quantitative profiling of single formalin fixed tumour sections: proteomics for translational research. Sci Rep. 2016;6:34949.
50. Seyfried NT, Dammer EB, Swarup V, Nandakumar D, Duong DM, Yin L, Deng Q, Nguyen T, Hales CM, Wingo T, et al. A multi-network approach identifies protein-specific co-expression in asymptomatic and symptomatic Alzheimer's disease. Cell Syst. 2017;4:60–72 e64.
51. Karran E, Mercken M, De Strooper B. The amyloid cascade hypothesis for Alzheimer's disease: an appraisal for the development of therapeutics. Nat Rev Drug Discov. 2011;10:698–712.
52. Martin L, Latypova X, Wilson CM, Magnaudeix A, Perrin ML, Yardin C, Terro F. Tau protein kinases: involvement in Alzheimer's disease. Ageing Res Rev. 2013;12:289–309.
53. Takashima A, Noguchi K, Sato K, Hoshino T, Imahori K. Tau protein kinase I is essential for amyloid beta-protein-induced neurotoxicity. Proc Natl Acad Sci U S A. 1993;90:7789–93.
54. Li G, Yin H, Kuret J. Casein kinase 1 delta phosphorylates tau and disrupts its binding to microtubules. J Biol Chem. 2004;279:15938–45.
55. Wagner U, Utton M, Gallo JM, Miller CC. Cellular phosphorylation of tau by GSK-3 beta influences tau binding to microtubules and microtubule organisation. J Cell Sci. 1996;109(Pt 6):1537–43.
56. Virdee K, Yoshida H, Peak-Chew S, Goedert M. Phosphorylation of human microtubule-associated protein tau by protein kinases of the AGC subfamily. FEBS Lett. 2007;581:2657–62.
57. Pooler AM, Polydoro M, Maury EA, Nicholls SB, Reddy SM, Wegmann S, William C, Saqran L, Cagsal-Getkin O, Pitstick R, et al. Amyloid accelerates tau propagation and toxicity in a model of early Alzheimer's disease. Acta Neuropathol Commun. 2015;3:14.
58. Tseng JH, Xie L, Song S, Xie Y, Allen L, Ajit D, Hong JS, Chen X, Meeker RB, Cohen TJ. The Deacetylase HDAC6 mediates endogenous Neuritic tau pathology. Cell Rep. 2017;20:2169–83.
59. Kook SY, Seok Hong H, Moon M, Mook-Jung I. Disruption of blood-brain barrier in Alzheimer disease pathogenesis. Tissue Barriers. 2013;1:e23993.
60. Marques F, Sousa JC, Sousa N, Palha JA. Blood-brain-barriers in aging and in Alzheimer's disease. Mol Neurodegener. 2013;8:38.
61. Laurent C, Dorothee G, Hunot S, Martin E, Monnet Y, Duchamp M, Dong Y, Legeron FP, Leboucher A, Burnouf S, et al. Hippocampal T cell infiltration promotes neuroinflammation and cognitive decline in a mouse model of tauopathy. Brain. 2017;140:184–200.
62. Baik SH, Cha MY, Hyun YM, Cho H, Hamza B, Kim DK, Han SH, Choi H, Kim KH, Moon M, et al. Migration of neutrophils targeting amyloid plaques in Alzheimer's disease mouse model. Neurobiol Aging. 2014;35:1286–92.
63. Zenaro E, Pietronigro E, Della Bianca V, Piacentino G, Marongiu L, Budui S, Turano E, Rossi B, Angiari S, Dusi S, et al. Neutrophils promote Alzheimer's disease-like pathology and cognitive decline via LFA-1 integrin. Nat Med. 2015;21:880–6.
64. Hohsfield LA, Humpel C. Migration of blood cells to beta-amyloid plaques in Alzheimer's disease. Exp Gerontol. 2015;65:8–15.
65. Chesser AS, Pritchard SM, Johnson GV. Tau clearance mechanisms and their possible role in the pathogenesis of Alzheimer disease. Front Neurol. 2013;4:122.
66. Kim Y, Kim C, Son SM, Song H, Hong HS, Han SH, Mook-Jung I. The novel RAGE interactor PRAK is associated with autophagy signaling in Alzheimer's disease pathogenesis. Mol Neurodegener. 2016;11:4.
67. Saura CA, Valero J. The role of CREB signaling in Alzheimer's disease and other cognitive disorders. Rev Neurosci. 2011;22:153–69.
68. Thomas GM, Huganir RL. MAPK cascade signalling and synaptic plasticity. Nat Rev Neurosci. 2004;5:173–83.
69. LaFerla FM, Oddo S. Alzheimer's disease: Abeta, tau and synaptic dysfunction. Trends Mol Med. 2005;11:170–6.
70. Zhu Y, Hou H, Rezai-Zadeh K, Giunta B, Ruscin A, Gemma C, Jin J, Dragicevic N, Bradshaw P, Rasool S, et al. CD45 deficiency drives Amyloid-β peptide Oligomers and neuronal loss in Alzheimer's disease mice. J Neurosci. 2011;31:1355–65.
71. ElAli A, Rivest S. The role of ABCB1 and ABCA1 in beta-amyloid clearance at the neurovascular unit in Alzheimer's disease. Front Physiol. 2013;4:45.
72. Latasiewicz J, Artz A, Jing D, Blanco MP, Currie SM, Avila MV, Schnoor M, Vestweber D. HS1 deficiency impairs neutrophil recruitment in vivo and activation of the small GTPases Rac1 and Rap1. J Leukoc Biol. 2017;101: 1133–1142.
73. Ciavardelli D, Silvestri E, Del Viscovo A, Bomba M, De Gregorio D, Moreno M, Di Ilio C, Goglia F, Canzoniero LM, Sensi SL. Alterations of brain and cerebellar proteomes linked to Abeta and tau pathology in a female triple-transgenic murine model of Alzheimer's disease. Cell Death Dis. 2010;1:e90.
74. Rhein V, Song X, Wiesner A, Ittner LM, Baysang G, Meier F, Ozmen L, Bluethmann H, Drose S, Brandt U, et al. Amyloid-beta and tau synergistically impair the oxidative phosphorylation system in triple transgenic Alzheimer's disease mice. Proc Natl Acad Sci U S A. 2009;106:20057–62.
75. Martin B, Brenneman R, Becker KG, Gucek M, Cole RN, Maudsley S. iTRAQ analysis of complex proteome alterations in 3xTgAD Alzheimer's mice: understanding the interface between physiology and disease. PLoS One. 2008;3:e2750.
76. Vizcaino JA, Deutsch EW, Wang R, Csordas A, Reisinger F, Rios D, Dianes JA, Sun Z, Farrah T, Bandeira N, et al. ProteomeXchange provides globally coordinated proteomics data submission and dissemination. Nat Biotechnol. 2014;32:223–6.

13

Abnormal dendritic calcium activity and synaptic depotentiation occur early in a mouse model of Alzheimer's disease

Yang Bai[1,2], Miao Li[1], Yanmei Zhou[1,2], Lei Ma[1], Qian Qiao[1], Wanling Hu[1], Wei Li[1], Zachary Patrick Wills[3] and Wen-Biao Gan[1,2*]

Abstract

Background: Alzheimer's disease (AD) is characterized by amyloid deposition, tangle formation as well as synapse loss. Synaptic abnormalities occur early in the pathogenesis of AD. Identifying early synaptic abnormalities and their underlying mechanisms is likely important for the prevention and treatment of AD.

Methods: We performed in vivo two-photon calcium imaging to examine the activities of somas, dendrites and dendritic spines of layer 2/3 pyramidal neurons in the primary motor cortex in the APPswe/PS1dE9 mouse model of AD and age-matched wild type control mice. We also performed calcium imaging to determine the effect of Aβ oligomers on dendritic calcium activity. In addition, structural and functional two-photon imaging were used to examine the link between abnormal dendritic calcium activity and changes in dendritic spine size in the AD mouse model.

Results: We found that somatic calcium activities of layer 2/3 neurons were significantly lower in the primary motor cortex of 3-month-old APPswe/PS1dE9 mice than in wild type mice during quiet resting, but not during running on a treadmill. Notably, a significantly larger fraction of apical dendrites of layer 2/3 pyramidal neurons showed calcium transients with abnormally long duration and high peak amplitudes during treadmill running in AD mice. Administration of Aβ oligomers into the brain of wild type mice also induced abnormal dendritic calcium transients during running. Furthermore, we found that the activity and size of dendritic spines were significantly reduced on dendritic branches with abnormally prolonged dendritic calcium transients in AD mice.

Conclusion: Our findings show that abnormal dendritic calcium transients and synaptic depotentiation occur before amyloid plaque formation in the motor cortex of the APPswe/PS1dE9 mouse model of AD. Dendritic calcium transients with abnormally long durations and high amplitudes could be induced by soluble Aβ oligomers and contribute to synaptic deficits in the early pathogenesis of AD.

Keywords: Alzheimer's disease, Dendritic calcium activity, Two-photon imaging, APPswe/PS1dE9, Soluble Aβ oligomers, Synaptic depotentiation

* Correspondence: gan@saturn.med.nyu.edu
[1]Drug Discovery Center, Key Laboratory of Chemical Genomics, Peking University Shenzhen Graduate School, Shenzhen 518055, China
[2]Skirball Institute, Department of Neuroscience and Physiology, New York University School of Medicine, New York, NY 10016, USA
Full list of author information is available at the end of the article

Background

Amyloid plaques, neurofibrillary tangles and synapse loss are the pathological hallmarks of Alzheimer's disease (AD) [1, 2]. AD patients exhibit progressive cognitive impairments, memory deficits and dementia. Previous studies have shown that synapse loss occurs many years before dementia and is the best correlate of cognitive impairment in AD patients [1, 3–6]. A significant reduction in postsynaptic spine density is detected before β-amyloid deposition in Tg2576 APP and PDAPP mouse models of AD [7–9]. Furthermore, down-regulation of various synaptic proteins has been observed in both AD patients and mouse models of AD [7, 10, 11]. These various synaptic deficits may underlie memory loss [8, 12, 13], as well as changes of sensory and motor systems observed at the early stage of AD [14–16].

The mechanisms underlying synaptic abnormalities and loss in AD remain unclear. Recent studies have shown that abnormal neuronal activities occur early in hippocampal and cortical regions in AD patients as well as in animal models of AD [8, 17–19]. For example, hyperactive neurons have been observed in the hippocampal CA1 region in 1.5 month-old APP23xPS45 Tg mice [19]. It has also been reported that the number of hypoactive and hyperactive cells in layer 2/3 neocortex increase in AD mice as compared to wild type mice [20]. Given the important role of neuronal activities in regulating synaptic plasticity [21, 22], alterations in neuronal activities likely cause abnormal synaptic structure and function in AD. However, the potential link between neuronal activity and synaptic abnormalities during the pathogenesis of AD remains elusive.

Many lines of evidence strongly suggest that soluble Aβ oligomers are the most neurotoxic Aβ peptides with detrimental effects on neurons and synapses in AD [17, 23–28]. The level of Aβ peptides, but not amyloid plaques, is the earliest known marker of AD and correlates with disease severity in patients [29–33]. Exogenous Aβ application into wild type mice can induce neuronal hyperactivity [34]. Furthermore, Aβ oligomers have been shown to disrupt calcium homeostasis in neurons by interacting with NMDA receptors, reducing glutamate uptake at synapses, and regulating calcium release from ER [35–41]. Because calcium elevation is an important trigger for synaptic plasticity [42, 43], these findings suggest that soluble Aβ oligomers may cause early synaptic deficits by affecting neuronal activity and calcium homeostasis in AD.

To better understand early synaptic deficits in AD, we performed transcranial two-photon calcium imaging of layer 2/3 neuronal somas, dendrites and dendritic spines in the motor cortex of 3-month-old APPswe/PS1dE9 transgenic mice before amyloid plaque formation [44–47]. We found that a fraction of dendritic branches of layer 2/3 pyramidal neurons exhibited a significant increase in the duration and amplitude of dendritic calcium transients during treadmill running in 3-month-old AD mice as compared with age-matched wild type control mice. Exogenous application of soluble Aβ oligomers into wild type mouse brain also increased the duration and peak amplitude of dendritic calcium transients during treadmill running. Notably, dendritic spines exhibited a decrease in activity and size after abnormal long-duration dendritic calcium transients. Together, these findings suggest that abnormal dendritic calcium elevation and synaptic depotentiation represent early dendritic and synaptic deficits in the pathogenesis of AD.

Methods

Experimental animals

The APPswe/PS1dE9 mice were purchased from Guangdong Medical Laboratory Animal Center, China. They overexpressed the Swedish mutation of APP, together with PS1 deleted in exon 9. Three-month-old mice were used in all the experiments. Mice expressing GCaMP6s in layer 2/3 and layer 5 pyramidal neurons were generated under the Thy-1 promoter in the Gan lab. Age-matched non-transgenic littermates served as controls. Mice of both sexes were used in the experiments. All experimental protocols were conducted in accordance with the institutional guidelines.

Administration of soluble Aβ42 oligomers or monomers

Aβ peptides were synthesized and provided by Dr. Zachary Wills from University of Pittsburgh. High performance liquid chromatography (HPLC), size exclusion chromatography (SEC) and electron microscopy (EM) were used to determine the concentration and oligomeric status of Aβ peptides as described in a recent publication [48]. Synthesized Aβ42 was dissolved in DMSO and aliquoted before freezing at −80 °C. 24 h prior to the experiment, Aβ42 was thawed and vortexed for 30 s to initiate the oligomerization and then incubated at 4 °C overnight. Before use, Aβ oligomers were diluted with artificial cerebrospinal fluid (ACSF) and used within 48 h of preparation at the concentration of 20 μM. 0.5 μl solution of Aβ42 oligomers (or Aβ42 monomers and vehicle) were slowly injected into the cortex of WT mice over 50 min. The vehicle or Aβ42 monomer without overnight incubation at 4 °C was used as control groups. To assess the global effect of Aβ42, we performed calcium imaging of neurons ~ 1 h after Aβ42 injection in the motor cortex contralateral to the injection site.

MK801 application

For local application of the NMDA receptor antagonist, MK801 (200 μM in artificial cerebrospinal fluid (ACSF),

M107, Sigma-Aldrich), a glass microelectrode with a 20-μm outer diameter was inserted through a bone flap into the superficial layer of the cortex (20–30 μm below the pial surface) with an angle of 45° toward and ~100 μm away from the imaging area. The bone flap (~50 μm in diameter) for drug delivery was made adjacent to a thinned skull window for imaging.

Treadmill running

Mice were subjected to treadmill running with the same method as described in previous studies [43, 49]. Briefly, a custom built free-floating treadmill (101 cm × 58 cm × 44 cm) was used for motor training under a two-photon microscope. This free-floating treadmill allowed head-fixed mice to move their forelimbs freely to perform motor running tasks. To minimize motion artifact during imaging, the treadmill was constructed so that all the moving parts (motor, belt and drive shaft) were isolated from the microscope stage and the supporting air-table. Animals were positioned on a custom-made head-holder device that allowed micro-metal bars to be mounted. At the onset of a running trial, the treadmill motor driven by a DC power supply was turned on and the belt speed gradually increased from 0 cm/s to 8 cm/s within ~3 s. The speed of 8 cm/s was maintained for the rest of the trial. Each mouse was trained for 6–7 trials (5 min running and 1 min resting for each trial).

Surgery for two-photon imaging

Surgical procedures were performed similarly as described in previous studies [43, 50]. 24 h before imaging, surgery was performed to attach a head holder and to create a thinned-skull cranial window. First, mice were deeply anesthetized with an intraperitoneal injection of pentobarbital sodium (80 mg/kg). The mouse head was shaved and the skull surface was exposed with a midline scalp incision. The periosteum tissue over the skull surface was removed without damaging the temporal and occipital muscles. A head holder composed of two parallel micro-metal bars was attached to the animal's skull to help restrain the animal's head and reduce motion-induced artifact during imaging. A small skull region (~0.2 mm in diameter) was located over the primary motor cortex based on stereotaxic coordinates [51] (1.0 mm posterior from bregma and 1.5 mm lateral from the midline) and marked with a pencil. A thin layer of cyanoacrylate-based glue was first applied to the top of entire skull surface, and the head holder was then mounted on top of the skull with dental acrylic cement such that the marked skull region was exposed between the two bars. Precaution was taken not to cover the marked region with dental acrylic cement.

Before imaging of dendrites and dendritic spines, a high-speed micro-drill and microsurgical blade were used to thin a circular area over the marked region to a thickness of approximately 20 μm. The thinning procedure generally took less than 5 min.

To image somas at the depth of ~250 μm below the pial surface, the skull overlying the motor cortex of interest (1 mm × 1 mm) was removed and replaced with a glass window right before two-photon imaging as described previously [43].

Two-photon imaging of somas, dendrites and dendritic spines in the motor cortex

Genetically encoded calcium indicator GCaMP6s was used for calcium imaging in the primary motor cortex of awake, head-restrained mice. For calcium imaging of APPswe/PS1dE9 mice and wild type controls, a total amount of 0.1–0.2 μl of AAV-synapsin-GCaMP6s (AAV serotype 2/1; >2 × 10^{13} (GC/ml) titer; from the University of Pennsylvania Gene Therapy Program Vector Core) was diluted two times in ACSF and slowly injected (Picospritzer III; 20 p.s.i., 20 ms, 0.3 Hz) over 10–15 min into layer 2/3 of the motor cortex (0–1.5 mm posterior from bregma and 0–1.5 mm lateral from midline) using a glass microelectrode. Mice were prepared for calcium imaging ~18 days after virus injection.

For calcium imaging of mice injected with Aβ42 oligomers and monomers, we used wild type mice infected with AAV-synapsin-GCaMP6s, as well as transgenic mice expressing GCaMP6s in layer 2/3 and layer 5 pyramidal neurons under the Thy-1 promoter. This transgenic mouse line was generated in the Gan lab. Calcium imaging of dendrites and somas was performed in mice immediately after Aβ42 injection.

For simultaneous calcium and structural imaging, three viruses (AAV1.hSyn.Cre.WPRE.hGH, AAV1.CAG.Flex.td-Tomato.WPRE.bGH and AAV1.CAG.Flex.GCaMP6s.W-PRE.SV40 from the University of Pennsylvania Gene Therapy Program Vector Core) were mixed at 1:15:80 volume ratios, and ~0.1 μl of the three mixed viruses were injected into layer 2/3 of the primary motor cortex. Viruses were injected into the primary motor cortex ~18 days before calcium and dendritic spine imaging.

To image somas at the depth of ~250 μm below the pial surface, the skull overlying the motor cortex of interest (1 mm × 1 mm) was removed and replaced with a glass window right before two-photon imaging. Dendritic calcium transients and spine calcium transients were imaged at the depth of ~50 μm below the pial surface through a thinned skull window. Neuronal somas were imaged at the depth of ~250 μm below the pial surface via a glass window. The imaging window was immersed in ACSF and the head-restrained animal was placed on the stage of a two-photon laser scanning microscopy (Olympus Fluoview 1000 two-photon system equipped with MaiTai

DeepSee Ti:Sapphire laser from Spectra Physics). The laser was tuned to the wavelength of 920 nm with laser power of ~ 20 mW on the tissue sample. Calcium signals were recorded at 2 Hz using a 25X objective (N.A. 1.05, 3X digital zoom). Dendritic spine structures were imaged at 0 h and 1.5 h using a 25X objective (N.A. 1.05, 3X digital zoom).

During quiet resting state, we took images for 60 s. During running, we acquired images for 5 running trials. Each running trial lasted 60 s. After the completion of each trial, the treadmill was turned off and the next trial started after a 60-s rest period.

Image analysis

Neuronal, dendritic and spine calcium activity, indicated by GCaMP6 fluorescence changes, were analyzed post hoc using Image J software (NIH). The GCaMP6 fluorescence (F) during quiet resting and running was measured by averaging pixels within each identifiable area (Regions of interests, ROIs). Then $\Delta F/F_0$ was calculated as $\Delta F/F_0 = (F-F_0)/F_0$, in which ΔF was $F-F_0$ (all F values were subtracted a background fluorescence value of vessels), and F_0 was the average of 10% minimum F values over 1 min period, representing baseline fluorescence. The threshold for determining calcium transients was calculated as three times the standard deviation (SD) of baseline fluorescence. The frequency of calcium transients was calculated as the number of calcium transients per minute on each dendrite. The duration was calculated as the total time of calcium transients with $\Delta F/F_0$ above the threshold. The peak amplitude was the highest value of the calcium transient. The total calcium activity was the accumulated calcium activities above the threshold per minute.

Similar to previous studies [42], back-propagating action potential-related calcium component was removed from spine calcium signals by subtracting a scaled version of the dendritic shaft signal, $\Delta F/F_{0spine\_specific} = \Delta F/F_{0spine} - 0.7 \times \Delta F/F_{0dendrite}$. We defined active spines as those with spine-specific calcium transients that crossed 3 SD of baseline fluorescence and inactive spines as those less than 3 SD.

Spine head size was measured according to previous studies [43, 49]. After background subtraction, the fluorescence intensity of tdTomato in the spine (the intensity of all pixels covering the spine in the best focal plane) was divided by the fluorescence intensity of the adjacent dendritic shaft. tdTomato fluorescence intensity of a spine was measured as follows, where Area was the number of pixels in an oval surrounding the head of the spine and mean optical density (Mean OD) was the mean brightness of pixels in that area:

The ratio of spine head diameter to adjacent dendritic shaft diameter = (Area (of spine) × Mean OD (of spine) - Area (of spine) × Mean OD (of background))/(Area (of spine) × Mean OD (of dendrite) - Area (of spine) × Mean OD (of background)). The Mean OD of both the background and the dendrite was calculated from measurements taken next to each spine, averaged for each dendrite segment.

After spine head sizes were measured on the same dendritic segment, spine size changes were calculated by comparing spine size measurement between imaging sessions.

Statistics

All data were presented as mean ± s.e.m. The Kolmogorov-Smirnov test was used to test whether datasets were normally distributed. If so, we used a two-tailed Student's t test to compare two groups. If not, tests for differences between groups were performed using non-parametric tests. Two Independent-samples Mann-Whitney Test and Related-samples Wilcoxon Signed Rank Test ware used to compare differences between groups whose distributions did not pass Kolmogorov-Smirnov test. Significant levels were set at $p \leq 0.05$. All statistical analyses were performed using the IBM SPSS Statistics 23.

Results

Somatic calcium activities of layer 2/3 neurons are reduced in 3-month-old AD mice than in WT mice during quiet rest, but not treadmill running

To investigate early neuronal deficits in the mouse model of AD, we first performed in vivo two-photon imaging of somatic calcium activities of layer 2/3 (L2/3) neurons expressing a genetically encoded calcium indicator (GCaMP6s) in the primary motor cortex (M1) of 3-month-old APPswe/PS1dE9 mice (Fig. 1a). Expression of GCaMP6s was achieved by injecting recombinant adeno-associated virus (AAV) encoding GCaMP6s under the human synapsin-1 (SYN1) promoter into the M1 region. Three weeks after viral injection, ~80% GCaMP6-expressing somas were located between 120 and 460 μm below the pia surface (Fig. 1b; 500 somas from 5 mice), indicating that GCaMP6 was expressed mostly in L2/3 neurons.

We imaged somatic calcium activities of L2/3 neurons in M1 under both resting and running conditions (Fig. 1c, d). Under the quiet resting condition, the frequency of calcium transients was comparable between AD and WT mice (Fig. 1e; WT: $n = 185$ somas from 4 mice; AD: $n = 186$ somas from 5 mice; $P = 0.519$). The duration, peak $\Delta F/F_0$ and integrated somatic calcium activity over 1 min were significantly lower in AD mice compared to WT mice (Fig. 1f-h, $P < 0.05$). On the other hand, when

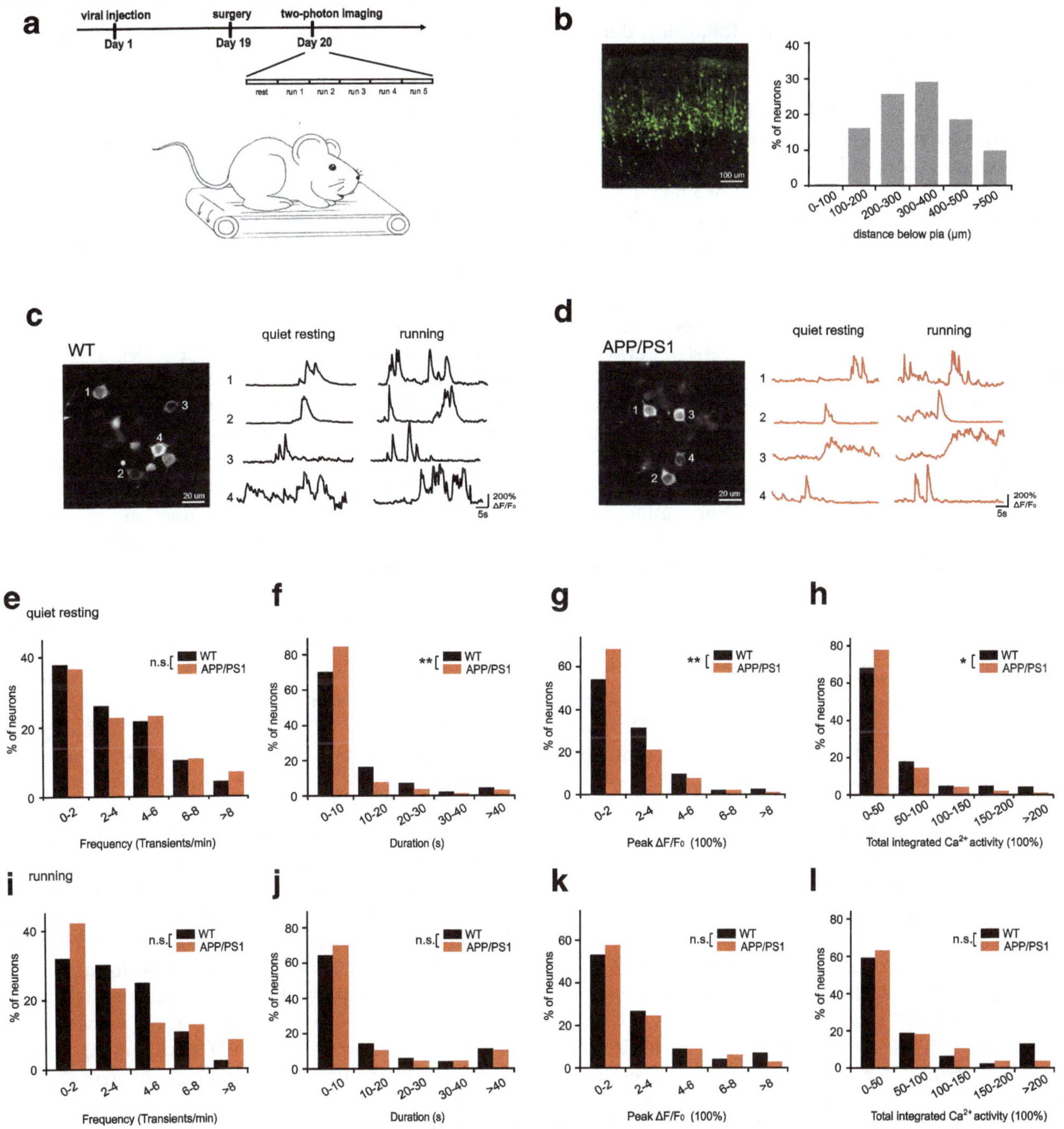

Fig. 1 Somatic calcium activities of APP/PS1 mice are lower than WT mice during quiet resting, but not during treadmill running. **a**. Experimental design. After viral infection and surgery, layer 2/3 neurons of the motor cortex were imaged over 1 min under quite resting and over 5 treadmill running trials (60 s each trial). **b**. The confocal image of neurons labeled by AAV-syn-GCaMP6s in the mouse primary motor cortex (left); Distance distribution of GCaMP6s-expressing somas shows most of the labeled cells are in layer 2/3 (right). **c**. A representative image of somatic calcium activity in WT mice (left). Fluorescence traces of 4 different somas during quiet resting and running states (right). **d**. A representative image of somatic calcium activity in APP/PS1 mice (left). Fluorescence traces of 4 different somas during quiet resting and running states (right). **e-h**. Distributions of the frequency (**e**), duration (**f**), peak $\Delta F/F_0$ (**g**) and total integrated activity (**h**) of somatic calcium transients in WT and APP/PS1 during quiet resting (WT: 4 mice, 185 somas; APP/PS1: 5 mice, 186 somas. Mann-Whitney U Test). **i-l**. Distributions of the frequency (**i**), duration (**j**), peak $\Delta F/F_0$ (**k**) and total integrated activity (**l**) of somatic calcium transients in WT and APP/PS1 during treadmill running (WT: 4 mice, 169 somas; APP/PS1: 5 mice, 180 somas. Mann-Whitney U Test). $^*P < 0.05$, $^{**}P < 0.01$, $^{***}P < 0.001$. n.s., not significant

the mice were performing a treadmill running task, there was no significant difference in the frequency, duration, peak $\Delta F/F_0$ and integrated somatic calcium transients between AD and WT mice (Fig. 1i-l; WT: n = 169 somas from 4 mice. AD: n = 180 somas from 5 mice. $P > 0.2$). Thus, different from hyperactivity reported in the hippocampus of 1.5-month-old APP23 × PS45 mice [19], L2/3 neurons in the M1 had a lower level of somatic calcium activity under quiet resting but not during treadmill running in 3-month-old APPswe/PS1dE9 mice when compared with WT mice.

The overall level of synaptic activities on apical dendrites of layer 2/3 pyramidal neurons is comparable between WT and AD mice

In addition to somatic calcium transients, we also examined calcium transients in dendritic spines on apical dendrites of layer 2/3 pyramidal neurons in WT and AD mice infected with GCaMP6s viruses (Fig. 2a, b). Under the quiet resting condition, we found no significant difference in the frequency, duration, peak $\Delta F/F_0$ and total integrated activity of spine calcium transients between WT and AD mice (Fig. 2c-f; WT: n = 4 mice, 32 spines; AD: n = 5 mice, 30 spines. $P > 0.1$).

When mice were subjected to treadmill running, the frequency of spine calcium transients was significantly higher in AD mice as compared to that in WT mice (Fig. 2g; WT: n = 33 spines from 4 mice; AD: n = 34 spines from 5 mice. $P = 0.002$). The duration, peak amplitude and total integrated activity of spine calcium transients were comparable between AD and WT mice (Fig. 2h - j; $P > 0.3$). Together, these results indicate that the overall level of synaptic activity is comparable between WT and AD mice under both quiet resting and running conditions.

The duration and peak $\Delta F/F_0$ of dendritic calcium transients are significantly higher during running in AD mice than in WT mice

Many lines of evidence indicate that dendritic calcium spikes are critical for synaptic plasticity of excitatory neurons [52–57]. Recent studies have shown that dendritic calcium spikes in apical dendrites of layer 5 pyramidal neurons are important for dendritic spine plasticity in the motor cortex [43]. To investigate potential dendritic deficits in AD mice, we examined dendritic calcium activity of L2/3 pyramidal neurons in WT and AD mice under both quiet resting and treadmill running conditions.

In the superficial layer of the motor cortex, we observed large dendritic calcium transients that occurred across long segments (> 30 μm) of apical tuft dendrites of layer 2/3 pyramidal neurons (Fig. 3a-c). The vast majority of these dendritic calcium transients lasted more than hundreds of milliseconds and had comparable $\Delta F/F_0$ across long stretches of dendrites, resembling NMDAR-activation-dependent dendritic calcium spikes described previously [43, 58–60] (Fig. 3c). Under the quiet resting condition, we found that the frequency and duration of such dendritic calcium transients were not significantly different between WT and AD mice (Fig. 3d, e; WT: n = 90 calcium transients from 4 mice; AD: n = 121 calcium transients from 5 mice; $P > 0.05$). However, the peak $\Delta F/F_0$ of dendritic calcium transients was significantly higher in AD mice than in WT mice (Fig. 3f; $P = 0.005$).

In mice running on the treadmill, we found that the frequency distribution of dendritic calcium transients was comparable between WT and AD mice (Fig. 3g; WT: n = 297 calcium transients from 4 mice; AD: n = 543 calcium transients from 5 mice. $P = 0.774$), whereas both the duration and peak amplitude distribution were significantly different (Fig. 3h, i; $P < 0.002$). Notably, a significantly larger fraction of dendritic calcium transients exhibited longer duration (> 8 s) and higher peak amplitude in AD mice than in WT mice (Fig. 3h, i).

Of all dendrites exhibiting dendritic calcium transients during a 5-min running period, ~47% and ~18% of dendrites exhibited at least one long-duration (> 8 s) dendritic calcium activity in AD mice and WT mice, respectively (Fig. 3j). In addition, 37.2% of dendrites showed at least one calcium transient with large peak amplitude (> 400%) in AD mice, higher than that (25.0%) in WT mice (Fig. 3k). There was a strong correlation between the duration and peak amplitude of dendritic calcium transients in both WT and AD, indicating that dendritic calcium transients with longer duration tended to have larger calcium peak amplitude (Fig. 3l, m; WT: n = 297 transients from 4 mice, r = 0.039, $P < 0.001$; AD: n = 543 transients from 5 mice, r = 0.052, $P < 0.001$). Together, these results indicate that even though overall dendritic spine activities were comparable between AD and WT mice (Fig. 2), a significantly larger fraction of dendrites exhibited dendritic calcium transients with abnormal long-duration and high peak amplitude in L2/3 pyramidal neurons in the M1 region of 3-month-old AD mice than in WT mice.

Exogenous soluble Aβ42 oligomers induce dendritic calcium transients with long duration and high peak amplitude during treadmill running

Many lines of evidence indicate that soluble Aβ42 oligomers can alter neuronal activity and lead to synaptic loss [61–65]. To investigate the effect of Aβ oligomers on neuronal activities in vivo, we injected Aβ oligomers into the motor cortex of wild type mice infected with AAV-hSyn-GCaMP6s virus. One hour after the injection of

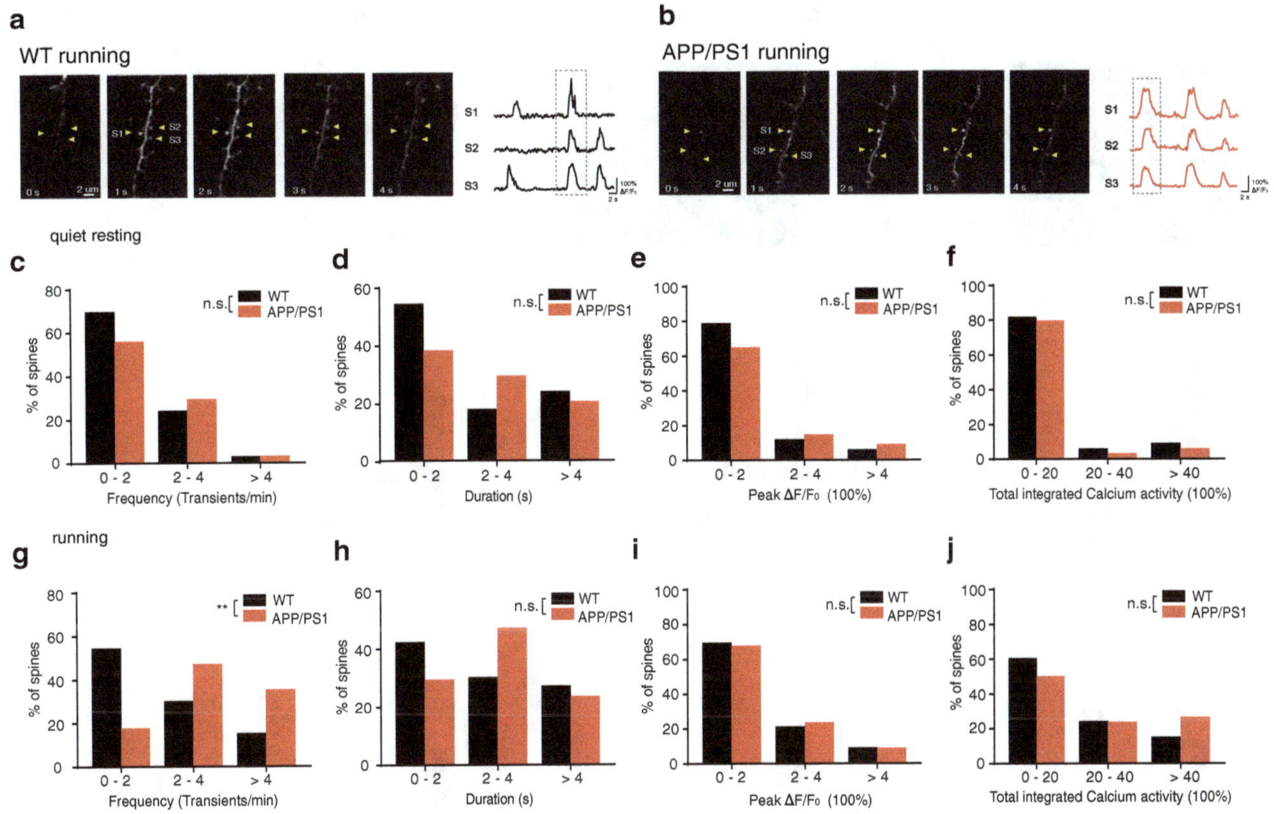

Fig. 2 The overall synaptic activity on apical dendrites is comparable between WT and APP/PS1 mice. **a**, **b**. Time-lapse images of dendritic spine calcium transients (left) and fluorescent traces of dendritic spines expressing GCaMP6s (right) in WT (**a**) and APP/PS1 mice (**b**). Calcium transients in three spines (arrowheads point to each spine) were shown. **c-f**. Distributions of the frequency (**c**), duration (**d**), peak $\Delta F/F_0$ (**e**) and total integrated activity (**f**) of spine calcium transients in WT and APP/PS1 mice under quiet resting state (WT:4 mice, 32 spines; APP/PS1: 5 mice, 30 spines. Mann-Whitney U Test). **g-j**. Distributions of the frequency (**g**), duration (**h**),peak $\Delta F/F_0$ (**i**) and total integrated activity (**j**) of spine calcium transientsin WT and APP/PS1 mice during treadmill running (WT: 4 mice, 33 spines; APP/PS1: 5 mice, 34 spines. Mann-Whitney U Test). $^{**}P < 0.01$; n.s., not significant

Aβ oligomers, we performed calcium imaging of somas, spines and apical dendrites of pyramidal neurons in the M1 contralateral to the site of Aβ injection (Fig. 4a-c). During treadmill running, we found that Aβ oligomers induced significantly higher somatic calcium activities (Additional file 1: Figure S1) but had no significant effect on the overall level of spine calcium activities of layer 2/3 pyramidal neurons (Additional file 2: Figure S2). Notably, while the frequency of dendritic calcium transients was not significantly different between vehicle and Aβ oligomer-injected mice (Fig. 4d; Vehicle: $n = 136$ calcium transients from 4 mice; Aβ42 oligomer: $n = 99$ calcium transients from 4 mice; $P = 0.034$), the injection of Aβ oligomers caused a significantly longer duration and higher peak amplitude of dendritic calcium transients as compared to vehicle injection (Fig. 4e-f; $P < 0.05$). These findings indicate that during treadmill running, Aβ oligomers cause a rapid increase in neuronal somatic calcium activities, as well as abnormally long duration of dendritic calcium transients in layer 2/3 neurons of the motor cortex.

To investigate the effects of Aβ oligomers further, we also examined dendritic calcium activities of pyramidal neurons in the motor cortex of transgenic mice expressing GCaMP6s after injecting either Aβ oligomers or Aβ monomers. During treadmill running, the frequency of dendritic calcium transients was not significantly different among Aβ oligomer, monomer and vehicle-injected mice (Fig. 4g; Vehicle: $n = 148$ dendritic calcium transients from 4 mice; Aβ monomer: $n = 176$ calcium transients from 4 mice; Aβ42 oligomer: $n = 152$ calcium transients from 4 mice. $P > 0.3$). However, administration of Aβ oligomers significantly increased the duration and peak amplitude of dendritic calcium transients when compared to control mice (Fig. 4h-i; $P < 0.001$). Taken together, these findings using mice infected with GCaMP6-expressing AAV or GCaMP6 transgenic mice suggest that exogenous soluble Aβ oligomers, but not Aβ monomers, cause abnormal dendritic calcium transients with long duration and high amplitude in mice during treadmill running.

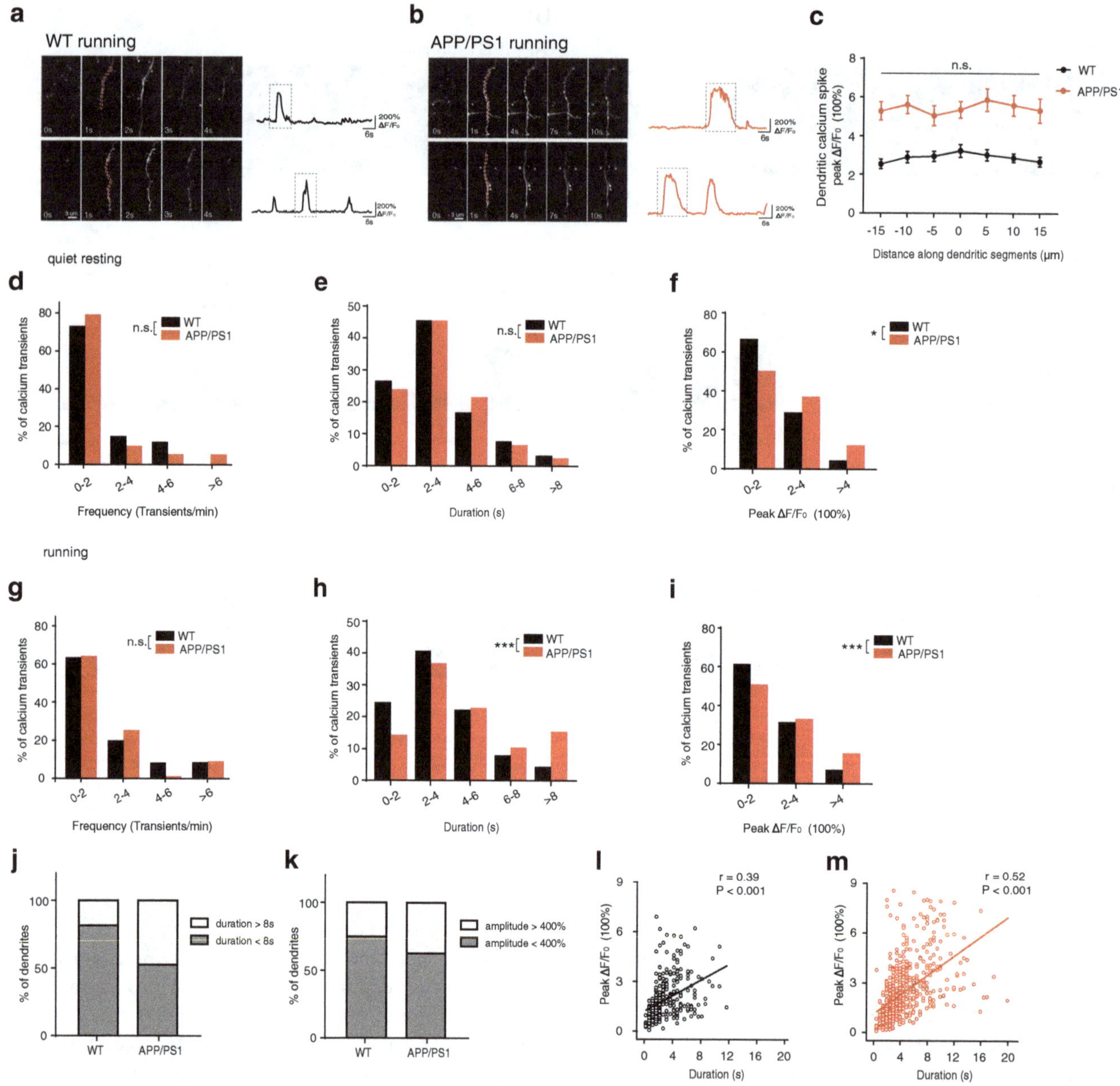

Fig. 3 The duration and peak $\Delta F/F_0$ of dendritic calcium transients are higher in APP/PS1 mice than in WT mice during running. **a**-**b**. Time-lapse images of dendritic calcium transients in WT (**a**) and APP/PS1 mice (**b**) during running. Apical dendrites of layer 2/3 pyramidal neurons exhibiting large calcium transients at time point 1 s were shown in red. Their calcium fluorescence traces were shown on the right. **c**. Measurements of calcium fluorescence along long dendritic segments in the plane of imaging. Comparable fluorescent signals were observed across dendritic segments in both WT (n = 10) and APP/PS1 mice (n = 10). **d**-**f**. Distributions of the frequency (**d**), duration (**e**) and peak $\Delta F/F_0$ (f) of dendritic calcium transients in WT and APP/PS1 mice under quiet resting state (WT:4 mice, 90 dendritic calcium transients; APP/PS1: 5 mice, 121 dendritic calcium transients. Mann-Whitney U Test). **g**-**i**. Distributions of the frequency (**g**), duration (**h**) and peak $\Delta F/F_0$ (**i**) of dendritic calcium transients in WT and APP/PS1 mice during treadmill running (WT: 4 mice, 297 dendritic calcium transients; APP/PS1: 5 mice, 543 dendritic calcium transients. Mann-Whitney U Test). **j**. The percentage of dendrites with at least one prolonged dendritic calcium transient (duration >8 s) during running in WT and APP/PS1 mice. **k**. The percentage of dendrites with at least one dendritic calcium transient with large peak amplitude (amplitude >400%) during running in WT and APP/PS1 mice. **l**-**m**. The duration of individual dendritic calcium transients correlates with the peak amplitude of calcium transients in both WT (**l**) and APP/PS1 mice (**m**) during running (WT: 4 mice, 297 dendritic calcium transients; APP/PS1: 5 mice, 543 dendritic calcium transients). Data in c are represented as the mean ± s.e.m. $^*P < 0.05$, $^{**}P < 0.01$, $^{***}P < 0.001$. n.s., not significant

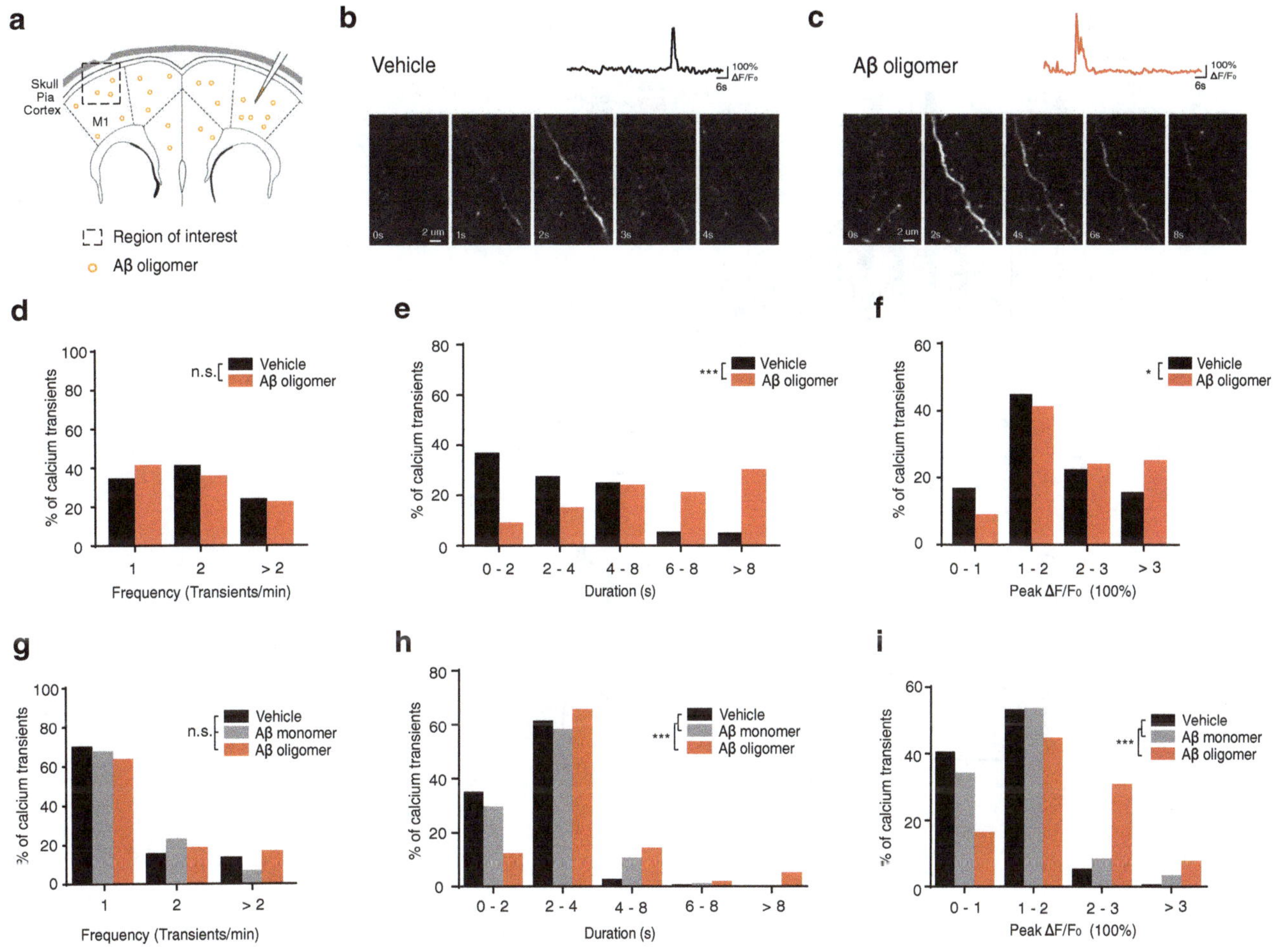

Fig. 4 Soluble Aβ oligomer injection induces dendritic calcium transients with abnormally long duration and high peak amplitude during running. **a**. Schematic showing the injection of soluble Aβ oligomers in the brain and the imaging area contralateral to the inject site. **b**-**c**. Time-lapse images of dendritic calcium transients in vehicle (**b**) and Aβ injected mice (**c**) during running. Top, traces of calcium transient fluorescence during running. **d**-**f**. Distributions of the frequency (**d**), duration (**e**) and peak $\Delta F/F_0$ (**f**) of dendritic calcium transients between vehicle and Aβ oligomer-injected mice during treadmill running. Mice were infected with AAV to express GCaMP6s in layer 2/3 neurons in the motor cortex (Vehicle: 4 mice, 136 dendritic calcium transients; Aβ oligomer: 4 mice, 99 dendritic calcium transients. Mann-Whitney U Test). **g**-**i**. Distributions of the frequency (**g**), duration (**h**) and peak $\Delta F/F_0$ (**i**) of dendritic calcium transients in Aβ oligomer, Aβ monomer and vehicle-injected mice during treadmill running in Thy-1 GCaMP6 transgenic mice (Vehicle: 4 mice, 148 dendritic calcium transients; Aβ monomer: 4 mice, 176 dendritic calcium transients; Aβ oligomer: 4 mice, 152 dendritic calcium transients. Mann-Whitney U Test). $^{***}P < 0.001$. n.s., not significant

The prolonged dendritic calcium transients reduce the peak $\Delta F/F_0$ of dendritic spine calcium transients in AD mice

Previous studies have shown that the level of dendritic calcium and the relative time windows between synaptic activity and dendritic calcium spikes are important for the induction of synapse potentiation or depotentiation [43, 55, 66–70]. To investigate whether and how abnormal dendritic calcium transients might affect synaptic activity and strength of L2/3 pyramidal neurons, we divided dendritic calcium transients into two groups based on their durations (0 – 8 s and longer than 8 s) (Fig. 5a). We then analyzed the peak $\Delta F/F_0$ of spine calcium transient before and after dendritic calcium transients in mice subjected to treadmill running (Fig. 5b). We found no significant difference in the peak $\Delta F/F_0$ of spine calcium transients before and after dendritic calcium transients with 0 – 8 s durations in either WT mice (Fig. 5c; n = 79 spine calcium transients from 4 mice. P = 0.135) or AD mice (Fig. 5e; n = 139 spine calcium transients from 5 mice. P = 0.858). Furthermore, we found a slight but not significant reduction in the peak amplitudes of spine calcium after long-duration (> 8 s) dendritic calcium transients in WT mice (Fig. 5d; n = 8 spine calcium transients from 4 mice. P = 0.076). Importantly, the peak $\Delta F/F_0$ of spine calcium transients was significantly reduced after the occurrence of long-duration (> 8 s) dendritic calcium transients in AD mice (Fig. 5f; n = 31 spine calcium transients from 5

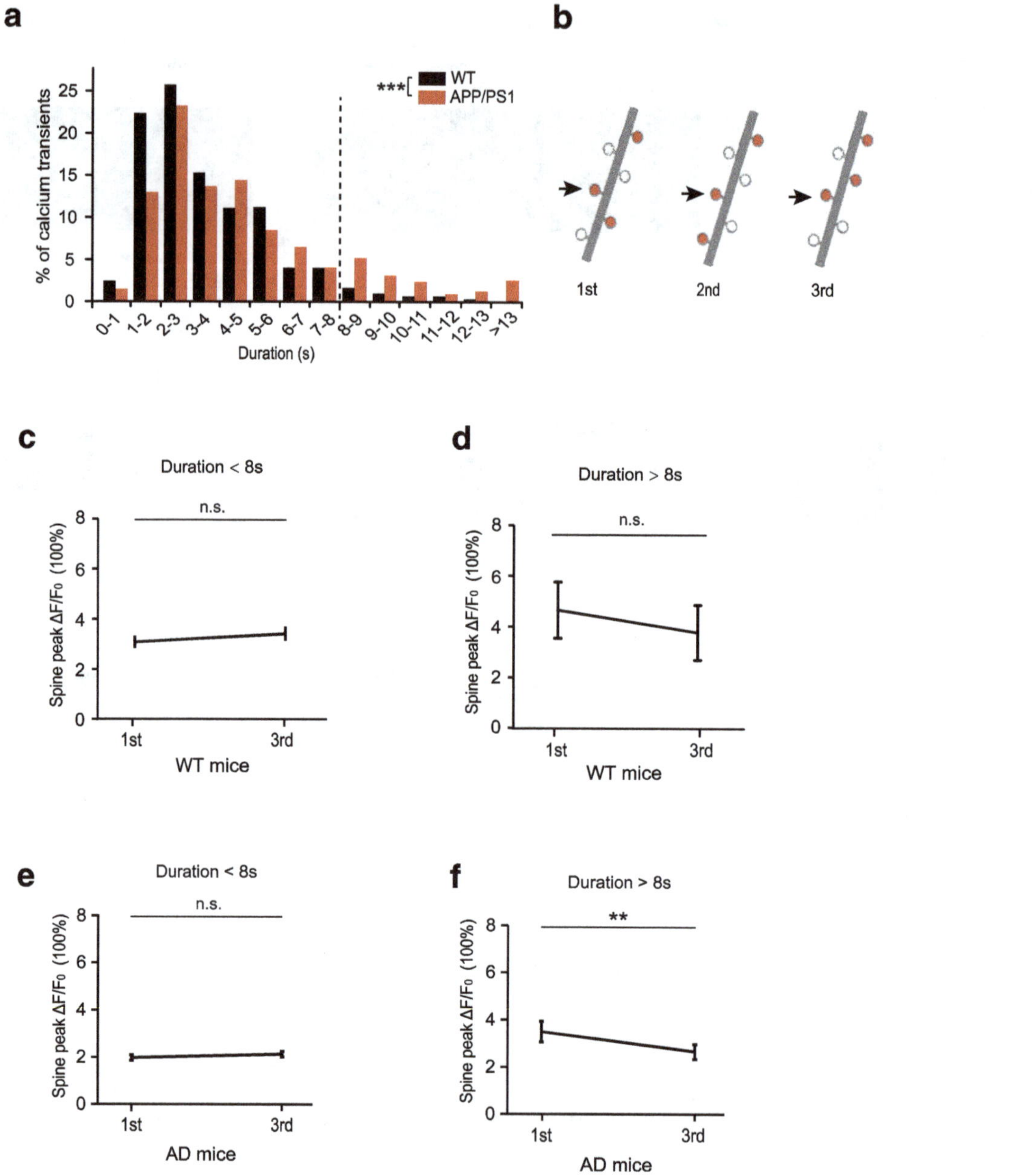

Fig. 5 Dendritic calcium transients with abnormal long-durations reduce peak amplitudes of spine calcium transients in APP/PS1 mice. **a**. Distributions of individual dendritic calcium transients in WT and APP/PS1 mice during running (WT: 4 mice, 297 calcium transients; APP/PS1:5 mice, 543 calcium transients. Mann-Whitney U Test). **b**. Schematic showing a dendritic branch exhibiting three dendritic calcium transients (1st, 2nd and 3rd) during a running trial. The peak $\Delta F/F_0$ of spine calcium transients was compared between 1st and 3rd image to examine the potential effect of the 2nd dendritic calcium activity. **c-d**. Changes of spine peak $\Delta F/F_0$ after the 2nd dendritic calcium transient in WT mice.The groups are divided according to the duration of the 2nd dendritic calcium transient: 0–8 s (c) and >8 s (d) respectively (0–8 s, 79 spine calcium transients; > 8 s, 8 spine calcium transients). **e-f**. Changes of spine peak $\Delta F/F_0$ after the 2nd dendritic calcium transient in APP/PS1 mice.The groups are divided by the duration of the 2nd dendritic calcium transients: 0–8 s (**c**) and > 8 s (d) respectively (0–8 s, 139 spine calcium transients; > 8 s, 31 spine calcium transients). Data are mean ± s.e.m. *P < 0.05, **P < 0.01. n.s., not significant

mice. P = 0.005). Taken together, these findings suggest that prolonged dendritic calcium transients lead to a significant depotentiation in the peak $\Delta F/F_0$ of spine calcium activity in AD mice.

The size of dendritic spines associated with long-duration dendritic calcium transients is reduced in AD mice

To further investigate the impact of long-duration dendritic calcium transients in AD mice, we examined changes in dendritic spine number and size on apical tuft dendrites of L2/3 pyramidal neurons expressing both GCaMP6s and a structural maker, tdTomato, in the M1 region (Fig. 6a). In this experiment, we first imaged dendritic spines at 0 h, trained mice on the treadmill for ~1.5 h, and performed imaging again at 1.5 h. Over the period of 1.5 h running, we found no formation or elimination of dendritic spines in both WT and AD mice (Additional file 3: Figure S3: 72 and 89 spines examined in WT and AD mice, respectively).

Next, we examined whether long-duration dendritic calcium transients may affect spine size by comparing the size of spines before and after 1.5 h treadmill running. Previous studies of layer 5 pyramidal neurons have shown that dendritic spines active at dendritic spike generation are potentiated [43]. Furthermore, the ratio of GCaMP6 fluorescence intensity in spine head to neighboring shaft for active spines was 1.56 ± 0.13 and for inactive spines was 0.46 ± 0.02 [43]. Based on similar criteria (see also Methods), we classified active and non-active spines of layer 2/3 pyramidal neurons according to the ratio of GCaMP6 fluorescence intensity between spine heads and adjacent dendritic shafts at the time of dendritic calcium transient generation. We found that active spines showed an increase in size on dendrites with short-duration (< 8 s) calcium transients, but a reduction in size on dendrites with long-duration (> 8 s) calcium transients over 1.5 h in both WT mice (Fig. 6b, c; n = 33 spines from 4 mice, duration <8 s; n = 10 spines, duration >8 s; P = 0.04) and AD mice (Fig. 6b, e; n = 30 spines from 4 mice, duration <8 s; n = 13 spines, duration >8 s; P < 0.001). Furthermore, spines that were not active during dendritic calcium transients did not exhibit significant changes over 1.5 h, regardless of the durations of dendritic calcium transients in WT mice (Fig. 6b, d; n = 9 spines, duration <8 s; n = 5 spines, duration >8 s. P = 0.792) and in AD mice (Fig. 6b, f; n = 15 spines, duration <8 s; n = 11 spines, duration >8 s. P = 0.899). Taken together, these results indicate that dendritic spines active on dendritic branches with frequently-occurring, long-duration dendritic calcium transients are reduced in size in AD mice. Because dendritic spine size strongly correlates with synaptic strength, these findings also suggest that prolonged dendritic calcium transients observed in AD mice lead to abnormal reduction in synaptic strength in the motor cortex.

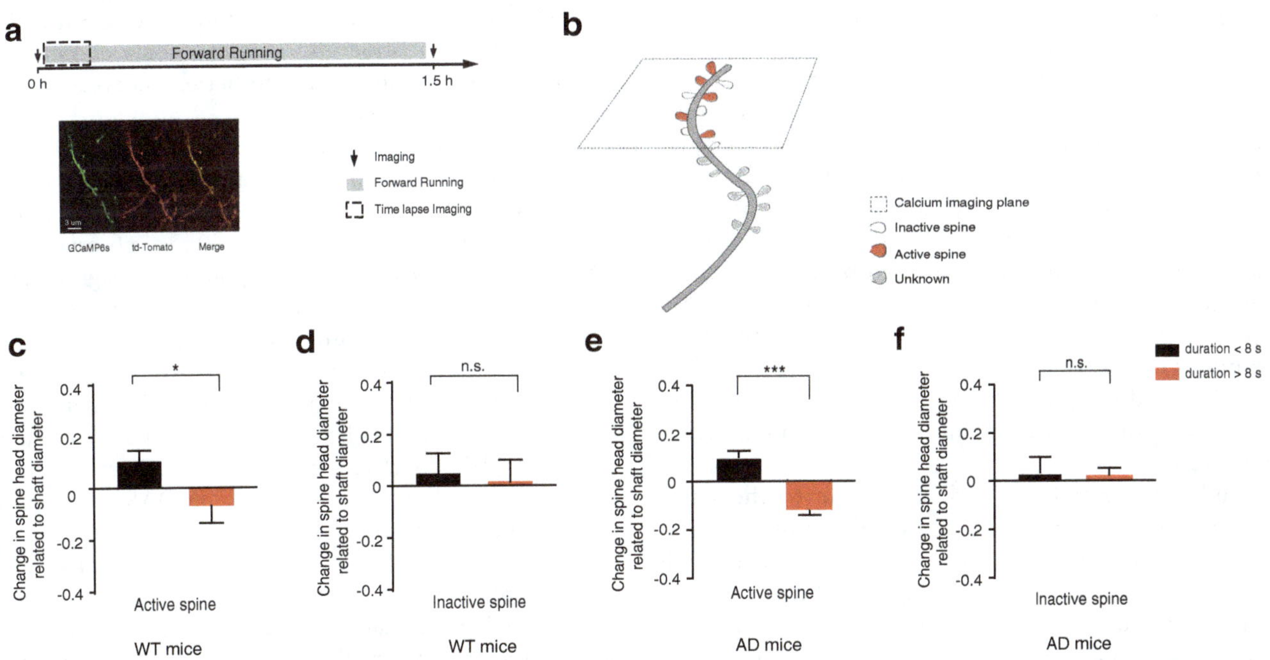

Fig. 6 Dendritic calcium transients with abnormal long-durations reduce dendritic spine size in APP/PS1 mice. **a**. Schematic of experimental design and imaging spine structure and calcium transients. Top, time course of imaging and treadmill running. Bottom, images of dendrites labeled with GCaMP6s (green) and Td-tomato (red). **b**. Schematic showing inactive (blank) and active (red) spines on the calcium imaging plane. **c-d**. Size change of active (**c**) and inactive (**d**) spines on dendrites with short and prolonged dendritic calcium transients in WT mice (active spine number: duration <8 s, n = 33 and duration >8 s, n = 10; inactive spine number: duration <8 s, n = 9 and duration >8 s, n = 5. Wilcoxon signed rank test). **e-f**. Size change of active (**e**) and inactive (**f**) spines on dendrites with short and prolonged dendritic calcium transients in APP/PS1 mice (active spine number: duration <8 s, n = 30 and duration >8 s, n = 13; inactive spine number: duration <8 s, n = 15 and duration >8 s, n = 11. Wilcoxon signed rank test). Data are mean ± s.e.m. ***P < 0.001. n.s., not significant

Discussion

In this study, we report that before amyloid plaque deposition, dendritic calcium transients with abnormally long durations and high peak amplitudes occur on apical dendrites of layer 2/3 pyramidal neurons in the motor cortex of 3 month-old APPswe/PS1dE9 transgenic mice. These abnormally long dendritic calcium transients could be induced after administration of soluble Aβ oligomers. Furthermore, long-duration dendritic calcium transients are associated with the reduction of dendritic spine calcium peak amplitude and spine size. Together, these results show that prolonged dendritic calcium transients and increased synaptic depotentiation are early neuronal deficits that occur before amyloid plaque formation in AD mice.

Previous studies have shown that L2/3 cortical neurons exhibit both hyperactivity and hypoactivity in aged APP23 × PS45 mice [20]. These hyperactive neurons are mostly clustered around amyloid plaques, suggesting that the microenvironment near amyloid plaques play an important role in triggering hyperactivity of nearby neurons [20]. Our findings indicate that prior to amyloid plaque deposition, calcium activities of L2/3 neuronal somas during the quiet resting state are lower in 3-month-old APPswe/PS1dE9 AD mice than in WT mice. Furthermore, somatic calcium activities of these cells during treadmill running have no significant difference between AD and age-matched WT mice. Thus, unlike the hyperactivity of cortical neurons near amyloid plaques in aged APP23 × PS45 mice, there is no overall increase in the activities of cortical neurons in the plaque-free motor cortex of 3-month-old APPswe/PS1dE9 mice. It is worth to note that neuronal hyperactivity has been observed in the hippocampus of 1.5 month APP23 × PS45 mice before the formation of amyloid plaques [19]. Further studies are needed to investigate whether neuronal hyperactivity may occur in the hippocampus, but not in the motor cortex, of 3-month-old APPswe/PS1dE9 mice. If so, it would suggest that alterations of neuronal activities in AD mice occur at different stages in different brain regions.

One key finding of our study is that during the active running state, a fraction of apical dendrites of L2/3 pyramidal neurons exhibit dendritic calcium transients with abnormal long-duration and high-amplitude in the motor cortex of APPswe/PS1dE9 mice, prior to amyloid plaque formation. Recent studies have shown that dendritic calcium spikes are critical for changes of spine calcium activity and spine size in the motor cortex [43]. Consistent with the fundamental role of dendritic calcium elevation in synaptic plasticity, we found that peak amplitudes of dendritic spines decrease after prolonged dendritic calcium transients (> 8 s). Furthermore, long-duration dendritic calcium transients are associated with a reduction in the size of active spines, but not inactive spines, at the generation of dendritic calcium transients. Because calcium activities of neuronal somas were comparable between APPswe/PS1dE9 and WT mice during running, these results suggest the dysregulation of dendritic calcium and spine plasticity are among the earliest-occurring neuronal deficits (prior to the neuronal somatic hyperactivity and plaque formation) in the pathogenesis of AD.

We found that administration of Aβ oligomers in WT mice causes abnormal long-duration dendritic calcium transients. This finding is consistent with the detrimental roles of soluble Aβ oligomers in disrupting calcium homeostasis and synaptic plasticity in AD. Aβ oligomers and PS1 mutations can disrupt calcium release from ER [71–77]. Soluble Aβ oligomers can also disrupt dendritic calcium by interacting with NMDA receptors, modulating glutamate uptake and regulating calcium release from ER [35–41]. Such alterations of dendritic and spine calcium activity would likely have detrimental impacts on synaptic function and may lead to a progressive loss of synapses in AD. It is important to note that although we found synaptic depotentiation associated with prolonged dendritic calcium activity, we did not observe an increase of spine loss over 1.5 h of treadmill running. Future studies are therefore needed to investigate the relationship among long-duration dendritic calcium activity, spine depotentiation and potential spine elimination over extended periods of time to better understand synapse loss in AD pathogenesis.

Many lines of evidence indicate that NMDAR activation plays important roles in the generation of dendritic calcium spikes and synaptic plasticity [43, 58–60]. Consistent with these previous studies [43, 58–60], we observed that NMDAR antagonist MK801 application significantly reduced the frequency, duration and peak amplitude of dendritic and spine calcium transients (Additional file 4: Figure S4 a-f). Furthermore, after MK801 application, there were no significant changes in the peak amplitude of spine calcium transients before and after dendritic calcium transients (Additional file 4: Figure S4 g). These findings raise the possibility that the use of NMDAR antagonists such as memantine may slow down AD progression in part by reducing prolonged dendritic calcium activity and synaptic abnormalities. Future studies are needed to investigate whether memantine and other pharmacological agents targeting abnormal dendritic calcium activities and their signaling may help the treatment of AD by alleviating synaptic depotentiation and loss.

Conclusion

Our findings show that abnormal long-duration dendritic calcium transients and decreases in spine size occur prior to amyloid plaque formation and overall changes of neuronal somatic activity in the APPswe/PS1dE9 mouse model of AD. The abnormal long-duration and high-amplitude dendritic calcium transients can be induced by soluble Aβ oligomers and may contribute to synaptic deficits during the early pathogenesis of AD.

Additional files

Additional file 1: Figure S1. Soluble Aβ oligomer injection induces higher neuronal calcium activity in virus injected WT mice during running. **a**. Distributions of the frequency, duration, peak $\Delta F/F_0$ and total integrated activity of somatic calcium transients in vehicle-injected mice and Aβ oligomer-injected mice during quiet resting (Vehicle: 4 mice, 80 somas; Aβ oligomer: 4 mice, 89 somas. Mann-Whitney U Test). **b**. Distributions of the frequency, duration, peak $\Delta F/F_0$ and total integrated activity of somatic calcium transients in vehicle-injected mice and Aβ oligomer-injected mice during running (Vehicle: 4 mice, 80 somas; Aβ oligomer: 4 mice, 89 somas. Mann-Whitney U Test). **P* < 0.05, ***P* < 0.01. n.s., not significant.

Additional file 2: Figure S2. The overall spine calcium activities are comparable between vehicle and soluble Aβ oligomer-injected mice. **a**. Distributions of the frequency, duration, peak $\Delta F/F_0$ and total integrated activity of spine calcium transients in vehicle and Aβ oligomer-injected mice during quiet resting state (Vehicle: 4 mice, 53 spines; Aβ oligomer: 4 mice, 62 spines. Mann-Whitney U Test). **b**. Distributions of the frequency, duration, peak $\Delta F/F_0$ and total integrated activity of spine calcium transients in vehicle and Aβ oligomer-injected mice during running (Vehicle: 4 mice, 66 spines; Aβ oligomer: 4 mice, 56 spines. Mann-Whitney U Test). **P* < 0.05. n.s., not significant.

Additional file 3: Figure S3. Spine turnover rate is comparable in WT and AD mice during 1.5 h treadmill running. Spine turnover rate (stable, elimination and formation rate) in WT mice (*n* = 4) and AD mice (*n* = 4). No spine formation or elimination was found over a 1.5 h period of treadmill running.

Additional file 4: Figure S4. The dendritic calcium activities decrease after MK801 application during running. **a-c**. The frequency (a), duration (b) and peak amplitude (c) of dendrite calcium transients before and after MK801 application (10 min). (60 dendrites from 4 mice, Student's T test). **d-f**. The frequency (d), duration (e) and peak amplitude (f) of spine calcium transients before and after MK801 application (10 min). (58 spines from 4 mice, Student's T test). **g**. No changes of spine peak $\Delta F/F_0$ before and after dendritic calcium transients after MK801 application (26 spines from 4 mice, Student's T test). Data are mean ± s.e.m. ****P* < 0.001. n.s., not significant.

Abbreviations
AD: Alzheimer's disease; APP/PS1: APPswe/PSEN1dE9; Aβ: β-amyloid

Acknowledgements
We thank all the members of Gan lab for critical comments and helpful discussions on this manuscript.

Funding
This work was supported by NIH 5R01 NS087198 and 5R01NS047325 to W.-B.G., Shenzhen Science and Technology Innovation Funds KQTD2015032709315529 and JSGG20140703163838793 to W. L., Shenzhen Science and Technology Innovation Funds JCYJ20160428154351820 to L.M., NIMH R21-MH107966 to Z.P.W.

Authors' contributions
YB and WBG designed the experiments and wrote the manuscript; YB, ML, YMZ and LM performed in vivo imaging experiments with the help of WL; WLH bred transgenic mice and performed genotyping; YB analyzed the data with the help of LM. ML, QQ and WL. All authors read and approved the final manuscript.

Authors' information
Information for all the co-authors is listed in the title page.

Competing interests
The authors declare that they have no competing interests.

Author details
[1]Drug Discovery Center, Key Laboratory of Chemical Genomics, Peking University Shenzhen Graduate School, Shenzhen 518055, China. [2]Skirball Institute, Department of Neuroscience and Physiology, New York University School of Medicine, New York, NY 10016, USA. [3]Department of Neurobiology, University of Pittsburgh, Pittsburgh, PA 15213, USA.

References
1. Terry RD, Masliah E, Salmon DP, Butters N, DeTeresa R, Hill R, Hansen LA, Katzman R. Physical basis of cognitive alterations in Alzheimer's disease: synapse loss is the major correlate of cognitive impairment. Ann Neurol. 1991;30:572–80.
2. Masliah E, Crews L, Hansen L. Synaptic remodeling during aging and in Alzheimer's disease. J Alzheimers Dis. 2006;9:91–9.
3. Scheff SW, Price DA. Synapse loss in the temporal lobe in Alzheimer's disease. Ann Neurol. 1993;33:190–9.
4. Selkoe DJ. Alzheimer's disease is a synaptic failure. Science. 2002;298:789–91.
5. Scheff SW, Price DA, Schmitt FA, Mufson EJ. Hippocampal synaptic loss in early Alzheimer's disease and mild cognitive impairment. Neurobiol Aging. 2006;27:1372–84.
6. Scheff SW, Price DA, Schmitt FA, DeKosky ST, Mufson EJ. Synaptic alterations in CA1 in mild Alzheimer disease and mild cognitive impairment. Neurology. 2007;68:1501–8.
7. Honer WG. Pathology of presynaptic proteins in Alzheimer's disease: more than simple loss of terminals. Neurobiol Aging. 2003;24:1047–62.
8. Jacobsen JS, CC W, Redwine JM, Comery TA, Arias R, Bowlby M, Martone R, Morrison JH, Pangalos MN, Reinhart PH, Bloom FE. Early-onset behavioral and synaptic deficits in a mouse model of Alzheimer's disease. Proc Natl Acad Sci U S A. 2006;103:5161–6.
9. CC W, Chawla F, Games D, Rydel RE, Freedman S, Schenk D, Young WG, Morrison JH, Bloom FE. Selective vulnerability of dentate granule cells prior to amyloid deposition in PDAPP mice: digital morphometric analyses. Proc Natl Acad Sci U S A. 2004;101:7141–6.
10. Reddy PH, Mani G, Park BS, Jacques J, Murdoch G, Whetsell W Jr, Kaye J, Manczak M. Differential loss of synaptic proteins in Alzheimer's disease: implications for synaptic dysfunction. J Alzheimers Dis. 2005;7:103–17. discussion 173-180
11. Ingelsson M, Fukumoto H, Newell KL, Growdon JH, Hedley-Whyte ET, Frosch MP, Albert MS, Hyman BT, Irizarry MC. Early Abeta accumulation and progressive synaptic loss, gliosis, and tangle formation in AD brain. Neurology. 2004;62:925–31.
12. Maras PM, Molet J, Chen Y, Rice C, Ji SG, Solodkin A, Baram TZ. Preferential loss of dorsal-hippocampus synapses underlies memory impairments provoked by short, multimodal stress. Mol Psychiatry. 2014;19:811–22.
13. Vanleeuwen JE, Penzes P. Long-term perturbation of spine plasticity results in distinct impairments of cognitive function. J Neurochem. 2012;123:781–9.
14. Albers MW, Gilmore GC, Kaye J, Murphy C, Wingfield A, Bennett DA, Boxer AL, Buchman AS, Cruickshanks KJ, Devanand DP, et al. At the interface of sensory and motor dysfunctions and Alzheimer's disease. Alzheimers Dement. 2015;11:70–98.
15. Chainay H, Louarn C, Humphreys GW. Ideational action impairments in Alzheimer's disease. Brain Cogn. 2006;62:198–205.
16. Hebert LE, Bienias JL, McCann JJ, Scherr PA, Wilson RS, Evans DA. Upper and lower extremity motor performance and functional impairment in Alzheimer's disease. Am J Alzheimers Dis Other Demen. 2010;25:425–31.

17. Minkeviciene R, Rheims S, Dobszay MB, Zilberter M, Hartikainen J, Fulop L, Penke B, Zilberter Y, Harkany T, Pitkanen A, Tanila H. Amyloid beta-induced neuronal hyperexcitability triggers progressive epilepsy. J Neurosci. 2009;29:3453–62.
18. Quiroz YT, Budson AE, Celone K, Ruiz A, Newmark R, Castrillon G, Lopera F, Stern CE. Hippocampal hyperactivation in presymptomatic familial Alzheimer's disease. Ann Neurol. 2010;68:865–75.
19. Busche MA, Chen X, Henning HA, Reichwald J, Staufenbiel M, Sakmann B, Konnerth A. Critical role of soluble amyloid-beta for early hippocampal hyperactivity in a mouse model of Alzheimer's disease. Proc Natl Acad Sci U S A. 2012;109:8740–5.
20. Busche MA, Eichhoff G, Adelsberger H, Abramowski D, Wiederhold KH, Haass C, Staufenbiel M, Konnerth A, Garaschuk O. Clusters of hyperactive neurons near amyloid plaques in a mouse model of Alzheimer's disease. Science. 2008;321:1686–9.
21. Lefort S, Tomm C, Floyd Sarria JC, Petersen CC. The excitatory neuronal network of the C2 barrel column in mouse primary somatosensory cortex. Neuron. 2009;61:301–16.
22. Petreanu L, Mao T, Sternson SM, Svoboda K. The subcellular organization of neocortical excitatory connections. Nature. 2009;457:1142–5.
23. Grutzendler J, Helmin K, Tsai J, Gan WB. Various dendritic abnormalities are associated with fibrillar amyloid deposits in Alzheimer's disease. Ann N Y Acad Sci. 2007;1097:30–9.
24. Perez-Cruz C, Nolte MW, van Gaalen MM, Rustay NR, Termont A, Tanghe A, Kirchhoff F, Ebert U. Reduced spine density in specific regions of CA1 pyramidal neurons in two transgenic mouse models of Alzheimer's disease. J Neurosci. 2011;31:3926–34.
25. del Valle J, Bayod S, Camins A, Beas-Zarate C, Velazquez-Zamora DA, Gonzalez-Burgos I, Pallas M. Dendritic spine abnormalities in hippocampal CA1 pyramidal neurons underlying memory deficits in the SAMP8 mouse model of Alzheimer's disease. J Alzheimers Dis. 2012;32:233–40.
26. Tsai J, Grutzendler J, Duff K, Gan WB. Fibrillar amyloid deposition leads to local synaptic abnormalities and breakage of neuronal branches. Nat Neurosci. 2004;7:1181–3.
27. Palop JJ, Chin J, Roberson ED, Wang J, Thwin MT, Bien-Ly N, Yoo J, Ho KO, GQ Y, Kreitzer A, et al. Aberrant excitatory neuronal activity and compensatory remodeling of inhibitory hippocampal circuits in mouse models of Alzheimer's disease. Neuron. 2007;55:697–711.
28. Koukouli F, Rooy M, Maskos U. Early and progressive deficit of neuronal activity patterns in a model of local amyloid pathology in mouse prefrontal cortex. Aging (Albany NY). 2016;8:3430–49.
29. Lue LF, Kuo YM, Roher AE, Brachova L, Shen Y, Sue L, Beach T, Kurth JH, Rydel RE, Rogers J. Soluble amyloid beta peptide concentration as a predictor of synaptic change in Alzheimer's disease. Am J Pathol. 1999;155:853–62.
30. Naslund J, Haroutunian V, Mohs R, Davis KL, Davies P, Greengard P, Buxbaum JD. Correlation between elevated levels of amyloid beta-peptide in the brain and cognitive decline. JAMA. 2000;283:1571–7.
31. Allsop D, Mayes J. Amyloid beta-peptide and Alzheimer's disease. Essays Biochem. 2014;56:99–110.
32. Moechars D, Dewachter I, Lorent K, Reverse D, Baekelandt V, Naidu A, Tesseur I, Spittaels K, Haute CV, Checler F, et al. Early phenotypic changes in transgenic mice that overexpress different mutants of amyloid precursor protein in brain. J Biol Chem. 1999;274:6483–92.
33. Mucke L, Masliah E, GQ Y, Mallory M, Rockenstein EM, Tatsuno G, Hu K, Kholodenko D, Johnson-Wood K, McConlogue L. High-level neuronal expression of abeta 1-42 in wild-type human amyloid protein precursor transgenic mice: synaptotoxicity without plaque formation. J Neurosci. 2000;20:4050–8.
34. Busche MA, Kekus M, Adelsberger H, Noda T, Forstl H, Nelken I, Konnerth A. Rescue of long-range circuit dysfunction in Alzheimer's disease models. Nat Neurosci. 2015;18:1623–30.
35. Texido L, Martin-Satue M, Alberdi E, Solsona C, Matute C. Amyloid beta peptide oligomers directly activate NMDA receptors. Cell Calcium. 2011;49:184–90.
36. Pellistri F, Bucciantini M, Relini A, Nosi D, Gliozzi A, Robello M, Stefani M. Nonspecific interaction of prefibrillar amyloid aggregates with glutamatergic receptors results in Ca2+ increase in primary neuronal cells. J Biol Chem. 2008;283:29950–60.
37. Snyder EM, Nong Y, Almeida CG, Paul S, Moran T, Choi EY, Nairn AC, Salter MW, Lombroso PJ, Gouras GK, Greengard P. Regulation of NMDA receptor trafficking by amyloid-beta. Nat Neurosci. 2005;8:1051–8.
38. Li S, Hong S, Shepardson NE, Walsh DM, Shankar GM, Selkoe D. Soluble oligomers of amyloid Beta protein facilitate hippocampal long-term depression by disrupting neuronal glutamate uptake. Neuron. 2009;62:788–801.
39. Green KN, Demuro A, Akbari Y, Hitt BD, Smith IF, Parker I, LaFerla FM. SERCA pump activity is physiologically regulated by presenilin and regulates amyloid beta production. J Cell Biol. 2008;181:1107–16.
40. Cheung KH, Shineman D, Muller M, Cardenas C, Mei L, Yang J, Tomita T, Iwatsubo T, Lee VM, Foskett JK. Mechanism of Ca2+ disruption in Alzheimer's disease by presenilin regulation of InsP3 receptor channel gating. Neuron. 2008;58:871–83.
41. Christensen RA, Shtifman A, Allen PD, Lopez JR, Querfurth HW. Calcium dyshomeostasis in beta-amyloid and tau-bearing skeletal myotubes. J Biol Chem. 2004;279:53524–32.
42. Chen TW, Wardill TJ, Sun Y, Pulver SR, Renninger SL, Baohan A, Schreiter ER, Kerr RA, Orger MB, Jayaraman V, et al. Ultrasensitive fluorescent proteins for imaging neuronal activity. Nature. 2013;499:295–300.
43. Cichon J, Gan WB. Branch-specific dendritic ca(2+) spikes cause persistent synaptic plasticity. Nature. 2015;520:180–5.
44. Jankowsky JL, Slunt HH, Ratovitski T, Jenkins NA, Copeland NG, Borchelt DR. Co-expression of multiple transgenes in mouse CNS: a comparison of strategies. Biomol Eng. 2001;17:157–65.
45. Borchelt DR, Davis J, Fischer M, Lee MK, Slunt HH, Ratovitsky T, Regard J, Copeland NG, Jenkins NA, Sisodia SS, Price DL. A vector for expressing foreign genes in the brains and hearts of transgenic mice. Genet Anal. 1996;13:159–63.
46. Garcia-Alloza M, Robbins EM, Zhang-Nunes SX, Purcell SM, Betensky RA, Raju S, Prada C, Greenberg SM, Bacskai BJ, Frosch MP. Characterization of amyloid deposition in the APPswe/PS1dE9 mouse model of Alzheimer disease. Neurobiol Dis. 2006;24:516–24.
47. Heiss JK, Barrett J, Yu Z, Haas LT, Kostylev MA, Strittmatter SM. Early activation of experience-independent dendritic spine turnover in a mouse model of Alzheimer's disease. Cereb Cortex. 2017;27:3660–74.
48. Zhao YJ, Sivaji S, Chiang MC, Ali H, Zukowski M, Ali D, Kennedy B, Sklyar A, Cheng A, Guo ZH, et al. Amyloid Beta peptides block new synapse assembly by Nogo receptor-mediated inhibition of T-type calcium channels. Neuron. 2017;96:355–72.
49. Li W, Ma L, Yang G, Gan WB. REM sleep selectively prunes and maintains new synapses in development and learning. Nat Neurosci. 2017;20:427–37.
50. Yang G, Lai CSW, Cichon J, Ma L, Li W, Gan WB. Sleep promotes branch-specific formation of dendritic spines after learning. Science. 2014;344:1173–8.
51. Li CX, Waters RS. Organization of the mouse motor cortex studied by retrograde tracing and intracortical microstimulation (ICMS) mapping. Can J Neurol Sci. 1991;18:28–38.
52. Helmchen F, Imoto K, Sakmann B. Ca2+ buffering and action potential-evoked Ca2+ signaling in dendrites of pyramidal neurons. Biophys J. 1996;70:1069–81.
53. Svoboda K, Helmchen F, Denk W, Tank DW. Spread of dendritic excitation in layer 2/3 pyramidal neurons in rat barrel cortex in vivo. Nat Neurosci. 1999;2:65–73.
54. Myoga MH, Beierlein M, Regehr WG. Somatic spikes regulate dendritic signaling in small neurons in the absence of backpropagating action potentials. J Neurosci. 2009;29:7803–14.
55. Golding NL, Staff NP, Spruston N. Dendritic spikes as a mechanism for cooperative long-term potentiation. Nature. 2002;418:326–31.
56. Humeau Y, Luthi A. Dendritic calcium spikes induce bi-directional synaptic plasticity in the lateral amygdala. Neuropharmacology. 2007;52:234–43.
57. Waters J, Helmchen F. Boosting of action potential backpropagation by neocortical network activity in vivo. J Neurosci. 2004;24:11127–36.
58. NL X, Harnett MT, Williams SR, Huber D, O'Connor DH, Svoboda K, Magee JC. Nonlinear dendritic integration of sensory and motor input during an active sensing task. Nature. 2012;492:247–51.
59. Grienberger C, Chen X, Konnerth A. NMDA receptor-dependent multidendrite ca(2+) spikes required for hippocampal burst firing in vivo. Neuron. 2014;81:1274–81.
60. Palmer LM, Shai AS, Reeve JE, Anderson HL, Paulsen O, Larkum ME. NMDA spikes enhance action potential generation during sensory input. Nat Neurosci. 2014;17:383–90.
61. Lesne S, Koh MT, Kotilinek L, Kayed R, Glabe CG, Yang A, Gallagher M, Ashe KH. A specific amyloid-beta protein assembly in the brain impairs memory. Nature. 2006;440:352–7.
62. Shankar GM, Li S, Mehta TH, Garcia-Munoz A, Shepardson NE, Smith I, Brett FM, Farrell MA, Rowan MJ, Lemere CA, et al. Amyloid-beta protein dimers

isolated directly from Alzheimer's brains impair synaptic plasticity and memory. Nat Med. 2008;14:837–42.
63. Woods NK, Padmanabhan J. Neuronal calcium signaling and Alzheimer's disease. Adv Exp Med Biol. 2012;740:1193–217.
64. Arbel-Ornath M, Hudry E, Boivin JR, Hashimoto T, Takeda S, Kuchibhotla KV, Hou S, Lattarulo CR, Belcher AM, Shakerdge N, et al. Soluble oligomeric amyloid-beta induces calcium dyshomeostasis that precedes synapse loss in the living mouse brain. Mol Neurodegener. 2017;12:27.
65. Dinamarca MC, Colombres M, Cerpa W, Bonansco C, Inestrosa NC. Beta-amyloid oligomers affect the structure and function of the postsynaptic region: role of the Wnt signaling pathway. Neurodegener Dis. 2008;5:149–52.
66. Holthoff K, Kovalchuk Y, Yuste R, Konnerth A. Single-shock LTD by local dendritic spikes in pyramidal neurons of mouse visual cortex. J Physiol. 2004;560:27–36.
67. Kampa BM, Letzkus JJ, Stuart GJ. Requirement of dendritic calcium spikes for induction of spike-timing-dependent synaptic plasticity. J Physiol. 2006;574:283–90.
68. Lisman J, Spruston N. Postsynaptic depolarization requirements for LTP and LTD: a critique of spike timing-dependent plasticity. Nat Neurosci. 2005;8:839–41.
69. Nevian T, Sakmann B. Single spine Ca2+ signals evoked by coincident EPSPs and backpropagating action potentials in spiny stellate cells of layer 4 in the juvenile rat somatosensory barrel cortex. J Neurosci. 2004;24:1689–99.
70. Sheffield ME, Dombeck DA. Calcium transient prevalence across the dendritic arbour predicts place field properties. Nature. 2015;517:200–4.
71. Berridge MJ. Dysregulation of neural calcium signaling in Alzheimer disease, bipolar disorder and schizophrenia. Prion. 2013;7:2–13.
72. Zeiger W, Vetrivel KS, Buggia Prevot V, Nguyen PD, Wagner SL, Villereal ML, Thinakaran G. Ca2+ influx through store-operated Ca2+ channels reduces Alzheimer disease beta-amyloid peptide secretion. J Biol Chem. 2013;288: 26955–66.
73. Supnet C, Bezprozvanny I. The dysregulation of intracellular calcium in Alzheimer disease. Cell Calcium. 2010;47:183–9.
74. Jensen LE, Bultynck G, Luyten T, Amijee H, Bootman MD, Roderick HL. Alzheimer's disease-associated peptide Abeta42 mobilizes ER ca(2+) via InsP3R-dependent and -independent mechanisms. Front Mol Neurosci. 2013;6:36.
75. Mattson MP. ER calcium and Alzheimer's disease: in a state of flux. Science signaling 2010;3:pe10.
76. Small DH. Dysregulation of calcium homeostasis in Alzheimer's disease. Neurochem Res. 2009;34:1824–9.
77. Popugaeva E, Bezprozvanny I. Role of endoplasmic reticulum Ca2+ signaling in the pathogenesis of Alzheimer disease. Front Mol Neurosci. 2013;6:29.

14

Prevention of C5aR1 signaling delays microglial inflammatory polarization, favors clearance pathways and suppresses cognitive loss

Michael X. Hernandez[1], Shan Jiang[2], Tracy A. Cole[3,6], Shu-Hui Chu[4], Maria I. Fonseca[4], Melody J. Fang[4], Lindsay A. Hohsfield[3], Maria D. Torres[3], Kim N. Green[3], Rick A. Wetsel[5], Ali Mortazavi[2] and Andrea J. Tenner[1,3,4*]

Abstract

Background: Pharmacologic inhibition of C5aR1, a receptor for the complement activation proinflammatory fragment, C5a, suppressed pathology and cognitive deficits in Alzheimer's disease (AD) mouse models. To validate that the effect of the antagonist was specifically via C5aR1 inhibition, mice lacking C5aR1 were generated and compared in behavior and pathology. In addition, since C5aR1 is primarily expressed on cells of the myeloid lineage, and only to a lesser extent on endothelial cells and neurons in brain, gene expression in microglia isolated from adult brain at multiple ages was compared across all genotypes.

Methods: C5aR1 knock out mice were crossed to the Arctic AD mouse model, and characterized for pathology and for behavior performance in a hippocampal dependent memory task. CX3CR1^{GFP} and CCR2^{RFP} reporter mice were bred to C5aR1 sufficient and knockout wild type and Arctic mice to enable sorting of microglia (GFP-positive, RFP-negative) isolated from adult brain at 2, 5, 7 and 10 months of age followed by RNA-seq analysis.

Results: A lack of C5aR1 prevented behavior deficits at 10 months, although amyloid plaque load was not altered. Immunohistochemical analysis showed no CCR2$^+$ monocytes/macrophages near the plaques in the Arctic brain with or without C5aR1. Microglia were sorted from infiltrating monocytes (GFP and RFP-positive) for transcriptome analysis. RNA-seq analysis identified inflammation related genes as differentially expressed, with increased expression in the Arctic mice relative to wild type and decreased expression in the Arctic/C5aR1KO relative to Arctic. In addition, phagosomal-lysosomal gene expression was increased in the Arctic mice relative to wild type but further increased in the Arctic/C5aR1KO mice. A decrease in neuronal complexity was seen in hippocampus of 10 month old Arctic mice at the time that correlates with the behavior deficit, both of which were rescued in the Arctic/C5aR1KO.

(Continued on next page)

* Correspondence: atenner@uci.edu
[1]Department of Pathology and Laboratory Medicine, School of Medicine, University of California, Irvine, CA, USA
[3]Department of Neurobiology and Behavior, University of California, Irvine, CA, USA
Full list of author information is available at the end of the article

(Continued from previous page)

Conclusions: These data are consistent with microglial polarization in the absence of C5aR1 signaling reflecting decreased induction of inflammatory genes and enhancement of degradation/clearance pathways, which is accompanied by preservation of CA1 neuronal complexity and hippocampal dependent cognitive function. These results provide links between microglial responses and loss of cognitive performance and, combined with the previous pharmacological approach to inhibit C5aR1 signaling, support the potential of this receptor as a novel therapeutic target for AD in humans.

Keywords: C5a, C5a receptor, Alzheimer's disease, Complement, Microglia, Mouse models, Behavior, Gene expression, Inflammation, Phagosome

Background

Alzheimer's disease is a neurodegenerative disorder associated with the loss of cognitive function and characteristic neuropathological changes that include synaptic and neuronal loss, neurofibrillary tangles and extracellular senile plaques composed of amyloid beta (Aß) protein deposits. The association of complement proteins and reactive glia with senile plaques suggests that inflammatory processes may play a role in the disease and that complement activation may contribute to the inflammatory environment [1–5].

Inflammation is a fundamental response to infection and injury. In the brain, the primary immune cells are microglia (reviewed in [6]). In AD, activated microglia have been found to be associated with fibrillar (beta sheet) Aß (fAß) plaques in both human brains and mouse models of AD [7, 8]. Microglia are of particular interest in Alzheimer's disease since microglial dysfunction has been implicated as a factor in the progression of AD [9]. Indeed, Zhang and colleagues in an unbiased systems approach identified the immune modulatory functions of microglia, such as cytokines, Fc receptors, toll-like receptors (TLRs) and complement to be key nodes and networks of late onset Alzheimer's disease [10].

The complement system is a well-known powerful effector mechanism of the immune system that normally contributes to protection from infection and resolution of injury [11]. Complement activation generates activation fragments C3a and C5a that interact with cellular receptors to recruit and/or activate phagocytes (including microglia) [12, 13]. While complement activation in the brain can be beneficial and indeed crucial at times, it can also be detrimental. Recently it has been shown that early components of the classical complement pathway are essential for proper synaptic pruning during development [14]. However, excessive complement-dependent synapse elimination seen during aging and in certain neurodegenerative disorders is correlated with loss of, or aberrant, neuronal function [15–18]. Fibrillar Aß can activate the classical complement pathway (in the absence of antibody) or the alternative complement pathway in vitro [19, 20] and in vivo as evidenced by the association of complement components with fAß plaques in human AD and mouse models of AD [2, 21, 22]. Potential consequences of this activation include opsonization (with C3b and/or iC3b) of fAß for engulfment by phagocytes, leukocyte recruitment (by C3a and C5a) and potential bystander lysis on neuronal cells by the membrane attack complex (C5b-9) (reviewed in [23]). In addition, in vitro cultures of C57BL6/J cortical neurons express C5aR1 and, upon binding, C5a is reported to injure neurons [24, 25]. Microglia also express C5aR1 leading to C5a-induced chemotactic functions [26]. In addition, microglia express TLRs. TLR stimulation has been shown to synergize with C5aR1 signaling in the periphery in mice, increasing the pro-inflammatory cytokine production over TLR signaling alone [27, 28]. Thus, strategic therapeutic targeting, such as through pharmacologic treatment with C5aR1 antagonists, could retain the beneficial effects of complement (such as enhanced clearance and neuroprotection) while inhibiting some of the detrimental aspects of complement activation.

Previous studies in our lab have demonstrated that treatment of mouse models of AD with a specific C5aR1 antagonist, PMX205, decreased fibrillar plaque accumulation and microglial CD45 expression and enhanced behavioral performance [7]. To validate C5aR1 as a therapeutic target, we investigated the effect of C5aR1 gene ablation on behavior, pathology and microglial gene expression in wild type and the Arctic AD mouse model. The Arctic mouse model has the human APP transgene containing three mutations (Swedish, Indiana, and Arctic) that increase risk of AD in humans [29]. The Arctic mutation results in the increased rate of fibril formation upon generation of the cleaved Aß42 peptide, resulting in a quite aggressive rate of fibrillar amyloid plaque deposition, initiating as early as 2 months of age in these mice [30, 31]. Since the fibrillar form of Aß is known to activate complement, C5a should be generated. Therefore, we crossed Arctic mice [30] with C5aR1KO [32] mice to test the hypothesis that the absence of C5aR1 would suppress microglial inflammatory responses and behavior deficits. Subsequently, both Arctic and Arctic/C5aR1KO mice were crossed to the

$CX3CR1^{GFP}$ and $CCR2^{RFP}$ reporter mice [33, 34] to enable fluorescence-activated cell sorting (FACS) of adult microglia (GFP+ RFP-) from monocytes/macrophages (GFP+ RFP+) isolated from brain at different ages for microglial specific gene expression analysis.

Our findings demonstrate that deletion of C5aR1 prevents the loss of neuronal complexity in hippocampal CA1 and protects from spatial cognitive deficits even in the presence of fibrillar amyloid plaques. Moreover, microglial transcriptome analysis revealed increased expression of inflammatory genes, including chemokines and members of the NF-κB pathway, in the Arctic mouse as early as 5 months of age that remained elevated through 10 months of age but were not so upregulated in the Arctic/C5aR1KO. Additionally, clearance and degradation pathways, such as the phagosome and lysosome pathways, were increased in the Arctic/C5aR1KO relative to the Arctic mice as early as 2 months of age and persisted through 10 months. Taken together, the data suggest that a lack of C5aR1 signaling prevents the C5a-induced polarization to more inflammatory, less phagocytic microglia. The absence of C5a-C5aR1 signaling also protected from cognitive deficits. The data supports further investigation of the use of antagonists for C5aR1 as part of a novel therapeutic strategy to slow the progression of Alzheimer's disease cognitive decline.

Methods

Animals

All animal experimental procedures were reviewed and approved by the Institutional Animal Care and Use Committee of University of California at Irvine, and performed in accordance with the NIH Guide for the Care and Use of Laboratory Animals. The AD mouse model used was the Arctic48, which carry the human APP transgene with the Indiana (V717F), Swedish (K670 N + M671 L), and Arctic (E22G) mutations (under the control of the platelet-derived growth factor-ß promoter), and thus produce Aß protofibrils and fibrils as early as 2–4 months old [30], graciously provided by Dr. Lennart Mucke (Gladstone Institute, San Francisco, CA, USA). C5aR1 knockout mice generated by target deletion of the C5a receptor gene [32], were crossed with $Arctic^{+/-}$ mice to produce Arctic mice lacking C5aR1 (Arctic/C5aR1KO) and wild type littermate mice lacking the C5a receptor (C5aR1KO) that were assessed for behavioral deficits and pathology in comparison to the C5aR1 sufficient animals. To enable isolation of microglia distinct from any infiltrating myeloid cells for differential gene expression studies, homozygous breeding pairs of CX3CR1-GFP and CCR2-RFP mice were obtained from Jackson Laboratories and bred to produce double homozygous reporter mice ($CX3CR1^{GFP/GFP}CCR2^{RFP/RFP}$). Double homozygous reporter mice were bred with Arctic model mice to generate $Arctic^{+/-}CX3CR1^{GFP/+}CCR2^{RFP/+}$ (Arctic) and littermates lacking the APP transgene that were used as controls (WT). $CX3CR1^{GFP/GFP}CCR2^{RFP/RFP}$ mice were bred to C5aR1 knockout to produce $CX3CR1^{GFP/GFP}CCR2^{RFP/RFP}$ mice lacking C5aR1. Then these mice were bred to Arctic+/- mice lacking the C5a receptor (Arctic/C5aR1KO), to generate wild type and Arctic/C5aR1KO all heterozygotic for $CX3CR1^{GFP}$ and $CCR2^{RFP}$. None of the mice generated exhibited any gross abnormalities. Both males and females were used in all experimental assessments.

Behavior testing

Mice were handled for two minutes each for five consecutive days prior to all behavior testing. After handling, mice were acclimated (allowed to explore) to a behavior chamber for five minutes/day, for four consecutive days. On the training day (24 h following the last day of habituation), mice were exposed to two of the same objects (e.g. 100 mL glass beakers, blue legos, or opaque light bulbs) in fixed positions within the context chamber near one wall. Twenty-four hours later mice were tested in a hippocampal independent novel object recognition task (iNOR), or in a hippocampal dependent object location memory task (OLM). The iNOR paradigm involved exchanging one of the objects for a novel object (e.g. blue lego or 100 mL beaker). Testing for spatial memory (OLM) was performed by moving one of the objects to the center of the context, thus changing the spatial relationship of that object within the context. Animals' preference for novelty was tested by determining the time spent with familiar and novel objects or locations. Objects used, sizes of objects, and dimensions of the contexts were as described [35]. To prevent olfactory distractions, all objects were cleaned with ethanol and the bedding stirred after each trial. Testing was scored blind by two independent observers using stopwatches and results correlated. There were no significant differences found in performance of mice of any of the genotypes during habituation to the context, using ANY-maze video tracking system software (version 4.82, Stoelting Co.) to assess video recordings on Day 4 (the day preceding training) during which speed, distance traveled, % time spent in an inner zone of the chamber, and % time spent in an outer zone of the chamber were scored (see Additional file 1). This demonstrates that there were no motor or motivational impairments in the different genotypes. Data from behavior performance were converted with the formula (time spent with novel object minus time spent with familiar object)/time spent with both objects) × 100 to obtain a percent (%) discrimination index [36]. Data are presented as mean +/− SEM. Results were compared with two-tailed non-parametric Mann-Whitney *U* test or unpaired t-test or

ANOVA followed by Tukey's post hoc tests. Differences were considered significant when p was < 0.05. Mice were removed from the analysis if they spent less than 1 s/min with the objects during training and/or testing, or if the performance of mice was +/− 2 standard deviations from the mean.

Microglia isolation and FACS

Adapted from [37], mice from WT, C5aR1KO, Arctic and Arctic/C5aR1KO genotypes were perfused with PBS at 2, 5, 7 and 10 months, and the brains (without olfactory bulbs, cerebellum, or midbrain) collected for microglia isolation. Brains were treated with Dispase II (Roche) at 37 °C for 1 h and passed through a 70 μM nylon cell mesh strainer (BD Biosciences) to obtain a single cell suspension. The cell suspension was washed in Hanks' balanced salt solution (HBSS; ThermoFisher) and spun at 1000 x g for 10 min at 4 °C. The cell pellet was resuspended in 70% Percoll (Sigma; diluted in HBSS), and 35% Percoll (diluted in HBSS) was carefully layered over to create a discontinuous Percoll gradient. After centrifugation at 800 x g for 45 min at 4 °C, the cells at the interphase were quickly collected, washed with HBSS +2% heat-inactivated fetal bovine serum (Gibco) and passed through a 40 μM nylon mesh cell strainer. Using a FACS Aria II, the viable cell population was gated based on forward and side scatter properties of a propidium iodide stained control. Using these forward and side scatter parameters, the GFP^+RFP^+ and the GFP^+RFP^- cells were sorted and collected directly into RA-1 lysis buffer (Illustra RNAspin mini isolation kit, GE Healthcare).

Immunohistochemistry

Some cohorts of mice were perfused with phosphate buffered saline (PBS). The brain was dissected at 4 °C with half of the tissue immediately frozen on dry ice for biochemical analysis, and the other half drop-fixed in 4% paraformaldehyde-PBS at 4 °C for immunohistochemistry. After 24 h, the fixed tissue was placed in PBS/0.02% sodium azide at 4 °C until use. Vibratome sections (coronal, 40 μm) were incubated sequentially with 3%H_2O_2/10% Methanol/Tris buffer saline (TBS) to block endoperoxidase and with 2% BSA/0.1%Triton X-100/TBS to block nonspecific binding. Tissues were incubated overnight at 4 °C with anti mouse CD45 antibodies (rat monoclonal anti CD45, 1 μg/mL, Serotec, or goat anti CD45 0.2 μg/mL, R&D systems, Minneapolis, MN), anti Aß antibody (rabbit polyclonal 1536 [38] gift from N.R Cooper) or appropriate control IgG in blocking solution. Primary antibodies were detected with biotinylated secondary antibodies against the corresponding species, followed by ABC complex and DAB (VECTOR, Burlingame, CA). In animals lacking GFP constructs, fibrillar Aß was stained with 1% thioflavine as previously described [39]. For immunofluorescence staining of total Aß, samples were incubated with blocking solution followed by rabbit polyclonal anti Aß (1536) and labeling detected with Alexa 405 anti rabbit secondary antibody (1:300, Invitrogen). For Iba1/Thioflavine double label, sections were washed with 50% ethanol for 3 min., incubated with 0.5% thioflavine for 10 min, and after washing were blocked with PBS + 0.2% TritonX-100 + 5% goat serum for 1 h and subsequently incubated with anti IBA1 (Wako, I μg/ml in blocking buffer) 4 °C overnight. After washing, anti-rabbit Alexa 647 (1:200, Invitrogen) was added for one hour room temperature.

Stained sections were observed under a Zeiss Axiovert-200 inverted microscope (Carl Zeiss, Thornwood, NY) and images were acquired with a Zeiss Axiocam high-resolution digital color camera (1300 × 1030 pixels) and analyzed using Axiovision 4.6 software. Percent of immunopositive area (% Field Area) (immunopositive area / total image area × 100) was determined for all the markers studied by averaging 2–4 images per section for Aß and thioflavine or 6 images per section for CD45 of the hippocampal area. Digital images were obtained using the same settings, and the segmentation parameters were constant as previously reported [40]. The mean value of the % Field Area for each marker in each animal was averaged per genotype group with the number of animals per group indicated in figure legends. Double labelled IBA1 and thioflavine images were collected on Leica DM5500 Q Confocal Microscope. IBA1+ microglial cell numbers and ThioS+ plaque numbers and sizes were determined using the spots and surfaces modules in Bit-plane Imaris 7.5 software, respectively. Data were analyzed using one-way ANOVA statistical analysis. Staining of all genotypes that were compared by image analysis in an experiment was done simultaneously per given marker.

Golgi staining and Sholl analysis

Mice were perfused as above, and half brains were fixed and, after sectioning (150 μm), stained using the super-Golgi Kit (Bioenno Lifesciences, Santa Ana, CA), following the instructions of the manufacturer. All sections were coded, such that the analysis was done blinded. The stained tissues were then quantified using a stereology Zeiss Axio Imager M2 with NeuroLucida software Version 11.03. The soma and apical dendrites along with its dendritic branching were traced under 100× magnification for 5 pyramidal neurons in the CA1 region of the hippocampus for each animal followed by Sholl analysis, determining the average number of branching for a given distance from the soma (μm) of each neuron. The average number of branchings for a given distance from the soma for the neurons of each animal and genotype

+/– SEM were generated using GraphPad Prism. Significance is defined as $p < 0.05$.

RNA extraction and RNA-Seq

Total RNA from $GFP^{+}RFP^{-}$ cells was extracted using the Illustra RNAspin mini isolation kit. RNA was quantified using the NanoDrop ND-1000 spectrophotometer (ThermoFisher) and the quality checked using the Agilent Bioanalyzer 2100 (Agilent Technologies). Sequencing was performed by the University of California at Irvine Genomics High Throughput Facility. The SMARTer Stranded Total RNA-Seq Kit - Pico Input Mammalian (Clontech Laboratories) was used to generate Illumina-compatible RNA-seq libraries. Briefly, total RNA was converted into cDNA and then adapters with barcodes for Illumina sequencing were added by PCR. The PCR products were then purified and the ribosomal cDNA depleted with sequence specific probes and RNaseH. The resulting cDNA fragments were further amplified (12 cycles) and the PCR products were purified once again to yield the final cDNA libraries. The barcoded cDNA libraries were multiplexed on the Illumina HiSeq 2500 platform to yield 100-bp paired-end reads.

Read alignment and expression quantification

Pair-end RNA-seq reads were aligned using STAR v.2.5.1b [41] with parameters '–outFilterMismatchNmax 10 –outFilterMismatchNoverReadLmax 0.1 –outFilterMultimapNmax 10' to the reference genome GRCm38/mm10. We used STAR to then convert to transcriptome-based mapping with gene annotation Gencode v.M8. Gene expression was measured using RSEM v.1.2.25 [42] with expression values normalized into transcripts per million (TPM).

Building of gene expression matrix for time-course gene expression and pathway analysis

Libraries with uniquely mapping percentages higher than 65% were considered to be of good quality and kept for downstream analysis. Protein coding and long non-coding RNA genes, with expression TPM > =0.5 in at least one of the duplicates for each genotype, were collected and quantile normalized for subsequent time-course and pathway analysis. Fastq files and processed data matrices were deposited in GEO with the accession ID GSE93824.

Time-course gene expression analysis

Quantile normalized gene expression (TPM) profiles were analyzed with maSigPro [43] to identify distinct gene expression profiles across time points whose expression differed in at least one other age in one other genotype with multiple cluster sizes. A cluster size of k = 9 gave the best set of profiles. An alpha of 0.05 for multiple hypothesis testing and $r^2 = 0.7$ for regression model were used to acquire significant genes for each cluster.

Gene ontology and pathway analysis

Gene clusters were analyzed for Gene ontology (GO) enrichment by Metascape (http://metascape.org) [44] using a hypergeometric test corrected p-value lower than 0.05. maSigPro clusters were also analyzed for KEGG pathway enrichments using PaintOmics 3 [45] with significant pathways selected based on Fisher's exact test p-value lower than 0.05.

qRT-PCR

RNA was converted to cDNA using Superscript III reverse transcriptase (Life Technologies) following manufacturer's instructions and quantified using the NanoDrop ND-1000 spectrophotometer (ThermoFisher). Quantitative RT-PCR was performed using the StepOne-Plus Real-Time PCR System, the StepOne software v2.3 (Applied Biosystems) with the following FAM dye and MGB quencher TaqMan probes (ThermoFisher): Mm00443111_m1 (Ccl4), Mm00436450_m1 (Cxcl2), Mm00437306_m1 (Vegfa), Mm00515586_m1 (Ctsd), Mm00487585_m1 (Man2b1, Mm00499230_m1 (Npc2). All genes were multiplexed with the VIC dye and MGB quencher probe Mm01545399_m1 (Hprt) to allow for normalization of housekeeping gene in the same well. For each gene, cDNA from three samples (unique animals) of each genotype was tested in triplicate. Two of the samples were from the same samples as the RNA-seq dataset and one was from a sample not analyzed by RNA-seq at ages 5 and 10 months. P values are calculated using one way ANOVA followed by Sidak's multiple comparison test.

Results

C5aR1 deficiency prevents deficits in spatial specific object location memory

Since a C5aR1 antagonist had previously been shown to suppress AD-like pathology in mouse models of AD [7], we evaluated the effect of C5aR1 gene ablation on the ability to perform memory tasks. Spatial memory cognitive deficits are observed in AD patients and the Arctic AD mouse model has been shown to recapitulate specifically hippocampal dependent spatial impairments [31]. Our hypothesis was that knocking out C5aR1 would lead to less inflammation and, thus, to better performance. To confirm that the behavior deficit is spatial and hippocampal-dependent we used both the traditional hippocampus independent novel object recognition (iNOR) and a modification of the iNOR paradigm that assessed spatial memory and was hippocampal dependent, the object location memory (OLM) task [46, 47]. Mice of all 4 genotypes (WT, C5aR1KO,

Arctic, Arctic/C5aR1KO) spent about 50% of their time with each object during the training phase demonstrating no preference for a certain side of the chamber or one of the objects within the chamber indicating that memory retrieval 24 h later would not be confounded by inherent spatial or object preferences (Additional file 1E). As expected, at 7 (data not shown) and 9 (Fig. 1a,b) months of age, all genotypes performed well, and there were no differences in performance between genotypes in the hippocampal independent iNOR task demonstrating that the Arctic mice as well as C5aR1 deficient mice were not impaired.

When tested in the spatial OLM task (Fig. 1c), WT and C5aR1KO mice at both 7 and 10 months of age exhibited a discrimination index greater than 30% during the first two minutes of testing, indicating that they had a strong preference for exploring the object in the new location and that genetic deletion of C5aR1 alone is not detrimental or beneficial (Fig. 1d,e). The C5aR1 sufficient Arctic mice did not exhibit significant behavioral deficits at 7 months, although there were 2 animals that were noticeably performing worse than all other mice (Fig. 1d, right). However, at 10 months of age, there was a significant deficit ($p < .001$) in performance of Arctic mice in comparison to wild type mice, while importantly, Arctic/C5aR1KO did not differ from wild type or C5aR1KO. A statistically significant difference in behavior ($p < .05$) was observed between the Arctic mice

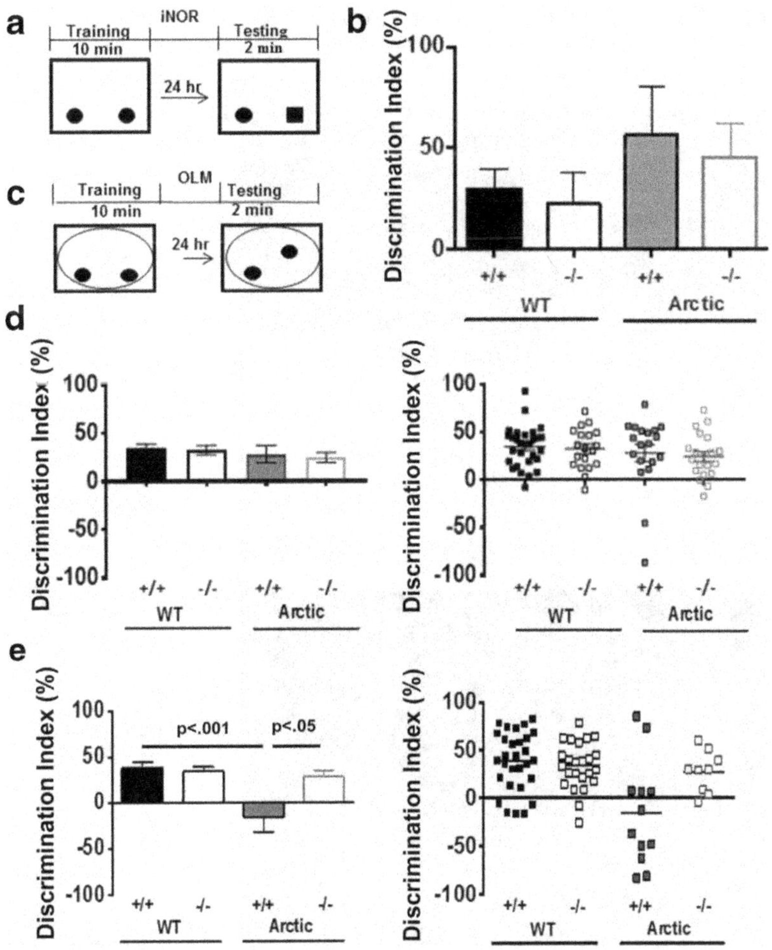

Fig. 1 Performance in Novel Object and Object Location Memory Tasks. Animals were tested in novel object recognition test (**a,b**) and novel object location memory test (**c-e**) after 5 days of handling and 4 days of habituation to the testing chamber. Paradigm schematics are presented for iNOR (**a**) and OLM (**c**). Solid oblongs or circles in the boxes represent identitcal objects. After Day 1 training, one familiar object was replaced with a novel object (solid square) (**a**) or a familiar object was moved to the center of the context (**c**). The novel object replacement or the object moved was counter balanced among all trials. Performance was evaluated using the first two minutes of testing at 9 months for iNOR (**b**), and either 7 months (**d**) or 10 months (**e**) for OLM. (**b**) WT $n = 11$, C5aR1KO $n = 6$, Arctic $n = 4$, Arctic/C5aR1KO $n = 5$. Right plots in **d** and **e** are the scatter plots for left bar graphs, respectively. (**d**) $n = 29$ (WT), 19 (C5aR1KO), 19 (Arctic) and 20 (Arctic/C5aR1KO). (**e**) $n = 29$ (WT), 25 (C5aR1KO), 12 (Arctic) and 9 (Arctic/C5aR1KO). (**b,d,e**) Data is expressed as the average +/− SEM. *P* values were determined by ANOVA followed by Tukey's post hoc test

lacking C5aR1 compared to the C5aR1 sufficient Arctic mice indicating protection from deficit in the Arctic/C5aR1KO mice relative to the Arctic mouse (Fig. 1e), consistent with the hypothesis that blocking C5aR1-mediated events prevents or slows the progression of cognitive defects.

Plaque accumulation and microglia marker CD45 immunoreactivity are not necessarily indicative of cognitive loss

Arctic mice at 7 and 10 months of age have abundant fibrillar plaque pathology in the hippocampus. Genetic deletion of C5aR1 did not alter the extent of fibrillar plaque pathology at either 7 or 10 months of age (Fig. 2; Additional file 2). IBA1 is a myeloid/ microglia specific marker in the brain. While CD45 is expressed on other cell types (T cells and endothelial cells), in the brain microglia are the dominant cells expressing this molecule, and it is also upregulated upon activation. Quantitative image analysis of these two markers revealed a slight but statistically significant decrease in CD45 immunoreactivity at 7 m in the Arctic/C5aR1KO mice compared to the C5aR1 sufficient Arctic mice (20%, p = .03) (Fig. 2b), while the number of IBA1 microglia was slightly greater (Additional file 2). However, those differences were not sustained in the 10 month mice (Fig. 2d; Additional file 2). Furthermore, neither fibrillar plaque pathology nor CD45 correlated with behavioral parameters of individual animals (data not shown). These data suggest that neither plaque load nor induction of CD45 is sufficient for neurotoxic effects that impact behavior in this model.

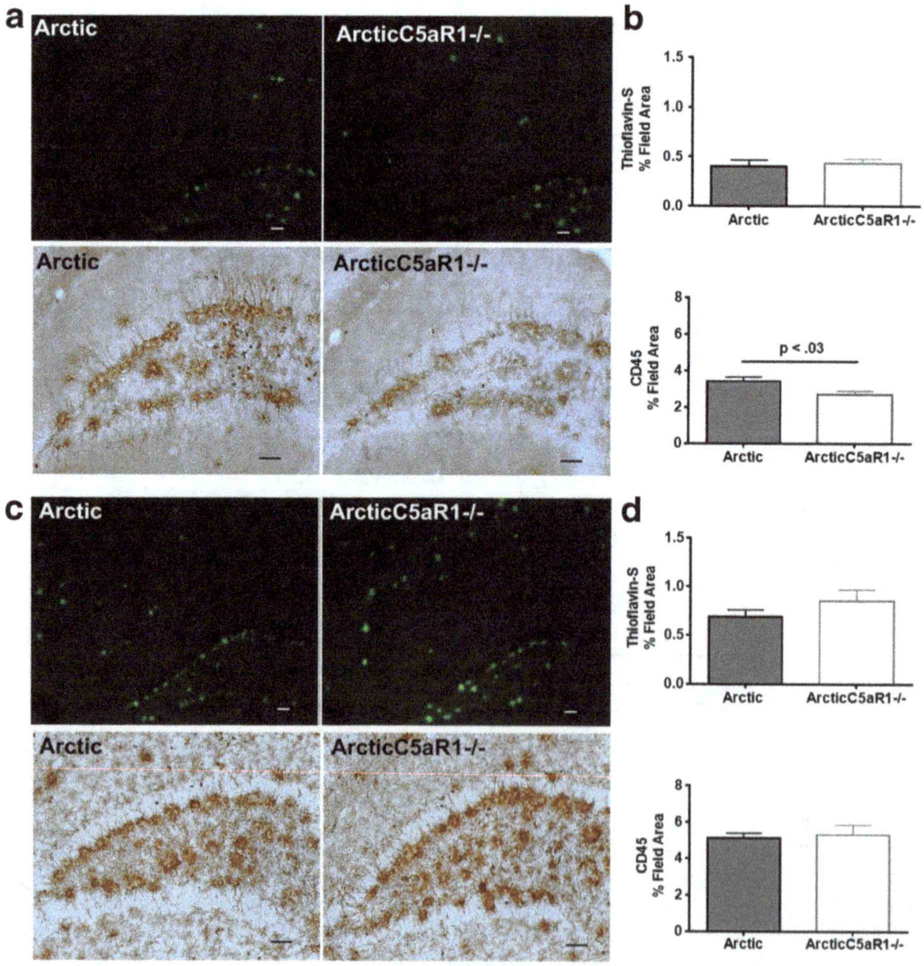

Fig. 2 Fibrillar plaque and CD45 microglial expression in hippocampus. Representative pictures of thioflavine-S staining (fibrillar plaques) (top panels) and CD45 staining (microglia) (lower panels) at 7 (**a**) and 10 months (**c**). Scale bar: 50 um. (**b**) Image analysis of 7 month thioflavine-S (upper) and CD45 (lower) staining (Arctic n = 9, Arctic/C5aR1KO n = 9) (**d**) Image analysis of 10 mo thioflavine (Arctic n = 12, Arctic/C5aR1KO n = 9) (upper) and CD45 (Arctic n = 11, Arctic/C5aR1KO n = 7) lower). Bars represent group means +/− SEM of n animals per genotype. Data represent the average of 2 to 4 sections per animal. P value was calculated using one- way ANOVA

Lack of CCR2-positive infiltrating monocytes around plaques

In the Arctic AD mouse model, we used the $CX3CR1^{GFP}$ and $CCR2^{RFP}$ reporter mice to differentiate microglia from infiltrating CCR2-positive monocytes [48]. Crossing $CX3CR1^{GFP/GFP}CCR2^{RFP/RFP}$ mice with Arctic or Arctic/C5aR1KO mice ultimately generated $CX3CR1^{+/GFP}CCR2^{+/RFP}Arctic^{-/-}$ (WT) and $CX3CR1^{+/GFP}CCR2^{+/RFP}Arctic^{+/-}$ (Arctic), $CX3CR1^{+/GFP}CCR2^{+/RFP}C5aR1^{-/-}$(C5aR1KO) and $CX3CR1^{+/GFP}CCR2^{+/RFP}Arctic^{+/-}C5aR1^{-/-}$ (Arctic/C5aR1KO) mice. While some studies with Alzheimer's disease mouse models have suggested that CX3CR1 and CCR2 play a role in the progression of disease [49–51], we determined that having a single copy of either gene does not alter plaque deposition or microglial CD45 reactivity (Additional file 3 A-E).

We next proceeded to age wild type (WT), C5aR1KO, Arctic, and Arctic/C5aR1KO mice to 2, 5, 7, and 10–11 months. As expected, no plaque pathology nor microglia clustering was observed in wild type mice or C5aR1KO mice (Fig. 3a,c). Plaque deposition increased with age and microglia clustered around the plaques, but was similar in the Arctic and Arctic/C5aR1KO mice across the different ages (Fig. 3b,d). Strikingly, no RFP-positive cells were found in areas near the plaques at any age. No RFP-positive cells were found anywhere in the parenchyma, while a few RFP-positive cells were localized around the surface of the brain, possibly meningeal macrophages (Fig. 3b,d insets).

Percoll gradient isolated cells, from brains of mice in the same cohort as that analyzed by IHC, when sorted by RFP and GFP showed a small population of GFP and RFP-positive cells. RFP-positive cells (which could represent the meningeal macrophages) represented 2–6% of the total sorted GFP-positive population (Fig. 3e), while RFP-negative microglia made up 94–98% of the GFP-positive cells (Fig. 3f). The absolute number of cells recovered varied, with means among all genotypes and ages between 700 and 2000 for RFP-positive cells (Fig. 3g) and between 27,000 and 55,000 for RFP-negative GFP-positive microglia (Fig. 3h).

Analysis of age dependent patterns of gene expression

To identify transcriptome changes in microglia in Arctic/C5aR1KO mice relative to Arctic mice, the FACS-sorted GFP-positive/RFP-negative cells of WT, C5aR1KO, Arctic, and Arctic/C5aR1KO mice at 2, 5, 7, and 10 or 11 months of age were collected and RNA extracted for RNA-seq analysis (Fig. 4a). RNA quality and quantity was sufficient for RNA sequencing and analysis (Additional file 4). RNA-seq libraries that

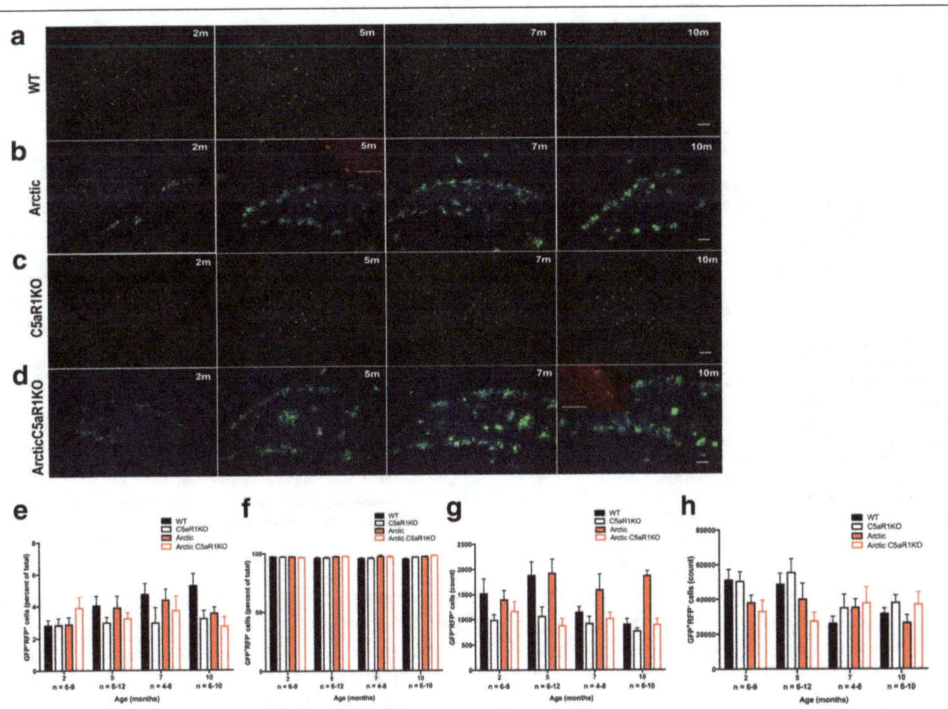

Fig. 3 Glia clustering around plaques are $CX3CR1^{+}CCR2^{-}$. Brain sections of (**a**) WT, (**b**) Arctic, (**c**) C5aR1KO, and (**d**) Arctic/C5aR1KO mice (all $CX3CR1^{+/GFP}CCR2^{+/RFP}$) at 2, 5, 7, and 10 months were fluorescently labelled in blue with anti-Aß antibody (1536). Staining was performed at separate times for cohort one (**a,b**) and cohort 2 (**c,d**). Representative pictures of cohorts one and two were taken at a close but slightly different bregma levels. Inset shows $CCR2^{+/RFP}$ macrophages. Scale bar:50 um (**e**) Percoll purified brain cells from WT, Arctic, C5aR1KO and Arctic/C5aR1KO mice (all $CX3CR1^{+/GFP}CCR2^{+/RFP}$; n = 4–12 per genotype, per age) were FACS-sorted as $GFP^{+}RFP^{+}$ (**e,g**) and $GFP^{+}RFP^{-}$ cells (**f,h**) and quantified as a percentage of total GFP+ cells (**e,f**) and total cell count (**g,h**)

passed our quality filters were used to estimate gene expression level. By doing time-course analysis with maSigPro [43] we identified 2156 differentially expressed genes that showed dynamic expression patterns over time with age and disease progression. The genes were partitioned into nine clusters, ranging in size from 125 genes to 445 genes, to show distinct temporal and genotype-specific profiles (Fig. 4b, Additional file 5). To identify clusters of interest to study further, we did the following: 1) Assessed the gene expression patterns of each cluster (generated by maSigPro) to identify differences in gene expression between the Arctic and Arctic/C5aR1KO (Fig. 4b, Additional file 5). 2) Performed gene ontology (GO) enrichment analysis using Metascape [44] to aid in the identification of clusters that had genes associated with biologically relevant processes (Additional file 6). 3) Used PaintOmics 3 for pathway analysis to identify significantly enriched KEGG pathways in each cluster (Additional file 7). Cluster 4 contained 125 genes (Additional file 8) that increased with age starting by 5 months in the Arctic relative to wild type. Those genes did not increase in the Arctic/C5aR1KO until 10 months of age and at that time showed levels similar to that seen in the 10 month wild type animals and still lower than the Arctic expression at 10 months (Fig. 4b). Cluster 2 consisted of 336 genes (Additional file 8) that were generally

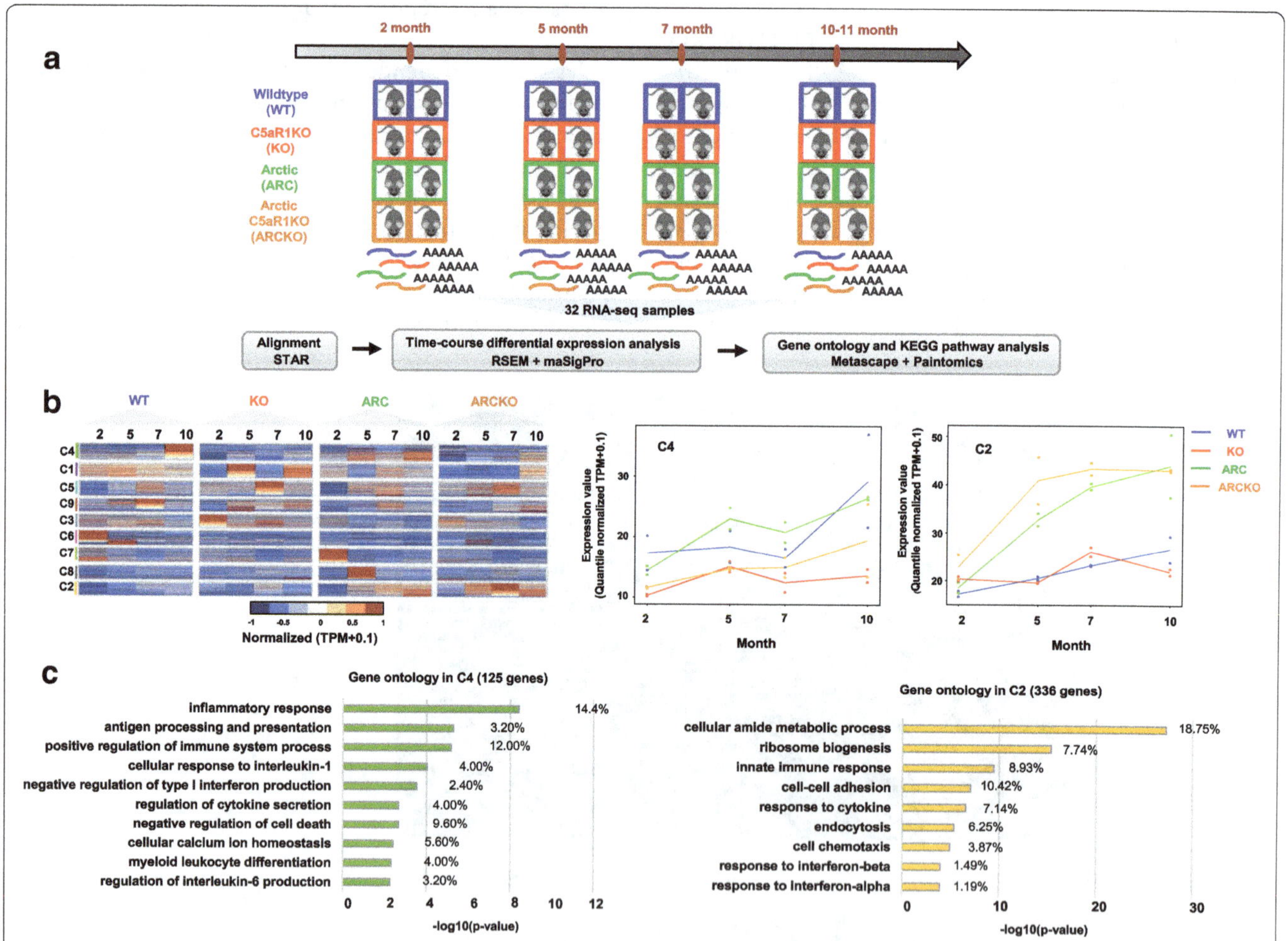

Fig. 4 Temporal gene expression profiles across four genotypes. (**a**) RNA-seq experiments were performed using duplicate samples from WT (blue), C5aR1KO (red), Arctic (green) and Arctic/C5aR1KO (orange) mice at 2, 5, 7 and 10–11 months. A total of 32 RNA-seq libraries were sequenced and analyzed. Reads were aligned to the reference genome with STAR. Gene expression level was estimated by RSEM and analyzed with maSigPro to identify distinct gene expression profiles across time. Differentially expressed genes during the time-course were loaded into Metascape and PaintOmics 3 to acquire gene ontology (GO) and KEGG pathways enrichment. (**b**, left) Heatmap of 2156 differentially expressed genes across four genotypes and four ages. Nine gene expression clusters were derived from maSigPro and labeled with number and color on the side. Quantile normalized TPM plus 0.1 were transformed between −1 and 1 to present high (red) and low (blue) expression level within each cluster. (**b**, right) Gene expression profiles for cluster 4 and 2. Median profile are plotted across all replicates for all the genes in the corresponding cluster. WT (blue), C5aR1KO (red), Arctic (green) and Arctic/C5aR1KO (orange). (**c**) Gene ontology enrichment was measured on genes from cluster 4 (green) and 2 (yellow). Gene ontology terms were sorted based on *p*-value. The percentage of genes in the cluster that are contained in the GO term is listed to the right of each bar

unchanged in the C5aR1KO relative to wild type but increased in the Arctic after 2 months relative to WT. The same genes were further increased in the Arctic/C5aR1KO (Fig. 4b). Gene ontology enrichment analysis using Metascape identified the enriched GO terms for cluster 4 of which the top 3 were: inflammatory response, antigen processing and presentation, and positive regulation of immune system process (Fig. 4c, left), whereas the top 3 enriched GO terms in cluster 2 were cellular amide metabolic process, ribosome biogenesis, and innate immune response (Fig. 4c, right).

Pathway analysis reveals less inflammation and higher degradative capacity in Arctic/C5aR1KO

Pathway analysis of cluster 4 identified several inflammatory diseases pointing to inflammation as well as canonical inflammation pathways. Of interest were NF-κB signaling, cytokine-cytokine receptor interaction, TLR signaling and chemokine signaling due to their statistical significance as well as their biological significance in the context of AD (Additional file 7). These four pathways were then investigated further and the 16 differentially expressed genes between the Arctic and Arctic/C5aR1KO (found in these 4 pathways) were plotted on a heat map (Fig. 5a). These genes remained elevated in the Arctic relative to WT, C5aR1KO, and Arctic/C5aR1KO through 10 months of age (Fig. 5a). Increases in those genes appeared in both WT and Arctic/C5aR1KO only beginning at 10 months (consistent with the increase in inflammatory gene expression with age [52]) but remained significantly lower than in microglia from the Arctic mice. Most of the inflammatory genes shown in Fig. 5a were either NF-κB subunits, transcriptionally regulated by NF-κB or were upstream activators of NF-κB as shown color-coded in Fig. 5b. These differentially expressed genes included cytokines and growth factors or their receptors (*Il1a, Vegfa, Il3ra*), chemokines (*Ccl3, Ccl4, Cxcl2, Cxcl16*), signaling receptors (*Tlr4, Vcam1, Cd40*), NF- κb transcription factor subunits (*Rela, Nfkb1, Relb, Nfkb2) and Ptgs2* (COX2) (Fig. 5a). Representative genes were validated by RT-PCR for each genotype at ages 5 and 10 months. Ccl4 and Cxcl2 were both significantly increased in the Arctic relative to WT at 5 months (3.5× and 4.4× respectively) and were decreased in the Arctic/C5aR1KO by 35% and 23%, respectively relative to the Arctic. Although Vegfa was not significantly increased in the Arctic relative to the WT at 5 months, it was significantly decreased by 46% in the Arctic/C5aR1KO relative to the Arctic (Fig. 5c, left). At 10 months, only Cxcl2 was significantly decreased in the Arctic/C5aR1KO relative to the Arctic and all 3 genes validated by RT-PCR showed no difference in expression between the WT and Arctic (Fig. 5c, right). These data thus follow the same trend observed in the RNA-seq data where C5aR1 deficiency in the Arctic leads to reduced expression of inflammatory genes early in the progression of the disease. Aside from cluster 4, cluster 3 also included some of the same pathways as in Fig. 5, such as chemokine signaling and cytokine-cytokine receptor interaction (Additional file 7), however the genes in this cluster did not contain differences between the Arctic and Arctic/C5aR1KO, rather, the C5aR1KO mice were substantially upregulated relative to the other genotypes.

Like cluster 4, pathway analysis of cluster 2 genes identified pathways that were of statistical significance as well as biologically relevant for microglia. The lysosome, antigen processing and presentation, and phagosome pathways identified 22 genes that were differentially expressed between the Arctic and Arctic/C5aR1KO. Trem2 and Tyrobp, also included in cluster 2, were added to the heat map due to known roles in microglial phagocytosis (Fig. 6a). In general, the genes in these pathways increased in the Arctic relative to WT at 5 mo but were further increased in the Arctic/C5aR1KO relative to Arctic (and as early as 2 months of age) and generally remained elevated through 10 months (Fig. 6a). The genes included phagocytosis-promoting receptors (*Tlr2, Fcgr4, Colec12, Trem2, Tyrobp*), lysosomal membrane proteins (*Lamp1, Npc2*), cathepsins (*Ctsb, Ctsd, Ctss, Ctsz*), glycosidases (*Gusb, Gba, Hexa, Naglu, Man2b1*) and MHCIb genes (*H2-d1, H2-m3, H2-t23, H2-q7*), all upregulated in the Arctic/C5aR1KO (Fig. 6b). *Cd63, Cd68, Ctsl,* and *Gaa* were increased at 2 mo in the Arctic/C5aR1KO relative to the Arctic levels. As with the Cluster 4 genes, representative genes were selected to validate the RNA-seq differential expression by RT-PCR. Genes expression of Cathepsin D and Mannosidase 2b1 were strikingly decreased in the Arctic at 5 months relative to WT (21% and 28% of WT respectively), something not seen in our RNA-seq data, however, both were increased in the Arctic/C5aR1KO relative to the Arctic (6.4× and 4.4× respectively) as seen in our RNA-seq analysis. NPC intracellular cholesterol transporter 2 (Npc2) expression was also greater in the Arctic/C5aR1KO relative to Arctic (1.4×) although no significant difference was seen between the WT and Arctic at 5 months (Fig. 6c, left). At 10 months of age, both Ctsd and Npc2 were upregulated in the Arctic relative to WT, however, only Npc2 was further increased in the Arctic/C5aR1KO (Fig. 6c, right).

Loss of neuronal complexity in the Arctic model is rescued in the absence of C5aR1

To assess the effect of the C5aR1-deficient environment on neurons, Golgi staining was performed and individual neurons in the CA1 region of the hippocampus were traced and analyzed for the number of branches at

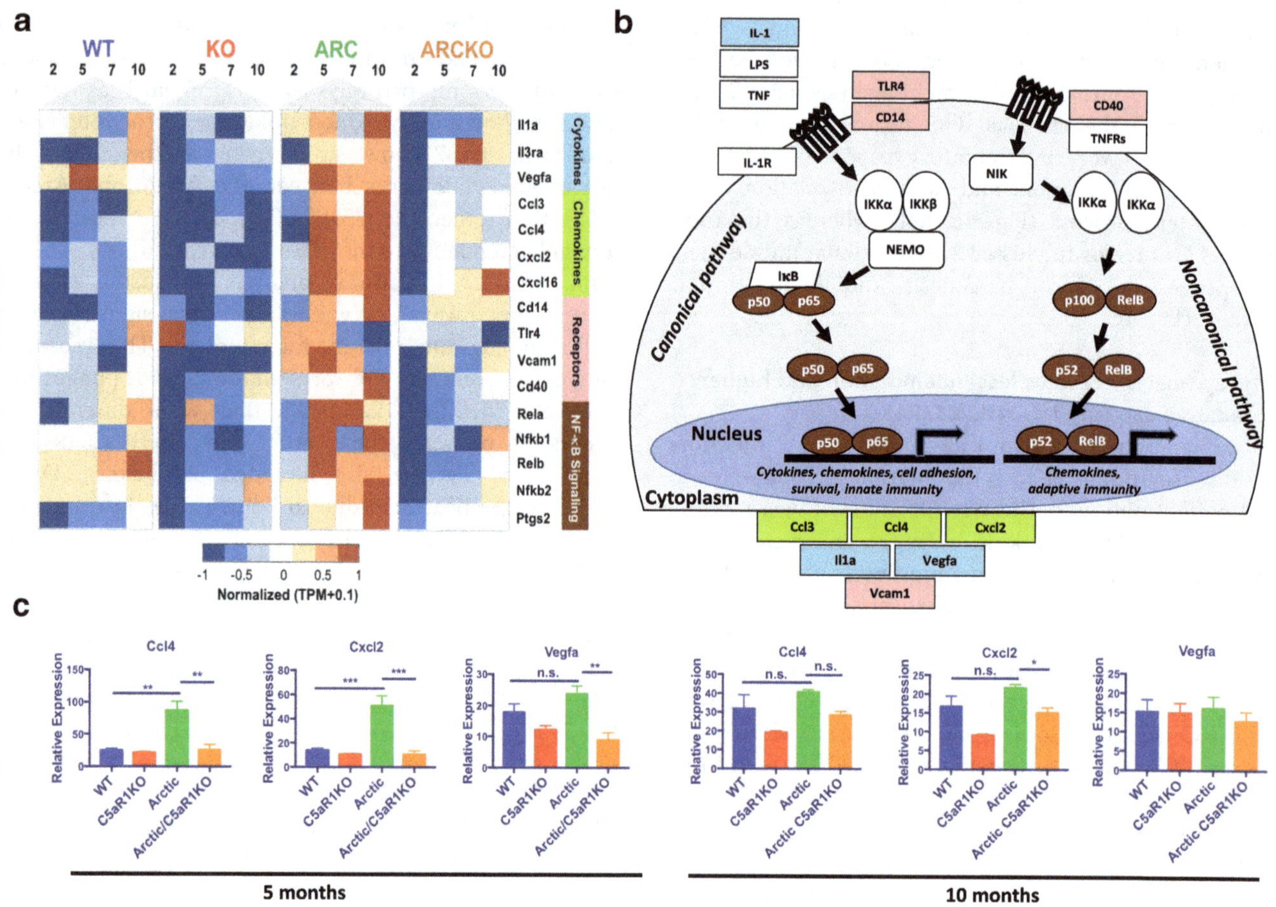

Fig. 5 Gene expression profiles of selected genes in inflammation pathways. All genes in heat map were present in cluster 4 and found in the NF-kB signaling pathway, cytokine-cytokine receptor interaction, and/or chemokine signaling KEGG pathways. (**a**) Selected genes were clustered based on molecule functions: cytokines (sky blue), chemokines (yellow green), receptors (pink), NF-kB signaling (brown). Quantile normalized TPM plus 0.1 were transformed between −1 and 1 to present high (red) and low (blue) expression level during time-course across four genotypes for each gene. (**b**) Schematic of the NF-kB pathway with genes present in heat map colored accordingly. (**c**) RT-PCR analysis on a subset of genes to validate the RNA-seq dataset. For each gene, 3 samples, two from the RNA-seq dataset and an additional sample not analyzed by RNA-seq, were analyzed for each genotype at ages 5 (left) and 10 months (right). Bars represent group mean expression +/− SEM. P value was calculated using one way ANOVA followed by Sidak's multiple comparison test

10 μm distances from the cell body. At 10 months of age the number of neuronal branches was significantly reduced in the Arctic mouse relative to the wild type, while the absence of C5aR1 in the Arctic model prevented the decrease, with Arctic/C5aR1KO similar to the wild type in this measure of neuronal complexity (Fig. 7a). This deficit correlated with loss of cognitive performance at 10 months of age (Fig. 1e) as at 7 month of age when no behavior differences are detected (Fig. 1d), neuronal branching in all animals were similar to each other (Fig. 7b). Only the Arctic mouse showed a decline in neurite branching between 7 month and 10 month of age (Fig. 7c). The rescue of the neuronal complexity in the CA1 area of the hippocampus in the Arctic/C5aR1KO aligns with the improvement in the OLM behavior test (hippocampal dependent) in this genotype compared to the Arctic.

Discussion

Genetic deletion of C5aR1 in the Arctic Alzheimer's disease mouse model resulted in protection from loss of neuronal complexity in CA1 neurons and prevented deficits in a hippocampal dependent spatial memory task relative to the C5aR1 sufficient Arctic animals. Significant and substantial loss of neuronal complexity and behavior deficits were pronounced at 10 months of age in the Arctic mouse. However, the gene expression profile of the microglia from Arctic/C5aR1KO brain showed a decrease in inflammatory pathways and greater induction of clearance and degradation pathways relative to the Arctic as early as 2–5 months of age. This gene expression profile indicates a polarization state of the microglia that is less inflammatory and more phagocytic that may prevent or delay behavior deficits. Such a timeline of events is consistent with current thought that the

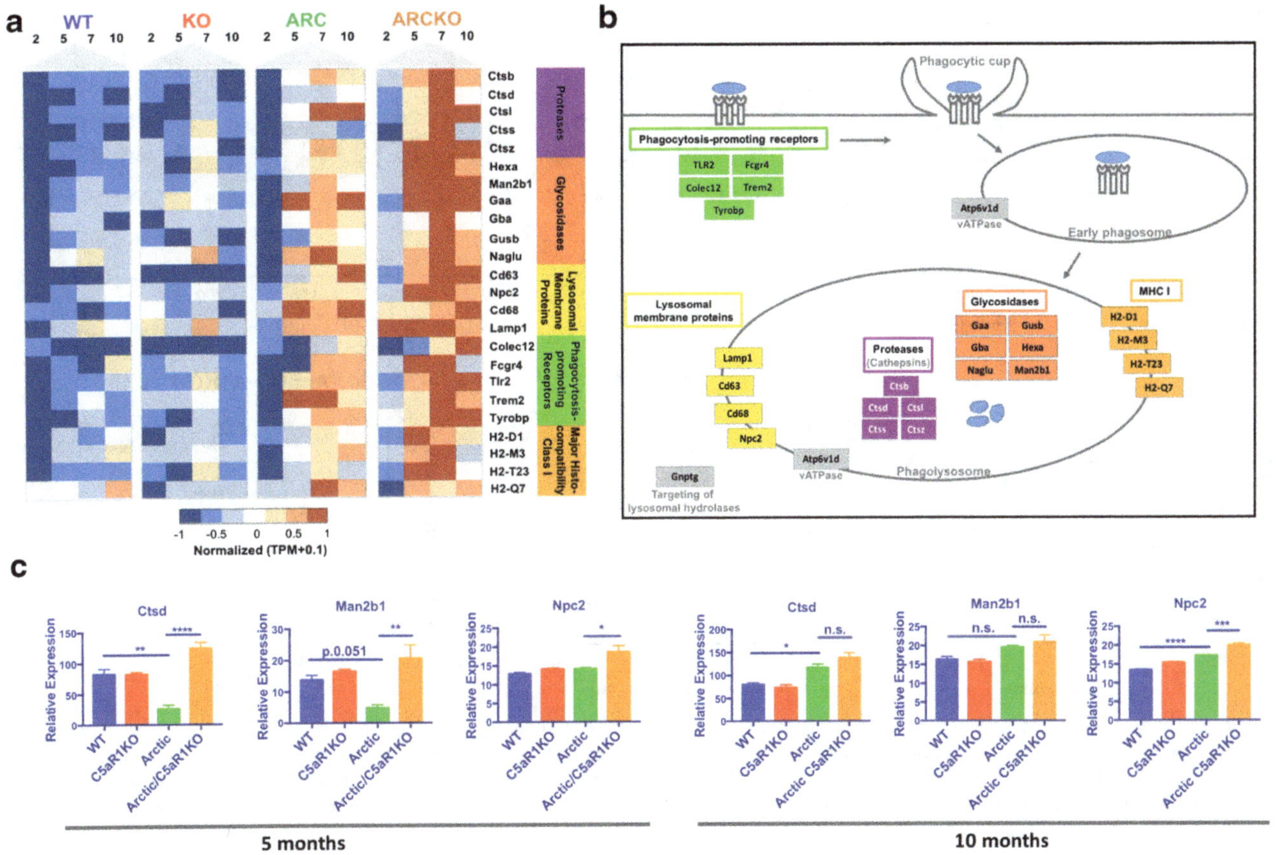

Fig. 6 Gene expression profiles of selected genes in lysosome and phagosome pathways. All genes in heat map were present in cluster 2. All but Trem2 and Tyrobp were also found in the phagosome or lysosome KEGG pathways. Trem2 and Tyrobp were added due to known roles in microglial phagocytosis. (**a**) Selected genes were clustered based on molecule functions: protease (purple), glycosidases (coral), lysosomal membrane proteins (yellow), phagocytosis-promoting receptors (green) and major histocompatibility class I (orange). Quantile normalized TPM plus 0.1 were transformed between −1 and 1 to present high (red) and low (blue) expression level during time-course across four genotypes for each gene. (**b**) Schematic of the phagolysosome pathway with genes present in heat map colored accordingly. (**c**). RT-PCR analysis on a subset of genes to validate the RNA-seq dataset, as described in Fig. 5 legend. Bars represent group mean expression +/− SEM (n = 3). P value was calculated using one way ANOVA followed by Sidak's multiple comparison test

disease process starts considerably prior to clinical signs of the disorder in humans. Consequently, treatment to suppress those detrimental processes may best be initiated substantially prior to clinical presentation.

Our previously published studies using a pharmacological approach to block function of C5aR1 in the Tg2576 and 3xTg AD mouse models [7] resulted in reduced fibrillar plaques and gliosis surrounding the plaques. In contrast, the genetic approach to eliminate C5aR1 function used in this Arctic model of AD did not result in reduced fibrillar plaque or microglial accumulation. However, this may due to the "Arctic" mutation in the Aß peptide that leads to rapid fibril formation upon generation of Aß [53]. These fibrils are highly resistant to degradation/clearance. Importantly, the prevention of cognitive loss is seen even in the presence of massive plaque accumulation, supporting the idea that neither the fibrillar plaque itself, nor global microglial markers per se are the major contributor to cognitive loss. Rather it is the specific inflammatory response to the plaque that leads to neurotoxicity [54], perhaps through activation of astrocytes as recently reported [55]. This preservation of cognitive performance in the presence of plaques was recently reported by Lemere and colleagues in another AD model in which C3 had been genetically ablated [16].

TLRs, other innate immune system sensors of danger/damage, when triggered have been found to synergize with C5a-C5aR1 signaling leading to greater proinflammatory cytokine release in models of inflammatory disease in the periphery (reviewed in [56]). Fibrillar Aß is a ligand for TLR2 and TLR4 [57–59] and these receptors have been shown to contribute to the detrimental effects of Aß. C5a may synergistically enhance microglial polarization to a more inflammatory state in response to Aß interactions (or other danger-associated signals) with

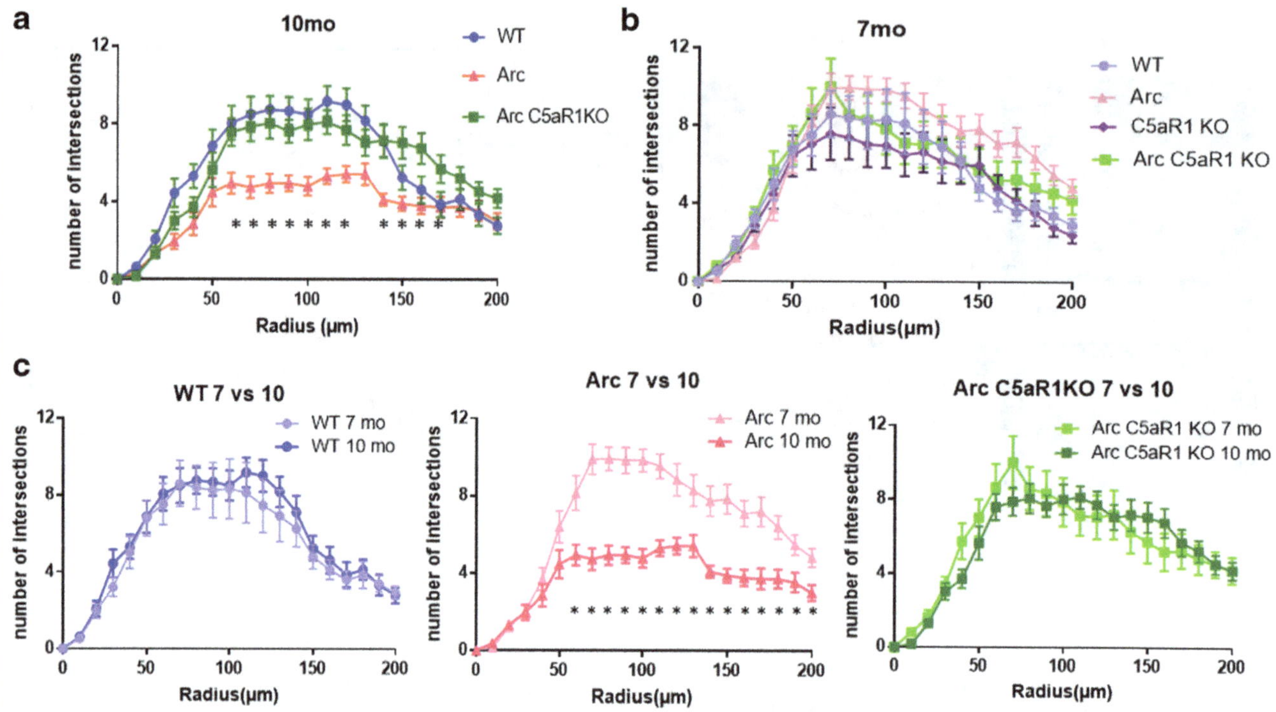

Fig. 7 Loss of neuronal complexity in the Arctic model is rescued in the absence of C5aR1. The average number of branchings for a given distance from the soma (um) of each neuron by Sholl analysis using the NeuroLucida software within the CA1 area of 10 mo (**a**) and 7 mo (**b**) mice (5 neurons/ animal, 3 mice per genotype) +/− SEM. * $p < .05$ for Arctic vs Arctic/C5aR1KO by 2 way ANOVA followed by Tukey's multiple comparison test. (**c**) The same data are plotted to compare the 7 and 10 mo branching in wild type (left), Arctic (middle) and Arctic/C5aR1KO (right) mice, *$p < .02$ by one way ANOVA

such receptors on plaque associated glia cells [60]. The increase in NFκB subunits may contribute to increased NF-κB signaling (Fig. 5) and greater expression of inflammatory cytokines and chemokines, all of which were seen in the Arctic mice, but not so elevated in the Arctic/C5aR1KO. In the literature, C5aR1 signaling is most often shown to involve activation of PI-3 K/AKT, PKC, phospholipase D, and MAP kinase (reviewed in [61]). However, instances of NF-κB activation by C5a have also been demonstrated in both human monocytes [62] and macrophages [63]. IL-1, Vegfa, Ccl3, Ccl4, Cxcl2 and Vcam1 are all regulated by the canonical NF-κB (p50/p65) signaling pathway, which can be activated via TLR4 [64]. It is likely that the increase in inflammatory components via NF-κB that we observed is due to a synergy between TLRs and C5aR1, since in the absence of C5aR1 the expression of several inflammatory genes is limited, even though fibrillar amyloid plaque, a TLR ligand, is unchanged.

Also consistent with differential polarization of the microglia in Arctic vs Arctic/C5aR1KO is the increase in phagosomal and lysosomal genes (Fig. 6). Phagocytosis-promoting receptors on microglia such as TREM2, FcγR's, TLR's and scavenger receptors have been associated with the clearance of amyloid beta in AD (reviewed in [65]). These genes showed higher expression in the Arctic/C5aR1KO either early in the disease (TREM2, TYROBP, Fcgr4) or later in the disease (TLR2, Colec12). Recent data suggest TREM2 is important in microgliosis and containment of Aß plaques over the progression of the disease [66, 67]. Gene network analysis by Zhang and colleagues identified a microglia specific module that includes TYROBP, the signaling adaptor protein of TREM2, as a key node of networks in late onset Alzheimer's disease [10].

Cathepsins, proteases that are involved in the endosomal-lysosomal pathway, were substantially and significantly increased in Arctic/C5aR1KO microglia relative to Arctic. Microglial cathepsins, particularly cysteine and aspartyl proteases, have been found to be upregulated with aging in rats (reviewed in [68]), though we did not see an increase in expression in our wild type mice from 2 to 10 months of age. Cathepsin B and D are Aß-degrading enzymes that have been implicated in clearance of amyloid beta in vivo (reviewed in ([69]). Early "activation" of microglia cells has been found to be beneficial in AD models, however, as Aß plaques form, the phagocytosis and clearance of Aß is reduced [70]. Hickman and colleagues found that gene expression of scavenger receptors and degradation enzymes decreased with age in AD mice [71]. C5aR1 deficiency prevents this decrease in phagocytosis and degradation enzymes seen relative to the aging AD mouse models. As mentioned above, fibrillar plaque load in this model is not decreased likely due to the inherent Arctic mutation that accelerates formation of amyloid protofibrils and fibrils, forms of amyloid resistant to ingestion and degradation. However, it is possible that toxic products could still be cleared resulting in the beneficial effects on behavior in the Arctic/C5aR1KO. Cheng and colleagues [31] demonstrated that the Arc48 model used here does show substantial levels of oligomeric (56kD) amyloid and thus it may be the clearance of these forms of Aß and/or neuronal blebs or apoptotic cells are enhanced in the Arctic/C5aR1KO. However, in the more general human AD population that does not have this APP mutation inducing rapid fibrillarization, the functional consequence of this differential gene expression may result in slower plaque accumulation as seen in the 3xTg and Tg2576 AD mouse models when treated with the C5aR1 antagonist, PMX205 [7]. Further investigation will be needed to determine whether or not the differential gene expression in inflammatory components or in clearance capacity or both contribute to the rescue of cognition.

It has been reported that CX3CR1 and CCR2 play a role in the pathogenesis of AD in some mouse models of the disease, either by affecting microglia or by limiting the infiltration of monocytes [49–51]. In the Arctic model we found no difference in amyloid plaque load in mice that possessed a single CX3CR1 or CCR2 allele compared to mice that had both copies of CX3CR1 or CCR2. In addition, no RFP+ myeloid cells were found in the parenchyma, though they were seen around the meninges and were observed (2–6% of FACS-sorted CX3CR1+ cells) by FACS analysis of whole brain suspensions. Given that RFP is expressed in the cytosol when the CCR2 promoter is activated (as in peripheral myeloid cells), and the estimated half-life of RFP in vivo is ~4.6 days [72], we would expect to visualize at least a fraction of RFP+ cells by immunohistochemistry at one of the ages analyzed if indeed CCR2+ monocytes were infiltrating the CNS. The difference between reported observations may be attributed to the different animal models used, which includes different kinetics of accumulation of various species of Aß among other differences.

Inflammation, as mentioned above, is recognized as having a complex role in the pathogenesis of AD (reviewed in [54]). The complement cascade is one aspect of the inflammatory response in AD, which results in both beneficial and detrimental outcomes and synergizes with other innate pathways (reviewed in [73]). Furthermore, epidemiologic and genetic evidence supports a role for complement in the etiology of late onset AD [74], although the GWAS CR1 protein likely has a primary role outside of the CNS on clearance of Aß [75, 76]. The consequences of genetic deletion of C5aR1 reported here support the contention that the mechanism by which the previously used small molecular weight cyclic hexapeptide C5aR1 antagonist, PMX205, was mediating its beneficial effects in AD mouse models [7] was via the inhibition of C5aR1 cell signaling, and support the continued assessment of C5aR1 antagonists for AD therapy. Such specific antagonists have been successfully utilized in acute and chronic inflammatory disease animal models such as sepsis, asthma, ischemia/reperfusion injury, and neurodegenerative diseases [77–80] and as reviewed in [81, 82]. In addition, blocking C5a in rodent CNS disease models has been shown to be beneficial, including in Huntington's disease [83, 84], traumatic brain injury [85], and ALS [86].

It is critical to note that several studies have demonstrated beneficial effects of complement in the brain (reviewed in [87]). In vitro, C1q has been shown to induce gene expression critical for neuronal survival and protection against oligomer and fibrillar Aß-induced neuronal death [88, 89]. Selective modulation of complement activation products or their receptors may therefore be a more effective strategy than global C1q or complement inhibition for retaining the neuroprotective, anti-inflammatory and phagocytic functions of complement, while dampening damaging excessive inflammation.

Given the inflammatory profile seen in microglia from Arctic mice with aging and the decrease in expression of the same genes in the Arctic/C5aR1KO, along with the activation of phagocytosis and protein degradation in the Arctic/C5aR1KO, we propose a model by which C5aR1 activation contributes to AD progression (Fig. 8). Complement is activated by fibrillar amyloid beta via the classical (or alternative) pathway and can have beneficial and detrimental effects. Phagocytosis-promoting components such as C1q, C4b, C3b, and iC3b (the latter 3 covalently bound via a thioester bond to plaques) could enhance clearance of Aß fibrils or protofibrils via microglial phagocytosis and/or in the periphery via the potential immune adherence mechanism [76, 90]. Continued downstream activation of the complement cascade leads to the generation of C5a which in the CNS can bind to microglial C5aR1 and synergize with TLR's when the microglia engage a plaque, polarizing the microglia to a more inflammatory state and suppressing upregulation of phagosomal and degradation pathways. The resulting inflammatory environment further damages neurons, perhaps via astrocyte activation [55], thereby contributing to cognitive deficits. If this model is correct, targeting C5aR1 will not disrupt the beneficial effects of the upstream complement activation products, but rather, it will suppress polarization of the microglia to an inflammatory state, allowing the phagocytosis and degradation promoting gene expression program of the cells to continue. Further in depth analysis is needed to test this proposed model.

Recent elegant studies have shown that excessive complement-mediated synapse pruning occurs in aging, AD, and other disorders leading to cognitive or behavior changes [17, 18, 91, 92]. Since the activation of complement in these scenarios could also result in the generation of C5a, it remains to be seen if it is the insult of C5a-mediated effects that directly results in the behavioral/cognitive dysfunction or if C5aR1 signaling influences synaptic pruning at the microglial or neuronal level, or if both mechanisms contribute independently to deficits. While additional studies in multiple animal models can be performed to discern this, what the balance is in human systems will require clinical trials. The lack of detrimental toxicity of the C5aR1 antagonist PMX53 and CCX168 in human clinical trials of refractory rheumatoid arthritis [93] and ANCA-associated vasculitis [94], and the clinical experience with FDA approved Eculizumab, an anti C5 monoclonal antibody that prevents the cleavage of C5 and thus the generation of C5a [95], suggests that suppression of C5a/C5aR1 signaling may not be harmful for extended clinical use in adults. In addition to the potential for greater access to the brain, an advantage of a selective C5aR1 antagonist vs Eculizumab for long term treatment of diseases such as AD is that, while it blocks effects of C5a, the generation of C5b by the uninhibited cleavage of C5 is still able to initiate the assembly of the bacteriolytic C5b-9 complex upon complement activation by pathogens. Thus, this protective bacteriolytic function of complement would not be systemically compromised by the antagonist as it is by Eculizumab. The preservation of CA1 neuronal complexity seen here provides proof of concept that blocking C5a-C5aR1 could prevent detrimental downstream effects of the complement cascade activation and thereby suppress damage to neurons, while preserving systemic protection from infection, which could be compromised by targeting other components in the complement cascade as treatment for this disease.

Conclusion

Genetic ablation of C5aR1 in a mouse model of AD resulted in microglial gene expression profile indicative of less inflammation and greater induction of clearance pathways, preserved neuronal complexity in the hippocampus and prevented deficits in a hippocampal dependent spatial memory task. These data, consistent with the increasingly proposed role of inflammation in neurodegenerative disorders, provide additional compelling rationale to pursue inhibition of C5aR1 as a strategic targeted therapy to slow the progression of AD in humans.

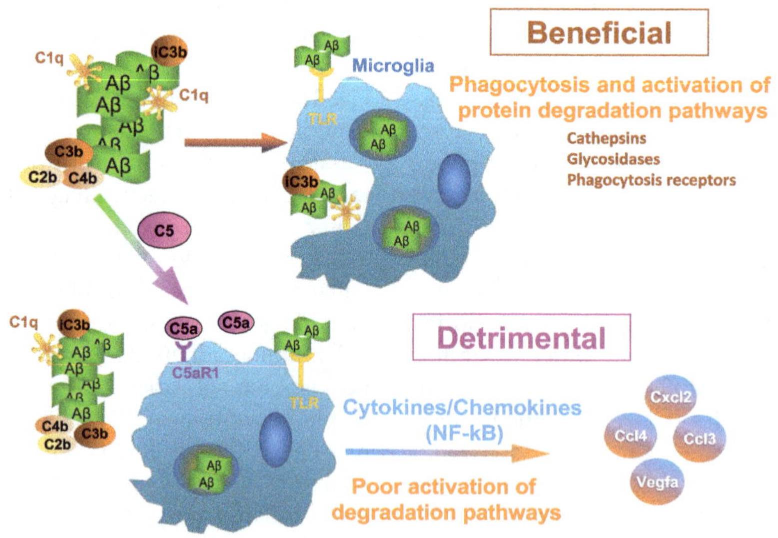

Fig. 8 Proposed mechanism by which C5aR1 stimulation contributes to AD progression. Aβ fibrils activate complement resulting in cleavage of C3 and C5. Amyloid deposited C3b/iC3b should lead to more efficient phagocytosis by microglia/macrophages, while generated C5a recruits and alters the function of microglia. C5a induces an inflammatory polarization of the microglia, potentially synergizing with TLRs, which results in production of neurotoxic inflammatory products while suppressing beneficial phagocytosis and degradation pathways thereby contributing to neuronal damage and cognitive deficits. Targeting C5a and its receptor C5aR1 will not interfere with the beneficial effects of upstream complement components

Additional files

Additional file 1: Representative habituation performance during testing and performance during training. Representative analysis of (A) Speed (B) distance traveled (C) percent of total time spent in an inner zone and (D) percent of total time spent in an outer zone quantified using the ANY-maze software. Data are from 10 months animals: $n = 19$ (WT), 16 (C5aR1KO), 7 (Arctic) and 8 (Arctic/C5aR1KO), representative of at least 2 experiments and similar assessments in 7 months animals. (E) During training, all genotypes were assessed for time spent with each object (left and right of the context). Bars show average percent time +/− SEM per object (left and right) for each genotype at 7 months. $n = 10$, 9, 9, and 10 for WT, C5aR1KO, Arctic, and Arctic/C5aR1KO respectively. No preference for left or right is detected by one- way AVOVA.

Additional file 2: Comparison of IBA1 microglia and Thioflavine S plaque size between Arctic and Arctic/C5aR1KO. (A-D) Representative images of the hippocampus stained for IBA1 and ThioS. (E) Quantification of the number of IBA1+ cells/field of view (FOV) using the spots modules in Bit-plane Imaris 7.5. (F) Quantification of the size of ThioS+ plaques/ FOV using the surfaces module in Bit-plane Imaris. Error bars represent SEM, ($n = 3$–4/group). *$p < 0.05$. Scale bar in D = 100 μm.

Additional file 3: Aβ plaque load and CD45 expression in Arctic heterozygous for CX3CR1 and CCR2. Brain sections from Arctic, Arctic-CX3CR1$^{+/GFP}$ or Arctic-CCR2$^{+/RFP}$ reporter mice at 6 or 7 months were stained with either thioflavine (A), or an anti-Aß antibody (1536) (C) to assess the plaque load (A, C). CD45 reactivity was probed to investigate microglial activation (B,D). Arctic mice were compared to Arctic mice heterozygous for CCR2-RFP (A, B) or heterozygous for Cx3CR1-GFP (C,D). Scale bar is 100 μm. (E). Bars represent the average Field Area % of 3–4 animals per genotype (2 sections per animal). No statistically significant difference was observed in Arctic compared to Arctic-CCR2$^{+/RFP}$ in thioflavine ($p < 0.75$) or CD45 ($p < 0.09$) or between Arctic and Arctic-CX3CR1$^{+/GFP}$ in Aß ($p < 0.67$) or CD45 ($p < 0.71$) by one-way ANOVA statistical analysis.

Additional File 4: RNA quality control. Amount of RNA extracted from FACS-sorted microglia isolated from adult mice was quantified by NanoDrop and the quality assessed by Agilent Bioanalyzer. All samples had greater than 1 ng/μl of RNA and RINs greater than 4, sufficient for the SMARTer Stranded Total RNA-Seq Kit - Pico Input Mammalian by Clontech.

Additional file 5: Dynamic gene expression profiles of 9 clusters. Gene expression clusters were derived from maSigPro. Median profile are plotted across all ages for all the genes in the corresponding cluster. WT (blue), C5aR1KO (red), Arctic (green) and Arctic/C5aR1KO (orange).

Additional file 6: Gene ontology enrichment analysis. Clusters were analyzed with Metascape (http://metascape.org) to identify the GO terms (biological processes) enriched in each cluster. The GO terms, their descriptions, logP, log(q-value), InTerm_InList (Genes in cluster/All genes from genome in GO term), and the gene and gene symbols are listed.

Additional file 7: Pathway analysis. Significantly enriched KEGG pathways were identified by PaintOmics 3. The pathway name, number of genes in the pathway, and the *p*-value of the enriched pathway is displayed for each cluster.

Additional file 8: Genes found in each maSigPro cluster. Genes present in each cluster are listed with Ensembl ID and gene symbol noted.

Abbreviations

AD: Alzheimer's disease; Aß: Amyloid beta peptide; C5aR1: C5a receptor 1, CD88; FACS: Fluorescence-activated cell sorting; fAß: Fibrillar amyloid beta peptide; GFP: Green fluorescent protein; GO: Gene ontology; HBSS: Hanks' balanced salt solution; iNOR: Hippocampal independent novel object recognition; KO: Genetic knock out; OLM: Object location memory; PBS: Phosphate buffered saline; PCR: Polymerase chain reaction; RFP: Red fluorescent protein; SEM: Standard error mean; TBS: Tris-buffered saline; TLR: Toll-like receptor; TPM: Transcripts per million; WT: Wild type

Acknowledgements

The authors thank Dr. Marcelo Wood for guidance in optimizing behavioral tasks. Drs. Melanie Oakes and Jenny Wu at the UCI GHTF for valuable insight and advice in designing and analyzing the RNA-Seq data, and Vanessa Scarfone for the expertise with the FACS Aria II at the Stem Cell FACS facility. The authors also thank Alice Berci, Samantha Harden, Eric Nguyen, Lila Modarresi, Andrew Pak, Pooja Selvan, Purnika Selvan, Amy Tran, Phuong (Remy) Vu, and Nathan Yu (UCI) for excellent technical assistance.

Funding

This work was supported by NIH grants NS 35144, AG 00538, and the Alzheimer's Association IIRG-1O-174,897 (AJT), NIH-IMSD TG GM055246 (MXH), NIH Training Grant T32 AG000096 (MXH, TAC), Alzheimer's Association Research Fellowship AARF-16-442,762 (LAH), NS083801 and AG0165573 (KNG), and NIH New Innovator Award to Ali Mortazavi (DP2 GM111100).

Authors' contributions

MXH, TAC, and AJT designed the experiments and overall project. SJ and AM performed bioinformatics and statistical analysis on RNA-seq data, TAC performed the behavioral studies, and MXH performed microglia isolations, RNA extractions and data analysis. MIF performed immunohistochemistry and image analysis, SC performed qPCR, designed and carried out all breeding and colony validation. MJF, performed imaging for Sholl analysis, and MT initiated, advised, provided verification of the analysis of neuronal complexity, LAH designed and performed the IBA1 studies and along with KNG provided conceptual guidance to the project. RAW provided the C5aR1 knockout animal, advised on the breeding, and contributed to the discussion of the data. MXH and AJT wrote the manuscript, with contributions from all co-authors. All authors approved of the final version of the paper.

Competing interests

The authors declare that they have no competing interests.

Author details

[1]Department of Pathology and Laboratory Medicine, School of Medicine, University of California, Irvine, CA, USA. [2]Department of Developmental and Cell Biology, University of California, Irvine, CA, USA. [3]Department of Neurobiology and Behavior, University of California, Irvine, CA, USA. [4]Department of Molecular Biology and Biochemistry, University of California, Irvine, CA, USA. [5]Research Center for Immunology and Autoimmune Diseases, Institute of Molecular Medicine for the Prevention of Human Diseases, University of Texas-Houston, Houston, TX, USA. [6]Present Address: Ionis Pharmaceuticals Inc., Carlsbad, CA 92010, USA.

References

1. Fonseca MI, Chu SH, Berci AM, Benoit ME, Peters DG, Kimura Y, Tenner AJ. Contribution of complement activation pathways to neuropathology differs among mouse models of Alzheimer's disease. J Neuroinflammation. 2011;8(1):4.
2. Afagh A, Cummings BJ, Cribbs DH, Cotman CW, Tenner AJ. Localization and cell association of C1q in Alzheimer's disease brain. ExpNeurol. 1996;138(1):22–32.
3. Cribbs DH, Berchtold NC, Perreau V, Coleman PD, Rogers J, Tenner AJ, Cotman CW. Extensive innate immune gene activation accompanies brain aging, increasing vulnerability to cognitive decline and neurodegeneration: a microarray study. JNeuroinflammation. 2012;9(1):179.
4. Meraz-Rios MA, Toral-Rios D, Franco-Bocanegra D, Villeda-Hernandez J, Campos-Pena V. Inflammatory process in Alzheimer's disease. Front IntegrNeurosci. 2013;7:59.
5. Heneka MT, Carson MJ, El KJ, Landreth GE, Brosseron F, Feinstein DL, Jacobs AH, Wyss-Coray T, Vitorica J, Ransohoff RM, et al. Neuroinflammation in Alzheimer's disease. Lancet Neurol. 2015;14(4):388–405.
6. Ransohoff RM, El Khoury J. Microglia in health and disease. Cold Spring Harb Perspect Biol. 2015;8(1):a020560.

7. Fonseca MI, Ager RR, Chu SH, Yazan O, Sanderson SD, LaFerla FM, Taylor SM, Woodruff TM, Tenner AJ. Treatment with a C5aR antagonist decreases pathology and enhances behavioral performance in murine models of Alzheimer's disease. J Immunol. 2009;183(2):1375–83.
8. El Khoury J, Luster AD. Mechanisms of microglia accumulation in Alzheimer's disease: therapeutic implications. Trends Pharmacol Sci. 2008; 29(12):626–32.
9. Huang KL, Marcora E, Pimenova AA, Di Narzo AF, Kapoor M, Jin SC, Harari O, Bertelsen S, Fairfax BP, Czajkowski J, et al. A common haplotype lowers PU.1 expression in myeloid cells and delays onset of Alzheimer's disease. Nat Neurosci. 2017;20(8):1052–61.
10. Zhang B, Gaiteri C, Bodea LG, Wang Z, McElwee J, Podtelezhnikov AA, Zhang C, Xie T, Tran L, Dobrin R, et al. Integrated systems approach identifies genetic nodes and networks in late-onset Alzheimer's disease. Cell. 2013;153(3):707–20.
11. Ricklin D, Lambris JD. Complement in immune and inflammatory disorders: pathophysiological mechanisms. J Immunol. 2013;190(8):3831–8.
12. Monk PN, Scola AM, Madala P, Fairlie DP. Function, structure and therapeutic potential of complement C5a receptors. Br J Pharmacol. 2007; 152(4):429–48.
13. Davoust N, Jones J, Stahel PF, Ames RS, Barnum SR. Receptor for the C3a anaphylatoxin is expressed by neurons and glial cells. Glia. 1999;26(3):201–11.
14. Stevens B, Allen NJ, Vazquez LE, Howell GR, Christopherson KS, Nouri N, Micheva KD, Mehalow AK, Huberman AD, Stafford B, et al. The classical complement cascade mediates CNS synapse elimination. Cell. 2007;131(6):1164–78.
15. Shi Q, Colodner KJ, Matousek SB, Merry K, Hong S, Kenison JE, Frost JL, Le KX, Li S, Dodart JC, et al. Complement C3-deficient mice fail to display age-related hippocampal decline. JNeurosci. 2015;35(38):13029–42.
16. Shi Q, Chowdhury S, Ma R, Le KX, Hong S, Caldarone BJ, Stevens B, Lemere CA. Complement C3 deficiency protects against neurodegeneration in aged plaque-rich APP/PS1 mice. Sci Transl Med. 2017:9(392).
17. Lui H, Zhang J, Makinson SR, Cahill MK, Kelley KW, Huang HY, Shang Y, Oldham MC, Martens LH, Gao F, et al. Progranulin deficiency promotes circuit-specific synaptic pruning by microglia via complement activation. Cell. 2016;165(4):921–35.
18. Hong S, Beja-Glasser VF, Nfonoyim BM, Frouin A, Li S, Ramakrishnan S, Merry KM, Shi Q, Rosenthal A, Barres BA, et al. Complement and microglia mediate early synapse loss in Alzheimer mouse models. Science. 2016;352(6286):712–6.
19. Jiang H, Burdick D, Glabe CG, Cotman CW, Tenner AJ. beta-amyloid activates complement by binding to a specific region of the collagen-like domain of the C1q a chain. J Immunol. 1994;152(10):5050–9.
20. Bradt BM, Kolb WP, Cooper NR. Complement-dependent proinflammatory properties of the Alzheimer's disease beta-peptide. J Exp Med. 1998; 188(3):431–8.
21. Matsuoka Y, Picciano M, Malester B, LaFrancois J, Zehr C, Daeschner JM, Olschowka JA, Fonseca MI, O'Banion MK, Tenner AJ, et al. Inflammatory responses to amyloidosis in a transgenic mouse model of Alzheimer's disease. AmJ Pathol. 2001;158(4):1345–54.
22. Zhou J, Fonseca MI, Pisalyaput K, Tenner AJ. Complement C3 and C4 expression in C1q sufficient and deficient mouse models of Alzheimer's disease. JNeurochem. 2008;106(5):2080–92.
23. Alexander JJ, Anderson AJ, Barnum SR, Stevens B, Tenner AJ. The complement cascade: yin-Yang in neuroinflammation–neuro-protection and -degeneration. J Neurochem. 2008;107(5):1169–87.
24. Pavlovski D, Thundyil J, Monk PN, Wetsel RA, Taylor SM, Woodruff TM. Generation of complement component C5a by ischemic neurons promotes neuronal apoptosis. FASEB J. 2012;26(9):3680–90.
25. Hernandez MX, Namiranian P, Nguyen E, Fonseca MI, Tenner AJ. C5a increases the injury to primary neurons elicited by fibrillar amyloid beta. ASN Neuro. 2017;9(1):1759091416687871.
26. Yao J, Harvath L, Gilbert DL, Colton CA. Chemotaxis by a CNS macrophage, the microglia. JNeurosciRes. 1990;27(1):36–42.
27. Zhang X, Kimura Y, Fang C, Zhou L, Sfyroera G, Lambris JD, Wetsel RA, Miwa T, Song WC. Regulation of toll-like receptor-mediated inflammatory response by complement in vivo. Blood. 2007;110(1):228–36.
28. Abe T, Hosur KB, Hajishengallis E, Reis ES, Ricklin D, Lambris JD, Hajishengallis G. Local complement-targeted intervention in periodontitis: proof-of-concept using a C5a receptor (CD88) antagonist. J Immunol. 2012; 189(11):5442–8.
29. Nilsberth C, Westlind-Danielsson A, Eckman CB, Condron MM, Axelman K, Forsell C, Stenh C, Luthman J, Teplow DB, Younkin SG, et al. The 'Arctic' APP mutation (E693G) causes Alzheimer's disease by enhanced Abeta protofibril formation. NatNeurosci. 2001;4(9):887–93.
30. Cheng IH, Palop JJ, Esposito LA, Bien-Ly N, Yan F, Mucke L. Aggressive amyloidosis in mice expressing human amyloid peptides with the Arctic mutation. NatMed. 2004;10(11):1190–2.
31. Cheng IH, Scearce-Levie K, Legleiter J, Palop JJ, Gerstein H, Bien-Ly N, Puolivali J, Lesne S, Ashe KH, Muchowski PJ, et al. Accelerating amyloid-beta fibrillization reduces oligomer levels and functional deficits in Alzheimer disease mouse models. J Biol Chem. 2007;282(33):23818–28.
32. Hollmann TJ, Mueller-Ortiz SL, Braun MC, Wetsel RA. Disruption of the C5a receptor gene increases resistance to acute gram-negative bacteremia and endotoxic shock: opposing roles of C3a and C5a. Mol Immunol. 2008;45(7): 1907–15.
33. Jung S, Aliberti J, Graemmel P, Sunshine MJ, Kreutzberg GW, Sher A, Littman DR. Analysis of fractalkine receptor CX(3)CR1 function by targeted deletion and green fluorescent protein reporter gene insertion. MolCell Biol. 2000; 20(11):4106–14.
34. Saederup N, Cardona AE, Croft K, Mizutani M, Cotleur AC, Tsou CL, Ransohoff RM, Charo IF. Selective chemokine receptor usage by central nervous system myeloid cells in CCR2-red fluorescent protein knock-in mice. PLoSONE. 2010;5(10):e13693.
35. Haettig J, Stefanko DP, Multani ML, Figueroa DX, McQuown SC, Wood MA. HDAC inhibition modulates hippocampus-dependent long-term memory for object location in a CBP-dependent manner. LearnMem. 2011;18(2):71–9.
36. Stefanko DP, Barrett RM, Ly AR, Reolon GK, Wood MA. Modulation of long-term memory for object recognition via HDAC inhibition. ProcNatlAcadSciUSA. 2009;106(23):9447–52.
37. Njie EG, Boelen E, Stassen FR, Steinbusch HW, Borchelt DR, Streit WJ. Ex vivo cultures of microglia from young and aged rodent brain reveal age-related changes in microglial function. NeurobiolAging. 2012;33(1):195–12.
38. Webster SD, Galvan MD, Ferran E, Garzon-Rodriguez W, Glabe CG, Tenner AJ. Antibody-mediated phagocytosis of the amyloid beta-peptide in microglia is differentially modulated by C1q. J Immunol. 2001;166(12):7496–503.
39. Fonseca MI, Head E, Velazquez P, Cotman CW, Tenner AJ. The presence of isoaspartic acid in beta-amyloid plaques indicates plaque age. Exp Neurol. 1999;157(2):277–88.
40. Fonseca MI, Zhou J, Botto M, Tenner AJ. Absence of C1q leads to less neuropathology in transgenic mouse models of Alzheimer's disease. J Neurosci. 2004;24(29):6457–65.
41. Dobin A, Davis CA, Schlesinger F, Drenkow J, Zaleski C, Jha S, Batut P, Chaisson M, Gingeras TR. STAR: ultrafast universal RNA-seq aligner. Bioinformatics. 2013;29(1):15–21.
42. Li B, Dewey CN. RSEM: accurate transcript quantification from RNA-Seq data with or without a reference genome. BMC Bioinformatics. 2011;12:323.
43. Nueda MJ, Tarazona S, Conesa A. Next maSigPro: updating maSigPro bioconductor package for RNA-seq time series. Bioinformatics. 2014; 30(18):2598–602.
44. Tripathi S, Pohl MO, Zhou Y, Rodriguez-Frandsen A, Wang G, Stein DA, Moulton HM, DeJesus P, Che J, Mulder LC, et al. Meta- and orthogonal integration of influenza "OMICs" data defines a role for UBR4 in virus budding. Cell Host Microbe. 2015;18(6):723–35.
45. Garcia-Alcalde F, Garcia-Lopez F, Dopazo J, Conesa A. Paintomics: a web based tool for the joint visualization of transcriptomics and metabolomics data. Bioinformatics. 2011;27(1):137–9.
46. Balderas I, Rodriguez-Ortiz CJ, Salgado-Tonda P, Chavez-Hurtado J, McGaugh JL, Bermudez-Rattoni F. The consolidation of object and context recognition memory involve different regions of the temporal lobe. LearnMem. 2008;15(9):618–24.
47. Mumby DG, Gaskin S, Glenn MJ, Schramek TE, Lehmann H. Hippocampal damage and exploratory preferences in rats: memory for objects, places, and contexts. LearnMem. 2002;9(2):49–57.
48. Mizutani M, Pino PA, Saederup N, Charo IF, Ransohoff RM, Cardona AE. The fractalkine receptor but not CCR2 is present on microglia from embryonic development throughout adulthood. J Immunol. 2012;188(1):29–36.
49. Lee S, Varvel NH, Konerth ME, Xu G, Cardona AE, Ransohoff RM, Lamb BT. CX3CR1 deficiency alters microglial activation and reduces beta-amyloid

deposition in two Alzheimer's disease mouse models. AmJ Pathol. 2010; 177(5):2549–62.
50. Liu Z, Condello C, Schain A, Harb R, Grutzendler J. CX3CR1 in microglia regulates brain amyloid deposition through selective protofibrillar amyloid-beta phagocytosis. JNeurosci. 2010;30(50):17091–101.
51. El Khoury J, Toft M, Hickman SE, Means TK, Terada K, Geula C, Luster AD. Ccr2 deficiency impairs microglial accumulation and accelerates progression of Alzheimer-like disease. Nat Med. 2007;13(4):432–8.
52. Giunta B, Fernandez F, Nikolic WV, Obregon D, Rrapo E, Town T, Tan J. Inflammaging as a prodrome to Alzheimer's disease. J Neuroinflammation. 2008;5:51.
53. Walsh DM, Klyubin I, Fadeeva JV, Cullen WK, Anwyl R, Wolfe MS, Rowan MJ, Selkoe DJ. Naturally secreted oligomers of amyloid beta protein potently inhibit hippocampal long-term potentiation in vivo. Nature. 2002;416(6880):535–9.
54. Wyss-Coray T, Rogers J. Inflammation in Alzheimer disease-a brief review of the basic science and clinical literature. Cold Spring HarbPerspectMed. 2012; 2(1):a006346.
55. Liddelow SA, Guttenplan KA, Clarke LE, Bennett FC, Bohlen CJ, Schirmer L, Bennett ML, Munch AE, Chung WS, Peterson TC, et al. Neurotoxic reactive astrocytes are induced by activated microglia. Nature. 2017;
56. Song WC. Crosstalk between complement and toll-like receptors. ToxicolPathol. 2012;40(2):174–82.
57. Jana M, Palencia CA, Pahan K. Fibrillar amyloid-beta peptides activate microglia via TLR2: implications for Alzheimer's disease. J Immunol. 2008; 181(10):7254–62.
58. Jin JJ, Kim HD, Maxwell JA, Li L, Fukuchi K. Toll-like receptor 4-dependent upregulation of cytokines in a transgenic mouse model of Alzheimer's disease. J Neuroinflammation. 2008;5:23.
59. Udan ML, Ajit D, Crouse NR, Nichols MR. Toll-like receptors 2 and 4 mediate Abeta(1-42) activation of the innate immune response in a human monocytic cell line. J Neurochem. 2008;104(2):524–33.
60. Tahara K, Kim HD, Jin JJ, Maxwell JA, Li L, Fukuchi K. Role of toll-like receptor signalling in Abeta uptake and clearance. Brain. 2006;129(Pt 11):3006–19.
61. Sarma JV, Ward PA. New developments in C5a receptor signaling. Cell Health Cytoskelet. 2012;4:73–82.
62. Pan ZK. Anaphylatoxins C5a and C3a induce nuclear factor kappaB activation in human peripheral blood monocytes. Biochim Biophys Acta. 1998;1443(1–2):90–8.
63. Kastl SP, Speidl WS, Kaun C, Rega G, Assadian A, Weiss TW, Valent P, Hagmueller GW, Maurer G, Huber K, et al. The complement component C5a induces the expression of plasminogen activator inhibitor-1 in human macrophages via NF-kappaB activation. J Thromb Haemost. 2006;4(8):1790–7.
64. Fitzgerald KA, Rowe DC, Barnes BJ, Caffrey DR, Visintin A, Latz E, Monks B, Pitha PM, Golenbock DT. LPS-TLR4 signaling to IRF-3/7 and NF-kappaB involves the toll adapters TRAM and TRIF. J Exp Med. 2003;198(7):1043–55.
65. Doens D, Fernandez PL. Microglia receptors and their implications in the response to amyloid beta for Alzheimer's disease pathogenesis. J Neuroinflammation. 2014;11:48.
66. Wang Y, Ulland TK, Ulrich JD, Song W, Tzaferis JA, Hole JT, Yuan P, Mahan TE, Shi Y, Gilfillan S, et al. TREM2-mediated early microglial response limits diffusion and toxicity of amyloid plaques. J Exp Med. 2016;213(5):667–75.
67. Jay TR, Hirsch AM, Broihier ML, Miller CM, Neilson LE, Ransohoff RM, Lamb BT, Landreth GE. Disease progression-dependent effects of TREM2 deficiency in a mouse model of Alzheimer's disease. J Neurosci. 2017; 37(3):637–47.
68. Stoka V, Turk V, Turk B. Lysosomal cathepsins and their regulation in aging and neurodegeneration. Ageing Res Rev. 2016;32:22–37.
69. Saido T, Leissring MA. Proteolytic degradation of amyloid beta-protein. Cold Spring Harb Perspect Med. 2012;2(6):a006379.
70. Krabbe G, Halle A, Matyash V, Rinnenthal JL, Eom GD, Bernhardt U, Miller KR, Prokop S, Kettenmann H, Heppner FL. Functional Impairment of Microglia Coincides with Beta-Amyloid Deposition in Mice with Alzheimer-Like Pathology. PLoS One. 2013:8(4).
71. Hickman SE, Allison EK, El KJ. Microglial dysfunction and defective beta-amyloid clearance pathways in aging Alzheimer's disease mice. JNeurosci. 2008;28(33):8354–60.
72. Verkhusha VV, Kuznetsova IM, Stepanenko OV, Zaraisky AG, Shavlovsky MM, Turoverov KK, Uversky VN. High stability of Discosoma DsRed as compared to Aequorea EGFP. Biochemistry. 2003;42(26):7879–84.
73. Veerhuis R, Nielsen HM, Tenner AJ. Complement in the brain. Mol Immunol. 2011;48:1592–603.
74. Eikelenboom P, Van EE, Veerhuis R, Rozemuller AJ, van Gool WA, Hoozemans JJ. Innate immunity and the etiology of late-onset Alzheimer's disease. NeurodegenerDis. 2012;10(1–4):271–3.
75. Fonseca MI, Chu S, Pierce AL, Brubaker WD, Hauhart RE, Mastroeni D, Clarke EV, Rogers J, Atkinson JP, Tenner AJ. Analysis of the putative role of CR1 in Alzheimer's disease: genetic association, Expression and Function. *PLoS ONE.* 2016;11(2):e0149792.
76. Brubaker WD, Crane A, Johansson JU, Yen K, Garfinkel K, Mastroeni D, Asok P, Bradt B, Sabbagh M, Wallace TL, et al. Peripheral complement interactions with amyloid beta peptide: erythrocyte clearance mechanisms. Alzheimers Dement. 2017;
77. Konteatis ZD, Siciliano SJ, Van RG, Molineaux CJ, Pandya S, Fischer P, Rosen H, Mumford RA, Springer MS. Development of C5a receptor antagonists. Differential loss of functional responses. J Immunol. 1994;153(9):4200–5.
78. Guo RF, Ward PA. C5a, a therapeutic target in sepsis. Recent Pat AntiinfectDrug Discov. 2006;1(1):57–65.
79. Kohl J. Drug evaluation: the C5a receptor antagonist PMX-53. CurrOpinMolTher. 2006;8(6):529–38.
80. Arumugam TV, Magnus T, Woodruff TM, Proctor LM, Shiels IA, Taylor SM. Complement mediators in ischemia-reperfusion injury. Clin Chim Acta. 2006; 374(1–2):33–45.
81. Holland MC, Morikis D, Lambris JD. Synthetic small-molecule complement inhibitors. CurrOpinInvestigDrugs. 2004;5(11):1164–73.
82. Woodruff TM, Nandakumar KS, Tedesco F. Inhibiting the C5-C5a receptor axis. Mol Immunol. 2011;48(14):1631–42.
83. Singhrao S, Neal JW, Morgan BP, Gasque P. Increased complement biosynthesis by microglia and complement activation on neurons in Huntington's disease. ExpNeurol. 1999;159:362–76.
84. Woodruff TM, Crane JW, Proctor LM, Buller KM, Shek AB, de VK, Pollitt S, Williams HM, Shiels IA, Monk PN, et al. Therapeutic activity of C5a receptor antagonists in a rat model of neurodegeneration. FASEB J. 2006;20(9):1407–17.
85. Sewell DL, Nacewicz B, Liu F, Macvilay S, Erdei A, Lambris JD, Sandor M, Fabry Z. Complement C3 and C5 play critical roles in traumatic brain cryoinjury: blocking effects on neutrophil extravasation by C5a receptor antagonist. J Neuroimmunol. 2004;155(1–2):55–63.
86. Woodruff TM, Costantini KJ, Crane JW, Atkin JD, Monk PN, Taylor SM, Noakes PG. The complement factor C5a contributes to pathology in a rat model of amyotrophic lateral sclerosis. J Immunol. 2008;181(12):8727–34.
87. Lucin KM, Wyss-Coray T. Immune activation in brain aging and neurodegeneration: too much or too little? Neuron. 2009;64(1):110–22.
88. Pisalyaput K, Tenner AJ. Complement component C1q inhibits beta-amyloid- and serum amyloid P-induced neurotoxicity via caspase- and calpain-independent mechanisms. JNeurochem. 2008;104(3):696–707.
89. Benoit ME, Hernandez MX, Dinh ML, Benavente F, Vasquez O, Tenner AJ. C1q-induced LRP1B and GPR6 proteins expressed early in Alzheimer disease mouse models, are essential for the C1q-mediated protection against amyloid-beta neurotoxicity. J BiolChem. 2013;288(1):654–65.
90. Rogers J, Li R, Mastroeni D, Grover A, Leonard B, Ahern G, Cao P, Kolody H, Vedders L, Kolb WP, et al. Peripheral clearance of amyloid beta peptide by complement C3-dependent adherence to erythrocytes. Neurobiol Aging. 2006;27(12):1733–9.
91. Sekar A, Bialas AR, de RH, Davis A, Hammond TR, Kamitaki N, Tooley K, Presumey J, Baum M, Van DV, et al. Schizophrenia risk from complex variation of complement component 4. Nature. 2016;
92. Vasek MJ, Garber C, Dorsey D, Durrant DM, Bollman B, Soung A, Yu J, Perez-Torres C, Frouin A, Wilton DK, et al. A complement-microglial axis drives synapse loss during virus-induced memory impairment. Nature. 2016; 534(7608):538–43.
93. Vergunst CE, Gerlag DM, Dinant H, Schulz L, Vinkenoog M, Smeets TJ, Sanders ME, Reedquist KA, Tak PP. Blocking the receptor for C5a in patients with rheumatoid arthritis does not reduce synovial inflammation. Rheumatology(Oxford). 2007;46(12):1773–8.

Depletion of adult neurogenesis exacerbates cognitive deficits in Alzheimer's disease by compromising hippocampal inhibition

Carolyn Hollands[1], Matthew Kyle Tobin[1], Michael Hsu[1], Kianna Musaraca[1], Tzong-Shiue Yu[2], Rachana Mishra[1], Steven G. Kernie[2] and Orly Lazarov[1*]

Abstract

Background: The molecular mechanism underlying progressive memory loss in Alzheimer's disease is poorly understood. Neurogenesis in the adult hippocampus is a dynamic process that continuously changes the dentate gyrus and is important for hippocampal plasticity, learning and memory. However, whether impairments in neurogenesis affect the hippocampal circuitry in a way that leads to memory deficits characteristic of Alzheimer's disease is unknown. Controversial results in that regard were reported in transgenic mouse models of amyloidosis.

Methods: Here, we conditionally ablated adult neurogenesis in APPswe/PS1ΔE9 mice by crossing these with mice expressing nestin-driven thymidine kinase (δ-HSV-TK).

Results: These animals show impairment in performance in contextual conditioning and pattern separation tasks following depletion of neurogenesis. Importantly, these deficits were not observed in age-matched APPswe/PS1ΔE9 or δ-HSV-TK mice alone. Furthermore, we show that cognitive deficits were accompanied by the upregulation of hyperphosphorylated tau in the hippocampus and in immature neurons specifically. Interestingly, we observed upregulation of the immediate early gene Zif268 (Egr-1) in the dentate gyrus, CA1 and CA3 regions of the hippocampus following learning in the neurogenesis-depleted δ-HSV-TK mice. This may suggest overactivation of hippocampal neurons in these areas following depletion of neurogenesis.

Conclusions: These results imply that neurogenesis plays an important role in the regulation of inhibitory circuitry of the hippocampus. This study suggests that deficits in adult neurogenesis may contribute to cognitive impairments, tau hyperphosphorylation in new neurons and compromised hippocampal circuitry in Alzheimer's disease.

Keywords: Alzheimer's disease, Hippocampal neurogenesis, Learning and memory, Hippocampal circuit, Tau phosphorylation

Background

The mechanism underlying cognitive deficits in Alzheimer's disease (AD) is not fully elucidated [1]. Normal age-related memory loss is thought to begin in the dentate gyrus (DG) [2]. This observation is supported by high-resolution fMRI [3–5] and cognitive studies [6–9]. In AD, neuronal loss in the entorhinal cortex is preceded by a long period of deficits in the connectivity of the hippocampal formation [10]. In the hippocampus there is an age-dependent decrease in the number of new neurons that are being continuously added to the dentate gyrus in rodents [11–16]. Similarly there is a decline in adult neurogenesis in humans [17–20]. This is compounded by changes in synaptic structure. In both rodents and humans the density of synaptic contacts formed onto granule cells of the DG is reduced with age [21, 22].

In familial Alzheimer's disease (FAD)-linked APPswe/PS1ΔE9 mice, hippocampal neurogenesis is impaired in

* Correspondence: olazarov@uic.edu
[1]Department of Anatomy and Cell Biology, College of Medicine, The University of Illinois at Chicago, 909 S Wolcott Ave, Chicago, IL 60612, USA
Full list of author information is available at the end of the article

young adults, prior to cognitive deficits or the appearance of amyloid plaque pathology [23]. Similar observations of neurogenic impairments were independently confirmed in the 3xTg-AD mouse [24, 25] (review [26, 27]). Additionally, in vitro studies of neural progenitor cells (NPCs), isolated from the subgranular layer of APPswe/PS1ΔE9 mice, show both expression of hyperphosphorylated tau and reduced proliferation [23]. Nevertheless, there have been contradicting reports about the fate of neurogenesis in FAD, and the contribution of neurogenesis to AD remains controversial [1, 28, 29].

Significantly, there is overlap between FAD related proteins and proteins regulating adult neurogenesis (review [26, 27]). In particular, presenilin 1 (PS1) regulates neural progenitor cell differentiation in vitro and in vivo [30]. Additionally, soluble amyloid precursor protein alpha (sAPPα), a cleavage product of the amyloid precursor protein (APP), acts as a proliferation factor on NPCs in the adult brain [31, 32]. PS1/γ-secretase regulates the metabolism of critical players in neurogenesis, such as notch-1, EGF, β-catenin and cAMP response element binding protein (CREB), all of which are important neurogenic signals. Changes in PS1 function could alter these signaling factors and thus affect neurogenesis. Importantly, we have shown that downregulation of PS1 compromises the maturation of new neurons, suggesting that defective neurons incorporate into the dentate gyrus [33].

In light of that, in this study we attempted to address three fundamental questions: 1. Does depletion of hippocampal neurogenesis promote cognitive decline observed in AD? 2. Does depletion of hippocampal neurogenesis promote AD-related neuropathology? and 3. Does depletion of hippocampal neurogenesis alter the hippocampal circuit? To address these questions, we conditionally ablated neurogenesis in APPswe/PS1ΔE9 mice using nestin-regulated expression of thymidine kinase (δ-HSV-TK). We show that depletion of adult neurogenesis in APPswe/PS1ΔE9 impaired performance in contextual conditioning and pattern separation tasks. These deficits were not observed in age-matched APPswe/PS1ΔE9 mice. Furthermore, depletion of neurogenesis induced hyperphosphorylation of tau in the hippocampus. However, we observed no effect of neurogenesis on level of oligomeric Aβ in the entorhinal cortex of these mice. Importantly, we show overactivation of neurons in the dentate gyrus, CA3 and CA1 regions of the hippocampus following depletion of neurogenesis, suggesting that neurogenesis plays an important role in regulating neuronal activation in the hippocampus. In summary, this is the first study to examine the effect of reduced neurogenesis on the development of cognitive deficits and AD. Combined, the results of this study suggest that reduced levels of hippocampal neurogenesis can induce cognitive dysfunction and tau pathology characterizing AD, and interfere with hippocampal function.

Methods

Animals

Animal care procedures were conducted according to the National Institutes of Health Guide for the Care and Use of Laboratory Animals. Our colony is maintained via group housing (≤5 mice per cage) in a high barrier facility under a 14:10 light:dark cycle with free access to food and water. FAD-linked APPswe/PS1ΔE9 mice [34] and Nestin-δ-HSV-TK mice [35] were generated as previously described. To maintain consistency of pathology progression and avoid gender-related disparate observations, mice used in this study were all females. Mouse euthanasia was performed using isofluorane and cervical dislocation.

Valganciclovir treatment

Valganciclovir powder was mixed into mouse chow (.09%, Valcyte, valganciclovir hydrochloride) and given ad libitum for an average dose of ~90 mg/kg/day (Custom Animal Diets, LLC (Easton, PA)). Animals were fed either Valganciclovir- containing chow or standard chow ("vehicle") right after weaning for 2 months. At the end of this period mice were subjected to behavioral tests, i.e., contextual fear conditioning and pattern separation sequentially. A separate group of mice was subjected to pattern separation followed by a single probe test, as described in Fig. 5. Following sacrifice, brains were analyzed as described below.

Contextual fear conditioning

Performed as previously described [36]. Conditioning was conducted in two distinct contexts: context A with the shock, and context C without the shock. Both test cages (17.8 × 17.8 × 30.5 cm) were encased by isolation cubicles. Context A had two plexiglass walls, two metal walls and a stainless steel grid floor (Coulbourn Instruments). The light and fan were turned on. A mild lemon blossom scent was used, and 70% ethanol for cleaning. Context C had the light and fan turned off, the chamber door ajar, a mild anise scent, and Clorox disinfecting wipes for cleaning. The shape of the chamber was altered with a plastic circular insert, and a plastic flooring was placed on top of the stainless steel grid floor with cage bedding added. Motion was recorded by a digital video camera mounted above the test cage. On day 0 mice were tested only in context A, then for 3 consecutive days in both A and C context with an hour separation. In test cage A the mice received a single 2 s foot shock (0.75 mA at the 185th second). FreezeFrame and FreezeView software (Actimetrics) were used for recording and analyzing freezing behavior. Percentage of freezing during the first 180 s in each context for each day was computed. Discrimination ratios were calculated using the formula:

$$\text{Discrimination Ratio} = (\text{Freezing}_A - \text{Freezing}_C)/(\text{Freezing}_A + \text{Freezing}_C).$$

Pattern separation

Performed as previously described [33]. Conditioning was conducted in two similar contexts: the shock context A, and the similar context B. Both cages had two clear Plexiglas walls, two grey metal walls and a stainless steel grid floor (Coulbourn Instruments). In cage A the house light and fan were turned on. A mild lemon blossom scent was used. Cages were cleaned with 70% ethanol prior to mouse placement. Test cage B differed from test cage A in that the metal walls had black and white inserts, the house light and fan were turned off and the chamber door was left ajar. A mild peppermint scent was used, and Clorox disinfecting wipes. On day 0 mice were exposed only to the training context A. For the next nine consecutive days mice were exposed to A and B in a randomized order. Discrimination ratios were calculated using the formula:

$$\text{Discrimination Ratio} = (\text{Freezing}_A - \text{Freezing}_B)/(\text{Freezing}_A + \text{Freezing}_B).$$

BrdU injections

Two doses of 5′-bromo-2′-deoxyuridine (BrdU; Sigma) were administered four hours apart intraperitoneally (100 mg/kg), in physiological saline. Animals were sacrificed four weeks later.

Brain tissue processing

For immunohistochemical staining, all mice were anesthetized using overdose of isofluorane and transcardially perfused with ice-cold PBS. Removed brains were halved on the sagittal plane, and half placed into 4% paraformaldehyde and half saved for western blot.

Immunohistochemistry

50 μm sagittal sections cut using a sliding freezing microtome (Leica Biosystems, Buffalo Grove, IL) were stored in cryoprotectant (glycerol, ethylene glycol, 1X PBS) at −20 °C. The following antibodies were used: rat anti-BrdU (1:400; Accurate Chemical & Scientific Corp., Westbury, NY), mouse anti-nestin (1:100; Millipore Corporation, Billerica, MA), goat anti-doublecortin (DCX; 1:400; Santa Cruz Biotechnology, Santa Cruz, CA), mouse anti-NeuN (1:400, Millipore, Temecula, CA), rabbit anti-Egr-1 (1:250, Santa Cruz Biotechnology, Santa Cruz, CA), goat anti-green fluorescent protein (GFP, 1:1000, Abcam, Inc. Cambridge, MA) and mouse anti-green fluorescent protein (GFP, 1:200; Santa Cruz Biotechnology, Santa Cruz, CA). Secondary antibodies from Jackson ImmunoResearch Laboratories (West Grove, PA): biotinylated species-specific anti-IgG (all used at 1:250), Cy3-conjugated Donkey anti-Rabbit (1:250), Cy3-conjugated Donkey anti-Rat (1:250), Alexa Fluor 647 (AF647)-conjugated Donkey anti-Mouse and anti-Rat (1:250), Cy2-conjugated Streptavidin (1:250), DAPI Nucleic Acid Stain (1:2500, Life Technologies, Grand Island, NY).

Stereological quantification

Cell counts were performed using design-based stereology (StereoInvestigator version 8, MBF Bioscience). For the analysis, every sixth section of brain tissue was quantified by applying the Nv × VRef method. Sections were traced using a Zeiss AX10 microscope (Carl Zeiss Ltd., Hertfordshire, England) in low magnification (5×) and counting was performed at high magnification (63×), counting frame = 100 μm × 100 μm, grid size 100 μm × 100 μm, and all sections were counted using 12.5-μm top and bottom guard zones.

Dot-blot for Oligomeric Aβ

Entorhinal cortex underwent extraction for isolating the water soluble Aβ fraction for dot-blot analysis as previously described [37]. Briefly, entorhinal cortex was homogenized in 1X PBS containing protease inhibitor cocktail (1:100, Sigma-Aldrich #P8340) followed by ultracentrifugation at 100,000 g for 1 h at 4 °C. The water-soluble fraction was quantified via the BCA method and 25 μg total protein was blotted onto prewet nitrocellulose membrane in the dot-blot apparatus (Bio-Rad Bio-Dot Microfiltration Apparatus). The membrane was then washed once in TBS and was blocked in 5% nonfat milk in 1X TBS + 0.01% Tween 20 (TBST) for 2 h at room temperature and incubated overnight at 4 °C in polyclonal rabbit anti-amyloid oligomer (A11; 1:5000; EMD Millipore #AB9234). The membrane was then washed three times in TBST and then incubated for 1 h at room temperature in IRDye 800CW donkey anti-rabbit IgG (1:20,000; Li-Cor #925–32213). The membrane was imaged using an Odyssey Fc (800 channel, 30 s acquisition) and protein expression levels were quantified using Image Studio Lite (version 5.2.5; Li-Cor).

Western blotting

Protein extraction of brain tissue was performed as previously [30]. Antibodies used for Western blot included mouse anti-actin (1:5000, Millipore, Temecula, CA), rabbit anti-amyloid precursor protein (APP, Abcam, Cambridge, MA), mouse anti-phospho-PHF-tau (AT8, 1:500, ThermoFisher Scientific) and mouse anti-tau (tau-5, 1:1000, Millipore, Temecula, CA). The following secondary antibodies were used, mouse anti-HRP (1:10,000, Thermo Scientific, Rockford, Il) and rabbit anti-HRP (1:15,000, Promega, Madison, WI). Protein expression was measured in ImageJ and was normalized to actin.

Statistical analysis

Stereological quantification was analyzed using two-tail or one-tail (Fig. 5), unpaired *t*-test, or Welch's unequal variance *t*-test where appropriate. Contextual fear conditioning, pattern separation, and discrimination ratios were analyzed using repeated measures, two-way ANOVA with Holm-Sidak multiple comparison testing. Western blot data was analyzed using two-tail, unpaired *t*-test, or Welch's unequal variance *t*-test where appropriate. All statistical analysis was done in GraphPad Prism (Version 7.01; GraphPad Software Inc., La Jolla, CA, USA). All data shown represent mean ± S.E.M. and a probability of less than 0.05 was considered statistically significant.

Results

Ablation of adult neurogenesis in a FAD mouse model

To address the hypothesis that decreased adult neurogenesis will exacerbate the cognitive deficits associated with Alzheimer's disease, we temporally ablated neural progenitor cells from the brains of FAD-linked APPswe/PS1ΔE9 transgenic mice. For this purpose, we bred the APPswe/PS1ΔE9 mice with the Nestin-δ-HSV-TK transgenic mouse line, [35]. The Nestin-δ-HSV-TK transgenic line contains a modified version of the herpes simplex virus thymidine kinase (TK), as well as an enhanced green fluorescent protein (GFP), driven by the nestin promoter and its second intron regulatory element (Fig. 1a). Administration of valganciclovir in mouse chow, which is specifically phosphorylated by Nestin-δ-HSV-TK, kills dividing nestin expressing cells in these mice by acting as a toxic thymidine analog. The number of GFP-expressing nestin positive cells in the subgranular layer of the hippocampus of Nestin-δ-HSV-TK treated with valganciclovir is reduced compared to vehicle-treated Nestin-δ-HSV-TK mice (Fig. 1b-f). Likewise, a dramatic decrease in GFP+ cells was observed in brain sections of APPswe/PS1ΔE9;Nestin-δ-HSV-TK treated with valganciclovir, compared to vehicle-treated APPswe/PS1ΔE9;Nestin-δ-HSV-TK mice (Fig. 1g-n). To determine the nature of neurogenic deficits in valganciclovir-treated Nestin-δ-HSV-TK and APPswe/PS1ΔE9;Nestin-δ-HSV-TK, we quantified the number of GFP+ neural progenitor cells (NPCs) by unbiased stereology following a two-month valganciclovir treatment. No change in the number of GFP + DCX- (nestin expressing NPCs; Fig. 1d) or GFP + DCX+ (neuroblasts; Fig. 1e) was observed between valganciclovir- and vehicle-treated Nestin-δ-HSV-TK mice. However, a significant reduction in the number of GFP-DCX+ (immature neurons) was observed in Nestin-δ-HSV-TK mice treated with valganciclovir (Fig. 1f; two-tailed, unpaired *t*-test; $t_7 = 5.589$, $P = 0.0008$). Taken together, this may suggest that in the tested conditions, reduced neurogenesis in the valganciclovir treated Nestin-δ-HSV-TK mice is manifested at the immature neuron stage. Interestingly, APPswe/PS1ΔE9;Nestin-δ-HSV-TK mice treated with valganciclovir displayed a significant decrease at earlier stages. Specifically, a significant reduction in total number of nestin expressing NPCs (GFP + DCX-, Fig. 1i; two-tailed, unpaired *t*-test; $t_9 = 3.253$, $P = 0.0099$), neuroblasts (GFP + DCX+, Fig. 1j, two-tailed, unpaired t-test; $t_9 = 3.305$, $P = 0.0092$) and immature neurons (GFP-DCX+, Fig. 1k, two-tailed, unpaired *t*-test; $t_9 = 2.932$, $P = 0.0167$) in the subgranular layer following treatment (Valganciclovir $N = 5$, Vehicle $N = 6$). This may suggest that in the APPswe/PS1ΔE9;Nestin-δ-HSV-TK mice, treatment with valganciclovir affects earlier neurogenic populations compared to the Nestin-δ-HSV-TK mice and is manifested by a significant reduction in the number of NPCs, neuroblasts and immature neurons. This may further support previous reports suggesting impairment of NPCs in FAD [30, 38]. To assess the impact on the number of newly born neurons we quantified the number of BrdU + NeuN+ cells in the granular cell layer of the DG of the APPswe/PS1ΔE9;Nestin-δ-HSV-TK mice. Unbiased stereology demonstrated a trending decrease in the total number of BrdU+ (Fig. 1l, two-tailed, Welch's unequal variance *t*-test; $t_{4.034} = 2.204$, $P = 0.0917$), BrdU + NeuN+ new neurons (Fig. 1m, two-tailed, Welch's unequal variance *t*-test; $t_{4.062} = 2.077$, $P = 0.1054$), as well as in the number of new glia BrdU + NeuN- cells (Fig. 1n, two-tailed, Welch's unequal variance t-test; $t_{4.137} = 2.457$, $P = 0.0679$) following valganciclovir treatment (Valganciclovir $N = 4$, Vehicle $N = 5$). Combined, this data demonstrates a successful ablation of adult neurogenesis in APPswe/PS1ΔE9;Nestin-δ-HSV-TK animals, resulting in less new neurons and glia in the granular cell layer of the DG. In addition, these results may imply that NPCs and neuroblasts are more vulnerable in the brains of APPswe/PS1ΔE9;Nestin-δ-HSV-TK mice compared to the Nestin-δ-HSV-TK mice.

Ablation of adult neurogenesis in FAD mice induces deficits in the contextual fear conditioning task

To determine cognitive performance of FAD mice following depletion of neurogenesis, mice were tested in the contextual fear conditioning and the DG-specific pattern separation tasks as previously described [36, 39]. In the contextual fear-conditioning task (Fig. 2a), age matched wild type (Nontransgenic, $N = 11$, Fig. 2b) and APPswe/PS1ΔE9 (Fig. 2d, $n=14$) mice that were fed with vehicle chow, were able to successfully distinguish between the two contexts, based on percentage freezing, by the end of the second day. Discrimination ratio shows no difference between vehicle- and valganciclovir-fed wild type (Fig. 2c) or APPswe/PS1ΔE9 mice (Fig. 2d), suggesting no side effect of the valganciclovir on animals' behavior. Similarly, Nestin-δ-HSV-TK animals fed with either vehicle- or valganciclovir-containing chow were also able to successfully learn the task (vehicle-treated Nestin-δ-HSV-TK $N = 12$, valganciclovir- treated Nestin-δ-HSV-TK $N = 8$,

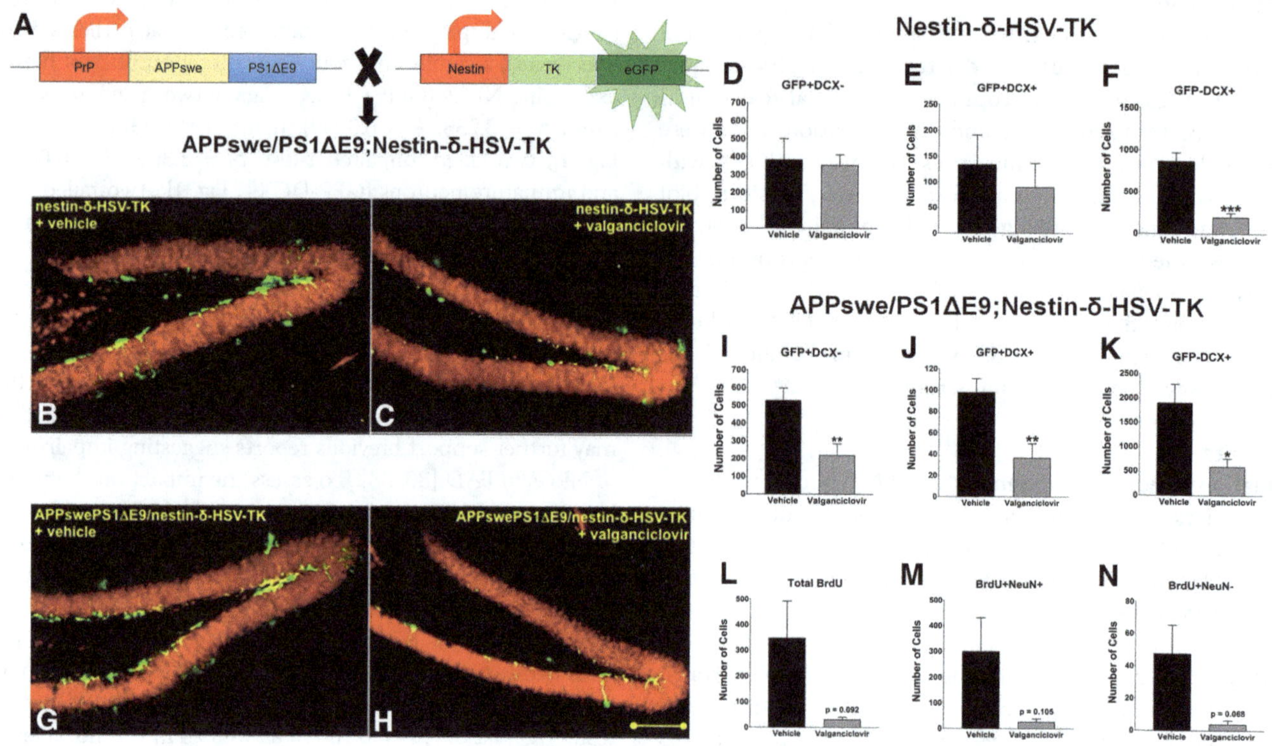

Fig. 1 Depletion of hippocampal neurogenesis following treatment of Nestin-δ-HSV-TK and APPswePS1ΔE9/Nestin-δ-HSV-TK mice with valganciclovir. **a** Breeding scheme of APPswe/PS1ΔE9 and Nestin-δ-HSV-TK transgenic mice, to produce transgenic FAD animals that can exhibit selectively ablated neurogenesis, i.e. APPswePS1ΔE9/Nestin-δ-HSV-TK mice. **b, c** Confocal images of hippocampal sections of Nestin-δ-HSV-TK transgenic mice stained with anti-NeuN and anti-green fluorescent protein (GFP) + antibodies. Images show less GFP+ neural stem and progenitor cells in the subgranular layer of valganciclovir-treated Nestin-δ-HSV-TK mice (**c**) compared to vehicle-treated Nestin-δ-HSV-TK transgenic mice (**b**). **d-f** Quantification of hippocampal neurogenesis in Nestin-δ-HSV-TK that either received vehicle (black bars) or valganciclovir chow (gray bars). There was no change in the number of GFP + DCX- (**d**) or GFP + DCX+ cells (**e**), but there was a significant decrease in the number of GFP-DCX+ cells [(**f**) two-tailed, unpaired *t*-test; $t_7 = 5.589$, $P = 0.0008$]. **g, h** Hippocampal sections of 4–5 month old APPswe/PS1ΔE9;Nestin-δ-HSV-TK fed with either vehicle (**g**) or valganciclovir (**h**) chow. Valganciclovir treated animals showed a significant decrease in GFP+ (nestin) and DCX+ expressing cells. **i-n** Quantification of hippocampal neurogenesis in APPswePS1ΔE9/Nestin-δ-HSV-TK that received vehicle- (black bar) or valganciclovir- chow (gray bar). Decrease in total number of (**i**) GFP + DCX- expressing neural progenitor cells (two-tailed, unpaired *t*-test; $t_9 = 3.253$, $P = 0.0099$), (**j**) GFP + DCX+ neuroblasts (two-tailed, unpaired *t*-test; $t_9 = 3.305$, $P = 0.0092$) and (**k**) GFP-DCX+ immature neurons (two-tailed, unpaired *t*-test; $t_9 = 2.932$, $P = 0.0167$) in the subgranular layer (valganciclovir $N = 5$, vehicle $N = 6$). Counts in the granular cell layer (valganciclovir $N = 4$, vehicle N = 5) show decrease in number of (**l**) total BrdU (two-tailed, Welch's unequal variance *t*-test; $t_{4.034} = 2.204$, $P = 0.0917$), (**m**) BrdU + NeuN+ (two-tailed, Welch's unequal variance *t*-test; $t_{4.062} = 2.077$, $P = 0.1054$) and (**n**) BrdU + NeuN- (two-tailed, Welch's unequal variance *t*-test; $t_{4.137} = 2.457$, $P = 0.0679$). Scale bar = 100 μm. $*P < 0.05$; $**P < 0.01$

Fig. 2f-h respectively), suggesting that ablation of adult neurogenesis alone is insufficient for the disruption of this behavioral task. Vehicle treated APPswe/PS1ΔE9;Nestin-δ-HSV-TK animals exhibited some difficulty learning the task on the first day, but successfully distinguished between the two contexts on day 2 and 3 ($N = 7$, Fig. 2i). Importantly, valganciclovir-fed APPswe/PS1ΔE9;Nestin-δ-HSV-TK mice were unable to distinguish between context A or C on any of the days of the test ($N = 9$, Fig. 2j). It is important to note that this deficit was only observed with the combination of ablated neurogenesis and the FAD mouse background. Nevertheless, discrimination ratios revealed no significant difference in the animal's ability to discriminate between contexts between days (Fig. 2k), which may suggest that the effect is very mild. However, valganciclovir-fed Nestin-δ-HSV-TK mice had a significant Context x Days interaction (Fig. 2l, repeated measures two-way ANOVA, Context x Days: $F_{2,36} = 3.56$ $P = 0.0388$). Furthermore, on Days 2 and 3 valganciclovir-fed Nestin-δ-HSV-TK exhibited significantly increased abilities to discriminate between contexts A and C compared to valganciclovir-fed APPswe/PS1ΔE9;-Nestin-δ-HSV-TK and APPswe/PS1ΔE9 mice (Fig. 2l; repeated measures two-way ANOVA, $*P < 0.05$, $^{\#}P < 0.05$, $^{\#\#}P < 0.01$) with the genotype having a significant influence on discrimination between contexts A and C (repeated measures two-way ANOVA, Genotype: $F_{2,22} = 7.00$ $P = 0.0044$). To examine whether freezing behavior is the result of anxiety rather than learning, mice were subjected to the Light/Dark box anxiety task. However we found no

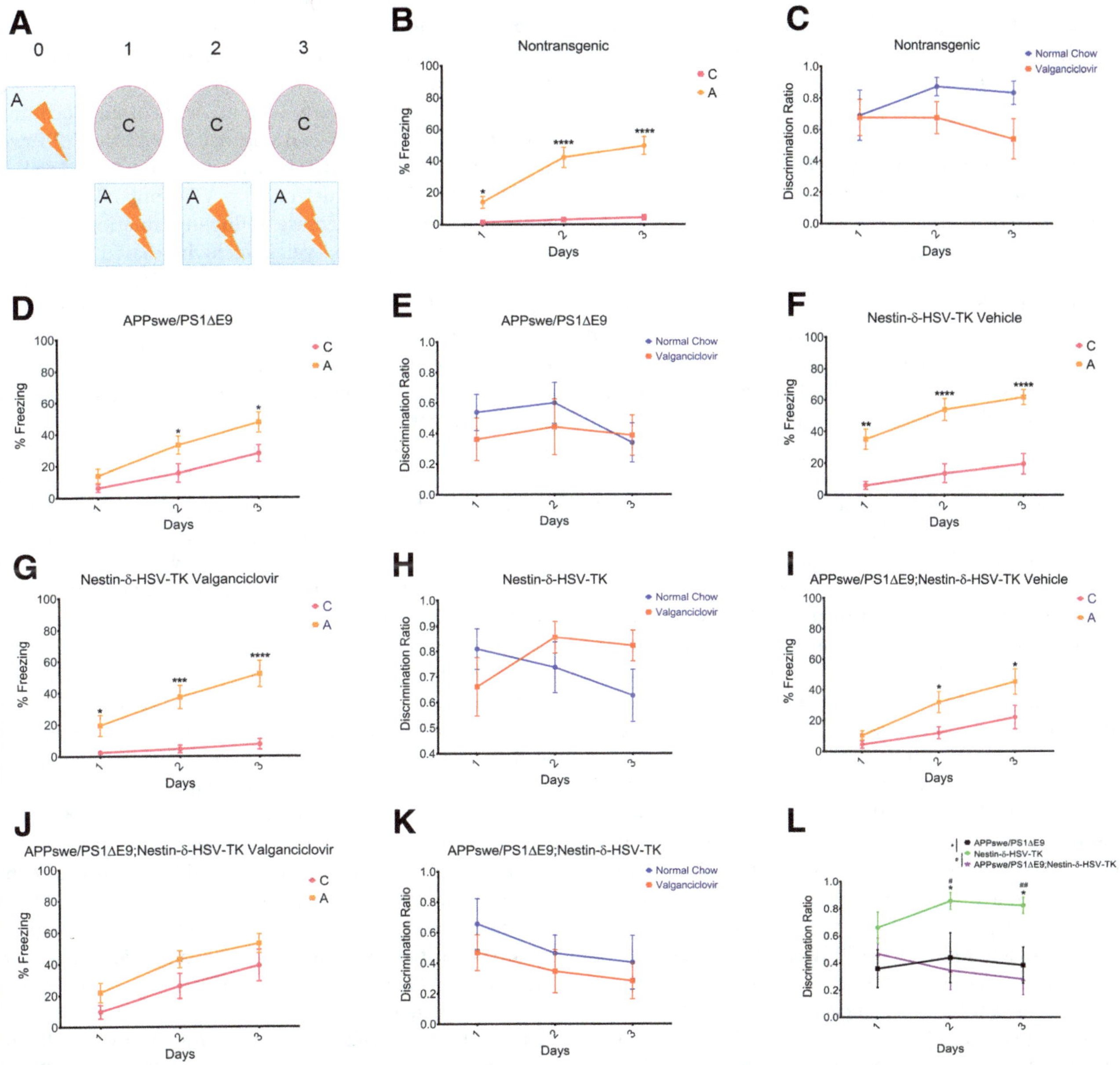

Fig. 2 Depletion in neurogenesis enhances impairments in contextual fear conditioning. **a** Schematic presentation of the experimental paradigm used. A (shock) and C (no shock) are distinct contexts. Mice were fed with either vehicle or valganciclovir chow after weaning for 1.5 months prior to the contextual fear conditioning task. **b**, **d**, **f**, **g** Based on anticipatory freezing behavior nontransgenic ($N = 11$) **b**), APPswePS1ΔE9 ($N = 14$) (**d**), vehicle-fed Nestin-δ-HSV-TK [((**f**), $N = 12$)] and valganciclovir-fed Nestin-δ-HSV-TK [(**g**), ($N = 8$)] mice are able to distinguish context A from C (repeated measures two-way ANOVA, **b**. Context: $F_{1,20} = 46.64$, $P < 0.0001$; **d**. Context: $F_{1,26} = 6.36$, $P = 0.0182$; **f**. Context: $F_{1,22} = 31.40$, $P < 0.0001$; **g**. Context: $F_{1,14} = 19.72$, $P = 0.0006$). **i** vehicle- treated APPswe/PS1ΔE9;Nestin-δ-HSV-TK ($N = 7$) are able to distinguish between the contexts (repeated measures two-way ANOVA, **i**. Context: $F_{1,12} = 7.90$, $P = 0.0157$). **j** valganciclovir-treated APPswe/PS1ΔE9;Nestin-δ-HSV-TK ($N = 9$) mice are unable to distinguish between the two contexts (repeated measures two-way ANOVA, **j**. Context: $F_{1,16} = 2.82$, $P = 0.1125$) .**c**, **e**, **h**, **k** Discrimination ratios in (**c**) nontransgenic, (**e**) APPswe/PS1ΔE9, (**h**) Nestin-δ-HSV-TK, and (**k**) APPswe/PS1ΔE9;Nestin-δ-HSV-TK revealed no significant differences in the animal's ability to discriminate between contexts between days; however, (**h**) Nestin-δ-HSV-TK mice had a significant Context x Days interaction (repeated measures two-way ANOVA, Context x Days: $F_{2,36} = 3.56$ $P = 0.0388$). **l** Valganciclovir-fed Nestin-δ-HSV-TK exhibited significantly better abilities to discriminate between contexts A and C compared to valganciclovir-fed APPswe/PS1ΔE9 and APPswe/PS1ΔE9;Nestin-δ-HSV-TK mice (repeated measures two-way ANOVA, *Nestin-δ-HSV-TK vs. APPswe/PS1ΔE9;, #Nestin-δ-HSV-TK vs. APPswe/PS1ΔE9;Nestin-δ-HSV-TK) with the genotype having a significant influence on discrimination between contexts A and C (repeated measures two-way ANOVA, Genotype: $F_{2,22} = 7.00$ $P = 0.0044$). $^{*}P < 0.05$; $^{**}P < 0.01$; $^{***}P < 0.001$; $^{****}P < 0.0001$; $^{\#}P < 0.05$; $^{\#\#}P < 0.01$

differences in anxiety level between any of the groups (data not shown), suggesting that these observed deficits are not a result of increased anxiety in the APPswe/PS1ΔE9; Nestin-δ-HSV-TK animals.

Ablation of adult neurogenesis in FAD mice induces deficits in the pattern separation task

We next asked whether depletion of neurogenesis in the FAD mice would induce difficulty learning in a known DG-specific task, pattern separation. The challenge in this task is the high similarity between the two contexts, and typically the learning process is longer compared to the contextual fear conditioning (Fig. 3a).

Vehicle chow-fed age matched wild type (Nontransgenic, N = 11, Fig. 3b) or APPswe/PS1ΔE9 animals (N = 13, Fig. 3d) were able to successfully distinguish between the two contexts, based on percentage freezing, by the end of the pattern separation task (repeated measures two-way ANOVA, $**P < 0.01$, $***P < 0.001$). Discrimination ratios of vehicle and valganciclovir-treated wild type (Fig. 3c) and APPswe/PS1ΔE9 (Fig. 3e) show no difference between the treatment groups, excluding the possibility of side effect of valganciclovir on mouse behavior. Unexpectedly, Nestin-δ-HSV-TK animals fed with either vehicle or valganciclovir containing chow were able to successfully learn the task (Vehicle-treated N = 12, valganciclovir-treated N = 7, Fig. 3f-h; repeated measures two-way ANOVA, $*P < 0.05$, $**P < 0.05$, $***P < 0.001$, $****P < 0.0001$), suggesting that either ablation of adult neurogenesis using the Nestin-δ-HSV-TK transgenic line is insufficient for the disruption of this behavioral task, or that our specific contexts were not sufficiently challenging, masking the deficit. Interestingly, vehicle-fed APPswe/PS1ΔE9;Nestin-δ-HSV-TK were able to discriminate between the tasks albeit not all days were statistically significant (N = 7, Fig. 3i; repeated measures two-way ANOVA, $*P < 0.05$, $**P < 0.05$, $***P < 0.001$). This may suggest a genetic background effect in comparison to vehicle-fed APPswe/PS1ΔE9 mice. Importantly, ablation of neurogenesis in the APPswe/PS1ΔE9;Nestin-δ-HSV-TK mice completely disrupted the performance of mice in the first three days of the task (N = 8, Fig. 3j; repeated measures two-way ANOVA, $*P < 0.05$). Discrimination ratios within genotype revealed no significant differences in the animal's ability to discriminate between contexts between days (Fig. 3k), suggesting a mild behavioral effect of neurogenesis in this task. Additionally, when comparing discrimination ratios between valganciclovir-fed Nestin-δ-HSV-TK, APPswe/PS1ΔE9 and APPswe/PS1ΔE9;Nestin-δ-HSV-TK mice there was no significance within days but there was an overall days effect among the groups (Fig. 3l; repeated measures two-way ANOVA, Days: $F_{5,100} = 10.50$ $P < 0.0001$).

Ablation of adult neurogenesis enhances tau hyperphosphorylation in FAD mice

Next, we asked whether, in addition to learning and memory, hippocampal neurogenesis would affect AD neuropathology. Western blot analysis of hippocampal protein lysate of vehicle- and valganciclovir-treated APPswe/PS1ΔE9;Nestin-δ-HSV-TK animals showed that the levels of phosphorylated tau, as detected by AT8 antibodies, demonstrated a trending increase following ablation of adult neurogenesis in the valganciclovir-treated APPswe/PS1ΔE9;Nestin-δ-HSV-TK (Fig. 4a,b). Total tau expression levels did not change (tau-5, Fig. 4a,c), while the ratio of phosphorylated tau to total tau was significantly increased (Fig. 4d; two-tailed, unpaired t-test; $t_4 = 4.368$, $P = 0.0120$). This observation suggests that ablation of adult neurogenesis induces upregulation of tau hyperphosphorylation in the hippocampus. Immunohistochemical analysis of hippocampal sections stained for phosphorylated tau (p-tau) and doublecortin (DCX) clearly show AT8 immunoreactivity in DCX+ neuroblasts and new neurons in valganciclovir-treated APPswe/PS1ΔE9;Nestin-δ-HSV-TK, but not in vehicle-treated APPswe/PS1ΔE9;-Nestin-δ-HSV-TK mice (Fig. 4e). This may suggest that depletion of neurogenesis compromises the regulation of tau phosphorylation in newly differentiated neurons. Given the critical role of tau in neuronal maturation, this may suggest that the reduced level of neurogenesis may lead to the incorporation of aberrant new neurons into the hippocampus. To make sure that the observed alterations in tau phosphorylation are not a side effect of the valganciclovir treatment, we examined p-tau expression in vehicle- and valganciclovir- treated wild type mice and observed no change in p-tau expression (Additional file 1: Figure S1). This suggests that induction of hyperphosphorylated tau observed in the valganciclovir-treated APPswe/PS1ΔE9;Nestin-δ-HSV-TK was due to the depletion of neurogenesis.

To address the effect of neurogenesis on the amyloidogenic pathway we examined levels of full length APP in hippocampal protein lysates of vehicle- and valganciclovir-treated APPswe/PS1ΔE9;Nestin-δ-HSV-TK animals. We observed that APP levels do not change after ablation of neurogenesis (N = 3, Fig. 4a). In addition, the level of oligomeric Aβ was comparable in water-soluble protein extracts prepared from the entorhinal cortices of these mice (Fig. 4f). These results suggest that the effect of depletion of neurogenesis on tau may not be modulated by amyloidosis.

Ablation of adult neurogenesis modifies hippocampal circuit activity

To assess the impact of loss of neurogenesis on the activity of the hippocampal circuitry we examined expression of the immediate early gene Egr-1 (zif268), as

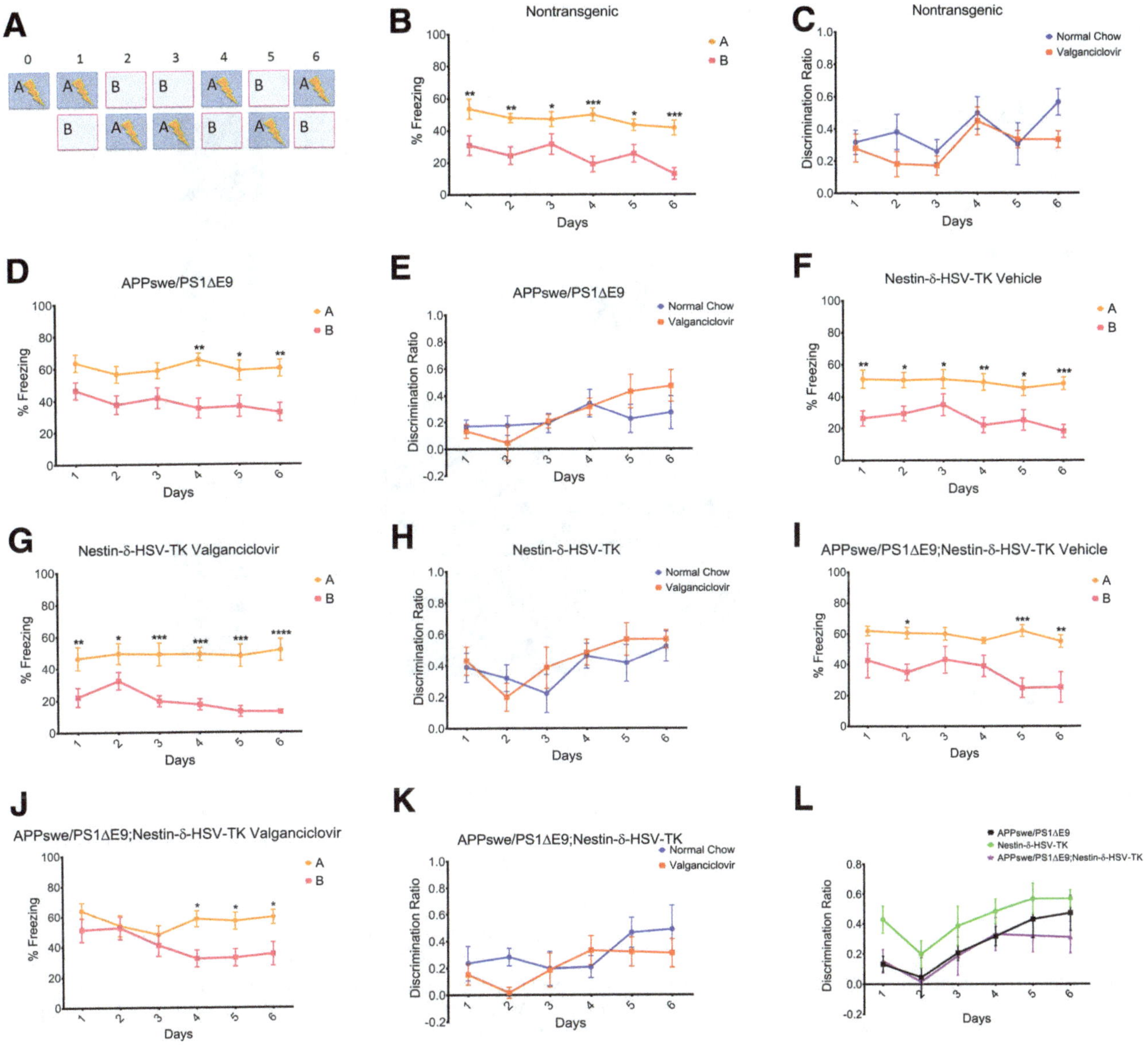

Fig. 3 Ablation of neurogenesis compromises pattern separation in APPswe/PS1ΔE9;Nestin-δ-HSV-TK mice. **a** Schematic presentation of the experimental paradigm used to test pattern separation. Two very similar contexts, A (shock) and B (no shock). Nontransgenic [$N = 11$, (**b**)], APPswe/PS1ΔE9 [$N = 13$, (**d**)], vehicle- treated Nestin-δ-HSV-TK [$N = 12$, (**f**)] and valganciclovir- treated Nestin-δ-HSV-TK [$N = 7$, (**g**)] mice are able to distinguish context A from B (repeated measures two-way ANOVA, **b**. Context: $F_{1,20} = 18.20$, $P = 0.0004$; **d**. Context: $F_{1,16} = 7.06$, $P = 0.0172$; **f**. Context: $F_{1,22} = 13.24$, $P = 0.0014$; **g**. Context: $F_{1,12} = 22.87$, $P = 0.0004$). **i** vehicle-treated APPswe/PS1ΔE9;Nestin-δ-HSV-TK mice ($N = 7$) exhibit similar but not identical learning patterns to APPswe/PS1ΔE9 mice (repeated measures, two-way ANOVA, $F_{1,10} = 18.09$, $P = 0.0017$). **j** Valganciclovir-treated APPswe/PS1ΔE9;Nestin-δ-HSV-TK ($N = 8$) mice are unable to distinguish between the two contexts for the first three days (repeated measures, two-way ANOVA, $F_{1,14} = 4.45$, $P = 0.0534$). **c**, **e**, **h**, **k** Discrimination ratios in (**c**) nontransgenic, (**e**) APPswe/PS1ΔE9, (**h**) Nestin-δ-HSV-TK, and (**k**) APPswe/PS1ΔE9;Nestin-δ-HSV-TK revealed no significant difference in the animal's ability to discriminate between contexts between days. **l** There were no significant differences in discrimination ratios between days for valganciclovir-fed Nestin-δ-HSV-TK, APPswe/PS1ΔE9, and APPswe/PS1ΔE9;Nestin-δ-HSV-TK mice but there was a significant effect overall across days (repeated measures two-way ANOVA, Days: $F_{5,100} = 10.50$ $P < 0.0001$). $^{*}P < 0.05$; $^{**}P < 0.01$; $^{***}P < 0.001$; $^{****}P < 0.0001$

an indicator of neuronal activation following learning. For this purpose, Nestin-δ-HSV-TK mice fed with vehicle or valganciclovir were subject to pattern separation, as above. To assess the neuronal population activated by the long-term memory of context A, ten days after task completion, a single probe trial of only the shock context was performed, and mice were immediately sacrificed and examined for Egr-1 expression (Fig. 5a). Using unbiased stereology the number of Egr-1 expressing cells was quantified in the granular cell layer of the DG, the CA1 region,

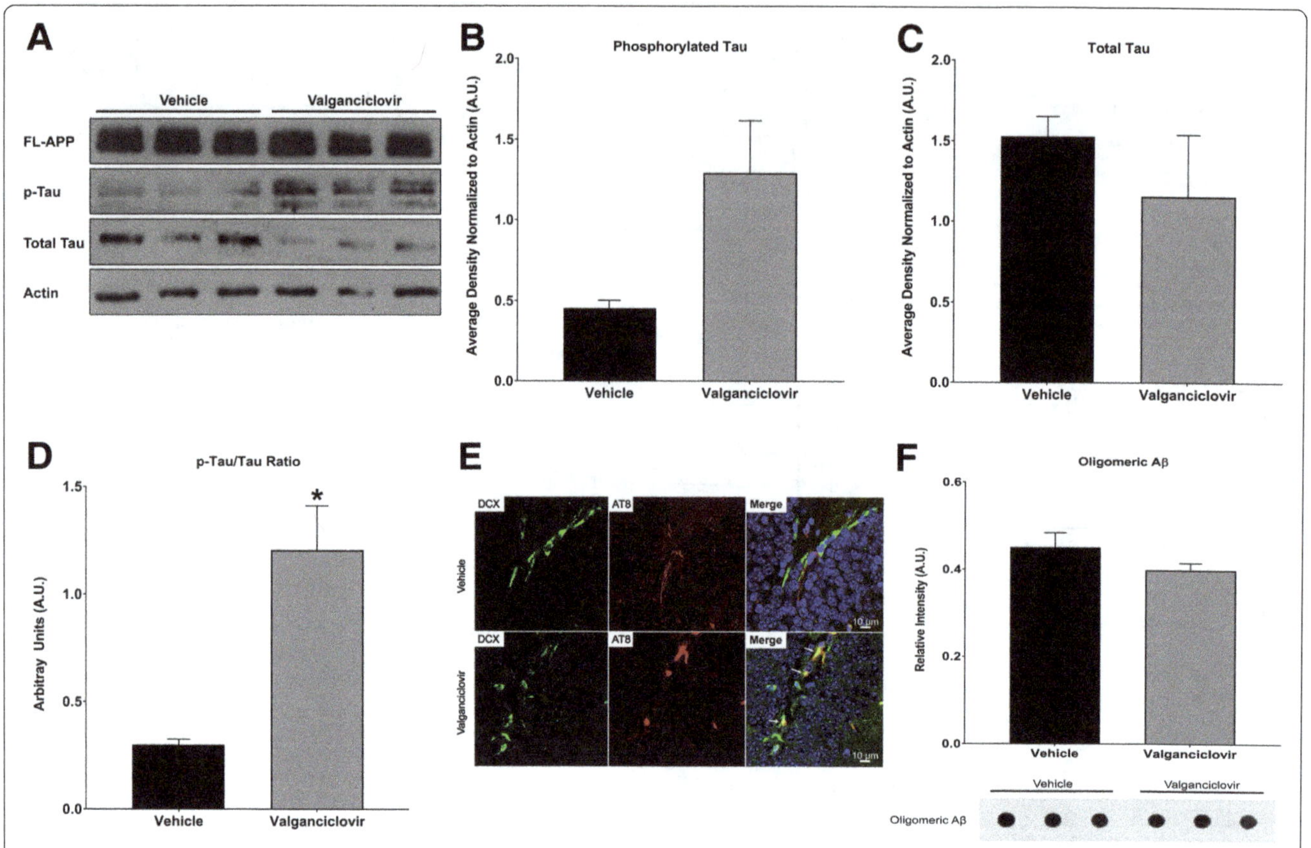

Fig. 4 Ablation of neurogenesis increases the expression of phosphorylated tau in the hippocampus of APPswe/PS1ΔE9;Nestin-δ-HSV-TK mice. **a** Western blot of hippocampal protein extract from 4 month old APPswe/PS1ΔE9;Nestin-δ-HSV-TK mice fed with vehicle or valganciclovir chow for 3 months ($N = 3$) shows that the expression level of full length amyloid precursor protein (APP) is comparable between the groups. However, there was a decrease in level of total tau and an increase in level of AT8-positive hyperphosphorylated tau (p-tau) in the valganciclovir-treated APPswe/PS1ΔE9;Nestin-δ-HSV-TK mice. **b-d** Semi-quantitative analysis of Western blot using Image J normalized to actin. There was a trending increase in levels of (**b**) p-tau (AT8; two-tail, Welch's unequal variance *t*-test, $t_{2.094} = 2.553$, $P = 0.1197$), with no change in (**c**) total tau (Tau-5, two-tail, unpaired t-test, $t_4 = 0.9195$, $P = 0.4099$) and (**d**) a significant increase in the ratio of p-tau to total tau (two-tailed, unpaired *t*-test; $t_4 = 4.368$, $P = 0.0120$) in the brains of valganciclovir-treated APPswe/PS1ΔE9;Nestin-δ-HSV-TK. $^*P < 0.05$. **e** Doublecortin (DCX) positive neuroblasts and immature neurons in the dentate gyrus of APPswe/PS1ΔE9;Nestin-δ-HSV-TK mice fed with valganciclovir chow are immunoreactive for the anti-p-tau antibodies AT8. Immunoreactivity was not detected in APPswe/PS1ΔE9;Nestin-δ-HSV-TK mice fed with vehicle. Scale bar = 10 μm. **f** Dot blot analysis of water soluble protein extract of the entorhinal cortex of APPswe/PS1ΔE9;Nestin-δ-HSV-TK mice fed with valganciclovir or normal chow reveals no difference in the level of A11 immunoreactive oligomeric Aβ between the groups ($N = 3$)

and the CA3 region of these mice ($N = 4$). Ablation of adult neurogenesis caused a trending increase in the number of Egr-1 expressing cells in the granular cell layer of the DG (Fig. 5b), with a significant increase in the CA3 region (Fig. 5c,e,f; one-tailed, unpaired *t*-test; $t_4 = 2.302$, $P = 0.0414$), and the CA1 region (Fig. 5d,g,h; one-tailed, unpaired *t*-test; $t_6 = 2.039$, $P = 0.0438$). These results suggest that eliminating the presence of new neurons relieves inhibitory circuitry in the DG-CA3-CA1. Alternatively, this may be the result of decreased excitatory synapses onto interneurons in the hilus.

Discussion

This study addresses three fundamental questions. First, we examined the role of neurogenesis in cognitive deficits in AD. We show that depletion of neurogenesis induces mild learning and memory impairments in APPswe/PS1ΔE9 mice. Previous reports show that in the APPswe/PS1ΔE9 mouse model cognitive deficits can develop as early as six months, including impairment in the fear-conditioning task [40]. We show that depletion of neurogenesis in the brains of APPswe/PS1ΔE9 mice exacerbates performance deficits in this task inducing deficits at 4 months of age. It should be noted that APPswe/PS1ΔE9 mice exhibit impairments in neurogenesis as early as 2 months of age characterized by both reduction in neurogenesis as well as defective neuronal differentiation [33]. Thus, the comparison between vehicle- and valganciclovir-treated APPswe/PS1ΔE9; Nestin-δ-HSV-TK mice is between defective and ablated neurogenesis, respectively. That said, in contrast to vehicle-treated, valganciclovir-treated APPswe/PS1ΔE9; Nestin-δ-HSV-

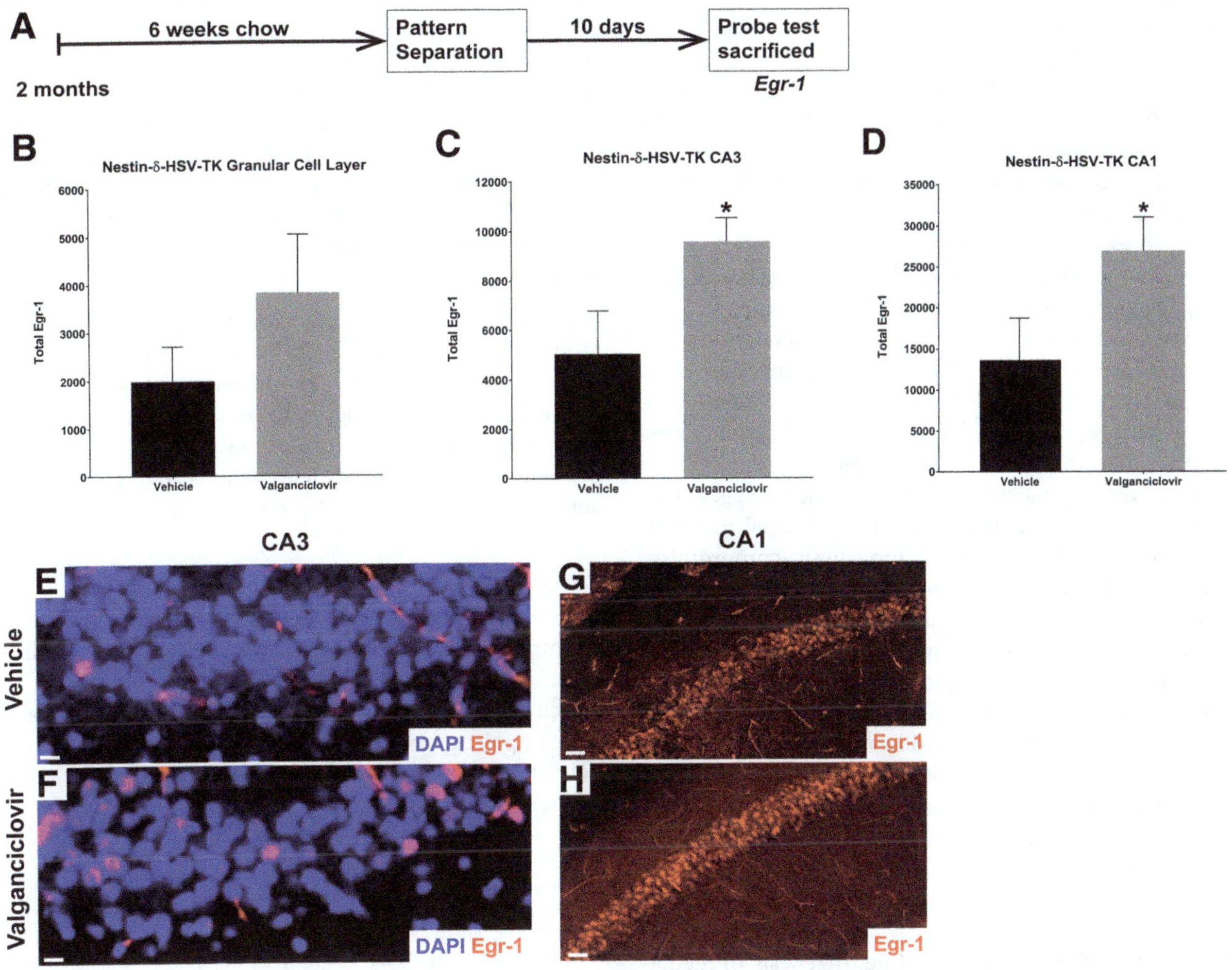

Fig. 5 Over-activation of hippocampal neurons following long term memory retrieval in neurogenesis-depleted Nestin-δ-HSV-TK mice (**a**) Experimental design. Nestin-δ-HSV-TK mice ($N = 4$) were fed with vehicle or valganciclovir chow following weaning for six weeks before performing pattern separation testing. Ten days after behavioral testing, a single probe test, where the mouse was placed only in the shock context A, was performed. Then, the animals were sacrificed for analysis of changes in Egr-1 (*zif268*) expression in the hippocampal circuitry. **b-d** Quantification of Egr-1 positive cells in the hippocampus. The total number of Egr-1 positive cells showed a trending increase in the granular cell layer of the dentate gyrus (**b**), with significant increases in the CA3 region (**c**) (one-tailed, unpaired *t*-test; $t_4 = 2.302$, $P = 0.0414$), and the CA1 region (**d**) (one-tailed, unpaired *t*-test; $t_6 = 2.039$, $P = 0.0438$). **e-h** Images of DAPI + Egr-1+ cells in the CA3 (**e**, **f**) and Egr-1+ cells in the CA1 (**g**, **h**) regions of vehicle- or valganciclovir-treated Nestin-δ-HSV-TK mice reveal more Egr-1+ cells in the valganciclovir-treated Nestin-δ-HSV-TK mice. Scale bar = 15 μM (E,F), 75 μM (**g**, **h**)

TK mice were unable to learn the contextual fear conditioning task at all. In the case of pattern separation, valganciclovir-treated APPswe/PS1ΔE9; Nestin-δ-HSV-TK mice were unable to learn the task for the first three days. These results are the first evidence that learning and memory impairments in AD can be induced by compromising neurogenesis. It should be noted that mice were subjected to pattern separation following contextual fear conditioning. Thus, we cannot exclude the possibility that the former played a role in training them better for the latter. In such case, this may mask the true level of the learning deficits of the valganciclovir-treated APPswe/PS1ΔE9; Nestin-δ-HSV-TK mice, who without training would likely have taken longer to learn the task.

Notably, Valganciclovir-treated Nestin-δ-HSV-TK mice, not on an AD background, did not exhibit deficits in either contextual conditioning or pattern separation. While neurogenesis has not been directly implicated in contextual fear conditioning, its role in pattern separation is well established [39, 41]. This may suggest that either ablation of adult neurogenesis using the Nestin-δ-HSV-TK transgenic line is not sufficient to disrupt learning and memory, or that our specific contexts were not sufficiently challenging to unravel deficits. While previous lesion studies of the hippocampus have shown deficits in pattern separation, more specific genetic modulation of adult neurogenesis demonstrates mixed results [1]. For example, [42] found deficits in pattern separation after ablation of nestin expressing cells using the Nestin-rtTA, TRE-BAX transgenic line, while [43] ablated proliferating GFAP expressing cells in the hippocampus and observed no deficits in pattern separation [42, 43]. Further studies will need to be done to determine if our result is due to the specific transgenic line used or if aspects of our study such as duration of feeding with valganciclovir chow, age/gender of the animals or specific aspects of our contextual paradigm are underlying this difference.

Second, we addressed the role of neurogenesis in modulation of tau pathology. We show that ablation of neurogenesis upregulates levels of hyperphosphorylated tau, and that this effect is neurogenesis- rather than valganciclovir-dependent. This may strongly suggest that neurogenesis plays a major role in hippocampal maintenance, and that depletion of neurogenesis compromises neuronal viability. In addition, induction of hyperphosphorylated tau in neural progenitor cells suggests that depletion of neurogenesis may compromise the integrity and functionality of new neurons in the hippocampus. In contrast, we did not detect any effect of neurogenesis on the level of full length APP or oligomeric Aβ. Our results are in agreement with studies reporting lack of direct association between amyloidosis and neurogenesis. For instance, previous studies suggest that enhanced neurogenesis does not alter amyloid plaque load [44]. In turn, amyloid does not play a major role in impairments of neurogenesis in FAD [45].

Third, we addressed the role of neurogenesis in regulation of the hippocampal circuit. It is thought that the DG regulates pattern separation either by encoding similar inputs with differential firing rates of place cells (rate remapping) or through the recruitment of non-overlapping engrams (global remapping) [46, 47]. However, the exact mechanism is not fully elucidated. A recent study suggests that neurogenesis modifies the excitability of mature DG neurons without affecting excitability in the CA3 [48]. Another study shows that genetic suppression of adult neurogenesis impairs pattern separation by increasing overlap between engrams of differing contexts in CA3 cells [49]. The latter study, in agreement with ours, examined neuronal activation following a learning task, which enhanced neuronal response in the hippocampus. We show that depletion of neurogenesis in valganciclovir-treated Nestin-δ-HSV-TK mice induces the activation of more neurons in the hippocampus, and that this neuronal over-activation takes place in the DG, CA3 and CA1. This result suggests that following depletion of neurogenesis, more neurons get activated, thus increasing the chance of coding overlap, which would subsequently impair pattern separation. Notably, our results suggest that the effect of ablation of neurogenesis on the hippocampal circuit is broader than previously reported. Our result may also suggest that neurogenesis plays a major role in memory storage and recall by regulating inhibitory networks in the hippocampus. One possibility is that new neurons affect the circuit by modulating the activity of the older mature granular neurons and affecting their feedback inhibition, which in turn, affects the CA3. Alternatively, they may directly affect feedforward excitation and inhibition to the CA3.

In summary, this study implies that depletion of hippocampal neurogenesis, as occurs in the adult brain as a function of age, may compromise hippocampal function and induce learning and memory deficits and some neuronal pathology. Future studies should address the possibility that enhanced neurogenesis may be protective and reduce the risk for AD.

Conclusions

The results of this study imply that neurogenesis plays an important role in the regulation of inhibitory circuitry of the hippocampus. In addition, this study suggests that deficits in adult neurogenesis may contribute to cognitive impairments, tau hyperphosphorylation in new neurons and compromised hippocampal circuitry in Alzheimer's disease.

Abbreviations

APPswe/PS1ΔE9: Coexpression of Amyloid Precursor Protein mutated at KM670/671NL (APPswe) and presenilin-1 lacking exon 9 (PS1ΔE9).; 3xTg-AD: Familial Alzheimer's disease mouse model carrying three mutant transgenes: APP KM670/671NL (Swedish), MAPT P301L, PSEN1 M146V; AD: Alzheimer's Disease; APP: Amyloid Precursor Protein; BrdU: 5′-bromo-2′-deoxyuridine; CA1,3: *Cornu Ammonis*, Hippocampal subfield 1,3; CREB : cAMP response element binding protein; DAPI: 4′,6-diamidino-2-phenylindole; DCX: Doublecortin; DG: Dentate Gyrus; FAD: Familial Alzheimer's Disease; GFP: Green Fluorescent Protein; IgG: Immunoglobulin G; NeuN: Neuronal Nuclear antigen; NPC: Neural Progenitor Cell; PS1: Presenilin 1; p-tau: Phosphorylated tau; sAPPα: Soluble Amyloid Precursor Protein Alpha; TBST: Tris Buffered Saline with 0.01% Tween 20; Zif268 (Egr-1): Zinc Finger Transcription Factor 268; δ-HSV-TK: Modified version of the Herpes Simplex Virus Thymidine Kinase

Acknowledgements

The study was supported by NIH grant R01AG033570, R01AG033570-S2, BRF SG 2010-10 and 2011-08 (OL).

Authors' contributions

CH study design, experiment execution, data collection and analysis and paper writing; MKT and RM experiment execution, data collection and analysis; MH and KM data collection and analysis; TSY and SGK transgenic mice generation; OL study design, data analysis and paper writing. All authors read and approved the final manuscript.

Competing interests

The authors declare that they have no competing interests.

Author details

[1]Department of Anatomy and Cell Biology, College of Medicine, The University of Illinois at Chicago, 909 S Wolcott Ave, Chicago, IL 60612, USA. [2]Department of Pediatrics and Pathology & Cell Biology, Columbia University College of Physicians and Surgeons, New York, NY 10032, USA.

References

1. Lazarov O, Hollands C. Hippocampal neurogenesis: learning to remember. Prog Neurobiol. 2016;138-140:1–18.
2. Pavlopoulos E, Jones S, Kosmidis S, Close M, Kim C, Kovalerchik O, Small SA, Kandel ER. Molecular mechanism for age-related memory loss: the histone-binding protein RbAp48. Sci Transl Med. 2013;5:200ra115.
3. Small SA, Chawla MK, Buonocore M, Rapp PR, Barnes CA. Imaging correlates of brain function in monkeys and rats isolates a hippocampal subregion differentially vulnerable to aging. Proc Natl Acad Sci U S A. 2004;101:7181–6.
4. Small SA, Tsai WY, DeLaPaz R, Mayeux R, Stern Y. Imaging hippocampal function across the human life span: is memory decline normal or not? Ann Neurol. 2002;51:290–5.
5. Moreno H, Wu WE, Lee T, Brickman A, Mayeux R, Brown TR, Small SA. Imaging the Abeta-related neurotoxicity of Alzheimer disease. Arch Neurol. 2007;64:1467–77.
6. Toner CK, Pirogovsky E, Kirwan CB, Gilbert PE. Visual object pattern separation deficits in nondemented older adults. Learn Mem. 2009;16:338–42.
7. Stark SM, Yassa MA, Stark CE. Individual differences in spatial pattern separation performance associated with healthy aging in humans. Learn Mem. 2010;17:284–8.
8. Brickman AM, Stern Y, Small SA. Hippocampal subregions differentially associate with standardized memory tests. Hippocampus. 2011;21:923–8.
9. Yassa MA, Lacy JW, Stark SM, Albert MS, Gallagher M, Stark CE. Pattern separation deficits associated with increased hippocampal CA3 and dentate gyrus activity in nondemented older adults. Hippocampus. 2011;21:968–79.
10. Selkoe DJ. Alzheimer's Disease is a synaptic failure. Science. 2002;298:789–91.
11. Demars MP, Hollands C, Zhao Kda T, Lazarov O. Soluble amyloid precursor protein-alpha rescues age-linked decline in neural progenitor cell proliferation. Neurobiol Aging. 2013;34:2431–40.
12. Seki T, Arai Y. Age-related production of new granule cells in the adult dentate gyrus. Neuroreport. 1995;6:2479–82.
13. Kuhn HG, Dickinson-Anson H, Gage FH. Neurogenesis in the dentate gyrus of the adult rat: age-related decrease of neuronal progenitor proliferation. J Neurosci. 1996;16:2027–33.
14. Tropepe V, Craig CG, Morshead CM, van der Kooy D. Transforming growth factor-alpha null and senescent mice show decreased neural progenitor cell proliferation in the forebrain subependyma. J Neurosci. 1997;17:7850–9.
15. Kempermann G, Kuhn HG, Gage FH. Experience-induced neurogenesis in the senescent dentate gyrus. J Neurosci. 1998;18:3206–12.
16. Kempermann G, Gast D, Gage FH. Neuroplasticity in old age: sustained fivefold induction of hippocampal neurogenesis by long-term environmental enrichment. Ann Neurol. 2002;52:135–43.
17. Bayer SA. Neuron production in the hippocampus and olfactory bulb of the adult rat brain: addition or replacement? Ann N Y Acad Sci. 1985;457:163–72.
18. Kempermann G, Gast D, Kronenberg G, Yamaguchi M, Gage FH. Early determination and long-term persistence of adult-generated new neurons in the hippocampus of mice. Development. 2003;130:391–9.
19. Ninkovic J, Mori T, Gotz M. Distinct modes of neuron addition in adult mouse neurogenesis. J Neurosci. 2007;27:10906–11.
20. Imayoshi I, Sakamoto M, Ohtsuka T, Takao K, Miyakawa T, Yamaguchi M, Mori K, Ikeda T, Itohara S, Kageyama R. Roles of continuous neurogenesis in the structural and functional integrity of the adult forebrain. Nat Neurosci. 2008;11:1153–61.
21. Geinisman Y, deToledo-Morrell L, Morrell F, Persina IS, Rossi M: Age-related loss of axospinous synapses formed by two afferent systems in the rat dentate gyrus as revealed by the unbiased stereological dissector technique. Hippocampus 1992, 2:437–444.
22. Flood DG. Critical issues in the analysis of dendritic extent in aging humans, primates, and rodents. Neurobiol Aging. 1993;14:649–54.
23. Demars M, Hu YS, Gadadhar A, Lazarov O. Impaired neurogenesis is an early event in the etiology of familial Alzheimer's disease in transgenic mice. J Neurosci Res. 2010;88:2103–17.
24. Rodriguez JJ, Jones VC, Tabuchi M, Allan SM, Knight EM, LaFerla FM, Oddo S, Verkhratsky A. Impaired adult neurogenesis in the dentate gyrus of a triple transgenic mouse model of Alzheimer's disease. PLoS One. 2008;3:e2935.
25. Hamilton LK, Aumont A, Julien C, Vadnais A, Calon F, Fernandes KJ. Widespread deficits in adult neurogenesis precede plaque and tangle formation in the 3xTg mouse model of Alzheimer's disease. Eur J Neurosci. 2010;32:905–20.
26. Lazarov O, Marr RA. Neurogenesis and Alzheimer's disease: at the crossroads. Exp Neurol. 2010;223:267–81.
27. Lazarov O, Marr RA. Of mice and men: neurogenesis, cognition and Alzheimer's disease. Front Aging Neurosci. 2013;5:43.
28. Lazarov O, Mattson MP, Peterson DA, Pimplikar SW, van Praag H. When neurogenesis encounters aging and disease. Trends Neurosci. 2010;33:569–79.
29. Jin K, Galvan V, Xie L, Mao XO, Gorostiza OF, Bredesen DE, Greenberg DA. Enhanced neurogenesis in Alzheimer's disease transgenic (PDGF-APPSw,Ind) mice. Proc Natl Acad Sci USA. 2004;101(36):13363-7. Epub 2004 Aug 30. PMID: 15340159.
30. Gadadhar A, Marr R, Lazarov O. Presenilin-1 regulates neural progenitor cell differentiation in the adult brain. J Neurosci. 2011;31:2615–23.
31. Demars MP, Bartholomew A, Strakova Z, Lazarov O. Soluble amyloid precursor protein: a novel proliferation factor of adult progenitor cells of ectodermal and mesodermal origin. Stem Cell Res Ther. 2011;2:36.
32. Baratchi S, Evans J, Tate WP, Abraham WC, Connor B. Secreted amyloid precursor proteins promote proliferation and glial differentiation of adult hippocampal neural progenitor cells. Hippocampus. 2012;22:1517–27.
33. Bonds JA, Kuttner-Hirshler Y, Bartolotti N, Tobin MK, Pizzi M, Marr R, Lazarov O. Presenilin-1 dependent neurogenesis regulates hippocampal learning and memory. PLoS One. 2015;10:e0131266.
34. Jankowsky JL, Slunt HH, Ratovitski T, Jenkins NA, Copeland NG, Borchelt DR. Co-expression of multiple transgenes in mouse CNS: a comparison of strategies. Biomol Eng. 2001;17:157–65.
35. Yu TS, Zhang G, Liebl DJ, Kernie SG. Traumatic brain injury-induced hippocampal neurogenesis requires activation of early nestin-expressing progenitors. J Neurosci. 2008;28:12901–12.
36. Kheirbek MA, Tannenholz L, Hen R. NR2B-Dependent plasticity of adult-born granule cells is necessary for context discrimination. J Neurosci. 2012;32: 8696–702.
37. Hu YS, Xu P, Pigino G, Brady ST, Larson J, Lazarov O. Complex environment experience rescues impaired neurogenesis, enhances synaptic plasticity, and attenuates neuropathology in familial Alzheimer's disease-linked APPswe/ PS1{Delta}E9 mice. FASEB J. 2010;24:1667–81.
38. Wen PH, Hof PR, Chen X, Gluck K, Austin G, Younkin SG, Younkin LH, DeGasperi R, Gama Sosa MA, Robakis NK, Haroutunian V, Elder GA. The presenilin-1 familial Alzheimer disease mutant P117L impairs neurogenesis in the hippocampus of adult mice. Exp Neurol. 2004;188(2):224-37. PMID: 15246822.
39. Sahay A, Scobie KN, Hill AS, O'Carroll CM, Kheirbek MA, Burghardt NS, Fenton AA, Dranovsky A, Hen R. Increasing adult hippocampal neurogenesis is sufficient to improve pattern separation. Nature. 2011;472:466–70.
40. Kilgore M, Miller CA, Fass DM, Hennig KM, Haggarty SJ, Sweatt JD, Rumbaugh G. Inhibitors of class 1 histone deacetylases reverse contextual memory deficits in a mouse model of Alzheimer's disease. Neuropsychopharmacology. 2010;35:870–80.
41. Sahay A, Wilson DA, Hen R. Pattern separation: a common function for new neurons in hippocampus and olfactory bulb. Neuron. 2011;70:582–8.
42. Tronel S, Belnoue L, Grosjean N, Revest JM, Piazza PV, Koehl M, Abrous DN. Adult-born neurons are necessary for extended contextual discrimination. Hippocampus. 2012;22:292–8.
43. Groves JO, Leslie I, Huang GJ, McHugh SB, Taylor A, Mott R, Munafo M, Bannerman DM, Flint J. Ablating adult neurogenesis in the rat has no effect on spatial processing: evidence from a novel pharmacogenetic model. PLoS Genet. 2013;9:e1003718.
44. Pan H, Wang D, Zhang X, Zhou D, Zhang H, Qian Q, He X, Liu Z, Liu Y, Zheng T, et al. Amyloid beta is not the major factor accounting for impaired adult hippocampal neurogenesis in mice overexpressing amyloid precursor protein. Stem Cell Reports. 2016;7:707–18.
45. Ager RR, Davis JL, Agazaryan A, Benavente F, Poon WW, LaFerla FM, Blurton-Jones M. Human neural stem cells improve cognition and promote synaptic

growth in two complementary transgenic models of Alzheimer's disease and neuronal loss. Hippocampus. 2015;25:813–26.

46. Leutgeb JK, Leutgeb S, Moser MB, Moser EI. Pattern separation in the dentate gyrus and CA3 of the hippocampus. Science. 2007;315:961–6.
47. Neunuebel JP, Knierim JJ. CA3 Retrieves coherent representations from degraded input: direct evidence for CA3 pattern completion and dentate gyrus pattern separation. Neuron. 2014;81:416–27.
48. Ikrar T, Guo N, He K, Besnard A, Levinson S, Hill A, Lee HK, Hen R, Xu X, Sahay A. Adult neurogenesis modifies excitability of the dentate gyrus. Front Neural Circuits. 2013;7:204.
49. Niibori Y, Yu TS, Epp JR, Akers KG, Josselyn SA, Frankland PW. Suppression of adult neurogenesis impairs population coding of similar contexts in hippocampal CA3 region. Nat Commun. 2012;3:1253.

Permissions

All chapters in this book were first published in MN, by BioMed Central; hereby published with permission under the Creative Commons Attribution License or equivalent. Every chapter published in this book has been scrutinized by our experts. Their significance has been extensively debated. The topics covered herein carry significant findings which will fuel the growth of the discipline. They may even be implemented as practical applications or may be referred to as a beginning point for another development.

The contributors of this book come from diverse backgrounds, making this book a truly international effort. This book will bring forth new frontiers with its revolutionizing research information and detailed analysis of the nascent developments around the world.

We would like to thank all the contributing authors for lending their expertise to make the book truly unique. They have played a crucial role in the development of this book. Without their invaluable contributions this book wouldn't have been possible. They have made vital efforts to compile up to date information on the varied aspects of this subject to make this book a valuable addition to the collection of many professionals and students.

This book was conceptualized with the vision of imparting up-to-date information and advanced data in this field. To ensure the same, a matchless editorial board was set up. Every individual on the board went through rigorous rounds of assessment to prove their worth. After which they invested a large part of their time researching and compiling the most relevant data for our readers.

The editorial board has been involved in producing this book since its inception. They have spent rigorous hours researching and exploring the diverse topics which have resulted in the successful publishing of this book. They have passed on their knowledge of decades through this book. To expedite this challenging task, the publisher supported the team at every step. A small team of assistant editors was also appointed to further simplify the editing procedure and attain best results for the readers.

Apart from the editorial board, the designing team has also invested a significant amount of their time in understanding the subject and creating the most relevant covers. They scrutinized every image to scout for the most suitable representation of the subject and create an appropriate cover for the book.

The publishing team has been an ardent support to the editorial, designing and production team. Their endless efforts to recruit the best for this project, has resulted in the accomplishment of this book. They are a veteran in the field of academics and their pool of knowledge is as vast as their experience in printing. Their expertise and guidance has proved useful at every step. Their uncompromising quality standards have made this book an exceptional effort. Their encouragement from time to time has been an inspiration for everyone.

The publisher and the editorial board hope that this book will prove to be a valuable piece of knowledge for researchers, students, practitioners and scholars across the globe.

List of Contributors

Ruohe Zhao, Wei Li and Wen-Biao Gan
Drug Discovery Center, Peking University Shenzhen Graduate School, Shenzhen 518055, China
Skirball Institute, New York University School of Medicine, New York, NY 10016, USA

Julia Tsai
Skirball Institute, New York University School of Medicine, New York, NY 10016, USA

Wanling Hu
Drug Discovery Center, Peking University Shenzhen Graduate School, Shenzhen 518055, China

Yoonhee Kim, Chaeyoung Kim, Sung Min Son, Hyundong Song, Hyun Seok Hong, Sun-ho Han and Inhee Mook-Jung
Department of Biochemistry and Biomedical Sciences, Seoul National University College of Medicine, 103 Daehak-ro, Jongro-gu, Seoul 110-799, Korea

Brendan P. Lucey, Anne M. Fagan, David M. Holtzman, John C. Morris and Randall J. Bateman
Department of Neurology, Washington University School of Medicine, 660 South Euclid Avenue, Campus St Louis, MO 63110, USA

Heesun Choi, Haeng Jun Kim, Jisoo Kim, Jinhee Yang, Wonik Lee and Inhee Mook-Jung
Department of Biochemistry and Biomedical Sciences, Seoul National University, College of Medicine, Seoul, Korea

Soohyun Kim and Junho Chung
Department of Biochemistry and Molecular Biology, Seoul National University, College of Medicine, Seoul, Korea
Cancer Research Institute, Seoul National University College of Medicine, Seoul, Korea

Yeonju Park and Dong-Sup Lee
Department of Biomedical Sciences, Laboratory of Immunology and Cancer Biology, Seoul National University College of Medicine, Seoul, Korea

Hoon Ryu
VA Boston Healthcare System, Boston University Alzheimer's Disease Center, and Department of Neurology, Boston University School of Medicine, Boston MA02130, USA
Center for Neuromedicine, Brain Science Institute, Korea Institute of Science and Technology, Seoul, Korea

Seung Jae Hyeon
Center for Neuromedicine, Brain Science Institute, Korea Institute of Science and Technology, Seoul, Korea

Francesc X. Guix, Ragna Sannerud, Amaia M. Arranz, Katrien Horré, An Snellinx, Enrico Radaelli, Nikky Corthout, Sebastian Munck, Isabel H. Salas and Wim Annaert
VIB Center for Brain and Disease research - VIB, Leuven, Belgium
Center of Human Genetics and Leuven Institute for Neurodegenerative Diseases (LIND), KULeuven, Leuven, Gasthuisberg O&N, Belgium

Fedor Berditchevski and Sundaresan Rajesh
School of Cancer Sciences, University of Birmingham, Edgbaston, Birmingham B15 2TT, UK

Amantha Thathiah
Department of Neurobiology, University of Pittsburgh Brain Institute, Pittsburgh Institute for Neurodegenerative Disease, University of Pittsburgh School of Medicine, Biomedical Science Tower 3, Room 6062, 3501 Fifth Avenue, Pittsburgh, PA 15213-3301, USA

Takaomi Saido and Takashi Saito
Laboratory for Proteolytic Neuroscience, RIKEN Brain Science Institute, Wako-shi, 351-0198 Saitama, Japan

Pascal Millet
Aix Marseille Université, CNRS, NICN UMR 7259, Marseille 13916, France
APHP, Groupe hospitalier universitaire Saint Louis-Lariboisière-Fernand Widal, Centre Mémoire de Ressources et de Recherche, Hôpital Fernand Widal, Paris, France

Michael Overduin
Department of Biochemistry, Faculty of Medicine & Dentistry, University of Alberta, Edmonton, Canada

Samir Kumar-Singh
Molecular Pathology Group, Cell Biology & Histology, Faculty of Medicine, University of Antwerp, Antwerp, Belgium

Julien Colombelli and Sébastien Tosi
Institute for Research in Biomedicine (IRB Barcelona), The Barcelona Institute of Science and Technology, c. Baldiri Reixac 10, 08028 Barcelona, Spain

Bart De Strooper
VIB Center for Brain and Disease research - VIB, Leuven, Belgium
Center of Human Genetics and Leuven Institute for Neurodegenerative Diseases (LIND), KULeuven, Leuven, Gasthuisberg O&N, Belgium
Dementia Research Institute (DRI-UK), University College London, Queen Square, WC1N 3BG London, UK

Michael X. Hernandez
Department of Pathology and Laboratory Medicine, School of Medicine, University of California, Irvine, CA, USA

Andrea J. Tenner
Department of Pathology and Laboratory Medicine, School of Medicine, University of California, Irvine, CA, USA
Department of Neurobiology and Behavior, University of California, Irvine, CA, USA
Department of Molecular Biology and Biochemistry, University of California, Irvine, CA, USA

Shan Jiang and Ali Mortazavi
Department of Developmental and Cell Biology, University of California, Irvine, CA, USA

Lindsay A. Hohsfield, Maria D. Torres and Kim N. Green
Department of Neurobiology and Behavior, University of California, Irvine, CA, USA

Shu-Hui Chu, Maria I. Fonseca and Melody J. Fang
Department of Molecular Biology and Biochemistry, University of California, Irvine, CA, USA

Rick A. Wetsel
Research Center for Immunology and Autoimmune Diseases, Institute of Molecular Medicine for the Prevention of Human Diseases, University of Texas-Houston, Houston, TX, USA

Tracy A. Cole
Department of Neurobiology and Behavior, University of California, Irvine, CA, USA
Ionis Pharmaceuticals Inc., Carlsbad, CA 92010, USA

Miao Li, Lei Ma, Qian Qiao, Wanling Hu and Wei Li
Drug Discovery Center, Key Laboratory of Chemical Genomics, Peking University Shenzhen Graduate School, Shenzhen 518055, China

Yang Bai, Yanmei Zhou and Wen-Biao Gan
Drug Discovery Center, Key Laboratory of Chemical Genomics, Peking University Shenzhen Graduate School, Shenzhen 518055, China
Skirball Institute, Department of Neuroscience and Physiology, New York University School of Medicine, New York, NY 10016, USA

Zachary Patrick Wills
Department of Neurobiology, University of Pittsburgh, Pittsburgh, PA 15213, USA

Dong Kyu Kim, Jinhee Yang, Ahbin Kim and Jongmin Woo
Department of Biomedical Sciences, Seoul National University, College of Medicine, 103 Daehak-ro, Seoul 110-799, South Korea

Joonho Park and Youngsoo Kim
Interdisciplinary Program in Bioengineering, College of Engineering, Seoul National University, 1 Gwanak-ro, Seoul 151-742, South Korea

Dohyun Han
Biomedical Research Institute, Seoul National University Hospital, 101 Daehak-ro, Seoul 110-744, South Korea

Inhee Mook-Jung
Department of Biomedical Sciences, Seoul National University, College of Medicine, 103 Daehak-ro, Seoul 110-799, South Korea
Neuroscience Research Institute, Seoul National University, College of Medicine, Seoul 110-799, South Korea

Tom Van Dooren, Katrien Princen, Koen De Witte and Gerard Griffioen
reMYND NV, Gaston Geenslaan 1, Leuven-Heverlee 3001, Belgium

Michael Dumbacher
reMYND NV, Gaston Geenslaan 1, Leuven-Heverlee 3001, Belgium
Cell Biology, Department of Biology, Faculty of Science, Utrecht University, 3584CH Utrecht, The Netherlands

Mélissa Farinelli
E-Phy-Science, IPMC, 660 route des Lucioles, 06560 Sophia Antipolis, France

Sam Lievens
Orionis Biosciences, Technologiepark 12B, Zwijnaarde-Ghent 9052, Belgium
Cytokine Receptor Lab, Flanders Institute of Biotechnology, Medical Biotechnology Center, Faculty of Medicine and Health Sciences, Ghent University, Albert Baertsoenkaai 3, 9000 Ghent, Belgium

Jan Tavernier
Cytokine Receptor Lab, Flanders Institute of Biotechnology, Medical Biotechnology Center, Faculty of Medicine and Health Sciences, Ghent University, Albert Baertsoenkaai 3, 9000 Ghent, Belgium

Wim Dehaen
Department of Chemistry, KU Leuven, Celestijnenlaan 200f - Leuven-Heverlee 3001, Belgium

Stefaan Wera
ViroVet NV, Ambachtenlaan 1, Leuven-Heverlee 3001, Belgium

Joris Winderickx
Department of Biology, Functional Biology, KU Leuven, Kasteelpark Arenberg 31 Leuven-Heverlee 3001, Belgium

Sara Allasia, Amuri Kilonda, Stéphane Spieser and Arnaud Marchand
Cistim Leuven vzw, Gaston Geenslaan 2, Leuven-Heverlee 3001, Belgium

Patrick Chaltin
Cistim Leuven vzw, Gaston Geenslaan 2, Leuven-Heverlee 3001, Belgium
Center for Drug Design and Development (CD3), KU Leuven, Waaistraat 6, 3000 Leuven, Belgium

Casper C. Hoogenraad
Cell Biology, Department of Biology, Faculty of Science, Utrecht University, 3584CH Utrecht, The Netherlands

Aaron D. Thome, Alireza Faridar, David R. Beers, Jason R. Thonhoff, Weihua Zhao, Shixiang Wen, Belen Pascual, Joseph C. Masdeu and Stanley H. Appel
Department of Neurology, Houston Methodist Neurological Institute, 6560 Fannin St. Suite 802, Houston, TX 77030, USA

Ramon Velazquez and Antonella Caccamo
Neurodegenerative Disease Research Center, Biodesign Institute, School of Life Sciences, Arizona State University, 727 E. Tyler Street, Tempe, AZ 85287-5001, USA

Darren M. Shaw and Salvatore Oddo
Neurodegenerative Disease Research Center, Biodesign Institute, School of Life Sciences, Arizona State University, 727 E. Tyler Street, Tempe, AZ 85287-5001, USA
School of Life Sciences, Arizona State University, Tempe, AZ 85287, USA

Khalid Iqbal
Department of Neurochemistry, and SUNY Downstate/NYSIBR Program in Developmental Neuroscience, New York State Institute for Basic Research (NYSIBR), 1050 Forest Hill Road, Staten Island, NY 10314, USA

Syed Faraz Kazim
Department of Neurochemistry, and SUNY Downstate/NYSIBR Program in Developmental Neuroscience, New York State Institute for Basic Research (NYSIBR), 1050 Forest Hill Road, Staten Island, NY 10314, USA
Graduate Program in Neural and Behavioral Science, and Department of Physiology and Pharmacology, State University of New York (SUNY) Downstate Medical Center, 450 Clarkson Avenue, Brooklyn, NY 11203, USA

Se Hoon Choi, Luisa Quinti, Rudolph E. Tanzi and Doo Yeon Kim
Genetics and Aging Research Unit, MassGeneral Institute for Neurodegenerative Disease, Massachusetts General Hospital, Harvard Medical School, 02129 Charlestown, MA, USA

Young Hye Kim
Biomedical Omics Group, Korea Basic Science Institute, Cheongju-si, Chungbuk 363-883, Republic of Korea

Véréna Landel, Kévin Baranger and François Féron
Aix Marseille Université, CNRS, NICN UMR 7259, Marseille 13916, France

Béatrice Loriod
Aix Marseille Université, INSERM UMR 1090, TAGC, Marseille, France, Marseille 13288, France

Carolyn Hollands, Matthew Kyle Tobin, Michael Hsu, Kianna Musaraca, Rachana Mishra and Orly Lazarov
Department of Anatomy and Cell Biology, College of Medicine, The University of Illinois at Chicago, 909 S Wolcott Ave, Chicago, IL 60612, USA

Tzong-Shiue Yu and Steven G. Kernie
Department of Pediatrics and Pathology & Cell Biology, Columbia University College of Physicians and Surgeons, New York, NY 10032, USA

Index

A

Activated Protein Kinase, 50-51, 57, 59-60, 96, 98, 105, 142

All-trans Retinoic Acid, 137, 153

Alzheimer' S Disease, 123

Amyloid Precursor Protein, 2, 10, 12, 30-31, 34, 43, 45, 47, 49, 60-61, 68, 72, 90-91, 93, 110, 121-122, 154, 156-157, 172, 188, 209-210, 216, 218-219

Anti-green Fluorescent Protein, 210, 212

Apolipoprotein E, 10, 47, 92, 95, 105-106, 173

Axonal Transport, 33-35, 39-46, 155

B

Bicinchoninic Acid, 58, 158

Blood Brain Barrier, 29, 90, 110, 115, 125

Brain-derived Neurotrophic Factor, 94, 105, 108-109, 154

C

Casein, 14, 174

Central Nervous System, 1, 47-49, 91, 99, 105-107, 124, 133-134, 206

Cerebrospinal Fluid, 47-49, 109, 125, 134, 138, 153, 176

Ciliary Neurotrophic Factor, 94, 98, 105, 108

Colonystimulating Factor 1 Receptor, 2

Cyclin-dependent Kinase 5, 105

Cytosolic Calcium, 135

Cytosolic Domain, 50-51

D

Dementia, 10, 12, 50, 63-64, 66, 69-70, 90, 92, 94-96, 105-107, 123-127, 129, 131-134, 154, 171, 173, 176

Dendritic Calcium Activity, 175, 180, 184, 186

Dentate Gyrus, 30, 46, 94, 97, 102-106, 109, 131, 208-209, 216-220

Differentially Expressed Proteins, 156-157, 159, 164-166, 168, 172

Dimethyl Sulfoxide, 35, 137, 153, 155

Diphtheria Toxin, 1-3, 9

Doublecortin, 103, 210, 214, 216, 218

E

Eculizumab, 204

Entorhinal Cortex, 34, 36, 97-98, 107, 170, 208-210, 216

Enzyme-linked Immunosorbent Assay, 47, 121

Escherichia Coli, 17, 57

Ethanol, 16-17, 36, 88, 192-193, 209-210

Extracellular Amyloid Plaques, 156, 171

F

Fibrillar Plaque, 191, 196, 201, 203

Fluorescence-activated Cell Sorting, 65, 192, 205

Foetal Calf Serum, 137, 153

G

Geranylgeranylated, 145-146

H

High-throughput Drug Screening, 61

Hippocampal Neurogenesis, 95, 97-98, 106-107, 109, 208-209, 212, 214, 218-219

Hippocampal Proteome, 156-157, 160, 162, 164, 169, 172

Histone Deacetylase 6, 33, 44-46

Hyperexcitability, 135-136, 152, 154-155, 188

I

Immunoprecipitation, 14, 24, 34-36, 44, 51-53, 58-59, 142

Interleukin, 76, 81, 91-92, 99, 105, 125

Intraluminal Vesicles, 12-13, 19, 22, 30

L

L-glutamine, 14

Lactate Dehydrogenase, 137, 153

Leukemia Inhibitory Factor, 94, 99, 105

Lipofectamine, 34, 58

Lysosomal Genes, 202

M

Microglia, 1-11, 70, 86, 93, 124-125, 129, 131, 133-134, 158, 171, 173, 190-193, 196-197, 199-200, 202-207

Mitogen-activated Protein Kinase, 51, 60, 98, 105, 142

Motor Cortex, 99, 175-181, 183, 185-186, 188

Multivesicular Bodies, 12-13, 19, 22, 30

Myeloid Cells, 8-10, 124-132, 192, 203, 206

Myeloid-derived Suppressor Cells, 124-125, 133-134

N

Nestin-driven Thymidine Kinase, 208

Neurofibrillary Tangles, 33, 50, 61, 94-95, 105, 110, 115, 121, 132, 136, 156, 171, 173, 176, 191

Neuroprotection, 45, 83, 85, 108, 135-136, 152-153, 155, 191

O

Oxidative Stress, 33, 40-46, 64, 84, 155

P

Peroxdiredoxin1, 33

Phosphate Buffered-saline, 35

Phosphatidylinositol 3-kinase, 93, 118

Pim1 Inhibitor, 110-112, 114-115, 117, 119-120

Presenilin 1, 2, 28-29, 32, 34, 45-46, 61, 69, 88, 90, 95, 105, 209, 218

Pyramidal Neurons, 2, 6, 138, 146, 149, 158, 162, 175-177, 180-183, 185-186, 188-189, 193

R

Rapamycin, 51, 59-60, 110-111, 121-122

Reactive Oxygen Species, 33, 45-46, 50

Ribosomal, 122, 194

S

Senile Plaques, 61, 95, 191

Surface Plasmon Resonance, 51, 58-59

Synaptic Depotentiation, 175-176, 186

T

Tamoxifen, 2-5, 8-9

Tandem Mass Tag, 156, 158, 172

Threonine Protein Kinase, 111

Toll-like Receptors, 191, 207

Transcriptome Analysis, 190, 192

Tris Buffer Solution, 158

Two-photon Imaging, 1-2, 175, 177-178

V

Vibratome, 3, 121, 138, 193

W

Western Blotting, 35, 41, 52-53, 58, 157, 210

www.ingramcontent.com/pod-product-compliance
Lightning Source LLC
LaVergne TN
LVHW080703210926
848485LV00003B/412